Renal Transplantation

Renal Transplantation

Ron Shapiro, MD
Director, Renal Transplantation
Thomas E. Starzl Transplantation Institute
Associate Professor of Surgery
University of Pittsburgh School of Medicine
Pittsburgh, Pennsylvania

Richard L. Simmons, MD
Distinguished Service Professor
George Vance Foster Professor and Chair
Department of Surgery
University of Pittsburgh
Medical Director
University of Pittsburgh Medical Center
Pittsburgh, Pennsylvania

Thomas E. Starzl, MD, PhD
Director
Thomas E. Starzl Transplantation Institute
Distinguished Service Professor of Surgery
University of Pittsburgh School of Medicine
Pittsburgh, Pennsylvania

Appleton & Lange
Stamford, Connecticut

97 98 99 00 01 / 10 9 8 7 6 5 4 3 2 1

Prentice Hall International (UK) Limited, *London*
Prentice Hall of Australia Pty. Limited, *Sydney*
Prentice Hall Canada, Inc., *Toronto*
Prentice Hall Hispanoamericana, S.A., *Mexico*
Prentice Hall of India Private Limited, *New Delhi*
Prentice Hall of Japan, Inc., *Tokyo*
Simon & Schuster Asia Pte. Ltd., *Singapore*
Editora Prentice Hall do Brasil Ltda., *Rio de Janeiro*
Prentice Hall, *Upper Saddle River, New Jersey*

Library of Congress Cataloging-in-Publication Data

Renal transplantation / [edited by] Ron Shapiro.
p. cm.
ISBN 0-8385-8383-0 (case : alk. paper)
1. Kidneys—Transplantation. I. Shapiro, Ron. 1954-
[DNLM: 1. Kidney Transplantation. WJ 368 R392058 1997]
RD575.R4582 1997
617.4'610592—dc20
DNLM/DLC
for Library of Congress 96-28894

Acquisitions Editor: Michael Medina
Production Editor: Jeanmarie M. Roche
Designer: Libby Schmitz

ISBN 0-8385-8383-0

PRINTED IN THE UNITED STATES OF AMERICA

To our families
and our patients

Contents

Contributors

Mark Bellinger, MD
Chief, Pediatric Urology
Children's Hospital of Pittsburgh
Professor of Surgery (Urology)
University of Pittsburgh
School of Medicine
Pittsburgh, Pennsylvania

Brian C. Bennett, MD
Chief Resident
Division of Urology
University of Pittsburgh
School of Medicine
Pittsburgh, Pennsylvania

Donald V. Cramer, DVM, PhD
Director, Transplantation Research
Saint Vincent Medical Center
Los Angeles, California

Anthony J. Demetris, MD
Director, Division of Transplant
Pathology
University of Pittsburgh
Medical Center
Associate Professor of Pathology
University of Pittsburgh
School of Medicine
Pittsburgh, Pennsylvania

Benjamin Eidelman, MD, PhD
Professor and Vice Chairman for
Clinical Affairs
Department of Neurology
University of Pittsburgh
School of Medicine
Pittsburgh, Pennsylvania

Demetrius Ellis, MD
Director, Pediatric Nephrology
Professor of Pediatrics
University of Pittsburgh
School of Medicine
Pittsburgh, Pennsylvania

John J. Fung, MD, PhD
Chief, Division of Transplantation
Thomas E. Starzl
Transplantation Institute
Associate Professor of Surgery
University of Pittsburgh
School of Medicine
Pittsburgh, Pennsylvania

Nisan Gilboa, MD
Associate Professor of Pediatrics
Department of Pediatric
Nephrology
University of Pittsburgh
School of Medicine
Pittsburgh, Pennsylvania

Carl G. Groth, MD, PhD
Senior Staff, Department of
Transplantation Surgery
Huddinge Hospital
Professor of Transplantation Surgery
Karolinska Institute
Stockholm, Sweden

Yuichi Iwaki, MD, PhD
Director
University of Southern California
Hepatic Transplantation Laboratory
Professor of Urology and Pathology
University of Southern California
Los Angeles, California

Mark L. Jordan, MD
Associate Professor of Surgery
(Urology/Renal Transplantation)
University of Pittsburgh
School of Medicine
Pittsburgh, Pennsylvania

Yoogoo Kang, MD
Director, Hepatic Transplantation
Anesthesiology
Professor of Anesthesiology
University of Pittsburgh
School of Medicine
Pittsburgh, Pennsylvania

Shimon Kusne, MD
Division of Transplantation Medicine
Thomas E. Starzl
Transplantation Institute
Associate Professor of Medicine
and Surgery
University of Pittsburgh
School of Medicine
Pittsburgh, Pennsylvania

Leonard Makowka, PhD
Executive Director
Comprehensive Liver Disease and
Treatment Center
Saint Vincent Medical Center
Los Angeles, California

Rafael Manez, MD, PhD
Director of Transplantation Medicine
Juan Canalejo Medical Center
La Coruna, Spain

Susan A. McCarthy, PhD
Associate Professor of Surgery,
Molecular Genetics and Biochemistry
University of Pittsburgh
School of Medicine
Pittsburgh, Pennsylvania

Jerry McCauley, MD
Director, Transplantation Nephrology
Thomas E. Starzl
Transplantation Institute
Associate Professor of Medicine
and Surgery
University of Pittsburgh
School of Medicine
Pittsburgh, Pennsylvania

Noriko Murase, MD
Associate Professor of Surgery
Thomas E. Starzl
Transplantation Institute
University of Pittsburgh
School of Medicine
Pittsburgh, Pennsylvania

Robert M. Naraghi, MD
Resident, Urological Surgery
University of Pittsburgh
Medical Center
Pittsburgh, Pennsylvania

James H. Oliver, III, MD
Assistant Professor of Radiology
University of Pittsburgh
School of Medicine
Pittsburgh, Pennsylvania

Philip D. Orons, DO
Assistant Professor of Radiology and Surgery
University of Pittsburgh School of Medicine
Pittsburgh, Pennsylvania

Abdul S. Rao, MD, DPhil
Director, Section of Cellular Transplantation
Thomas E. Starzl Transplantation Institute
Assistant Professor of Surgery and Pathology
University of Pittsburgh School of Medicine
Pittsburgh, Pennsylvania

Parmjeet S. Randhawa
Assistant Professor, Pathology
University of Pittsburgh School of Medicine
Pittsburgh, Pennsylvania

Camillo Ricordi, MD
Co-Director
Diabetes Research Institute
Chief, Division of Cellular Transplantation
Professor of Surgery
University of Miami School of Medicine
Miami, Florida

Velma P. Scantlebury, MD
Associate Professor of Surgery
Thomas E. Starzl Transplantation Institute
University of Pittsburgh School of Medicine
Pittsburgh, Pennsylvania

Ajit N. Shah, MD
Director, Nuclear Medicine Residency Program
Assistant Professor of Radiology
University of Pittsburgh School of Medicine
Pittsburgh, Pennsylvania

Ron Shapiro, MD
Director, Renal Transplantation
Thomas E. Starzl Transplantantion Institute
Associate Professor of Surgery
University of Pittsburgh School of Medicine
Pittsburgh, Pennsylvania

Thomas E. Starzl, MD, PhD
Director, Thomas E. Starzl Transplantation Institute
Distinguished Service Professor of Surgery
University of Pittsburgh School of Medicine
Pittsburgh, Pennsylvania

Angus W. Thomson, PhD, DSc
Director, Transplant Immunology
Research Professor of Surgery
University of Pittsburgh School of Medicine
Pittsburgh, Pennsylvania

Annika Tibell, MD, PhD
Senior Staff Member, Department of Transplantation Surgery
Huddinge Hospital
Karolinska Institute
Stockholm, Sweden

Massimo Trucco, MD
Director, Histocompatibility Laboratory for Tissue Typing

Professor of Pediatrics and Hellman
Professor of Pediatric Immunology
University of Pittsburgh
School of Medicine
Pittsburgh, Pennsylvania

Carlos A. Vivas, MD
Assistant Professor of Surgery
(Urology/Renal Transplantation)
University of Pittsburgh
School of Medicine
Pittsburgh, Pennsylvania

Albert B. Zajko, MD
Chief, Division of Vascular and
Interventional Radiology
Professor of Radiology and Surgery
University of Pittsburgh
School of Medicine
Pittsburgh, Pennsylvania

Adriana Zeevi, PhD
Associate Professor of Pathology
and Surgery
University of Pittsburgh
School of Medicine
Pittsburgh, Pennsylvania

Preface

This book represents an attempt to describe in detail the principles and practice of clinical renal transplantation. Although the chapter authors are mostly from one institution, the University of Pittsburgh, this book was not designed to reflect the dogmas or prejudices of a single group. Rather it represents an attempt to present, as clearly as possible, a comprehensive guide to the practice of kidney transplantation. Where there is more than one point of view on a certain subject, all views are discussed. Where applicable, the particulars of our institutional practice are mentioned, but only as part of a more broadly based presentation.

Chapter 1 is a discussion of outcomes after renal transplantation. Where appropriate, both large multicenter and single center experiences are presented.

Chapter 2 is a discussion of the early history of renal transplantation. For those relatively young students of transplantation, who only know of renal transplantation in the context of a well-established, successful clinical service, the description of this early time is illuminating.

Chapters 3 and 4 discuss recipient and donor evaluation, and Chapter 5 discusses anesthetic management during the transplant procedure. Chapter 6, on the technical aspects of renal transplantation, discusses in some detail the "back table" preparation of the cadaver kidney, as well as the details of implantation. A special mention is made regarding pediatric en-bloc kidneys.

Chapter 7 discusses the nonimmunologic aspects of postoperative care, while Chapter 8 describes the basic immunology of the immune response, immunologic monitoring, HLA matching, the mechanisms of action of immunosuppressive agents, and the clinical aspects of both conventional and new immunosuppressive agents.

Chapter 9 includes a special section on microchimerism, which has emerged as a new field of investigation in clinical transplantation.

Chapter 10 discusses the pathologic issues in renal transplantation. Chapter 11 discusses complications, and focuses on surgical, medical, infectious, neurologic, and malignancy issues.

Chapter 12 describes the medical and technical management of patients who require allograft nephrectomy.

Chapter 13 focuses on the radiologic evaluation of renal transplant patients.

Chapter 14 discusses issues of particular relevance to pediatric renal transplantation, and Chapter 15 discusses renal transplantation in conjunction with concomitant or staged extrarenal transplantation.

Chapter 16 discusses issues related to pregnancy after renal transplantation.

Although xenotransplantation is not, properly speaking, currently a part of clinical renal transplantation, it was felt important to introduce the reader to these issues in Chapter 17. Finally, Chapter 18 discusses issues of renal transplantation that may be of relevance in the future.

In any multiauthored text of this type, there are bound to be areas of overlap among the different chapters. Every attempt has been made to keep this to a minimum.

Renal transplantation as a clinical discipline has come a long way in a relatively short period of time. This book attempts to chronicle what has been accomplished in the field and what has yet to be achieved.

Acknowledgments

This type of multiauthored work represents the efforts of a great many individuals. We would like to thank all of the authors who contributed their time and energy to produce the many chapters that make up this book. Without them, it would simply not exist.

As anyone involved in transplantation knows, none of the work involved in the care of transplant patients is possible without the help and commitment of a large number of transplant coordinators, inpatient nurses, social workers, and other staff personnel involved in the care of renal transplant patients. Our heartfelt thanks go to all of these individuals, without whom the work of clinical renal transplantation would come to a screeching halt. They specifically are Regina Fenton, RN, BSN; Loraine Oczypok, RN, BSN; Deborah Good, RN, BSN; Holly Woods, RN; Jareen Flohr; RN, BSN; Sue Bauder, RN, BSN; Sharon Orlofske, RN; Jennifer Ovesney, RN; Mark Paynter, RN, BSN; Gerri James, RN; Lisa Fox-Hawranko, RN, MSN; Karen Tanase, RN, BSN; and Leebrun Johnson, MSW.

At Appleton & Lange, we offer our thanks and our appreciation to Edward H. Wickland, Jr., Vice President and Publisher, and Kathleen McCullough, Managing Editor, Development, for their patience and support during this entire process.

We would like to thank also our medical illustrator, John Coulter, and our photographer, Robert Coulter, for their help in illustrating this book.

To Karen Toler, our previous secretary, and Susan Shandor, our current secretary, we give our thanks for countless hours of retyping the many chapters and references.

Finally, to our families, whose patience has been tried by the long hours of commitment to finish this project, we offer our heartfelt gratitude.

1

Outcome After Renal Transplantation

Ron Shapiro

Over the past 40 years, clinical renal transplantation has evolved from a nearly hopeless enterprise to a broadly based, highly effective clinical service. It has become the treatment of choice for patients with end-stage renal disease. Renal transplantation is, however, in many ways an imperfect therapy in terms of both patient and graft survival and the side effects associated with immunosuppressive therapy.

This chapter focuses on the results of renal transplantation. It begins with a discussion of patient survival and the causes of death after transplantation and follows with an analysis of short- and long-term graft survival and the causes of graft failure. Both multicenter data and selected single-center reports are cited, as are data from recent work with a new immunosuppressive agent, tacrolimus. The chapter concludes with comments on the quality of life after renal transplantation. The goal is to provide both an accurate picture of current expectations and to point out the limitations of present therapies.

▲ PATIENT SURVIVAL

The first question asked about any therapy is how well the patient survives it. Analyses of patient survival after renal transplantation have been classified according to the type of donor (living or cadaveric), the causes of end-stage renal disease, and recipient demographic variables. A standard measurement has been the 1-year actuarial survival rate, but longer time frames have also been studied. Over the past 10 years, the 1-year actuarial patient survival rate after cadaveric transplantation has remained stable at 92%–95%.[1–6] This followed a 15-year period during which there had been a progressive improvement in the 1-year patient survival rate from 70% to 90%.[6–16] Parenthetically, whereas at the end of the azathioprine era, the patient survival rate after cadaveric transplantation was no better than that in equally good-risk dialysis patients, at present, the overall patient survival rate is clearly better in

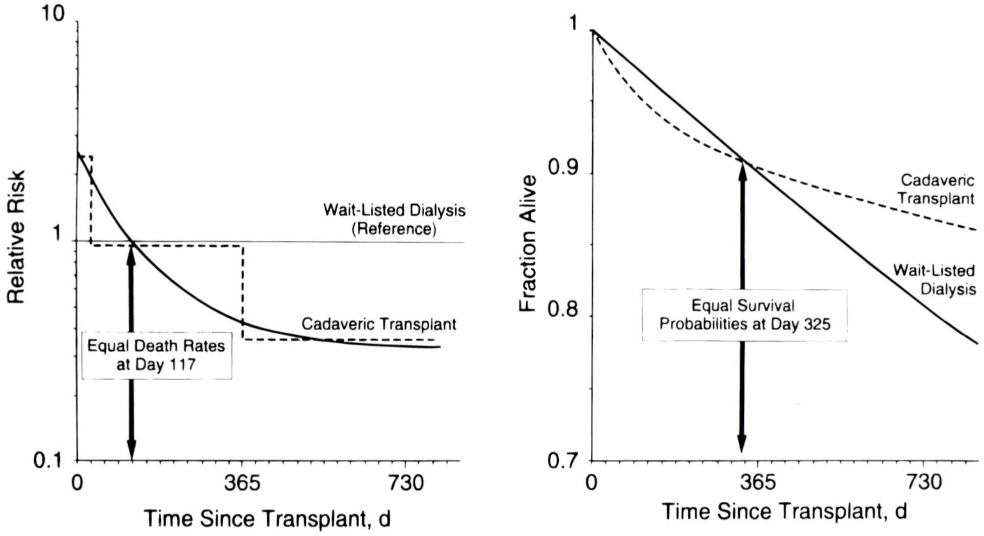

Figure 1–1. Patient survival rate after cadaveric transplantation and with dialysis. The dialysis group represents the subset of dialysis patients on the transplant waiting list (a group at better risk than and more appropriately comparable than the dialysis population at large). Patient survival rate after transplantation is better than with dialysis, particularly among patients with diabetes mellitus as the underlying cause of renal failure. (*From Port FK, et al: Comparison of survival probabilities for dialysis patients vs. cadaveric renal transplant recipients.* JAMA *270:1339–1343, 1993. Copyright 1993. American Medical Association.*)

patients undergoing transplantation (Fig. 1–1).[17,18] This holds true not only for the dialysis population as a whole[17] but also for dialysis patients who are on renal transplant waiting lists (the latter being a more directly comparable group).[18] There is some variability according to the cause of renal failure. For example, among patients with glomerulonephritis, the difference between transplantation and dialysis is less marked than in patients with diabetes mellitus, for whom the patient survival rate after transplantation is much better.[18,19]

In living related donor transplantation, the 1-year actuarial patient survival rate is 98%, somewhat superior to that after cadaveric transplantation (and clearly better than with dialysis).[1–8] This advantage has held throughout the history of renal transplantation, although the gap has narrowed considerably as results with cadaveric transplantation have improved.

In our own experience using tacrolimus as the primary immunosuppressive agent after transplantation, we have seen, in an adult patient population at relatively high risk, overall 1- and 3-year actuarial patient survival rates of 95% and 92%, respectively (Fig. 1–2).[20,20a] In living donor recipients, the 1-year patient survival rate has been 99%[21]; in children, it has been 100%.[22]

As the results with renal transplantation have improved, older patients have begun to be referred, and a fair number of recipients have been older than 60 or even 70 years of age. Although there may be a slight disadvantage in terms of

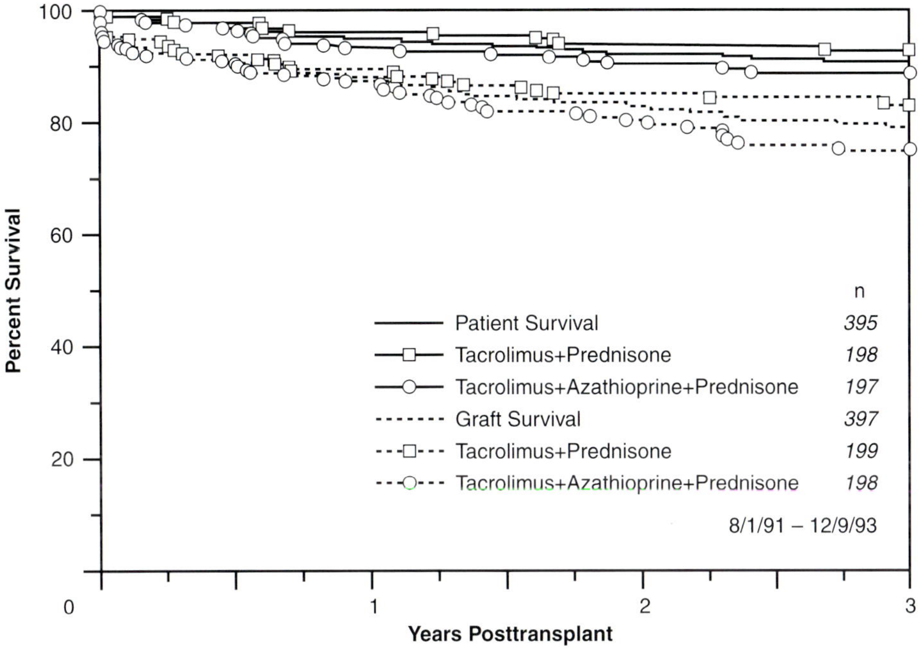

Figure 1–2. Patient (n = 395) and graft (n = 397) survival rates for patients receiving tacrolimus-based immunosuppression. One- and three-year actuarial survival rates were 95% and 92%, respectively. One- and three-year actuarial graft survival rates were 89% and 80%, respectively. The 1-year actuarial graft survival rate for first cadaveric transplants was 91%. Azathioprine was associated with a worse 3-year survival (76% versus 84%, P = .031). *(From Shapiro R, et al: The superiority of tacrolimus in renal transplant recipients—the Pittsburgh experience. In: Teraski PI (ed):* Clinical Transplants 1995. *Los Angeles, UCLA Tissue Typing Laboratory, 1996:199–205.)*

patient survival rate, this is perhaps 5%, and the overall results have been quite gratifying.[23–26]

Renal transplantation thus is associated with a high degree of success, at least in terms of patient survival. Unfortunately, although 1-year results have demonstrated a low mortality, the patient survival rate after the first year has not leveled off. The 5-year actuarial patient survival rate after cadaveric transplantation is 80%–90%.[27,28]

It is important to understand the early and late causes of death after transplantation. In virtually all published series, the most important causes of death after renal transplantation have been infection or cardiac disease.[9,10,29–33] Beyond these two reasons, there have been numerous etiologic factors, such as gastrointestinal problems, pulmonary disorders, malignancy, and cerebrovascular disease (Table 1–1). In addition, a late cause of death has been liver disease.[33,34] These causes of death have been similar throughout the history of transplantation.[9,10,33]

An additional important principle in mortality after renal transplantation is that, in many cases, death has occurred with a nonfunctioning graft; either graft function was never achieved, or it was lost after initial function (Table 1–2).[9,29,31] Tables of

TABLE 1–1 ▲ CAUSES OF DEATH AFTER KIDNEY TRANSPLANTATION

Cause	
Infection	38%
Cardiovascular disease	21%
Gastrointestinal disease	7%
Cerebrovascular disease	6%
Malignant disease	5%
Other	23%

Data from references 29–32.

mortality after transplantation are designed to include deaths from any cause, even if death occurs years after graft failure. This requirement has resulted in a relative paucity of long-term studies of mortality.

▲ GRAFT SURVIVAL

In contrast to studies of patient survival, there are numerous publications that discuss graft survival. Rather than attempt to be encyclopedic, the goal here will be to describe the factors that are associated with better or worse outcomes.

Cadaveric Kidneys

As a baseline, the overall 1-year actuarial graft survival rate after first cadaveric transplantation under some form of cyclosporine-based immunosuppression is about 84%.[1] This represents an incremental improvement over the past few years and remains much better than the 50%–60% 1-year results in the azathioprine-prednisone era[2–6] (Fig. 1–3). In our experience with tacrolimus, the 1-year actuarial graft survival rate for first cadaveric transplants in adults has been 91%[20]; in children, it has been 100%.[22] In addition, two recent multicenter analyses of renal transplant patients receiving tacrolimus also showed a 1-year graft survival rate of 91%.[35,35a]

TABLE 1–2 ▲ STATUS OF ALLOGRAFT AT TIME OF DEATH

Status	
Functioning	37%
Not Functioning	63%

Data from references 30 and 31.

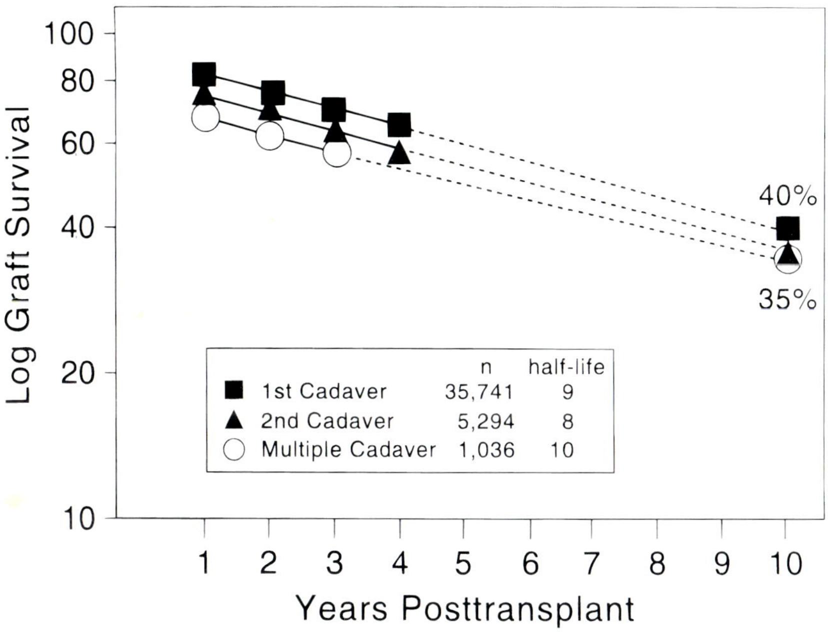

Figure 1–3. Graft survival rate after transplantation. The 1-year actuarial graft survival rates in 1992 for first, second, and multiple transplants were 84%, 82%, and 69%, respectively. *(From Cecka JM, Terasaki PI: The UNOS Scientific Renal Transplant Registry. In: Terasaki PI, Cecka JM (eds),* Clinical Transplants 1993. *Los Angeles, UCLA Tissue Typing Laboratory, 1994:2.)*

A number of variables affect this general outcome. Patients undergoing a second or subsequent retransplantation have had inferior graft survival rates in the past, but there have been recent improvements in outcome.[1–6,36–40] Second transplants have a 1-year graft survival rate of 82% and third or greater transplants have a 1-year graft survival rate of 69%.[1] Essentially all the differences are related to rejection during the first 3 months.[1–2] Among patients undergoing retransplantation who received tacrolimus, the 1- and 3-year actuarial graft survival rates were 83% and 75%, respectively.[20a]

Patients with high levels of preformed antibodies spend more time waiting for a transplant than do patients with lower levels of or no antibodies, and the 1-year graft survival rate also is inferior, 70%–75%.[1] This difference holds for patients undergoing first transplants and patients undergoing retransplantation.[1–6,41–43] Individual centers sometimes have been able to achieve better results.[40,44] Our experience with tacrolimus in patients with preformed antibody levels greater than 40% demonstrated 1- and 3-year actuarial graft survival rates of 87% and 78%, respectively, nearly as good as in patients with pre-formed antibody levels less than 40%.[20a]

The presence or absence of immediate allograft function is an enormously important factor. Kidneys that do not function immediately have a 15%–20% lower 1-year graft survival rate than kidneys without delayed graft function[1–6,27,45] (Fig. 1–4). In our experience with tacrolimus, delayed graft function was the most important fac-

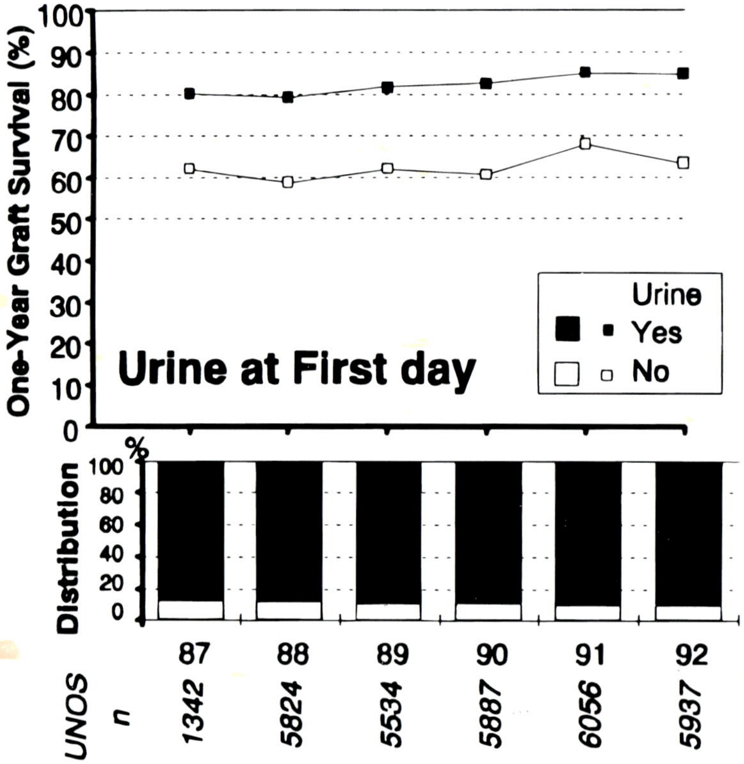

Figure 1–4. Effect of early non-function on graft survival. Delayed graft function is associated with a 15%–20% worse 1-year actuarial graft survival rate. *(From Cecka JM, Terasaki PI: The UNOS Scientific Renal Transplant Registry. In: Terasaki PI, Cecka JM (eds),* Clinical Transplants 1993. *Los Angeles, UCLA Tissue Typing Laboratory, 1994:560.)*

tor associated with inferior graft survival. The 1- and 3-year actuarial graft survival rates were 95% and 86%, respectively, in patients with immediate function and 78% and 69%, respectively, in patients with delayed function.[20a] Initial lack of function is the result of many factors, including cold and warm ischemia time, type of preservation solution and modality, prerecovery condition of the donor, immunologic status of the recipient, and type of immunosuppression used. In general, shorter ischemia times, better donor condition before recovery, and lower recipient preformed antibodies are all more likely to be associated with immediate function.[46] The use of the University of Wisconsin preservation solution is also associated with less delayed graft function.[47] In addition, several centers have demonstrated very low rates of early nonfunction when pulsatile perfusion preservation is used.[48–54] However, many large studies have reported no difference in the rate of delayed graft function between cold-storage and pulsatile preservation.[46,55–57]

A number of centers have used induction immunosuppression with antilymphocyte globulin (ALG) preparations.[58–65] The sequential four-drug immunosuppression regimen has the theoretical advantage of avoiding the use of nephrotoxic immunosuppressive agents until good graft function has been obtained. Additional goals include reducing the rate of early rejection and minimizing delayed graft function. The disadvantages of ALG induction therapy include exposing all patients to an increased risk of herpes virus complications and the increased expense. A course of any of these agents can easily range from $5,000 to $10,000. A multicenter analysis of induction ALG therapy suggests that 1-year graft survival rate is improved but only by 2% and that the rate of rejection is ultimately not much lower. Rejection is merely delayed.[66] For some subgroups, however, induction therapy may have profound advantages,[58] and the regimen is quite popular in the United States.

An additional general feature of induction regimens has been the implicit assumption that maintenance therapy with three immunosuppressive agents—cyclosporine, azathioprine, and prednisone—is preferable and superior to the double-drug regimen of cyclosporine and prednisone.[67–71] Although triple therapy has been routinely accepted almost as an article of faith (and we also,[31,72,73] on the basis of retrospective studies, advocated this line of reasoning in the past), several prospective trials have not found a benefit of triple over double therapy.[65,74,75] Our experience with tacrolimus actually has shown a disadvantage to adding azathioprine as a third agent, with a worse 3-year graft survival (76% vs 84%), although a slightly lower incidence of rejection was noted; see Chapter 8.[20,76] Recent studies with azathioprine substitutes, principally mycophenolate mofetil,[77] but also including preliminary work with sirolimus (rapamycin),[78] have suggested substantially less rejection in patients receiving these new third agents. These findings may have important implications for future therapies (see Chapter 8).

An important cause of deterioration in graft survival is the occurrence of episodes of acute rejection. Patients who never experience acute rejection have a significantly better 1-year graft survival rate (86%) than patients with one or more episodes of acute rejection (67%).[2,66,79–83] Long-term graft survival also is adversely affected.[84,85] Of interest, in our patients receiving tacrolimus, steroid-treated rejection was not associated with an early significant deterioration in graft survival, although steroid-resistant rejection was associated with a much worse graft survival. Among patients who never experienced rejection, the 1- and 3-year actuarial graft survival rates were 91% and 87%, respectively; in patients with steroid-treated rejection, they were 92% and 80%, whereas in patients with steroid-resistant rejection, they were 71% and 53%, respectively.[20a]

The impact of human leukocyte antigen (HLA) matching has been a source of some controversy in renal transplantation (see Chapter 8). There are widely accepted data suggesting that recipients of perfectly matched kidneys (six-antigen match) have a better 1-year graft survival rate (88%) than recipients of all other cadaveric kidneys.[1,2,86] Beyond that, however, there has been enormous controversy about the utility of matching. Two large retrospective multicenter registries have pointed to a benefit of matching,[87–89] whereas a number of single-center studies have not shown any benefit.[90–93] The disagreements at times have been remarkably acrimonious, and the issues are not merely academic. Matching is, at present, the dominant factor in the allocation of cadaveric kidneys.[94] The principle of equitable allo-

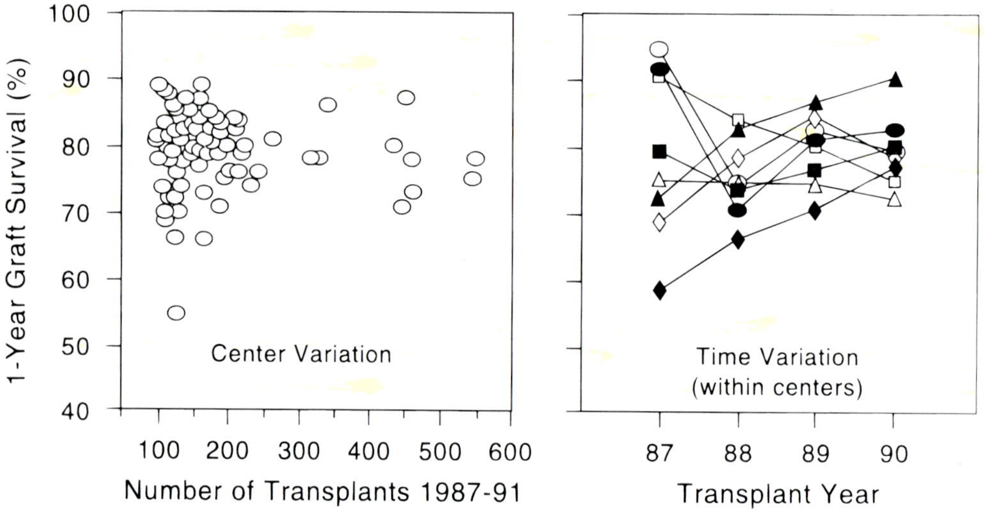

Figure 1–5. Variability in graft survival rates. Left. Among different centers. Right. Over time in particular centers. *(From Ogura K, Cecka JM: Center effects in renal transplantation. In: Terasaki PI, Cecka JM (eds),* Clinical Transplants 1992. *Los Angeles, UCLA Tissue Typing Laboratory, 1993:245.)*

cation of organs, particularly with regard to minority groups, has raised questions about the legitimacy of the current system, particularly in view of the unclear benefits of anything less than a perfect match. Thus the controversy about the value of matching is unlikely to disappear.

One of the most important prognostic factors in transplantation has been called the center effect.[95–104] There is a range of 1-year graft survival rates among different transplant centers, from 55% to about 90%[105] (Fig. 1–5). The center effect actually accounts for about 30% of the variability and may be the single most important factor in determining graft survival.[99,100,106] The causes of the center effect are more difficult to understand. Although there is a possibility that differences in surgical and medical expertise account for the center effect, centers with high-risk recipients and donors may have worse outcomes than more selective centers. Philosophic judgments about who should receive a kidney enter into this calculation. There are, in addition, many socioeconomic risk factors relating to compliance and reliability of follow-up therapy that are difficult to interpret.

The effect of the recipient race has been somewhat controversial in renal transplantation. Several single-center and multicenter registry reports have claimed that African-American recipients have lower graft survival rates after transplantation than white recipients.[107–113] Other centers, including ours, have noted no difference.[114–117] More recent multicenter registry reports have suggested that the differences are narrowing.[118]

Explanations for the worse outcomes among African-Americans have involved recipient risk factors such as a higher incidence of hypertension,[119] sensitization,[109,120] mismatching of particular antigens,[121,122] and compliance.[109,113,124] One analysis looked at the role of the center effect; centers with high rates of graft survival seemed to have fewer racial differences, whereas centers with lower graft survival rates had statistically significantly worse outcomes among minority recipients.[125]

Pretransplant blood transfusions have had a paradoxic effect on graft survival after kidney transplantation. Since the discovery that prior blood transfusion had a beneficial effect on graft survival toward the end of the azathioprine era,[126–128] many programs deliberately performed transfusions, with the goal of improving graft survival. With the advent of cyclosporine, however, the transfusion effect disappeared.[129,130] In recent years, transfusions have been associated with worse outcomes after transplantation, presumably because of sensitization (Fig. 1–6).[131,132]

In the past few years, new protocols of perioperative[133–136] or delayed[136–139] donor-specific bone marrow infusion have been developed. Conceptually descended from donor-specific blood transfusions,[140] the infusion of donor bone marrow represents an attempt to augment chimerism[141–144] in the recipient with the goal of improving long-term graft survival (see Chapter 9). Early reports have demonstrated both the safety and short-term efficacy of this approach; long-term outcome studies will require further follow-up.

A final important determinant of graft survival is the cause of end-stage renal disease. Immunoglobulin A (IgA) nephropathy has been associated with statistically higher 1- and 3-year graft survival rates than any other cause of renal failure.[145–148] The most recent report does not demonstrate marked differences at 1 year among

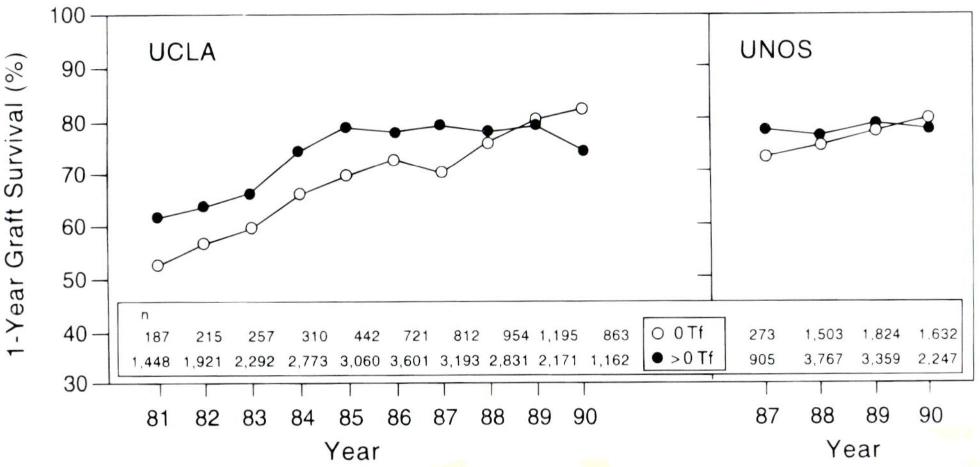

Figure 1–6. The effect of pretransplant transfusion over time. 0-Year survival rate was better among patients who underwent transfusions during the azathioprine era. In more recent years, however, the transfusion effect has disappeared, and now transfusion has a negative effect on graft survival. *(From Ogura K, Cecka JM: Center effects in renal transplantation. In: Terasaki PI, Cecka JM (eds),* Clinical Transplants 1992. *Los Angeles, UCLA Tissue Typing Laboratory, 1993:245.)*

other etiologies, but by 3 years after transplantation, patients with Alport's disease and polycystic kidney disease tend to have somewhat better graft survival rates than those with systemic lupus erythematosus (SLE) or hypertensive nephrosclerosis.[148,149] Specific interactions with race and HLA also have been noted. For example, white patients who have SLE with class II major histocompatibility (MHC) antigens DR2 or DR3, diabetes mellitus with DR3 or DR4, or chronic glomerulonephritis with DR1, or blacks with nephrosclerosis and DR2 or DR4 seem to have better outcomes than the same groups who do not carry the DR antigen in question.[148,149]

In addition to recipient characteristics, there are donor variables that can affect graft survival. Very young (less than 5 years of age) or old (greater than 60 years of age) donors have been associated with poorer graft survival, although with the organ shortage, the differences are not so great as to preclude the use of these donors.[1,150] Our results in patients receiving pediatric en bloc kidneys under tacrolimus therapy have been equivalent to those in patients receiving adult kidneys, with 1- and 3-year actuarial graft survival rates of 84% and 84% in en bloc recipients and 89% and 79% in other cadaveric recipients. Kidneys from donors dying as a result of trauma have been shown to have better outcomes than kidneys from donors dying of intracerebral hemorrhage.[150] Kidneys from black donors and female donors have been associated with worse outcomes, although the effect of donor sex has been diminishing.[1,150] Under tacrolimus-based therapy, outcomes with female donors have been equivalent to those with male donors.[150a] Longer ischemia times are also associated with slightly poorer outcomes, probably as a function of higher initial nonfunction rates.[1]

Living Donors

Graft survival in recipients of kidneys from living donors has always been better than that in recipients of cadaveric kidneys[1–6] (Fig. 1–7). Even as the results of cadaveric transplantation have improved, the results with living donors have remained better, with a 1-year graft survival rate of 94%. Living donors traditionally have been categorized into HLA-identical or one haplotype–matched relatives, and recipients of HLA-identical kidneys have had a slightly better 1-year outcome, 95% versus 88%–91%. Other single-center reports have demonstrated essentially equivalent results between two, one, and even zero haplotype–matched relatives[151] (Fig. 1–8). The 1-year graft survival rate in tacrolimus-treated recipients of living donor kidneys has been 96%, and over 80% of these patients have been able to have prednisone discontinued.[21]

An interesting recent phenomenon has been the rise of living unrelated donor transplantation. The donors have usually been emotionally related, mostly spouses. These transplants generally involve a low level of or zero HLA matching. The 1-year actuarial graft survival rate is 90%, as good as or better than with perfectly matched cadaveric kidneys[1,2,152–157] (Fig. 1–7). The benefit of early good function apparently overcomes the disadvantage of poor matching, at least in the short and medium term, and actually calls into question the benefit of matching.

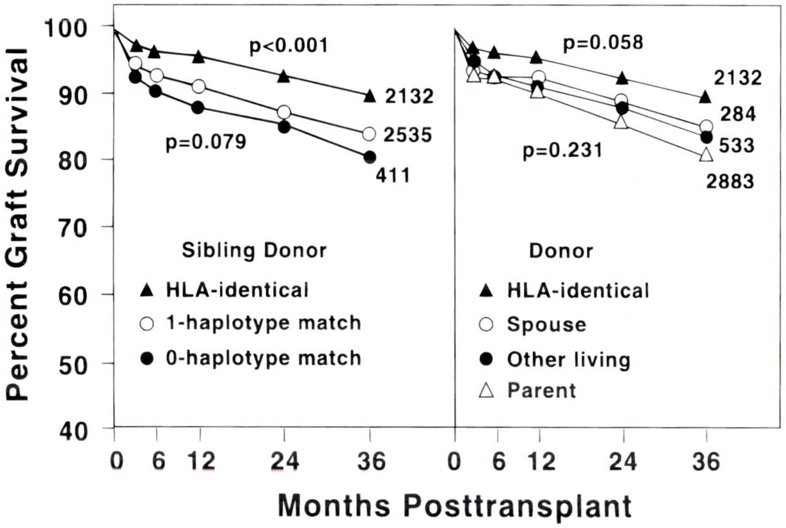

Figure 1–7. Graft survival rate with living related and living unrelated donors. HLA identical donors are associated with the best 1-year graft survival rate, 95%. However, the differences between one haplotype and zero haplotype–matched siblings and between one haplotype–related and poorly matched living unrelated donors are not significant. (*From Cecka JM, Terasaki PI: The UNOS Scientific Renal Transplant Registry. In: Terasaki PI, Cecka JM (eds),* Clinical Transplants 1993. *Los Angeles, UCLA Tissue Typing Laboratory, 1994:4.*)

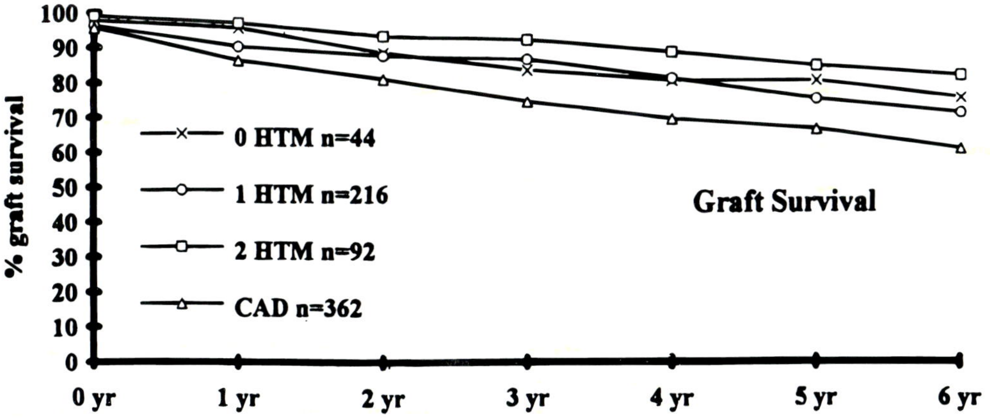

Figure 1–8. Single-center experience with zero, one, and two haplotype–matched (HTM) related living donors. This report shows no difference in outcome at 6 years among the three groups. CAD, Cadaveric kidney. (*From Jones JW, et al.: Successful long-term outcome with 0-haplotype-matched living-related kidney donors.* Transplantation *57:512–515, 1994.*)

Graft Loss

An important idea introduced by Terasaki and his co-workers has been the concept of graft half-life.[158–160] It describes the period of time, beginning 1 year after transplantation, until a graft survival rate of 50% has been achieved. The half-life of a cadaveric kidney is about 9 years, whereas that of a kidney from a related donor ranges from 12 to 24 years[1] (Fig. 1–9). The half-life of an HLA-identical sibling graft is longer than the expected life span of the recipient. To some extent, the half-life is the measurement of the rate of graft loss secondary to chronic rejection, although other factors (such as death with a functioning kidney or recurrence of the primary renal disease in the allograft) can play a role. Interestingly, half-life does not correlate with short-term graft survival[161] (Fig. 1–10). In addition, although short-term (ie, 1 year) graft survival has improved considerably with cyclosporine-based immunosuppression, the half-life has improved by only 2 years.[35] Finally, some early multicenter data suggest that the projected half-life with tacrolimus-based immunosuppression is 13.8 years, which is considerably longer than that seen with any other agent (Fig. 1–11).[35]

The first 3 months after transplantation are the highest risk for early graft loss. The causes of early graft loss, as shown in Figure 1–12, are related mainly to acute rejection and death. Technical causes, recurrence of native kidney disease, and infection can also be factors (it should be noted that infection is an important cause of death and thus accounts for a higher percentage of graft loss than is indicated in

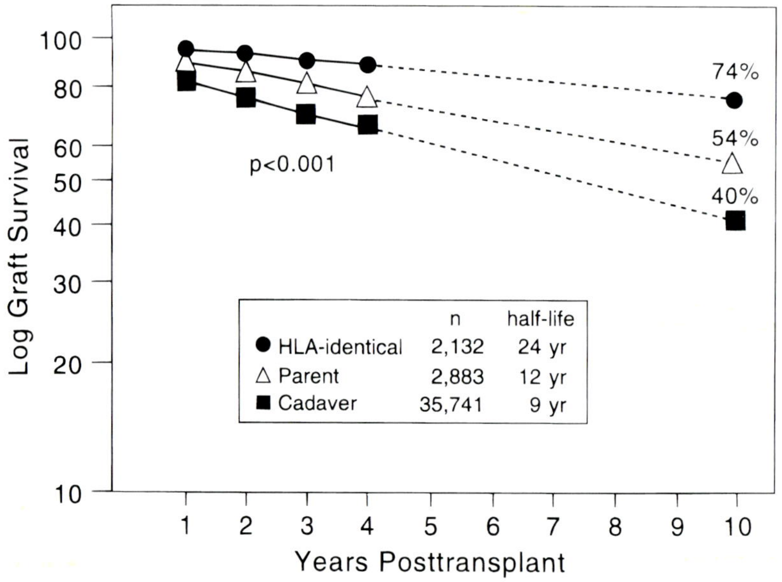

Figure 1–9. Long-term graft survival as a function of donor source. The half-life of kidneys from related donors is longer than that of kidneys from cadaveric donors. *(From Cecka JM, Terasaki PI: The UNOS Scientific Renal Transplant Registry. In: Terasaki PI, Cecka JM (eds),* Clinical Transplants 1993. *Los Angeles, UCLA Tissue Typing Laboratory, 1994:1.)*

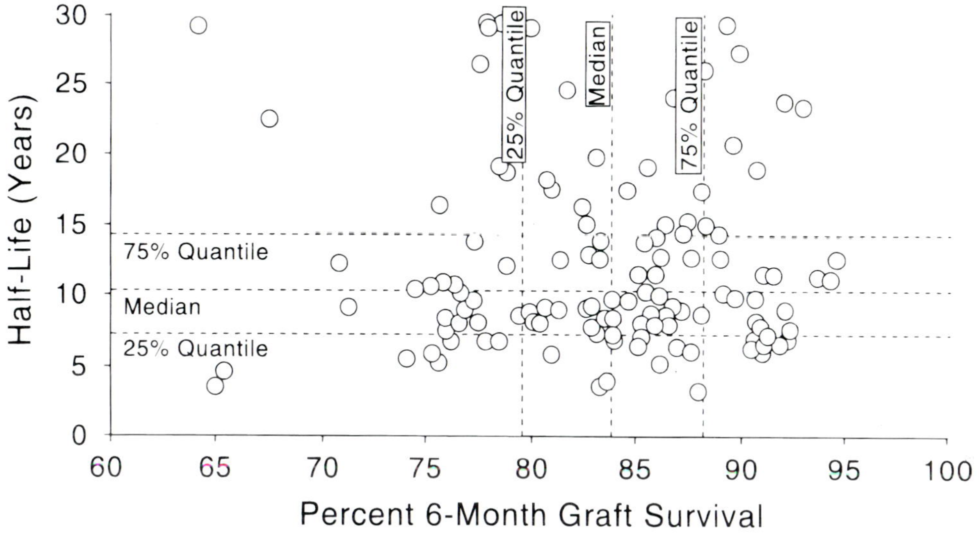

Figure 1–10. Lack of correlation between short-term and long-term graft survival. There is no relation between graft survival at 6 months and half-life. (*From Cho YW, Cecka JM: Center effects in the UNOS Scientific Renal Transplant Registry. In: Terasaki PI, Cecka JM (eds),* Clinical Transplants 1992. *Los Angeles, UCLA Tissue Typing Laboratory, 1993:333.*)

Figure 1–12 [see Table 1–1]). Late graft losses are primarily related to chronic rejection and/or chronic drug injury, mainly from cyclosporine. Death with a functioning allograft is also an important cause of late graft loss. Some investigators argue for recalculating graft survival to account for this factor and thereby obtain a more accurate assessment of immunologically mediated graft loss.[162] The occurrence of a de novo renal disease such as focal segmental glomerulosclerosis or membranous glomerulonephritis (see Chapter 10) occasionally leads to allograft failure.

Although the diagnosis and treatment of acute rejection are well understood at a practical level (see Chapter 8),[163,164] one of the failures of transplantation has been the inability to understand and deal with chronic rejection. Many investigators consider chronic rejection to be related directly to previous episodes of acute rejection,[81–85] but immunologic factors may only be partially responsible for the nonspecific changes that accompany gradual renal failure. For example, the primary maintenance immunosuppressive agent, cyclosporine (or, at some centers, tacrolimus), is nephrotoxic.

An alternative theory to explain chronic rejection has been proposed by Brenner et al.[165,166] He considers hyperfiltration to be responsible for many of the morphologic changes seen in chronic rejection, and the underlying problem is that insufficient renal mass, ie, one kidney instead of two, is being transplanted. His proposed solution, that both kidneys from a donor be transplanted into one recipient, is unfortunately not realistic at this time, when there are an insufficient number of donor kidneys to provide even one for every potential recipient.

If truly long-term success in renal transplantation is to be achieved, it will be nec-

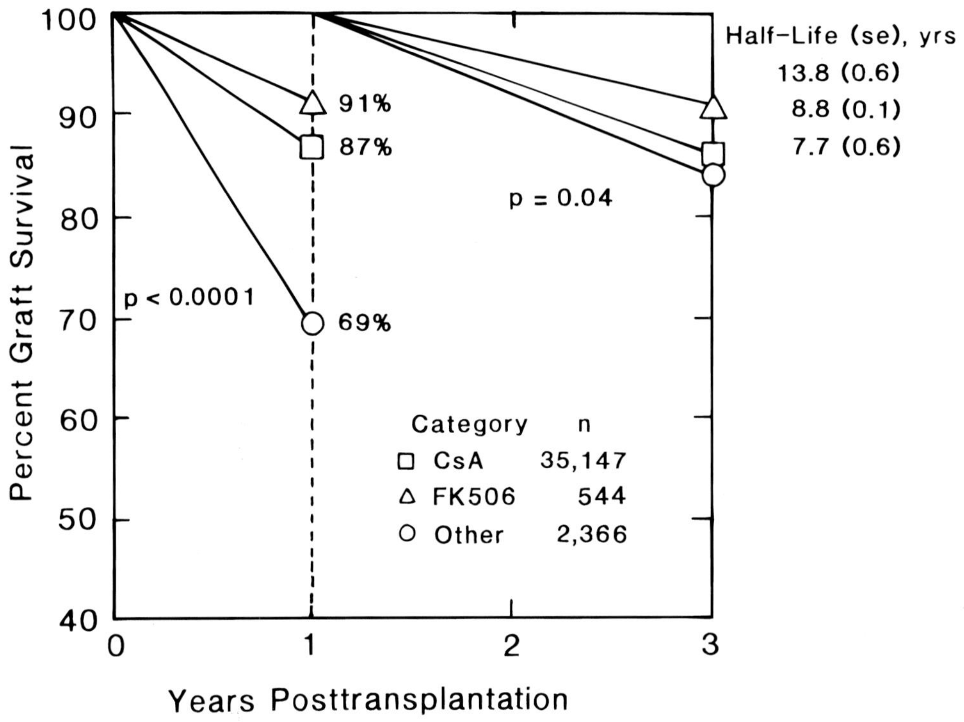

Figure 1–11. Plots of 1- and 3-year graft survival rates for first-time recipients of cadaveric kidneys grouped according to drug maintenance regimen after hospital discharge. One-year rates were based on recipients whose grafts survived at least 15 days, and 3-year rates were based on recipients whose grafts survived longer than 1 year. Drug half-lives were estimated with the assumption that there was a constant rate of graft failure beyond 1 year after transplantation. *(From Gjertson DW, Cecka JM, Terasaki PI: The relative effects of FK506 and cyclosporine on short- and long-term kidney graft survival.* Transplantation *60:1388, 1995.)*

essary to develop the ability to prevent or treat chronic rejection and use non-nephrotoxic maintenance immunosuppression. The large number of active research programs around the world that are studying tolerance induction (see Chapters 8 and 17) and the new immunosuppressive agents being investigated (see Chapter 8) are a testimony to these fundamental limitations of the current state of the art in renal transplantation.

▲ QUALITY OF LIFE

If renal transplantation is associated with very good but imperfect rates of patient and graft survival, there is little question that patients who undergo successful transplantation enjoy marked improvement in their quality of life compared with a life of dialytic therapy. Across a wide variety of measurements, in a number of different

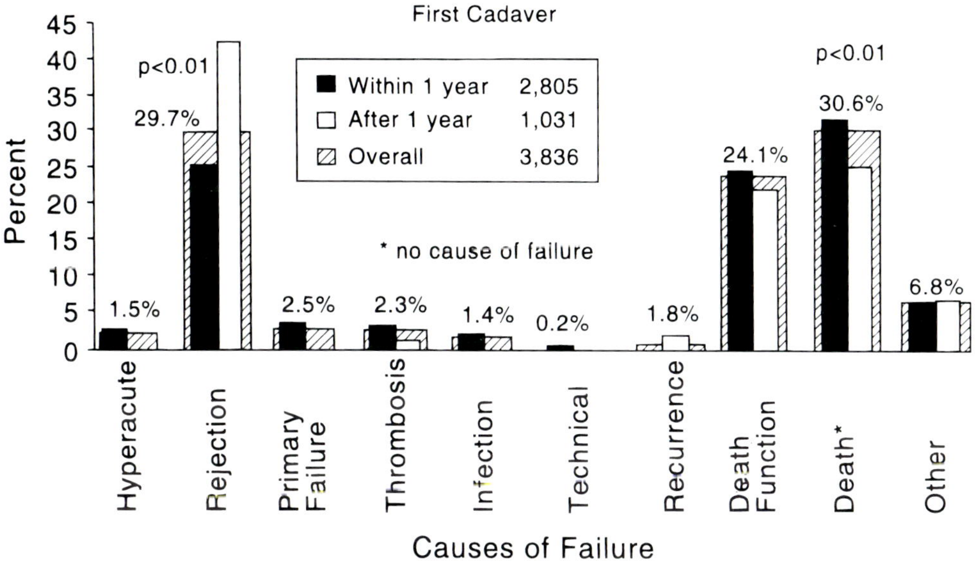

Figure 1–12. Causes of graft failure. The most common causes of graft failure are death, rejection, and infection (the last is an important cause of death [see Table 1-1]). (*From Cecka JA, Terasaki PI: The UNOS Renal Scientific Transplant Registry. In: Terasaki PI, Cecka JM (eds),* Clinical Transplants 1992. *Los Angeles, UCLA Tissue Typing Laboratory, 1993:13.*)

studies, patients who undergo successful transplantation attain a quality of life that is close to normal.[167–179] Objective measurements suggest that almost 75% are working and nearly 80% function at close to normal levels. Transplant recipients have more independence in daily activities, better physical well-being, and more health satisfaction than patients undergoing dialysis. Transplant patients also report more life satisfaction, emotional well-being, self-esteem, and happiness than dialysis patients. These differences persist when controlled for age, degree of illness, and cause of end-stage renal disease. This association of successful transplantation with a markedly improved quality of life is perhaps the most important benefit of transplantation. It explains the willingness of patients who have had failed transplants to undergo retransplantation and the continuing increase in the size of the waiting list.

Renal transplantation is generally successful therapy for end-stage renal disease, but it is neither always nor permanently so. The low but ongoing rate of patient loss and the higher and more progressive rate of graft loss suggest that there is still room for improvement. Recent experiences with new immunosuppressive agents, such as tacrolimus,[20–22,35,76] mycophenolate mofetil,[77] and possibly others[78] (see Chapter 8) suggest that some of these improvements are achievable today. When successful, renal transplantation is a remarkably effective therapy; the goals are to increase further the rate of this success and to make it last longer.

▲ REFERENCES

1. Cecka JM, Terasaki PI: The UNOS Scientific Renal Transplant Registry. In: Terasaki PI, Cecka JM (eds), *Clinical Transplants 1993.* Los Angeles, UCLA Tissue Typing Laboratory, 1994:1.
2. Cecka JM, Terasaki PI: The UNOS Scientific Renal Transplant Registry. In: Terasaki PI, Cecka JM (eds), *Clinical Transplants 1992.* Los Angeles, UCLA Tissue Typing Laboratory, 1993:1.
3. Cecka JM, Corcoran S, Takemoto S, et al: The UNOS Scientific Renal Transplant Registry. In: Terasaki PI (ed), *Clinical Transplants 1989.* Los Angeles, UCLA Tissue Typing Laboratory, 1989:1.
4. Cecka JM, Terasaki PI: The UNOS Scientific Renal Transplant Registry—1990. In: Terasaki PI (ed), *Clinical Transplants 1990.* Los Angeles, UCLA Tissue Typing Laboratory, 1991:1.
5. Cecka JM, Terasaki PI: The UNOS Scientific Renal Transplant Registry—1991. In: Terasaki PI, Cecka JM (eds), *Clinical Transplants 1991.* Los Angeles, UCLA Tissue Typing Laboratory, 1992:1.
6. Terasaki PI, Toyotome A, Mickey MR, et al: Patient, graft and functional survival rates: An overview. In: Terasaki, PI (ed), *Clinical Kidney Transplants 1985.* UCLA Tissue Typing Laboratory, 1985: 1–26.
7. Vollmer WM, Wahl PW, Blagg CR: Survival with dialysis and transplantation in patients with end stage renal disease. *N Engl J Med* 308:1553–1558, 1983.
8. Hutchinson TA, Thomas DC, Lemieux JC, Harvey CE: Prognostically controlled comparison of dialysis and renal transplantation. *Kidney Int* 26:44–51, 1984.
9. Starzl TE, Porter KA, Halgrimson CG, et al: A decade followup in early cases of renal homotransplantation. *Ann Surg* 180:4:606–616, 1974.
10. Starzl TE, Porter KA, Husberg BS, et al: Renal homotransplantation. I, II. *Curr Prob Surg* April, May:1975.
11. Henari FZ, Gower PE, Curtis JR, et al: Survival in 200 patients treated by hemodialysis and renal transplantation. *Br Med J* 1:409–412, 1977.
12. Higgins MR, Grace M, Dossetor JB: Survival of patients treated for end-stage renal disease by dialysis and transplantation. *Can Med Assoc J* 117:880–883, 1977.
13. Price JD, Ashby KM, Reeve CE: Results of 12 years' treatment of chronic renal failure by dialysis and transplantation. *Can Med Assoc J* 118:263–266, 1978.
14. Weller JM, Port FK, Swartz RD, et al: Analysis of survival of end-stage renal disease patients. *Kidney Int* 21:78–83, 1982.
15. Garcia-Garcia G, Deddens JA, D'Achiardi-Rey R, et al: Results of treatment in patients with end-stage renal disease: a multivariate analysis of risk factors and survival in 341 successive patients. *Am J Kidney Dis* 5:10–18, 1985.
16. Burton PR, Walls J: Selection-adjusted comparison of life-expectancy of patients on continuous ambulatory peritoneal dialysis, hemodialysis, and renal transplantation. *Lancet* 1:1115–1119, 1987.
17. The USRDS 1993 Annual Data Report: Methods of ESRD Treatment, 1993:29–38.
18. Port FK, Wolfe RA, Mauger EA, et al: Comparison of survival probabilities for dialysis patients vs. cadaveric renal transplant recipients. *JAMA* 270:1339–1343, 1993.
19. Basadonna G, Matas AJ, Gillingham K, et al: Kidney transplantation in patients with Type I diabetes: 26 year experience at the University of Minnesota. In: Terasaki PI, Cecka JM (eds), *Clinical Transplants 1992.* Los Angeles, UCLA Tissue Typing Laboratory, 1993:227.

20. Shapiro R, Jordan ML, Scantlebury VP, et al: A prospective, randomized trial of FK506/prednisone vs. FK506/azathioprine/prednisone in renal transplant patients. *Transpl Proc* 27:814–817, 1995.
20a. Shapiro R, et al: The superiority of tacrolimus in renal transplant recipients—the Pittsburgh experience. In: Terasaki PI (ed), *Clinical Transplants 1995.* Los Angeles, UCLA Tissue Typing Laboratory, 1996:199–205.
21. Scantlebury V, Shapiro R, Fung JJ, et al: Living donor kidney transplantation with Prograf. Presented at ASTP Annual Meeting, May, 1995.
22. Shapiro R, Scantlebury VP, Jordan ML, et al: FK506 in pediatric kidney transplantation: Primary and rescue experience. *Pediatr Nephrol* 1995; 9:543.
23. Vivas CA, Hickey DP, Jordan ML, et al: Renal transplantation in patients 65 years or older. *J Urol* 147:990, 1992.
24. Jordan ML, Novick AC, Steinmuller D, et al: Renal transplantation in the older recipient. *J Urol* 134:243–246, 1985.
25. Roza AM, Lepatk SG, Johnson CP, Adams MB: Renal transplantation in patients more than 65 years old. *Transplantation* 48:689–690, 1989.
26. Murie JA, Lauffer G, Gray D, et al: Renal transplantation in the older patient. *Transplant Proc* 21:2024–2025, 1989.
27. Morris PJ: Results of renal transplantation. In: *Kidney Transplantation: Principles and Practice.* Philadelphia, Saunders, 1988: 737.
28. Keown PA: Health status and rehabilitation following organ transplantation. *Literature scan: Transplantation* 9:23–24, 1993.
29. Smith AY, Van Buren CT, Lewis RM, et al: Factors determining renal transplant outcome at the University of Texas at Houston. In: Terasaki PI (ed), *Clinical Transplants 1987.* Los Angeles, UCLA Tissue Typing Laboratory, 1987:155.
30. Jeffrey JR, Downs H, Fong D, et al: Transplantation in Manitoba. In: Terasaki PI (ed), *Clinical Transplants 1988.* Los Angeles, UCLA Tissue Typing Laboratory, 1988:159.
31. Shapiro R, Tzakis A, Fung J, et al: The University of Pittsburgh: a three and three-quarter-year experience with cadaveric renal transplant under the point system. In: Terasaki PI (ed), *Clinical Transplants 1989.* Los Angeles, UCLA Tissue Typing Laboratory, 1989:287.
32. Perez RV, Matas AJ, Gillingham KJ, et al: Lessons learned and future hopes: three thousand and renal transplants at the University of Minnesota. In: Terasaki PI (ed), *Clinical Transplants 1990.* Los Angeles, UCLA Tissue Typing Laboratory, 1991:217.
33. Starzl TE, Schroter GPJ, Hartmann N, Barfield N, Taylor P, Mangan TL: Long-term (25-year) survival after renal homotransplantation: the world experience. *Transplant Proc* 22:2361–2365, 1990.
34. Venkateswara Rao K, Andersen RC, Lacombe MJ: Experience with renal transplantation in the second and third decades at the Hennepin County Medical Center. In: Terasaki PI (ed), *Clinical Transplants 1990.* Los Angeles, UCLA Tissue Typing Laboratory, 1991:223.
35. Gjertson DW, Cecka JM, Terasaki PI: The relative effects of FK506 and cyclosporine on short- and long-term kidney graft survival. *Transplantation* 60:1384–1388, 1995.
35a. Pirsch J for the FK506 US Kidney Transplant Multicenter Group: FK506 in Kidney Transplantation. Result of the US Randomized Cooperative Phase III Study. Joint ASTP/ASTS Plenary Session, May 29, 1996.
36. Ogura K, Cecka JM: Cadaver Retransplants. In: Terasaki PI (ed), *Clinical Transplants 1990.* Los Angeles, UCLA Tissue Typing Laboratory, 1991:471.
37. Mitsuishi Y, Cecka JM: Recent improvements in cadaver-donor kidney retransplantation. In: Terasaki PI, Cecka JM (eds), *Clinical Transplants 1991.* Los Angeles, UCLA Tissue Typing Laboratory, 1992:281.

38. Cabacungan C: Regrafts. In: Terasaki PI, Cecka JM (eds), *Clinical Transplants 1992.* Los Angeles, UCLA Tissue Typing Laboratory, 1993:471.
39. Schroeder TJ, Rirst MR, Mansour ME, et al: Prophylactic use of OKT3 in immunologic high-risk cadaver renal transplant recipients. *Am J Kidney Dis* 14:14, 1989.
40. Rosenthal JT, Danovitch G, Ettenger RB, Wilkenson A: Kidney transplantation at UCLA. In: Terasaki PI (ed), *Clinical Transplants 1991.* Los Angeles, UCLA Tissue Typing Laboratory, 1991:255.
41. Rankin GW, Wang X, Terasaki PI: Sensitization to kidney transplants. In: Terasaki PI (ed), *Clinical Transplants 1990.* Los Angeles, UCLA Tissue Typing Laboratory, 1991:417.
42. Zhou YC, Cecka JM: Sensitization in renal transplantation. In: Terasaki PI (ed), *Clinical Transplants 1991.* Los Angeles, UCLA Tissue Typing Laboratory, 1992:313.
43. Ogura K: Sensitization. In: Terasaki PI (ed), *Clinical Transplants 1992.* Los Angeles, UCLA Tissue Typing Laboratory, 1993:357.
44. Delmonico FL, Fuller TC, Cosimi AB: 1,000 Renal transplants at the Massachusetts General Hospital: Improved allograft survival for high-risk patients without regard to HLA matching. In: Terasaki PI (ed), *Clinical Transplants 1990.* Los Angeles, UCLA Tissue Typing Laboratory, 1991:247.
45. Lim EC, Terasaki PI: Early graft function. In: Terasaki PI, Cecka JM (eds), *Clinical Transplants 1991.* Los Angeles, UCLA Tissue Typing Laboratory, 1992:401.
46. Zhou YC, Cecka JM: Preservation. In: Terasaki PI, Cecka JM (eds), *Clinical Transplants 1992.* Los Angeles, UCLA Tissue Typing Laboratory, 1993:383.
47. Ploeg RJ: Kidney preservation with the UW and Euro-Collins solutions. *Transplantation* 49:281, 1990.
48. McClelland J, Cecka JM: Kidney preservation. In: Terasaki PI (ed), *Clinical Transplants 1987.* Los Angeles, UCLA Tissue Typing Laboratory, 1987:415.
49. Heil JE, Canafax DM, Sutherland DER, et al: A controlled comparison of kidney preservation by two methods: machine perfusion and cold storage. *Transplant Proc* 19:20–46, 1987.
50. Mendez R, Mendez RG, Koussa N, et al: Preservation effect on oligo-anuria in the cyclosporine era: a prospective trial with 26 paired cadaveric renal allografts. *Transplant Proc* 19:2047, 1987.
51. Manis T, Hong JH, Bronsther OL, et al: Superior results with machine-perfused kidneys in cyclosporine-treated transplant recipients. *Transplant Proc* 17:1483, 1985.
52. Hoffmann RM, Stratta RJ, D'Alessandro AM, et al: Combined cold storage-perfusion preservation with a new synthetic perfusate. *Transplantation* 47:1:32–37, 1989.
53. Barber WH, Laskow DA, Deierhoi MH, et al: Comparison of simple hypothermic storage, pulsatile perfusion with Belzer's gluconate-albumin solution, and pulsatile perfusion with UW solution for renal allograft preservation. *Transplant Proc* 23:2394–2398, 1991.
54. Tesi RJ, Elkhammas EA, Davies EA, et al: Pulsatile kidney perfusion for preservation and evaluation: use of high-risk kidney donors to expand the donor pool. *Transplant Proc* 25:3099–3100, 1993.
55. Halloran P, Aprile M: A randomized prospective trial of cold storage versus pulsatile perfusion for cadaver kidney preservation. *Transplantation* 43:827, 1987.
56. Opelz G, Terasaki PI: Advantage of cold storage over machine perfusion for preservation of cadaver kidneys. *Transplantation* 23:64, 1982.
57. Merion RM, Oh HK, Port FK, et al: A prospective controlled trial of cold-storage versus machine perfusion in cadaveric renal transplantation. *Transplantation* 50:230, 1990.
58. Gaston RS, Hudson SL, Deierhoi MH, et al: Improved survival of primary cadaveric renal

allografts in blacks with quadruple immunosuppression. *Transplantation* 53:103–109, 1992.
59. Ferguson RM for the Transplant Information Share Group: A multicenter experience with sequential ALG/cyclosporine therapy in renal transplantation. *Clin Transplant* 2:285, 1988.
60. Condie RM, Waskowsky KE, Hall BL, et al: Efficacy of Minnesota antilymphocyte globulin in renal transplantation: a multicenter placebo-controlled, prospective, randomized, double-blind study. *Transplant Proc* 17:1304, 1985.
61. Goldman M, Abramowicz D, De Pauw L, et al. Beneficial effects of prophylactic OKT3 in cadaver kidney transplantation: a comparison with cyclosporine A in a single center prospective randomized study. *Transplant Proc* 23:1046, 1991.
62. Shield CF: Effective induction immunosuppression for cadaver renal transplantation at the St. Francis Regional Medical Center. In: Terasaki PI (ed), *Clinical Transplants 1990.* Los Angeles, UCLA Tissue Typing Laboratory, 1991:265.
63. Matas AJ, Tellis VA, Quinn TA, et al: Individualization of immediate post-transplant immunosuppression: the value of antilymphocyte globulin in patients with delayed graft function. *Transplantation* 45:406, 1988.
64. Deierhoi MH, Sollinger HW, Kalayoglu M, Belzer FO: Quadruple immunosuppression in 305 consecutive cadaver renal allografts. *Clin Transplant* 1:71, 1987.
65. Sommer BG, Henry ML, Ferguson RM: Sequential antilymphoblast globulin and cyclosporine for renal transplantation. *Transplantation* 43:85, 1987.
66. Cecka JM, Young WC, Terasaki PI: Analyses of the UNOS scientific renal transplant registry at three years: early events affecting transplant success. *Transplantation* 53:59–64, 1992.
67. Squifflet J-P, Sutherdland DER, Rynasiewicz JJ, et al: Combined immunosuppressive therapy with cyclosporine-A and azathioprine. *Transplantation* 34:315–318, 1982.
68. Ilner WD, Land W, Habersetzer R, et al: Cyclosporine in combination with azathioprine and steroids in cadaveric renal transplantation. *Transplant Proc* 17:1181–1184, 1985.
69. Slapak M, Goeghegan T, Digard N, et al: The use of low-dose cyclosporine in combination with azathioprine and steroids in renal transplantation. *Transplant Proc* 17:1222–1226, 1985.
70. Fries D, Kechrid C, Charpentier B, et al: A prospective study of a triple association: cyclosporine, corticosteroids, and azathioprine in immunologically high-risk renal transplantation. *Transplant Proc* 17:1231–1234, 1985.
71. Simmons RL, Canafax DM, Strand M, et al: Management and prevention of cyclosporine nephrotoxicity after renal transplantation: Use of low doses of cyclosporine, azathioprine and prednisone. *Transplant Proc* 17:266–275, 1985.
72. Shapiro R, Tzakis AG, Hakala TR, et al: Cadaveric renal transplantation at the University of Pittsburgh: a two and one half year experience with the point system. In: Terasaki PI (ed), *Clinical Transplantation 1988.* Los Angeles, UCLA Tissue Typing Lab, 1989:181
73. Shapiro R, Tzakis A, Hakala T, et al: Cadaveric renal transplantation under the American organ allocation system. *Contrib Nephrol* 70:30, 1989.
74. Brinker KR, Dickerman RM, Gonwa TA, et al: A randomized trial comparing double-drug and triple-drug therapy in primary cadaveric renal transplants. *Transplantation* 50:43, 1990.
75. Lindholm A, Albrechtsen D, Tufveson G, et al: A randomized trial of cyclosporine and prednisone versus cyclosporine, azathioprine, and prednisolone in primary cadaveric renal transplantation. *Transplantation* 54:624, 1992.
76. Shapiro R, Jordan ML, Scantlebury VP, et al: A prospective randomized trial of FK506-

based immunosuppression after renal transplantation. *Transplantation* 59:4:485–490, 1995.
77. Sollinger HW, Deierhoi MH, Belzer FO, et al: RS-61443-A phase I clinical trial and pilot rescue study. *Transplantation* 53:428, 1992.
78. Kahan SD: Concentration-controlled immunosuppressive regimens using cyclosporine with sirolimus or brequinar in human renal transplantation. *Transplant Proc* 27:1:33–36, 1995.
79. Koyama H, Cecka JM: Rejection episodes. In: Terasaki PI (ed), *Clinical Transplants 1992.* Los Angeles, UCLA Tissue Typing Laboratory, 1993:391.
80. Cecka JM: Early rejection: analyses of the UNOS Scientific Renal Transplant Registry. In: Terasaki PI (ed), *Clinical Transplants 1990.* Los Angeles, UCLA Tissue Typing Laboratory, 1991:577.
81. Gulanikar AC, MacDonald AS, Sungurtekin U, Belitsky P: The incidence and impact of early rejection episodes on graft outcome in recipients of first cadaver kidney transplants. *Transplantation* 53:323, 1992.
82. Foster MC, Rowe PA, Dennis MJS, et al: Characteristics of cadaveric renal allograft recipients developing chronic rejection. *Ann R Coll Surg Engl* 72:23, 1990.
83. Cecka JM: Early rejection: determining the fate of renal transplants. *Transplant Proc* 23:1263, 1991.
84. Tesi RJ, Henry ML, Elkhammas EA, Ferguson RM: Predictors of long-term primary cadaveric renal transplant survival. *Clin Transplant* 7:345–352, 1993.
85. Almond PS, Matas A, Gillingham K, et al: Risk factors for chronic rejection in renal allograft recipients. *Transplantation* 55:752–757, 1993.
86. Takemoto S, Terasaki PI, Cecka JM, et al: Survival of nationally shared, HLA-matched kidney transplants from cadaveric donors. *N Engl J Med* 327:834, 1992.
87. Takiff H, Cook DJ, Himaya NS, et al: Dominant effect of histocompatibility on ten-year kidney transplant survival. *Transplantation* 48:410, 1988.
88. Terasaki PI, Cecka JM, Gjertson DW, et al: A ten-year prediction for kidney transplant survival. In Terasaki PI, Cecka JM (eds), *Clinical Transplants 1992.* Los Angeles, UCLA Tissue Typing Laboratory, 1993:501.
89. Opelz G, Wujciak T, Mytillineous J, Scherere S: Revisiting HLA matching for kidney transplantation. *Transplant Proc* 25:173, 1993.
90. Stratta RJ, D'Alessandro AM, Hoffman RM, et al: Cadaveric renal transplantation in the cyclosporine and OKT3 era. *Surgery* 104:606, 1988.
91. Greenstein SM, Schechner RS, Louis P, et al: Evidence that zero antigen matched cyclosporin-treated renal transplant recipients have graft survival equal to that of matched recipients. *Transplantation* 49:332, 1990.
92. Kahan BD, Van Buren CT, Flechner SM, et al: Cyclosporine immunosuppression mitigates immunologic risk factors in renal allotransplantation. *Transplant Proc* 17:1194, 1985.
93. Ferguson RM: Treatment protocols: is there a role for tissue typing in renal transplantation? *Transplant Proc* 20:242, 1988.
94. Halasz NA: Toward a more equitable and utilitarian distribution of kidneys. *Clin Transplant* 7:357–359, 1993.
95. Opelz G, Mickey MR, Terasaki PI: Comparison of kidney transplant survival among transplant centers. *Transplantation* 19:226, 1975.
96. Gilks WR, Selwood N, Bradley BA: The variation among transplant center results in the United Kingdom and Ireland from 1977 to 1981. *Transplantation* 38:235, 1984.
97. Taylor RM, Ting A, Briggs J: Renal transplantation in the UK and Ireland: the center effect. *Lancet* 1:798, 1985.

98. Mickey MR: Center effect. In: Terasaki PI (ed), *Clinical Kidney Transplants 1986.* Los Angeles, UCLA Tissue Typing Laboratory, 1986:165.
99. Mickey MR: Center variability. In: Terasaki PI (ed), *Clinical Transplants 1989.* Los Angeles, UCLA Tissue Typing Laboratory, 1990:435.
100. Gjertson D: Update: center effects. In: Terasaki PI (ed), *Clinical Transplants 1990.* Los Angeles, UCLA Tissue Typing Laboratory, 1991:375.
101. Cicciarelli J: Transplant center and kidney graft survival. In: Terasaki PI (ed), *Clinical Kidney Transplants 1985.* Los Angeles, UCLA Tissue Typing Laboratory, 1985:93.
102. Benlahrache C, Cecka M, Mickey MR, Cicciarelli J: The center effect. In: Terasaki PI (ed), *Clinical Kidney Transplants 1987.* Los Angeles, UCLA Tissue Typing Laboratory, 1988:325.
103. Ogura K, Cecka JM: Center effects in renal transplantation. In: Terasaki PI (ed), *Clinical Transplants 1991.* Los Angeles, UCLA Tissue Typing Laboratory, 1992:245.
104. Gjertson D, Terasaki PI: The large center variation in half-lives of kidney transplants. *Transplantation* 53:357, 1992.
105. Cho YW, Cecka JM: Center effects in the UNOS Renal Transplant Registry. In: Terasaki PI, Cecka JM (eds), *Clinical Transplants 1992.* Los Angeles, UCLA Tissue Typing Laboratory, 1993:333.
106. Gjertson DW. Multifactorial analysis of renal transplants reported to the UNOS Registry. In: Terasaki PI, Cecka JM (eds), *Clinical Transplants 1992.* Los Angeles, UCLA Tissue Typing Laboratory, 1993:299.
107. Takemoto S, Terasaki PI: A comparison of kidney transplant survival in white and black recipients. *Transplant Proc* 21:3865, 1989.
108. Yuge J, Cecka JM: The race effect. In Terasaki PI (ed), *Clinical Transplants 1987.* Los Angeles, UCLA Tissue Typing Laboratory, 1987:217.
109. Milgrom M, Gharagozloo H, Gomez C, et al: Results of renal transplantation in Miami analyzed by race. *Transplant Proc* 21:3934, 1989.
110. Opelz G, Pfarr E, Engelmann A, Keppel E, for the Collaborative Transplant Study: Kidney graft survival rates in black cyclosporine-treated recipients. *Transplant Proc* 21:3918, 1989.
111. Butkas DE, Kirchner KA, Krueger R, et al: Racial differences in primary renal cadaveric allograft survival. *Clin Transplant* 5:411, 1991.
112. Kasiske BL, Neylan JF, Riggio RR, et al: The effect of race on access and outcome in transplantation. *N Engl J Med* 324:302, 1991.
113. Barger BO, Hudson SL, Shroyer TW, et al: Influence of race on renal allograft survival in the pre- and postcyclosporine era. In: Terasaki PI (ed), *Clinical Transplants 1987.* Los Angeles, UCLA Tissue Typing Laboratory, 1987:217.
114. Matas AJ, Tellis VA, Perez L, et al: Does race affect renal transplant results? A single institution study. *Clin Transplant* 1:261, 1987.
115. Sommer BG, Sing DE, Henry ML: The influence of recipient race on renal allograft survival: a single institute analysis. *Transplant Proc* 21:3929, 1989.
116. Shapiro R, Tzakis AG, Hakala TR, et al: Renal transplantation in black recipients at the University of Pittsburgh. *Transplant Proc* 21:3921, 1989.
117. Sumrani NB, Hong JH, Hanson P, et al: Renal transplantation in blacks: impact of immunosuppressive regimens. *Transplant Proc* 21:3943, 1989.
118. Koyama H, Cecka JM: Race effects. In: Terasaki PI (ed), *Clinical Transplants 1991.* Los Angeles, UCLA Tissue Typing Laboratory, 1992:269–280.
119. White JC, Whelton PK, Seidler AJ, et al: Does racial variation in risk factors explain black-white differences in the incidence of hypertensive end-stage renal disease? *Arch Intern Med* 151:1359, 1991.

120. Kerman RH, Kimball PM, Van Buren CT, et al: Possible contribution of pretransplant immune responder status to renal allograft survival differences of black vs. white recipients. *Transplantation* 51:338, 1991.
121. Pfaff WW, Howard RJ, Ireland J, et al: The effect of Lewis antigen and race on kidney survival. *Transplant Proc* 15:1139, 1983.
122. Lee TD, Lee A, Shi WX: HLA-A, B-DR, -DQ antigens in black North Americans. *Tissue Antigens* 37:79, 1991.
123. Pirsch JD, Armburst MJ, D'Allessandro AM, et al: Kidney transplantation in blacks at the University of Wisconsin. *Transplant Proc* 21:3926, 1989.
124. Dunn J, Vathsala A, Golden D, et al: Impact of race on the outcome of renal transplantation under cyclosporine-prednisone. *Transplant Proc* 21:3946, 1989.
125. Yuge J, Cecka JM: The race effect. In: Terasaki (ed), *Clinical Transplants 1989.* Los Angeles, UCLA Tissue Typing Laboratory, 1990:407.
126. Opelz G, Sengar DPS, Mickey MR, Terasaki PI: Effect of blood transfusion on subsequent kidney transplants. *Transplant Proc* 4:253, 1973.
127. Cecka JM. The transfusion effect. In: Terasaki PI (ed), *Clinical Transplants 1987.* Los Angeles, UCLA Tissue Typing Laboratory, 1987:287.
128. Tiwari JL. Blood transfusion and kidney graft survival: A review. In: Terasaki PI (ed), *Clinical Transplants 1986.* Los Angeles, UCLA Tissue Typing Laboratory, 1986:341.
129. Opelz G: Improved kidney graft survival in non-transfused recipients. *Transplant Proc* 19:149, 1987.
130. Lundgren G, Albrechtson D, Flatmark A, et al: HLA-matching and pretransplant blood transfusions in cadaveric renal transplantation: a changing picture with cyclosporin. *Lancet* 1:66, 1986.
131. Cecka JM, Toyotome A. The transfusion effect. In: Terasaki PI (ed), *Clinical Transplants 1989.* Los Angeles, UCLA Tissue Typing Laboratory, 1990:335.
132. Ahmed Z, Terasaki PI. Effect of transfusions. In: Terasaki PI (ed), *Clinical Transplants 1991.* Los Angeles, UCLA Tissue Typing Laboratory, 1992:305.
133. Fontes P, Abdul R, Demetris AJ, et al: Bone marrow augmentation of donor-cell chimerism in kidney, liver, heart, and pancreas islet transplantation. *Lancet* 344:151–155, 1994.
134. Rao AS, Fontes P, Zeevi A, et al: Combined bone marrow and whole organ transplantation from the same donor. *Transplant Proc* 26:3377–3378, 1994.
135. Rao AS, Fontes P, Zeevi A, et al: Augmentation of chimerism in whole organ recipients by simultaneous infusion of donor bone marrow cells. *Transplant Proc* 27:210–212, 1995.
136. Shapiro R, Rao AS, Fontes P, et al: Combined kidney/bone marrow transplantation: evidence for augmentation of chimerism. *Transplantation* 59:306–309, 1995.
137. Monaco AP, Clark AW, Brown RW: Active enhancement of a human cadaver renal allograft with ALS and donor bone marrow: case report of an initial attempt. *Surgery* 79:384–392, 1976.
138. Barber WH, Mankin JA, Laskow DA, et al: Long-term results of a controlled prospective study with transfusion of donor specific bone marrow in 57 cadaveric renal allograft recipients. *Transplantation* 51:70–75, 1991.
139. McDaniel DO, Nafilan J, Hulvey K, et al: Peripheral blood chimerism in renal allograft recipients transfused with donor bone marrow. *Transplantation* 57:852–856, 1994.
140. Salvatierra O Jr, Melzer J, Potter D, et al: A seven-year experience with donor-specific blood transfusions: results and considerations for maximum efficacy. *Transplantation* 40:654–659, 1985.

141. Starzl TE, Demetris AJ, Trucco M, et al: Chimerism and donor-specific nonreactivity 27 to 29 years after kidney allotransplantation. *Transplantation* 55:1272–1277, 1993.
142. Starzl TE, Demetris AJ, Murase N, et al: Cell migration, chimerism, and graft acceptance. *Lancet* 339:1579–1582, 1992.
143. Starzl TE, Demetris AJ, Trucco M, et al: Cell migration and chimerism after whole organ transplantation: the basis of graft acceptance. *Hepatology* 17:1127–1152, 1993.
144. Starzl TE, Demetris AJ, Murase N, et al: Cell chimerism permitted by immunosuppressive drugs is the basis of organ transplant acceptance and tolerance. *Immunol Today* 14:326–332, 1993.
145. Lim EC, Terasaki PI: Outcome of kidney transplantation in different diseases. In: Terasaki PI (ed), *Clinical Transplants 1990.* Los Angeles, UCLA Tissue Typing Laboratory, 1991:461.
146. Lim EC, Terasaki PI: Outcome of renal transplantation in different primary diseases. In: Terasaki PI, Cecka JM (eds), *Clinical Transplants 1991.* Los Angeles, UCLA Tissue Typing Laboratory, 1992:293.
147. Mitsuishi Y, Cecka JM: Disease effects and associations. In: Terasaki PI, Cecka JM (eds), *Clinical Transplants 1992.* Los Angeles, UCLA Tissue Typing Laboratory, 1993:371.
148. Hirata M, Terasaki PI: The long-term effect of primary disease on cadaveric-donor renal transplant recipients. In: Terasaki PI, Cecka JM (ed), *Clinical Transplants 1993.* Los Angeles, UCLA Tissue Typing Laboratory, 1994:485.
149. Cicciarelli J: HLA-DR1 is a low responsiveness antigen in human kidney transplant recipients. In: Terasaki PI (ed), *Clinical Transplants 1987.* Los Angeles, UCLA Tissue Typing Laboratory, 1987:381.
150. Takiff H: Donor factors. In: Terasaki PI (ed), *Clinical Transplants 1989.* Los Angeles, UCLA Tissue Typing Laboratory, 1990:417.
150a. Shapiro R, Vivas C, Scantlebury VP, et al: Suboptimal kidney donors—the experience with tacrolimus-based immunosuppression. *Transplantation* 62:1242–1246, 1996.
151. Jones JW, Gilingham KJ, Sutherland DER, et al: Successful long-term outcome with 0-haplotype-matched living-related kidney donors. *Transplantation* 57:512–515, 1994.
152. Pirsch JD, Sollinger HW, Kalayoglu M, et al: Unrelated living donor kidney transplantation: results of 40 patients. *Am J Kidney Dis* 12:499, 1988.
153. Haberal M, Gulay H, Tokyay R, et al: Living unrelated donor kidney transplantation between spouses. *World J Surg* 16:1183, 1992.
154. Sollinger HW, Kalayoglu MK, Belzer FO: Use of the donor specific transfusion protocol in living-related donor-recipient combinations. *Ann Surg* 204:315, 1986.
155. Squifflet JP, Pirson Y, Poncelet A, et al: Unrelated living donor kidney transplantation. *Transplant Int* 3:32, 1990.
156. Elick BA, Sutherland DER, Gillingham K, et al: Use of distant relatives and living unrelated donors: a strategy to increase the application of kidney transplantation to treat chronic renal failure. *Transplant Proc* 22:343, 1990.
157. Park K, Kim YS, Lee EM, et al: Single center experience of living-unrelated donor renal transplantation in the cyclosporine era. *Clin Transpl* 249, 1993.
158. Takiff H, Mickey RM, Terasaki PI: Factors important in 10-year kidney transplant survival. *Clin Transpl* 157, 1986.
159. Cook DJ: Long-term survival of kidney allografts. *Clin Transpl* 277, 1987.
160. Mickey R, Yong WC, Carnahan E: Long-term graft survival. *Clin Transpl* 385, 1991.
161. Gjertson DW: Survival trends in long-term first cadaver-donor kidney transplants. *Clin Transpl* 225, 1992.

162. Matas AJ, Gillingham KJ, Sutherland DER: Half-life and risk factors for kidney transplant outcome: importance of death with function. *Transplantation* 55:757–761, 1993.
163. Shapiro R, Simmons RL: Renal transplantation. In: Starzl TE, Shapiro R, Simmons RL (eds), *Atlas of Organ Transplantation.* New York, Gower, 1992:4.2.
164. Danovitch G: Immunosuppressive medications and protocols for kidney transplantation. In: Danovitch GM (ed), *Handbook of Kidney Transplantation.* Boston, Little, Brown, 1992:67.
165. Brenner BM, Milford EL: Nephron underdosing: a programmed cause of chronic renal allograft failure. *Am J Kidney Dis* 21:66, 1993.
166. Brenner BM, Cohen RA, Milford EL: Renal transplantation, one size may not fit all. *J Am Soc Nephrol* 3:162, 1992.
167. De-Nour AK, Shannon J: Quality of life of dialysis and transplant patients. *Nephron* 25:117–120, 1980.
168. Simmons RG, Kamstra-Hennen L, Thompson CR: Psycho-social adjustment five to nine years posttransplant. *Transplant Proc* 13:40–43, 1981.
169. Simmons RG, Anderson CR: Related donors and recipients five to nine years posttransplant. *Transplant Proc* 14:9–12, 1982.
170. Simmons RG: Long-term reactions of renal recipients and donors. In: Levy NB (ed), *Psychonephrology*, ed 2. New York, Plenum, 1983:275–287.
171. Simmons RG, Marine SK, Simmons RL: *Gift of Life: The Effect of Organ Transplantation on Individual, Family, and Societal Dynamics.* New Brunswick, NJ, Transaction, 1987.
172. Simmons RG, Anderson CR, Kamstra LK: Comparison of quality of life of patients on CAPD, hemodialysis and transplantation. *Am J Kidney Dis* 4:253–255, 1984.
173. Evans RW, Manninen DL, Garrison JP Jr. et al: The quality of life of patients with end-stage renal disease. *N Engl J Med* 312:553–559, 1985.
174. Johnson JP, McCauley CR, Copely JB: The quality of life of hemodialysis and transplant patients. *Kidney Int* 22:286–291, 1982.
175. Churchill DN, Torrance GW, Taylor DW, et al: Measurement of quality of life end-stage renal disease: the time trade-off approach. *Clin Invest Med* 10:14–20, 1987.
176. Simmons RG, Abress L, Anderson CR: Quality of life after kidney transplantation: a prospective, randomized comparison of cyclosporine and conventional immunosuppressive therapy. *Transplantation* 45:415–421, 1988.
177. Simmons RG, Abress L, Anderson CR: Rehabilitation after kidney transplantation. In: Cerilli JG (ed), *Organ Transplantation and Replacement,* Philadelphia, Lippincott, 1988:481–489.
178. Julius M, Hawthorne VM, Carpentier-Alting P, Kneisley J, Wolfe RA, Port FK: Independence in activities of daily living for end-stage renal disease patients: biomedical and demographic correlates. *Am J Kidney Dis* 13:61–69, 1989.
179. Simmons RG, Abress L: Quality-of-life issues for end-stage renal disease patients. *Am J Kidney Dis* 25:201–208, 1990.

2

History of Renal Transplantation

Thomas E. Starzl / Anthony J. Demetris

Renal transplantation came from a series of steps that began to appear in the literature at the beginning of the 20th century. The steps were small, widely spread in time, and usually overlooked or condemned. As late as 1961, the Nobel Laureate, Macfarland Burnet, wrote in the *New England Journal of Medicine* that ". . . much thought has been given to ways by which tissues or organs not genetically and antigenetically identical with the patient might be made to survive and function in the alien environment. On the whole, the present outlook is highly unfavorable to success. . . ."[1] This opinion was published on the eve of the successful clinical renal transplantations in 1962 and 1963 that extended this procedure beyond the occasional identical and fraternal twin cases of the mid and late 1950s. Even then, these efforts provoked editorials questioning their inherent feasibility as well as their ethical basis.[2]

▲ TWENTIETH CENTURY BEGINNINGS

Heterotransplantation (Xenotransplantation)

In fact, the trials of the early 1960s were already late in a long, but at first slowly unfolding, story of whole-organ transplantation. The first known attempts at clinical renal transplantation by vascular anastomoses were made between 1906 and 1923 with pig, sheep, goat, and subhuman primate donors. The first of these efforts were in France[3] and Germany,[4] but others followed as summarized elsewhere.[5–7] None of the kidneys functioned for long, if at all, and the human recipients died a few hours to 9 days later. Although the biologic barrier to success was not understood, the applicability of vascular suture techniques (from Alexis Carrel) and even the possibility of using pelvic implantation sites were either envisioned or actually practiced. No further animal to human transplantations were tried again until 1963, when systematic and surprisingly successful clinical trials were made with chimpanzee[6] and baboon[7,8] kidneys. The eventual death of all of the recipients of animal organs ended renal xenotransplantation trials until the Baby Fae baboon heart xenotransplantation in the mid 1980s.[9]

Homotransplantation (Allotransplantation)

In 1936 Voronoy of Kiev, Russia,[10] reported the transplantation of a kidney from a cadaver donor of B+ blood type to a recipient of O+ blood type in violation of what have become accepted rules of tissue transfer.[11] In addition, the donor had been dead for 6 hours. The recipient died 48 hours later without making urine. Sporadic further efforts at renal allotransplantation were made in the ensuing 15 years without effective immunosuppression, as documented by Groth[5] and Hume et al.[12]

This was the dawn of renal transplantation. However, the stage was being set for the sunrise. Although renal transplantation lay largely dormant until 1951, Rene Kuss et al[13] and Charles Dubost et al[14] of Paris and Marceau Servelle et al of Strasbourg[15] carried out a series of cadaveric renal transplantations from convict donors after execution by guillotine. The next year, the French physician, Jean Hamburger, working with the urologist Louis Michon at the Hospital Necker, Paris, reported transplanting a kidney from a live volunteer donor.[16] The kidney, which was donated to a young man (named Marius) from his mother, functioned well and for 3 weeks before being rejected by the nonimmunosuppressed recipient. The kidney transplant procedure originally developed by Kuss and the other French surgeons was used for this patient. It has been performed hundreds of thousands of times since then, including for the celebrated identical (monozygotic) twin transplantations performed by Murray (Nobel Laureate, 1990) et al[17] in Boston.

Visitors flocked to France in the early 1950s to learn first hand from this experience, including John Merrill, who observed the extraperitoneal pelvic operation (often called the Kuss procedure in Europe). This was described in the classic account by Hume and Merrill et al[12] of their first clinical trials at the Peter Bent Brigham Hospital. In the Boston operations, all but one of the transplants were placed in the thigh and revascularized from the femoral vessels, with urine drainage by skin ureterostomies.[12] The extensive discussion of the French experience by Hume et al[12] included acknowledgment of the French source of the vascular surgical technology in the person of Alexis Carrel (Nobel Laureate, 1912),[18] who had spent much of his professional life in the United States in transplantation research. Carrel understood that transplanted organ allografts were not permanently accepted, but he did not know why.

Although the Peter Bent Brigham program postdated the early French efforts, the depth and serious intentions of the Harvard group were obvious in the report by Hume et al.[12] It contained observations on nine kidney allografts in nonimmunosuppressed recipients. The first of these kidneys was transplanted into the normal location in the recipient after its removal for a lower ureteral carcinoma on March 30, 1951, by Dr. L. H. Doolittle, of Springfield, Massachusetts. The patient had been undergoing short-term dialysis care at the Brigham, where the first artificial kidney in the United States had been brought from Holland by Wilhelm Kolff and modified by Harvard engineers, as described in detail by Moore.[19]

The next eight renal allografts, all placed in the thigh location, were transplanted between April 23, 1951, and December 3, 1952. Hume's description of this experience stands as one of the great medical classics of the 20th century. It provides a nearly complete clinical and pathologic profile of renal allograft rejection in an untreated human recipient. None of the European and American efforts to this time, however, or all together, would have had any lasting impact on medical practice were it not for what lay ahead. The principal ingredients of organ transplantation—immunosuppression, tissue matching, and organ procurement (and preservation)—were still unknown or undeveloped. The only examples of probable allograft function through 1954 were provided first by one of the nonimmunosuppressed patients of Hume et al[12] whose graft in the thigh location functioned for 5 months and an even earlier patient treated in Chicago by Lawler et al[20] about whom similar claims were considered implausible by later critics. Hume's career lasted well into the next era of transplantation, until his death in May, 1973, near Los Angeles in the crash of a private plane. John Merrill drowned off the beach of a Caribbean island in 1984.

The perception, if not the reality, of hopelessness was changed at the Peter Bent Brigham Hospital 2 days before Christmas 1954, when a kidney was removed from a healthy man by the urologist J. Hartwell Harrison and transplanted by Joseph E. Murray to the pelvic location of the donor's uremic identical twin brother; the nephrologist was John P. Merrill.[17,21] As in the earlier mother-to-son transplant in France,[16] no effort was made to preserve the transplanted kidney, which functioned promptly even though it underwent 82 minutes of warm ischemia time. According to Merrill et al,[17] the bold step of exploiting the principle of genetic identity for whole-organ transplantation had been suggested by the recipient's physician, David C. Miller, of the Public Health Service Hospital, Boston. It already was well known that identical twins did not reject each others' skin grafts.[22] To ensure identity, reciprocal skin grafting was performed on the Boston twins. Although the identical twin cases attracted worldwide attention, organ transplantation had reached a dead end. Further progress in the presence of an immunologic barrier would require effective immunosuppression.

THE CONCEPT OF IMMUNOSUPPRESSION

With Recipient Irradiation

For Bone Marrow Transplantation

The transition of tissue and organ transplantation from an exercise in futility to tenuous practicality was a slow process that began more than 10 years before Murray's identical twin case. The fundamental problem of transplantation was defined by Medawar (Nobel Laureate with Burnet, 1960) when he provided evidence in 1944 that rejection is an immunologic event.[23,24] In retrospect, every further development was a logical and inevitable extension of this concept. If rejection was an immune reaction, why not protect the organ transplant by weakening the immune system? This was done with adrenal corticosteroids[25,26] and total body irradiation,[27] both of which prolonged skin graft survival in animals.

However, the delay of rejection of rodent skin grafts was modest at best. Hopes were fanned when Billingham, Brent, and Medawar[28] accomplished permanent skin allograft acceptance in a special circumstance not involving any immunosuppression; namely, the inoculation of fetal or perinatal mice with immunocompetent spleen cells from adult donors. Instead of being rejected, these cells survived in the immunologically immature recipients, who were endowed with the ability in later life to accept skin from the original donor strain.[28,29] This was the first example of acquired transplantation tolerance.

The impetus and rationale for these experiments came originally from the observation by Owen[30] that freemartin cattle (the calf equivalents of human fraternal twins) were permanent hematopoietic chimeras if placental fusion and fetal cross circulation had existed in utero. Burnet and Fenner[31] predicted that such chimerism and the ability to exchange other tissues could be induced by the kind of experiment eventually performed with Medawar by Billingham and Brent. However, the surgical interest generated by the mouse tolerance experiments was quickly dampened when Billingham and Brent[32] learned that the penalty for the infusion of donor splenocytes was lethal graft versus host disease (GVHD) unless there was close histocompatibility between the donor and the immunologically defenseless recipients.

Immunosuppression was first exploited to achieve tolerance when in 1955 Main and Prehn[33] simulated in adult (as opposed to fetal) mice an environment they likened to that in the perinatal Billingham-Brent-Medawar animals. The three steps were: first, to cripple the immune system with supralethal total body irradiation, next to rescue it with allogeneic bone marrow (producing a hematolymphopoietic chimera), and finally to engraft skin from the bone marrow donor strain. Although these efforts were successful,[33,34] lethal GVHD could be avoided, as in the perinatal mouse model only by using histocompatible donors. Mannick et al[35] extended these observations by producing bone marrow chimerism in a single irradiated beagle dog, followed by kidney allotransplantation from the original marrow donor. The dog survived for 73 days.[35] Rapaport et al[36] later showed that, as in the rodent models, this strategy could not work unless perfectly tissue-matched canine marrow donors were used, usually litter mates. Efforts by Hume et al,[37] Rapaport et al,[36] and others to broaden the acceptable histocompatibility requirements were totally unsuccessful—leading to lethal GVHD, rejection, or both.

Appreciation of the dilemma posed by the administration of bone marrow to cytoablated recipients caused a break in ranks in 1959–1962 between those interested in the treatment of hematologic disorders and those for whom bone marrow was only the means to the end of transplantation of a needed whole organ. From this point onward, the therapeutic philosophies of bone marrow and solid organ transplantation took separate pathways—one dependent and the other seemingly independent of classic chimerism-associated tolerance induction as defined by the

Billingham, Brent, and Medawar model.[29] In spite of the fact that only perfectly matched siblings could be used, clinical bone marrow transplantation was accomplished in 1963 by Mathe et al in Paris[38] and in 1968 by Gatti et al in Minneapolis[39] and Bach at the University of Wisconsin.[40] Successes by Thomas (Nobel Laureate, 1990),[41] van Bekkum,[42] and others fueled the maturation of bone marrow transplantation into accepted clinical therapy for hematologic diseases and an assortment of other indications.

For Whole Organs

In contrast to the hematologists, Murray et al[43] attempted to use the Main-Prehn principle of recipient cytoablation with total body irradiation (TBI) plus bone marrow and kidney transplantation in two patients only, both in 1958. Sublethal TBI[43,44] without bone marrow was used for the next 10 kidney recipients. Although 11 of 12 irradiated recipients died after 0–28 days, the survivor (who was not given bone marrow) had adequate renal function from the time his fraternal twin brother's kidney was transplanted in January 1959 until he died of arteriosclerotic heart disease in 1979. The detailed description of this patient by Merrill et al in the *New England Journal of Medicine*[45] was arguably the single most influential clinical case report in the transplantation literature, because this was the first time that the genetic barrier to transplantation had been breeched.[43,44,46] Five months later, Hamburger et al[47–49] added a similar fraternal twin case. The second recipient had good renal function until his death 26 years later from carcinoma of the urinary bladder.

However, it was conceivable with these fraternal (dizygotic) twin recipients that their individual placentas had cross-circulated with those of their kidney donors during gestation, like the circumstances in Owen's freemartin cattle. This suspicion was put to rest with the further extraordinary kidney transplant experience in France during 1960–1962 in which TBI was used *without* bone marrow reconstitution. Hamburger et al[48,49] succeeded with kidney transplantation from a sibling and a first-cousin donor. The latter kidney (transplanted in February 1962) functioned for 18 years before retransplantation was performed (without interim dialysis) on a patient who now is a member of the French parliament. He is the longest surviving kidney allograft recipient (34 years) from that heroic era.[50]

Also in Paris, Rene Kuss et al[51,52] had long-term survival of three of six irradiated patients treated with kidney transplantation from January 1960 through 1961. This was a monumental achievement, because two of Kuss's long-surviving patients were given kidneys from nonrelated donors (the first in June 1960) that functioned for 17 and 18 months. During the critical period from January 1959 through the spring of 1962, the cumulative French experience was the principal (and perhaps the only) justification to continue clinical kidney transplantation trials (Table 2–1). By showing that bone marrow infusion was *not* a necessary condition for substantial prolongation of kidney grafts, the stage was set for the transition to drug therapy. In fact, Kuss was using 6-mercaptopurine (6-MP) and steroids as adjuvant therapy as early as 1960.[51]

Those examining this period historically have been inclined to consider

TABLE 2–1 ▲ LONG SURVIVING HUMAN KIDNEY ALLOGRAFTS (BEFORE MAY 1962)

Reported by	Reference	Date	Donor	Primary Immunosuppression	Kidney Survival (years)
Murray	43,44,46	January 24, 1959	Fraternal twin	X-ray	20.5[a]
Hamburger	47	June 29, 1959	Fraternal twin	X-ray	25[a]
Kuss	51	June 22, 1960	Unrelated	X-ray (also 6-MP, steroids)	1.5
Hamburger	48	December 19, 1960	Mother	Irradiation (also steroids)	>1
Kuss	51	March 12, 1961	Unrelated	Irradiation (also 6-MP, steroids)	1.5
Hamburger	49	February 12, 1962	Cousin	Irradiation (also steroids)	15[b]
Murray	53	April 5, 1962	Unrelated	Imuran (azathioprine)	1.5

6-MP, 6-mercaptopurine.
[a] Died of cancer.
[b] Patient alive after retransplantation of sister kidney (without interim dialysis) on March 28, 1977.

irradiation-induced and drug-induced graft acceptance as different phenomena.[5,44,46] However, it seems certain that the Boston and Paris fraternal twin kidney recipients, as well as the 5 long-surviving non-twin French recipients, had achieved to variable degrees the kind of graft acceptance that later was seen in tens of thousands of drug-treated humans after all kinds of whole-organ transplantation. The fact that the mechanism was the same has been appreciated only since it was discovered that extensive migration and survival of sessile tissue leukocytes (most obviously of dendritic cells) from graft to host (microchimerism) is the explanation of "acceptance" of all whole organs with any immunosuppressive modality.[54–58]

Chemical Immunosuppression

Because of the success (albeit limited) with kidney transplantation after TBI, it was not surprising that the search for immunosuppressive drugs was focused at first on myelotoxic agents that mimicked irradiation. They were viewed as "space makers" for donor marrow or for recovering recipient bone marrow. In September 1960, Goodwin et al produced profound bone marrow suppression with methotrexate and cyclophosphamide in a daughter recipient of a maternal kidney. The patient subsequently experienced several rejections that were temporarily reversed with prednisone during the 143 days of survival. This was the first example of protracted human kidney graft function with drug treatment alone.[59] However, the case was not reported until 1963.

Kidney transplant surgeons were quick to realize that myelotoxicity should be avoided, not deliberately imposed. The most important step in this appreciation followed the discovery by Schwartz and Dameschek[60] that 6-MP in nontransplant models was immunosuppressive without bone marrow depression. Within a few months, Schwartz and Dameschek[61] and Meeker et al[62] showed that 6-MP allowed a dose-related mitigation of skin-graft rejection in rats. Close behind, Calne[63] and Zukoski et al[64] independently demonstrated the same thing in dogs following kidney transplantation.

In June, 1960, Calne moved from the Royal Free Hospital, London, to Boston to be the team leader in Murray's Brigham laboratory for further preclinical development of 6-MP and its analogue, azathioprine.[65,66] What was achieved at first in Boston and in laboratories elsewhere with the canine kidney transplant model was delay of rejection or death of the animal from overimmunosuppression. However, occasional examples of long-term or seemingly permanent allograft acceptance were observed throughout 1962 and 1963[67–70]—defined as long survival of transplanted mongrel kidneys following completion of a 4- to 12-month course of 6-MP or azathioprine. The same thing has been observed since with each new major immunosuppressive agent (or drug cocktail regimen), including cyclosporine and tacrolimus (FK 506). Until the advent of cyclosporine and tacrolimus, the most potent agents for induction of this state have been the antilymphocyte sera (ALS) and antilymphocyte globulins (ALG) that at the beginning were polyclonal agents[71,72] and later the highly specific monoclonal preparations first used clinically by Cosimi et al.[73]

This new kind of graft acceptance in outbred dogs was easier to produce with drugs than with TBI, but the number of absolute examples was (and is) extremely small in contrast to what can be achieved in small rodents. In Murray's summary of his research with Calne and subsequent collaborators, a handful of long-surviving animals ($<5\%$) was the distillation from 1000 experiments with 6-MP or azathioprine performed in the Boston laboratories.[67] The same was true everywhere. The animals proudly displayed as long-term survivors in laboratories in Boston, Denver, Richmond, and Minneapolis were limited to a few who had run the gauntlet of therapy to the point where treatment was stopped. However, a unique observation was made at the University of Colorado. Adrenocortical steroids were shown to reverse rejection in 88% of dogs, sometimes in a spectacular way, before the steroids in this species almost always caused fatal peptic erosions of the gastrointestinal tract.[74]

It was on this dismal record that the clinical kidney transplant trials of the early 1960s were based. In a display of optimism that would not be tolerated in today's clinical research climate, the rare exceptional survival was given more weight than the customary failure. Thus the poor results came as no surprise when the drugs were first used for patients in the same way as had been tried in dogs.[44,53] However, one of the Boston patients whose transplantation under azathioprine had been performed in April, 1962, had functional graft survival for more than 18 months after receiving the kidney of a patient who could not be weaned from a heart-lung apparatus after open heart surgery[53,75] under conditions comparable to those of a "heart-beating cadaver."[76] Although the allograft failed after 18 months, this pioneer recipient was the first to achieve long survival with azathioprine, and this constituted the opening wedge into a new era.

▲ THE YEAR OF THE STAMPEDE: 1963

The Crucial Role of Steroids

The Reversibility of Rejection

At the University of Colorado, where the synergism of azathioprine and prednisone had been observed in dog experiments,[74] the two drugs were routinely used together from the origin of this program in early 1962. The results exceeded everyone's expectations[77,78] and precipitated a revolution in clinical transplantation. Acute rejection could readily be reversed with prednisone in almost all cases. The use of adrenocortical steroids in transplantation can be traced to the experimental work a decade earlier of Billingham et al[25] and Morgan.[26] Goodwin et al[59] had observed reversal of rejection in a kidney recipient whose primary treatment had been with methotrexate and cyclophosphamide. Hamburger et al[48] and Kuss et al[51] also had administered steroids to their irradiated patients under unknown circumstances. However, there was no hint in any of these reports suggesting either the profound effectiveness of prednisone or the indispensability of this dose-maneuverable drug, which remains an essential component of treatment regimens to the present day.

Host-Graft Nonreactivity

A second and equally fundamental observation in the Colorado kidney recipients was a subsequent diminution in the amount of drug treatment required to prevent rejection,[77] often allowing the life-time rehabilitation of many patients in an unrestricted environment. Of the first 64 patients in the Colorado series compiled between 1962 and March 1964,[78] 15 survived for the next 25 years, including the recipient with the longest surviving allograft in the world (now 33 years).[50] Two of the 15 patients stopped all immunosuppression without rejection for 28 and 30 years, recapitulating the phenomenon occasionally seen in dogs and in the irradiated Boston and Paris fraternal twins. Nine other patients from the era preceding early 1964, including three treated by Hume (who had moved to Richmond), were alive in six other centers in the summer of 1989. None of these quarter-century survivors had been given a kidney from a nonrelated donor. The first such example in the world passed the 25-year mark in October 1989.[50] This was a recipient of a cadaveric kidney treated in Paris by Hamburger et al in October 1964.

TABLE 2–2 ▲ THE FOUNDATION OF CLINICAL TRANSPLANTATION

Central Therapeutic Dogma	Principal Baseline Agents
Therapy with baseline drugs	Azathioprine
Secondary adjustments with steroids with or without antilymphoid agents	Cyclophosphamide
Case to case trial (and potential error) of weaning	Cyclosporine
	Tacrolimus (FK 506)

Evolution of a Treatment Dogma

The reversibility of rejection and change in the host-graft relationship eventually were verified with all other transplanted organs, beginning with the liver.[79,80] Although immunosuppression has improved, the central therapeutic dogma for solid-organ transplantation that had emerged by 1963[77,78] has changed very little in more than 30 years. The dogma calls for daily treatment with one or two baseline drugs with further immune modulation by the highly dose-maneuverable adrenocortical steroids to whatever level is required to maintain stable graft function (Table 2–2). This means that every recipient of a whole organ goes through a trial and potential error experience as drugs are weaned to maintenance levels.

When the news became known in 1963 of the successes with azathioprine and prednisone therapy, a proliferation of kidney transplant centers began on both sides of the Atlantic. In January 1963, there were only three active clinical kidney transplant centers in the United States. These were at the Brigham, the Medical College of Virginia (where Dave Hume moved from Boston in 1956), and the University of Colorado, where the first renal transplantation was performed in March 1962. Centers were equally scarce in Europe, where the two in Paris had been in existence for more than a dozen years. By year's end, more than 50 American kidney centers were gearing up, and some had already started. The same thing occurred in Europe. Trials with the liver, the next vital organ beyond the kidney, had started,[81] and clinical xenotransplantation with chimpanzee[6] and baboon[8] donors had been systematically tried with encouraging, although ultimately unsatisfactory results.

Failure to explain the reason for the empirically derived treatment regimen did not prevent its worldwide acceptance almost overnight and its refinement to an art form with each new agent beginning with the addition of ALG in 1966 as a third (adjuvant) agent[71] and continuing in 1989 with the addition of tacrolimus (FK 506).[82] The introduction of cyclosporine by Calne et al[83] in 1978 eventually led to a dramatic change in the field. However, the use of cyclosporine alone (or in combination with myelotoxic agents) was unacceptably toxic and suboptimally therapeutic. When combined with prednisone (with or without other agents),[84] the new drug narrowed the gap between the results of cadaveric versus living-related transplantation and opened the doors to further development of transplantation of the liver, heart, and other extrarenal organs.

▲ KIDNEY PROCUREMENT AND PRESERVATION

The sudden arrival of clinical kidney transplantation in 1963 was so unexpected that little collateral research or other formal preparation had been made to preserve the organs. The lack of insight 50 years ago about the requirements for successful kidney preservation was illustrated by the fact that Voronoy's first cadaveric kidney donor (in 1936) had been dead for 6 hours before procurement.[10] Even in the highly successful identical twin cases, kidneys were not protected from warm ischemia until 1962.

Yet the potential benefit of lowering the temperature of an excised organ was grasped instinctively by early workers, in part because cardiac surgeons were knowledgeable about hypothermia for open heart operations and had demonstrated a reduction of ischemic damage below the level of aortic cross clamping when the subdiaphagmatic organs were cooled.[85] Lillehei et al[86] simply immersed intestine in iced saline solution before its autotransplantation. The value of hypothermia for liver allografts was quantified chemically by Sicular and Moore,[87] who reported a slowed rate of enzyme degradation in cold hepatic slices. Thus the principle of hypothermia was understood, although not efficiently applied.

Hypothermia to protect human renal homografts was first systematically accomplished with the cumbersome and potentially dangerous method of ice-tub immersion of living volunteer donors.[88] Total body hypothermia was soon replaced by core (intravascular) cooling by means of infusion of chilled solutions into the renal artery after donor nephrectomy.[89] This technique (using lactated Ringer's solution) had been used for the first time during the development of experimental liver transplantation.[90] Its modification for the renal operation by the same team was an early example of the cross fertilization of procedures that continues today, despite the balkanization of transplantation along organ-defined specialty lines.

Core cooling remains the first step in the preservation of all whole-organ grafts. In cadaveric donors, this is most often done in situ by means of some variation of the technique described by Marchioro et al.[91] This method for the continuous hypothermic perfusion of cadaveric livers and kidneys was used clinically long before the acceptance of brain-death conditions.[92] Ackerman and Snell[93] and Merkel et al[94] popularized in situ cooling of cadaveric kidneys with simple infusion of cold electrolyte solutions into the distal aorta.

Until 1981, transplantation of the extrarenal organs was an unusual event. By late 1981, it had become clear that liver and thoracic-organ transplant procedures were going to be widespread. A method of multiple organ procurement was required by which the kidneys, liver, heart, and lungs or various combinations of these organs could be removed without jeopardizing any of the individual organs. Such a system, called the *flexible technique*,[95] was developed at the University of Colorado and the University of Pittsburgh. Aided by the efforts of C. Everett Koop, the Surgeon General of the United States, the technique was adopted as a worldwide standard almost overnight. All organs to be used are cooled in situ, and after cooling they are rapidly removed by means of dissection in a bloodless field. The sharing of organs from a common donor by recipient teams from widely separated centers became routine by the mid 1980s.

Extension of the safe period after initial cooling has followed one of two prototype strategies, developed in research conducted mainly with kidneys and applied secondarily to livers and other organs. One approach was to provide a limited and continuous renal arterial circulation, as was done by Ackerman and Barnard[96] with a perfusate primed with blood and oxygenated within a hyperbaric oxygen chamber. When Belzer et al[97] were able to eliminate the hemoglobin and hyperbaric chamber components, their asanguineous perfusion technique was immediately accepted but then slowly abandoned in most centers when it was learned that the quality of two-day preservation was not markedly better than with the simpler and less expensive infusion and slush methods. Nevertheless, it is expected that refinement of this approach will someday allow true organ banking.

The alternative strategy for the preservation of kidneys and other organs has been the instillation of special solutions such as that described by Collins et al[98] or plasma-like solutions.[99] The original Collins solution, or modifications of it, was used for almost 20 years for the so-called slush techniques of kidney preservation. The introduction of the University of Wisconsin (UW) solution was the first important development in kidney preservation in almost two decades.

The superiority of the UW solution to any of previous conventional solutions for preservation of kidney, liver, and other organs has been demonstrated in experimental kidney transplant test models[100–102] and confirmed in clinical trials.[103] The UW preservation allowed longer safe preservation (2 days), a higher rate of graft survival, and a lower rate of primary nonfunction. The day of economical and practical national organ sharing had finally arrived after 30 years of evolution.

▲ TISSUE TYPING

Antigen Matching

In the early 1960s, when the modern era of transplantation was in its infancy, it was predicted that tissue matching would have to be perfected if kidney grafting procedures were to succeed with any degree of reliability and predictability. The first prospective matching trials were started in 1964 by Terasaki et al,[104] of Los Angeles, in collaboration with the University of Colorado transplantation team.

The results were disappointing. Since then, the genetics of the human major histocompatibility complex (MHC), its overriding importance in human biology, and above all its complexity have been established. Although the value of tissue matching for transplantation between highly compatible family or nonrelated donor members (the perfect match) was established as early as 1970,[105] the complexity of the human histocompatibility system has militated against perfect matching between nonrelated people for cadaveric kidney transplantation. Lesser degrees of matching have not correlated well with outcome.[106–109]

Whether these expensive efforts at matching should continue has become a debated public policy because of the increasing use by the United Network of Organ Sharing (UNOS) of tissue matching as the overriding determinant of national distribution of cadaveric kidneys. Reports from two American and European multicenter case compilations with an overlapping database have consistently claimed a slight but statistically significant gain in survival of well-matched versus mismatched cadaveric kidneys, but most of the centers or consortia that contribute to these data pools are unable to see this trend in their own material. In the meanwhile, the results with modern-day immunosuppression have become almost as good with unmatched cadaveric kidneys as with kidneys from less than perfectly matched (double haplotype identical) blood relatives.

The most nagging intellectual concern to kidney transplant surgeons and others who wanted to but could not see an influence of human leukocyte antigen (HLA) matching in their own practices was the knowledge that only a perfect or near perfect match had a significant effect on outcome, and even then a small one. It was difficult to see why HLA matching was so critical for success with bone marrow transplantation[41,110] but so inconsequential for whole organs. A plausible explanation for this dichotomy was provided with the discovery of systemic chimerism in organ recipients many years after organ transplantation.[54–56] How this chimeric state, which is believed to be the basis of renal graft acceptance, explains the blindfolding of an HLA matching effect is discussed in Chapter 9.

Cross Matching

None of the immunosuppressive measures available today can prevent the immediate destruction of kidneys by preformed humoral antibodies in what has been called *hyperacute rejection.* This catastrophic complication was first seen with transplantation from ABO incompatible donors and ascribed to antidonor isoagglutinins.[11] After the description by Terasaki et al[111] of hyperacute kidney rejection by a recipient with antidonor lymphocytotoxic antibodies, Kissmeyer-Nielsen et al[112] and others[113–115] confirmed the etiologic role of these antigraft antibodies. Although hyperacute rejection usually can be avoided with the "cross match" originally recommended by Terasaki et al,[111] its exact pathogenesis remains mysterious 30 years later. Understanding and prevention of the process is believed to be the key to successful xenotransplantation.[116]

▲ REFERENCES

1. Burnet FM: The new approach to immunology. *N Engl J Med* 264:24–34, 1961.
2. Elkinton JR: Moral problems in the use of borrowed organs artificial and transplanted. *Ann Intern Med* 60:309–313, 1964.

3. Jaboulay M: Greffe du reins au pli du coude par soudures arterielles et veineuses. *Lyon Med* 107:575–577, 1906.
4. Unger E: Nierentransplantation. *Wien Klin Wochenschr* 47:573–578, 1910.
5. Groth CG: Landmarks in clinical renal transplantation. *Surg Gynecol Obstet* 134:323–328, 1972.
6. Reemstsma K, McCracken BH, Schlegel JU, et al: Renal heterotransplantation in man. *Ann Surg* 160:384–410, 1964.
7. Starzl TE: *Experience in Renal Transplantation.* Philadelphia, Saunders, 1964:262 298, 345–359.
8. Starzl TE, Marchioro TL, Peters GN, et al: Renal heterotransplantation from baboon to man: experience with 6 cases. *Transplantation* 2:752–776, 1964.
9. Bailey L, Nehlsen-Cannarella S, Concepcion W, Jolley W: Baboon to human cardiac xenotransplantation in a neonate. *JAMA* 254:3321–3329, 1985.
10. Voronoy U: Sobre bloqueo del aparato reticuloendotelial del hombre en algunas formas de intoxicacion por el sublimado y sobre la transplantacion del rinon cadaverico como metodo de tratamiento de la anuria consecutiva a aquella intoxicacion. *Siglo Medico* 97:296–297, 1937.
11. Starzl TE: Patterns of permissible donor-recipient tissue transfer in relation to ABO blood groups. In: *Experience in Renal Transplantation.* Philadelphia, Saunders, 1964:37–47.
12. Hume DM, Merrill JP, Miller BF, Thorn GW: Experiences with renal homotransplantation in the human: report of nine cases. *J Clin Invest* 34:327–382, 1955.
13. Kuss R, Teinturier J, Milliez P: Quelques essais de greffe rein chez l'homme. *Mem Acad Chir* 77:755–764, 1951.
14. Dubost C, Oeconomos N, Nenna A, Milliez P: Resultats d'une tentative de greffe renale. *Bull Soc Med Hop Paris* 67:1372–1382, 1951.
15. Servelle M, Soulie P, Rougeulle J: Greffe d'une rein de supplicie a une malade avec rein unique congenital, atteinte de nephrite chronique hypertensive azatemique. *Bull Soc Med Hop Paris* 67:99–104, 1951.
16. Michon L, Hamburger J, Oeconomos N, et al: Une tentative de transplantation renale chez l'homme: aspects medicaux et biologiques. *Presse Med* 61:1419–1423, 1953.
17. Merrill JP, Murray JE, Harrison JH, Guild WR: Successful homotransplantation of the human kidney between identical twins. *JAMA* 160:277–282, 1956.
18. Carrel A: The operative technique for vascular anastomoses and transplantation of viscera. *Lyon Medical* 98:859, 1902.
19. Moore FD: *Transplant: The Give and Take of Tissue Transplantation.* New York, Simon & Schuster, 1972:1–364.
20. Lawler RH, West JW, McNulty PH, et al: Homotransplantation of the kidney in the human. *JAMA* 144:844–845, 1950.
21. Murray JE, Merrill JP, Harrison JH: Renal homotransplantation in identical twins. *Surg Forum* 6:432, 1955.
22. Brown JB: Homografting of skin: with report of success in identical twins. *Surgery* 1:558–563, 1937.
23. Medawar PB: The behavior and fate of skin autografts and skin homografts in rabbits. *J Anat* 78:176–199, 1944.
24. Medawar PB: Second study of behavior and fate of skin homografts in rabbits. *J Anat* 79:157, 1945.
25. Billingham RE, Krohn PL, Medawar PB: Effect of cortisone on survival of skin homografts in rabbits. *Br Med J* 1:1157–1163, 1951.

26. Morgan JA: The influence of cortisone on the survival of homografts of skin in the rabbit. *Surgery* 30:506–515, 1951.
27. Dempster WJ, Lennox B, Boag JW: Prolongation of survival of skin homotransplants in the rabbit by irradiation of the host. *Br J Exp Pathol* 31:670–679, 1950.
28. Billingham RE, Brent L, Medawar PB: "Actively acquired tolerance" of foreign cells. *Nature* 172:603–606, 1953.
29. Billingham R, Brent L, Medawar P: Quantitative studies on tissue transplantation immunity. III. Actively acquired tolerance. *Philos Trans R Soc Lond Biol Sci* 239:357–412, 1956.
30. Owen RD: Immunogenetic consequences of vascular anastomoses between bovine twins. *Science* 102:400–401, 1945.
31. Burnet FM, Fenner F: *The Production of Antibodies,* ed 2. Melbourne, Macmillan, 1949:1–142.
32. Billingham R, Brent L: Quantitative studies on transplantation immunity. IV. Induction of tolerance in newborn mice and studies on the phenomenon of runt disease. *Philos Trans R Soc Lond Biol Sci* 242:439–477, 1956.
33. Main JM, Prehn RT: Successful skin homografts after the administration of high dosage X radiation and homologous bone marrow. *J Natl Cancer Inst* 15:1023–1029, 1955.
34. Trentin JJ: Mortality and skin transplantibility in X-irradiated mice receiving isologous or heterologous bone marrow. *Proc Soc Exp Biol Med* 92:688–693, 1956.
35. Mannick JA, Lochte HL, Ashley CA, et al: A functioning kidney homotransplant in the dog. *Surgery* 46:821–828, 1959.
36. Rapaport FT, Bachvaroff RJ, Mollen N, et al: Induction of unresponsiveness to major transplantable organs in adult mammals. *Ann Surg* 190:461–473, 1979.
37. Hume DM, Jackson BT, Zukoski CF, et al: The homotransplantation of kidneys and of fetal liver and spleen after total body irradiation. *Ann Surg* 152:354–373, 1960.
38. Mathe G, Amiel JL, Schwarzenberg L, et al: Haematopoietic chimera in man after allogenic (homologous) bone-marrow transplantation. *Br Med J* 1963:1633–1635.
39. Gatti RA, Meuwissen HJ, Allen HD, et al: Immunological reconstitution of sex-linked lymphopenic immunological deficiency. *Lancet* 2:1366–1369, 1968.
40. Bach FH: Bone-marrow transplantation in a patient with the Wiskott-Aldrich syndrome. *Lancet* 2:1364–1366, 1968.
41. Thomas ED: Allogeneic marrow grafting: a story of man and dog. In: Terasaki PI (ed), *History of Transplantation: Thirty-Five Recollections.* Los Angeles, UCLA Tissue Typing Laboratory, 1991:379–393.
42. van Bekkum DW: Bone marrow transplantation: a story of stem cells. In: Terasaki PI (ed), *History of Transplantation: Thirty-Five Recollections.* Los Angeles, UCLA Tissue Typing Laboratory, 1991:395–434.
43. Murray JE, Merrill JP, Dammin GJ, et al: Study of transplantation immunity after total body irradiation: clinical and experimental investigation. *Surgery* 48:272–284, 1960.
44. Murray JE, Merrill JP, Dammin GJ, et al: Kidney transplantation in modified recipients. *Ann Surg* 156:337–355, 1962.
45. Merrill JP, Murray JE, Harrison JH, et al: Successful homotransplantation of the human kidney between non-identical twins. *N Engl J Med* 262:1251–1260, 1960.
46. Murray JE: Nobel Prize Lecture: The first successful organ transplants in man. In: Terasaki PI (ed), *History of Transplantation: Thirty-Five Recollections.* Los Angeles, UCLA Tissue Typing Laboratory, 1991:121–143.

47. Hamburger J, Vaysse J, Crosnier J, et al: Transplantation of a kidney between nonmonozygotic twins after irradiation of the receiver: good function at the fourth month. *Presse Med* 67:1771–1775, 1959.
48. Hamburger J, Vaysse J, Crosnier J, et al: Renal homotransplantation in man after radiation of the recipient. *Am J Med* 32:854–871, 1962.
49. Hamburger J: Memories of old times. In: Terasaki PI (ed), *History of Transplantation: Thirty-Five Recollections.* Los Angeles, UCLA Tissue Typing Laboratory, 1991:71.
50. Starzl TE, Schroter GPJ, Hartmann NJ, et al: Long term (25 year) survival after renal homotransplantation: the world experience. *Transplant Proc* 22:2361–2365, 1990.
51. Kuss R, Legrain M, Mathe G, et al: Homologous human kidney transplantation: experience with six patients. *Postgrad Med J* 38:528–531, 1962.
52. Kuss R: Human renal transplantation memories, 1951 to 1981. In: Terasaki PI (ed), *History of Transplantation: Thirty-Five Recollections.* Los Angeles, UCLA Tissue Typing Laboratory, 1991:37–59.
53. Murray JE, Merrill JP, Harrison JH, et al: Prolonged survival of human-kidney homografts by immunosuppressive drug therapy. *N Engl J Med* 268:1315–1323, 1963.
54. Starzl TE, Demetris AJ, Murase N, et al: Cell migration, chimerism, and graft acceptance. *Lancet* 339:1579–1582, 1992.
55. Starzl TE, Demetris AJ, Trucco M, et al: Cell migration and chimerism after whole organ transplantation: the basis of graft acceptance. *Hepatology* 17:1127–1152, 1993.
56. Starzl TE, Demetris AJ, Trucco M, et al: Chimerism and donor specific nonreactivity 27 to 29 years after kidney allotransplantation. *Transplantation* 55:1272–1277, 1993.
57. Starzl TE, Demetris AJ, Trucco M, et al: Chimerism after liver transplantation for type IV glycogen storage disease and type I Gaucher's disease. *N Engl J Med* 328:745–749, 1993.
58. Starzl TE, Demetris AJ: Transplantation milestones: viewed with one- and two-way paradigms of tolerance. *JAMA* 273:876–879, 1995.
59. Goodwin WE, Kaufman JJ, Mims MM, et al: Human renal transplantation. I. Clinical experience with six cases of renal homotransplantation. *J Urol* 89:13–24, 1963.
60. Schwartz R, Damesheck W: Drug-induced immunological tolerance. *Nature* 183:1682–1683, 1959.
61. Schwartz R, Dameshek W: The effects of 6-mercaptopurine on homograft reactions. *J Clin Invest* 39:952–958, 1960.
62. Meeker W, Condie R, Weiner D, et al: Prolongation of skin homograft survival in rabbits by 6-mercaptopurine. *Proc Soc Exp Biol Med* 102:459–461, 1959.
63. Calne RY: The rejection of renal homografts: inhibition in dogs by 6-mercaptopurine. *Lancet* 1:417–418, 1960.
64. Zukoski CF, Lee HM, Hume DM: The prolongation of functional survival of canine renal homografts by 6-mercaptopurine. *Surg Forum* 11:470–472, 1960.
65. Calne RY: Inhibition of the rejection of renal homografts in dogs with purine analogues. *Transplant Bull* 28:445, 1961.
66. Calne RY, Murray JE: Inhibition of the rejection of renal homografts in dogs by Burroughs Wellcome 57-222. *Surg Forum* 12:118, 1961.
67. Murray JE, Sheil AGR, Moseley R, et al: Analysis of mechanism of immunosuppressive drugs in renal homotransplantation. *Ann Surg* 160:449, 1964.
68. Pierce JC, Varco RL: Effects of long term 6-mercaptopurine treatment upon kidney homotransplants in dogs. *Surgery* 54:1254, 1968.

69. Zukowski CF, Callaway JM: Adult tolerance induced by 6-methyl mercaptopurine to canine renal homografts. *Nature* 198:706, 1963.
70. Starzl TE: Host-graft adaptation. In: *Experience in Renal Transplantation*. Philadelphia, Saunders, 1964:164–170.
71. Starzl TE, Marchioro TL, Porter KA, et al: The use of heterologous antilymphoid agents in canine renal and liver homotransplantation and in human renal homotransplantation. *Surg Gynecol Obstet* 124:301–318, 1967.
72. Scanfield I, Wolf JS, Wren SF, et al: Mechanism of permanent survival of canine renal allografts following a limited course of ALS treatment. *Transplant Proc* 5:533–534, 1973.
73. Cosimi AB, Burton RC, Colvin RB, et al: Treatment of acute renal allograft rejection with OKT3 monoclonal antibody. *Transplantation* 32:535–539, 1981.
74. Marchioro TL, Axtell HK, LaVia MF, et al: The role of adrenocortical steroids in reversing established homograft rejection. *Surgery* 55:412–417, 1964.
75. Murray JE, Wilson RE, O'Connor NE: Evaluation of long-functioning human kidney transplants. *Surg Gynecol Obstet* 124:509–520, 1967.
76. Merrill JP, Murray JE, Takacs F: Successful transplantation of kidney from a human cadaver. *JAMA* 185:347–353, 1963.
77. Starzl TE, Marchioro TL, Waddell WR: The reversal of rejection in human renal homografts with subsequent development of homograft tolerance. *Surg Gynecol Obstet* 117:385–395, 1963.
78. Starzl TE: *Experience in Renal Transplantation*. Philadelphia, Saunders, 1964.
79. Starzl TE, Marchioro TL, Porter KA, et al: Factors determining short- and long-term survival after orthotopic liver homotransplantation in the dog. *Surgery* 58:131–155, 1965.
80. Starzl TE: *Experience in Hepatic Transplantation*. Philadelphia, Saunders, 1969.
81. Starzl TE, Marchioro TL, Von Kaulla KN, et al: Homotransplantation of the liver in humans. *Surg Gynecol Obstet* 117:659–676, 1963.
82. Starzl TE, Todo S, Fung J, et al: FK 506 for human liver, kidney and pancreas transplantation. *Lancet* 2:1000–1004, 1989.
83. Calne RY, Rolles K, White DJG, et al: Cyclosporin A initially as the only immunosuppressant in 34 recipients of cadaveric organs: 32 kidneys, 2 pancreases, and 2 livers. *Lancet* 2:1033–1036, 1979.
84. Starzl TE, Weil R III, Iwatsuki S, et al: The use of cyclosporin A and prednisone in cadaver kidney transplantation. *Surg Gynecol Obstet* 151:17–26, 1980.
85. Owens TC, Prevedel AE, Swan H: Prolonged experimental occlusion of thoracic aorta during hypothermia. *Arch Surg* 70:95–97, 1955.
86. Lillehei RC, Goott B, Miller FA: The physiological response of the small bowel of the dog to ischemia including prolonged in vitro preservation of the bowel with successful replacement and survival. *Ann Surg* 150:543–560, 1959.
87. Sicular A, Moore FD: The postmortem survival of tissues. *J Surg Res* 1:16, 1961.
88. Starzl TE, Brittain RS, Stonington OG, et al: Renal transplantation in identical twins. *Arch Surg* 865:600–607, 1963.
89. Starzl TE: Donor nephrectomy. In: *Experience in Renal Transplantation*. Philadelphia, Saunders, 1964:68–71.
90. Starzl TE, Kaupp HA Jr, Brock DR, et al: Reconstructive problems in canine liver homotransplantation with special reference to the postoperative role of hepatic venous flow. *Surg Gynecol Obstet* 111:733–743, 1960.
91. Marchioro TL, Huntley RT, Waddell WR, Starzl TE: Extracorporeal perfusion for obtaining postmorten homografts. *Surgery* 54:900–911, 1963.

92. Starzl TE: The role of cadaveric donors in homotransplantation. In: *Experience in Renal Transplantation.* Philadelphia, Saunders, 1964:54–57.
93. Ackerman JR, Snell MR: Cadaveric renal transplantation. *Br J Urol* 40:515–521, 1963.
94. Merkel FK, Jonasson O, Bergan JJ: Procurement of cadaver donor organs: evisceration technique. *Transplant Proc* 4:585–589, 1972.
95. Starzl TE, Hakala TR, Shaw BW Jr, et al: A flexible procedure for multiple cadaveric organ procurement. *Surg Gynecol Obstet* 158:223–230, 1984.
96. Ackerman JR, Barnard CN: A report on the successful storage of kidneys. *Br J Surg* 53:525–532, 1966.
97. Belzer FO, Ashby BS, Dunphy JE: 24-hour and 72-hour preservation of canine kidneys. *Lancet* 2:536–538, 1967.
98. Collins GM, Bravo-Shugarman M, Terasaki PI: Kidney preservation for transportation: initial perfusion and 30 hours ice storage. *Lancet* 2:1219–1224, 1969.
99. Schalm SW: A simple and clinically applicable method for the preservation of a liver homograft. Leyden, The Netherlands, University of Leyden, 1968. Thesis.
100. Hoffman B, Sollinger H, Kalayoglu M, Belzer FO: Use of UW solution for kidney transplantation. *Transplantation* 46:338–339, 1988.
101. Ploeg RJ, Goossens D, McAnulty JF, et al: Successful 72-hour cold storage of dog kidneys with UW solution. *Transplantation* 46:191–196, 1988.
102. Ueda Y, Todo S, Imventarza O, et al: The UW solution for canine kidney preservation: its specific effect on renal hemodynamics and microvasculature. *Transplantation* 48:913–918, 1989.
103. Belzer FO, Southard JH: Principles of solid-organ preservation by cold storage. *Transplantation* 45:673-676, 1988.
104. Terasaki PI, Porter KA, Marchioro TL, et al: Serotyping for homotransplantation. VII. Selection of kidney donors for thirty-two recipients. *Ann NY Acad Sci* 129:500–520, 1966.
105. Starzl TE, Porter KA, Andres G, et al: Long-term survival after renal transplantation in humans: with special reference to histocompatibility matching, thymectomy, homograft glomerulonephritis, heterologous ALG, and recipient malignancy. *Ann Surg* 172:437–472, 1970.
106. Tatemoto S, Terasaki PI, Cecka JM, et al: Survival of nationally shared HLA-matched kidney transplants from cadaveric donors. *N Engl J Med* 327:834–839, 1992.
107. Matas AJ, Sutherland DER, Najarian JS: The impact of HLA matching on graft survival. *Transplantation* 54:568–569, 1992.
108. Ferguson R for the Transplant Information Share Group (TISG): A multicenter experience with sequential ALG/cyclosporine therapy in renal transplantation. *Clin Transplant* 2:285–294, 1988.
109. Salvatierra O Jr: Optimal use of organs for transplantation. *N Engl J Med* 318:1329–1331, 1988.
110. Meuwissen HJ, Gatti RA, Terasaki PI, et al: Treatment of lymphopenic hypogammaglobulinemia and bone marrow aplasia by transplantation of allogeneic marrow: crucial role of histocompatibility matching. *N Engl J Med* 281:691–697, 1969.
111. Teraski PI, Marchioro TL, Starzl TE: Sero-typing of human lymphocyte antigens: preliminary trials on long-term kidney homograft survivors. In: Russell PS, Winn HJ, Amos DB (eds), *Histocompatibility Testing 1965.* Washington, DC, National Academy of Science, 1965:83–96.
112. Kissmeyer-Nielsen F, Olson S, Peterson VP, Fjeldborg O: Hyperacute rejection of kidney al-

lografts, associated with preexisting humoral antibodies against donor cells. *Lancet* 2:622–665, 1966.
113. Williams GM, Lee HM, Weymouth RF, et al: Studies in hyperacute and chronic renal homograft rejection in man. *Surgery* 62:204–212, 1967.
114. Starzl TE, Lerner RA, Dixon FJ, et al: Schwartzman reaction after human renal transplantation. *N Engl J Med* 278:642–648, 1968.
115. Ting A: The lymphocytotoxic crossmatch test in clinical renal transplantation. *Transplantation* 35:403–407, 1983.
116. Starzl TE, Valdivia LA, Murase N: The biological basis of and strategies for clinical xenotransplantation. *Immunol Rev* 141:213–244, 1994.

3

Evaluation of the Potential Renal Allograft Recipient

Jerry McCauley

Advances in patient care and immunosuppression have led to improved patient and graft survival after renal transplantation. As a result, the criteria for referral for transplantation of patients with end-stage renal disease (ESRD) have broadened. Candidates for renal transplantation are increasingly older and present with more complex medical problems. This development presents a challenge to those involved in the recipient evaluation process. Extrarenal medical problems must be identified and, if possible, treated before a patient is placed on the list for transplantation. At issue is the risk of morbidity and mortality after transplantation in patients with medical problems balanced against the potential for successful transplantation and the discontinuation of dialysis. This chapter discusses the details involved in the evaluation of potential recipients for renal transplantation and addresses both straightforward and complex situations.

▲ REFERRING PATIENTS FOR KIDNEY TRANSPLANTATION

Consideration for renal transplantation begins with referral by the nephrologist. Patients with ESRD have three options for renal replacement therapy: hemodialysis, chronic ambulatory peritoneal dialysis (CAPD), or transplantation. The decision to refer patients for transplantation is based on the relative risks and benefits of transplantation compared with dialysis. Most patients begin hemodialysis or CAPD before being referred for transplantation (although this is not absolutely necessary). In 1990, the mean time from initiation of dialysis until transplantation was 1 year for recipients of kidneys from living donors and 2 years for recipients of cadaveric organs.[1]

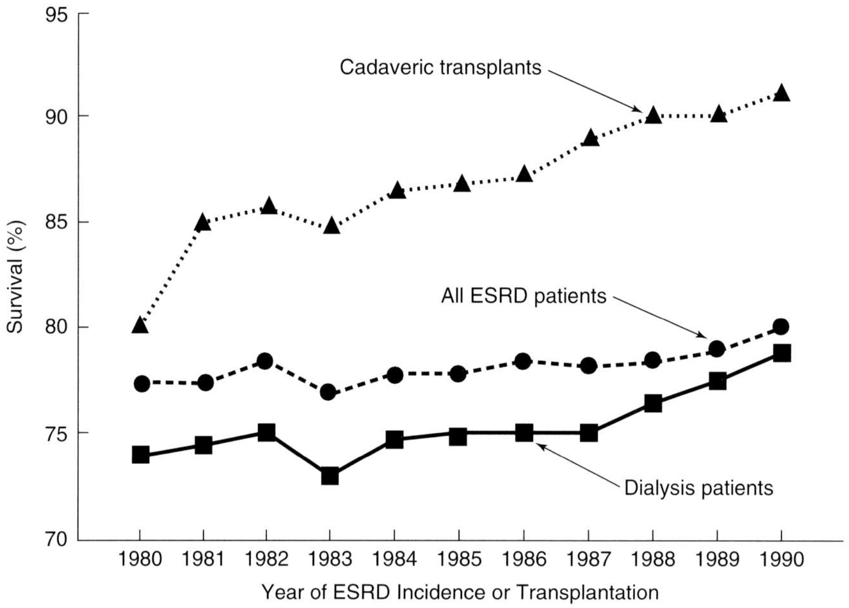

Figure 3–1. Changes in patient survival for dialysis, all other treatment modalities, and cadaveric renal transplants from 1980 to 1990. (*Data from USRDS Annual Report.*)

During the 1980s, patient survival for both dialysis and renal transplantation improved (Fig. 3–1). Many studies have suggested that patient survival is better after transplantation than with dialysis.[2–4] The main criticism of these studies has been that unselected dialysis patients generally have more severe coexisting disease than do transplant patients. Despite these concerns, most authors are convinced that transplantation reduces the risk of death for patients with ESRD. The best evidence for superior patient survival, in the absence of properly controlled, randomized studies, was reported by Port et al.[5] These investigators analyzed patient survival in recipients of cadaveric renal transplants. Transplantation candidates who continued dialysis acted as a comparison group. Despite an early postoperative increased risk of death in transplant patients, long-term patient survival was increased by 68%. The greatest reduction in risk occurred in patients with diabetes. There was little improvement in survival in patients with glomerulonephritis.

The causes of death are similar in both dialysis and transplant patients (Fig. 3–2). Myocardial infarction, other cardiac disorders, and cerebrovascular disease are important causes of death, and special attention should be given to these potential problems during the pretransplant evaluation. Infection is another important source of mortality. Active infection absolutely contraindicates transplantation until the patient has been treated and the infection has resolved. Cancer also is an absolute contraindication. For most patients, after initial treatment, a 2-year period without evidence of recurrence is necessary before renal transplantation can proceed.

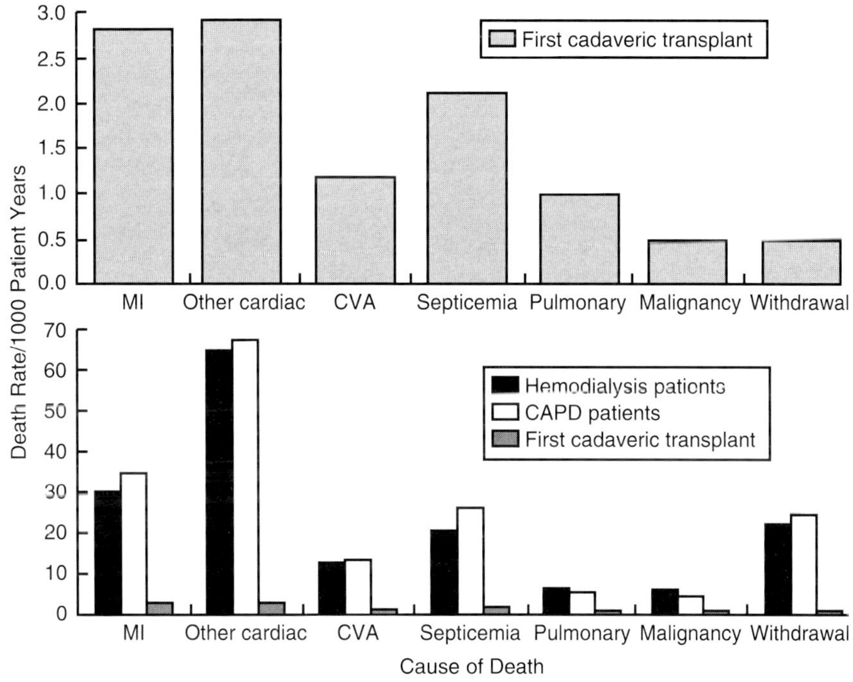

Figure 3–2. Causes of death for dialysis and transplant patients. **Bottom.** All modalities. **Top.** First cadaveric renal transplants. (*Data from USRDS 1993 Annual Report.*)

Recurrence of a preexisting malignant tumor, or cancer that develops after transplantation can be an important cause of death. Finally, withdrawal of treatment is a major cause of death in both the hemodialysis and CAPD dialysis populations (although it is uncommon in transplant patients).[1] The presence of a severe intercurrent illness often prompts this decision.

▲ RECIPIENT EVALUATION PROCESS

Once patients are referred for transplantation, they are seen at the transplant center, where they receive detailed evaluations by the social worker, transplant coordinator, surgeon, and nephrologist. The protocol for recipient evaluation at the University of Pittsburgh is outlined in Table 3–1.

At our center, the initial history is taken by the transplant coordinators. Their evaluation focuses on the primary renal disease, dialysis treatment and complications, history of previous transplantation (reason for graft loss, number of rejection episodes, previous treatment with antilymphocyte preparations), medical and surgical history, and medications and allergies. This history provides the foundation for

TABLE 3–1 ▲ RENAL TRANSPLANT EVALUATION PROTOCOL, UNIVERSITY OF PITTSBURGH

Service	Component
Professional evaluations	Interaction with social worker, nurse coordinator, dentist, surgeon, nephrologist
General laboratory studies	BUN, creatinine, electrolytes, AST, ALT, calcium, phosphorus, alkaline phosphatase, cholesterol, triglycerides, LDH, amylase, albumin, total protein, CBC, platelet count, PT, PTT, RPR
Viral infection screen	CMV (IgG and IgM), hepatitis B (HBsAg and HBsAb), hepatitis C, HIV, Epstein-Barr virus (IgG, IgM, EB early antigen, EBV nuclear antigen, restricted, diffuse), herpes zoster, herpes simplex (IgG and IgM), varicella
Other routine studies	Chest radiograph, ECG, PPD plus controls, urine C&S
Urologic	Ultrasound both kidneys and right upper quadrant
	VCUG (anuric ≥6 months, or history of urologic disease)
	PSA (men ≥ 40 years old)
Screening studies for women	Mammogram (35 years or older) Gynecologic examination + Pap smear
Immunology studies	ABO type and screen, HLA typing, DR typing, quick PRA, circulating antibodies, cross match
Gastrointestinal evaluation	Flexible sigmoidoscopy (50 years or older)

BUN, blood urea nitrogen; AST, aspartate aminotransferase; ALT, alanine aminotransferase; GGTP, gamma glutamyl transpeptidase; LDH, lactate dehydrogenase; CBC, complete blood count; PT, prothrombin time; PTT, partial thromboplastin time; RPR, rapid plasma reagent test; CMV, cytomegalovirus; HIV, human inmmunodeficiency virus; PPD, purified protein derivative; C&S, culture and sensitivity; VCUTG, voiding cystourethrogram; PSA, prostate-specific antigen; PRA, panel reactive antibodies.

the physician's history and saves time. The nephrologist's history and physical examination reviews all potential medical problems. Special attention is directed at identifying preexisting cardiac, pulmonary, and gastrointestinal disorders, which could complicate the perioperative and postoperative periods. The concurrent evaluation by the surgeon gives special attention to issues that might affect the technical performance of the transplant.

The social worker's evaluation looks at the patient's social and psychologic state. This includes screening for known psychopathologic conditions and behavioral styles that might prevent long-term success after transplantation. In particular, noncompliance with dialysis is explored. Patients with a history of noncompliance may be more likely to lose the kidney to acute or chronic rejection after transplantation; however, a history of noncompliance is not an absolute contraindication to transplantation. We have occasionally required noncompliant patients to spend a 6–12 month period of documented compliance with dialysis therapy before placement on the waiting list. Similarly, a history of drug or alcohol abuse generally requires completion of a drug or alcohol rehabilitation program and documentation of abstinence or sobriety before being accepted for transplantation. Other important issues, such as family support, living arrangements, and insurance coverage to pay for (often expensive) immunosuppressive drugs, are explored in detail.

A detailed dental examination is performed (generally by the patient's own dentist) to identify dental caries or other problems that might develop into infectious complications. Fever of unknown origin after transplantation can occasionally be caused by a dental abscess. All dental procedures needed are performed before the patient is placed on the waiting list. In addition, antibiotic prophylaxis is generally required for any dental procedures on patients with an arteriovenous fistula or after transplantation.

The usual laboratory tests can be performed at the patient's referring dialysis center. Similarly, mammograms, gynecologic evaluations, cardiac testing, and other studies can often be obtained by the referring nephrologist. Studies that generally need to be performed at the transplant center include immunologic testing and virologic screening.

▲ IDENTIFYING PATIENTS AT HIGH RISK

As the success of renal transplantation has increased, the number of absolute contraindications has diminished. Universally accepted contraindications include active infection and malignancy. A larger number of relative contraindications exist, but these can vary among centers. Advanced age (>70 years), a history of cancer, or certain causes of renal disease are no longer accepted by all centers as contraindications to transplantation. The goal of the pretransplant evaluation is to identify patients who are at high risk and, if possible, correct the problem(s) before transplantation. Table 3–2 shows the factors that increase the risk for morbidity and mortality after renal transplantation.

Age

During the past decade the number of elderly patients being treated for ESRD has steadily grown. In 1985, 35% of patients starting dialysis were at least 65 years of age; by 1989, this figure had increased to 40%. However, only 0.8% of these older patients received transplants.[6] Reports from the 1970s suggested that transplantation of cadaveric kidneys into patients older than 45 years resulted in dismal outcomes. This prompted the recommendation that these patients receive transplants from living related donors or not undergo transplantation at all.[7] Later studies in the precyclosporine era reported more encouraging results, with a patient survival rate of 57–75% and a graft survival rate of 49–62%.[8] Factors associated with improved results during this era included careful patient selection and the realization that elderly patients often need less immunosuppression. There is evidence that older patients are immunologically less reactive across a number of parameters, and clinical studies suggest that older people have a lower incidence of rejection than younger patients.[8]

TABLE 3–2 ▲ RISK FACTORS FOR RENAL TRANSPLANTATION

Factor	Indicator of High Risk
Age	Elderly
Race	African-American
Obesity	
Psychosocial factors	Known psychiatric illness Noncompliance
	Preexisting illness
Renal disease	Association with other diseases, such as polycystic kidney disease Recurrent renal disease
Diabetes	
Cardiovascular disease	Coronary and valvular heart disease
Chronic infections	Hepatitis B or C, CMV, EBV, and HIV
GI disorders	Peptic ulcers, pancreatitis, diverticulitis
Pulmonary disease	Chronic restrictive or obstructive pulmonary disease/fungal diseases
Carcinoma	

Approaches to immunosuppression that reflect a potentially diminished immune response in elderly patients have reduced the rate of infection-related death and have led to outcomes similar to those seen in younger adults.[9]

During the cyclosporine era, patient and graft survival rates among the elderly have continued to improve. Most centers now report 1-year patient survival rates of 80–85%, and graft survival rates are comparable to or only slightly lower than among younger patients.[9] When patients who die with functioning grafts are excluded, graft survival appproximates that seen in younger patients.[9] In elderly patients, the leading cause of graft loss is death, and most recipients die with excellent renal function.

The improvement in patient survival in elderly patients can be, at least in part, attributed to more careful patient selection and rigorous pretransplant medical evaluation. Paramount in the evaluation is a detailed cardiovascular and peripheral vascular examination. Elderly patients should undergo routine echocardiography and pharmacologic thallium studies. Coronary arteriography should be considered for patients in whom the noninvasive studies are less than definitively normal. Because peripheral vascular disease is also common among the elderly, part of the history and physical examination should screen for arterial insufficiency. Typical symptoms of claudication may not be reported by elderly dialysis patients who are inactive. For such patients, the physical examination and symptoms of nocturnal leg cramps can be very helpful. Severe atherosclerotic vascular disease may complicate the technical performance of the transplant and may also jeopardize blood flow to the lower extremity. Noninvasive vascular studies or angiography may be required to identify correctable lesions. Cerebrovascular disease is also prevalent in the elderly dialysis population and should be investigated as needed.

Identification and treatment of malignant disease is important. Carcinoma of the skin, lung, and gastrointestinal tract are common among the elderly and should be ruled out before transplantation.

Finally, the social aspect of dialysis should be considered for elderly dialysis patients. For some patients, dialysis three times a week provides a regular time for social interaction for otherwise isolated patients. In such patients, dialysis may be the preferred method of therapy for ESRD. Transplantation for most elderly patients improves their quality of life and frees them to enjoy their retirement years with family and friends. For others, it can return them to lonely lives without regular social contact or a caring touch. In such patients, the dialysis staff and other patients fill the emptiness of advancing years. Selection of the elderly should take this unique problem into consideration.

Race

Race is a factor in patient survival on dialysis and after transplantation. African-American patients with hypertension survive longer on dialysis than do whites; however, both patient and allograft survival are worse for African-Americans after transplantation.[4] The reasons for this are not clear. The rate of transplantation is lower for African-Americans, and the waiting time is longer.[10] This could have the effect of leaving relatively healthy African-American patients on dialysis, thus artificially improving their survival on dialysis. No studies have looked at the contribution of coexisting disease and presensitization on longer waiting times. Accurate tissue typing is more difficult in African-Americans[11,12] because of the high frequency of poorly defined or undefined human leukocyte antigens (HLA) in this population. These antigens may be seen as "blanks" when tissue typing is performed. Opelz et al[12] compared DNA to serologic tissue typing and found a 39% discrepancy for African-Americans, compared to 23% for whites. These factors may also play a part in the inferior allograft survival rates and longer waiting times.

Obesity

Obesity is a well-known risk factor; it increases the risk for cardiac, pulmonary, endocrine, and technical complications after any surgical procedure.[13] Several studies have examined obesity in the setting of renal transplantation. Two confirmed a higher rate of complications in obese patients.[14,15] Both groups of investigators used a body mass index $\left(\text{BMI} = \dfrac{\text{weight (kg)}}{\text{height}^2\ (\text{m}^2)}\right)$ greater than or equal to 30 as an indication of obesity. Morbid obesity is defined as a BMI greater than 35. Obese patients experienced a greater number of infections, wound complications, admissions to the intensive care unit, new-onset diabetes, and deaths than nonobese patients. Both initial and long-term graft function were also worse. These reports led to the recommendation that obese patients lose weight before transplantation. For patients who are morbidly obese, weight reduction should be attempted only in a structured program and under medical supervision. From a practical point of view, however, keeping obese patients who do not lose weight off the waiting list is problematic, particularly if they develop dialysis access problems. We have continued to perform transplantation in obese patients who have not fully met their weight-loss goals, as long as they understand the increased risk.

▲ THE PRIMARY RENAL DISEASE AND TRANSPLANTATION

Consideration of the patient's primary renal disease is an important aspect of the pretransplant evaluation. Table 3–3 summarizes the influence of primary renal diagnosis on the rate of renal transplantation and the risk of death during the first year of dialysis.[1] Diabetes (34.2%) is the leading cause of renal failure, followed by hypertensive nephropathy (29.4%) and various glomerular diseases (14.2%). This distribution reflects a trend that began in the 1970s of providing dialysis and transplantation for increasingly ill patients. From the inception of dialysis in the 1940s until approximately 1972, renal replacement therapy was offered to patients who were relatively healthy in all ways except for renal disease. Patients with diabetes and the elderly were considered to be too ill, with a limited life expectancy and quality of life. An amendment to the Social Security Act of 1972 provided Medicare coverage for all U.S. citizens with ESRD. This legislation provided financial support for hemodialysis and renal transplantation. With the introduction of this amendment, the criteria for acceptance into dialysis programs became more flexible, and with the increased number of dialysis patients came more potential transplant candidates. Despite the relaxation of criteria for dialysis, Kjellstrand,[16] in 1985, estimated that the number of patients dying with untreated ESRD was similar to the number being treated with dialysis and transplantation. Treatment of patients with diabetes, elderly patients, and those with other serious diseases has undoubtedly reduced the number of untreated patients but has made evaluation for renal transplantation more complex.

Patients with congenital and hereditary diseases are most likely to receive transplants during the first year of ESRD. Diseases such as congenital obstructive uropathy, dysgenesis, agenesis, Alport's syndrome, and others typically occur in children or young adults who are otherwise healthy. The pretransplant evaluation for such patients is usually not extensive, and the risk of death during the first year of ESRD is likewise relatively low. In contrast, patients with diabetes or hypertension tend to be older (mean age 60 years for patients with diabetes and 67 years for patients with hypertension) and to have extrarenal problems that necessitate detailed evaluation. The risk of death among such patients during the first year of ESRD is high, approximately 25%.

Patients with cancer and acquired immunodeficiency syndrome (AIDS) nephropathy are seldom referred for transplantation. The mortality rate is approximately 50%

TABLE 3–3 ▲ TRANSPLANT AND DEATH RATES FOR PATIENTS WITH END-STAGE RENAL DISEASE (1987–1990)

Primary Disease	Total No. of Patients	% Transplanted in First Year	% Died in First Year
Diabetes	51,665 (34.2)	6.5	23.3
Hypertension	44,305 (29.4)	2.9	26.5
Glomerulonephritis	21,435 (14.2)	15.4	14.1
Goodpasture's	615 (0.4)	6.2	21.5
Focal sclerosing	2343 (1.5)	20.3	9.5
Membranous	806 (0.5)	17.6	12
Membranoproliferative	638 (0.4)	29.8	8.5
Cystic kidney disease	5128 (3.4)	19.2	7.6
Interstitial disease	5176 (3.4)	9.6	19.4
Obstructive nephropathy	3536 (2.3)	6.1	27.6
Lupus nephropathy	2215 (1.4)	10.9	10.2
Scleroderma	402 (0.2)	3	38.1
Wegener's granulomatosus	318 (0.2)	9.4	21.7
Hemolytic-uremic syndrome	330 (0.2)	10.3	22.4
Polyarteritis	96 (<0.1)	7.3	29.2
Henoch-Schönlein purpura	57 (<0.1)	35.1	8.8
Multiple myeloma	1403 (0.9)	<0.1	49.7
Renal and urinary tract carcinoma	614 (0.4)	2.6	38.9
Lymphomas	43 (<0.1)	7	44.2
Amyloidosis	596 (0.3)	3	43.5
Oxalosis	59 (<0.1)	22	16.9
Cystinosis	31 (<0.1)	71	6.5
Fabry's disease	42 (<0.1)	35.7	4.8
Alport's syndrome	327 (0.2)	43.7	2.8
Sickle cell disease	154 (0.1)	5.2	15.6
AIDS-related nephropathy	297 (0.1)	0.7	45.1
All others	17,033 (11.3)	14.4	14.8

Numbers in parentheses are percentages.

in patients with malignant disease during the first year of ESRD. Although a growing number of patients with AIDS-related nephropathy are initiating dialysis, these patients are generally not considered candidates for transplantation. All transplant centers consider clinical manifestations of AIDS to be an absolute contraindication to transplantation. Before serologic studies were available to confirm exposure to the human immunodeficiency virus (HIV), a number of patients who were, in retrospect, HIV positive at the time of transplantation but did not have manifestations of AIDS underwent transplantation[17] with relatively encouraging results. Although a few centers (ours included) are willing to consider patients who are HIV positive but have no symptoms, patients with AIDS are considered to have an active infection and are not considered for transplantation. Even in programs willing to evaluate HIV-positive patients, the reality is that most patients have evidence of AIDS at the time of evaluation and are rejected as candidates.

In the past, primary hyperoxaluria (PHO) was considered to be an absolute contraindication to renal transplantation. PHO is a rare autosomal recessive disorder that results in increased conversion of glyoxylate to oxalate and glycolate.[18,19] Type 1 PHO is the most common form and is caused by a deficiency in the hepatic enzyme alanine glyoxylate aminotransferase.[20] Type 2 PHO is caused by a deficiency in the cytosolic enzyme glyoxylate reductase D-glycerate dehydrogenase. It has the same clinical presentation as type 1 PHO but has only been described in a small number of families. The enzyme deficiencies may be caused by reduced production, production of an abnormal protein, or an intracellular protein-trafficking abnormality that leads to accumulation of the enzyme in the mitochondria instead of the perioxisomes.[18] Deposition of oxalate causes nephrocalcinosis, renal calculi, and interstitial nephritis and progresses to ESRD. Systemic deposition of oxalate in the heart, bone, and other tissues may be fatal. The diagnosis of PHO is suggested by the constellation of recurrent calcium oxalate stones, severe hyperoxaluria, normal calcium and uric acid excretion without ingestion of large doses of vitamin C, and gastrointestinal disease causing increased oxalate absorption.[19] Liver biopsy may further confirm the diagnosis of alanine glyoxylate aminotransferase deficiency in type 1 PHO.

Kidney transplantation alone for type 1 PHO has been complicated by almost universal recurrence of oxalate deposition in the kidney, resulting in a 1-year graft survival rate of approximately 30%.[21,22] The introduction of measures to decrease the production and excretion of oxalate has improved graft survival somewhat, but these transplants are at very high risk (Table 3–4).[18] Treatment with orthophosphate or magnesium to prevent crystal formation in patients with good renal function may be useful but may lead to hyperphosphatemia, worsening hyperparathyroidism, and hypermagnesemia in patients with severe renal impairment.[18] After transplantation, it is vital that patients maintain a brisk diuresis to avoid oxalate deposition in the kidney. Some authors have advocated the use of living-related donor transplants, because early excellent renal function is more predictable.[23] If cadaveric grafts are used, organs likely to have delayed graft function should be avoided. The use of induction protocols without cyclosporine has been advocated by some authors.[18] Despite these measures, renal transplantation alone has yielded disappointing results regardless of the precautions taken to reduce oxalate production.[21,24] Isolated

TABLE 3–4 ▲ MANEUVERS TO IMPROVE RESULTS FOR PATIENTS WITH OXALOSIS

General measures for patients with good renal function
High urine output (>3 liters/day)
Decreases renal deposition
High dose pyridoxine (25–250 mg/day)
Increases conversion of glyoxalate to glycine instead of oxalate
Magnesium oxide or neutral phosphate
Reduces renal stone formation
Transplantation issues
Intensive dialysis before transplantation
If living related donor, daily dialysis for 1 week before transplant
Early transplantation
Glomerular filtration rate >30 mL/min (? before renal insufficiency)
Absent or minimal bone or heart disease
Living-related renal transplant
Cadaveric kidney with high likelihood of good function
Combined liver and kidney transplant
Liver has normal enzyme function
Consider sequential liver then kidney transplant
Wait 6 months to 1 year between procedures
High-dose pyridoxine (25–250 mg/day)
High urine output after transplantation

renal transplantation appears to be more successful if performed early in the course of renal insufficiency but does not prevent further oxalate deposition in the native kidneys, bones, or the new allograft, since the hepatic enzyme defect persists.[25]

Because the enzyme deficiency in type 1 PHO is confined to the liver, replacement of the defective organ by means of transplantation should be curative. Some authors have suggested that patients without substantial deposition of oxalate in the native kidneys, heart, or bones might benefit from early isolated hepatic transplantation.[26,27] If hepatic transplantation is performed after renal insufficiency or ESRD has developed, dialysis is incapable of removing much deposited oxalate from tissues.[28] Hemodialysis is, however, preferable to peritoneal dialysis, since the former removes quantatively more oxalate. After the initial report of combined liver and kidney transplantation by Watts et al., many centers attempted these operations with encouraging results.[29–32] Just as in isolated hepatic transplantation, reversal of oxalate deposition is possible with liver/kidney transplantation.[33] The most encouraging results were obtained with transplantation in patients without massive deposition of oxalate in the kidney and other organs.

The strategies for performing transplantation in patients with oxalosis are being developed, but some general recommendations can be made. Transplantation of patients with early evidence of oxalate deposition appears to be preferable to waiting until ESRD and other organ dysfunctions have developed. Isolated renal transplantation does not correct the primary metabolic defect and therefore can be expected to be unsuccessful in the long term. Isolated hepatic transplantation may be useful for patients with very early disease but should not be attempted in patients with moderate to severe renal insufficiency, since mobilized oxalate from tissues will be slowly excreted and may hasten progression of the renal failure. Combined hepatic and renal transplantation appears to be promising, and just as with isolated renal or hepatic transplantation, early transplantation also seems to be important. Once renal failure has developed, combined liver/kidney transplantation is probably best performed as a staged procedure. Hepatic transplantation is performed first, followed by kidney transplantation after 6 months to 1 year of aggressive dialysis. The optimal timing has not been determined, given the small series of cases accumulated thus far with isolated kidney, isolated liver, or combined simultaneous or staged liver and kidney transplantation.

▲ RECURRENCE OF PRIMARY RENAL DISEASE AFTER TRANSPLANTATION

The risk of recurrence of the primary renal disease is an important consideration in the recipient evaluation. Glomerular diseases are the most common lesions to recur. Table 3–5 shows the glomerular and nonglomerular diseases and the rates of recurrence and graft loss due to recurrence.[34] Recurrence of renal disease typically presents in a manner similar to that of the primary disease. Most patients with glomerulonephritis develop proteinuria. The initial presentation of most recurrences may be low-grade proteinuria, which can progress to nephrotic range in many patients. Fortunately, many patients may have histologic evidence of recurrence without clinical manifestations for the life of the allograft.

Focal Sclerosing Glomerulonephritis

The true rate of recurrence of focal sclerosing glomerulonephritis (FSGS) is not known, since de novo disease due to chronic rejection and/or chronic toxicity related to cyclosporine also can occur after transplantation. The estimated rate of recurrence is 20–30%, and the rate of graft loss in these patients is 30–40%.[35–37] These figures may require adjustment because of progressively improving allograft survival rates, which may allow enough time for the recurrent lesion to result in graft loss. Some workers place the rate of recurrence as high as 80–100% in patients at high risk.[38,39] Risk factors for recurrence include rapid progression of the disease in the native kidneys; age younger than 20 years; interval between diagnosis and ESRD of less than 3 years; and history of recurrence in a previous graft. Proteinuria may be demonstrated within hours of transplantation. In one study involving pediatric patients, the median time to development of proteinuria was 14 days after transplanta-

TABLE 3–5 ▲ THE PRIMARY RENAL DISEASE AND TRANSPLANTATION

Renal Disease	Recurrence Rate (%)	Graft Loss Rate (%)
	Idiopathic glomerular diseases	
FSGS	20–30	30–40
MGN	3–7	Rare
Type I MPGN	20–30	30–40
Type II MPGN	>80	>50
IgA nephropathy	~50	~10
Anti-GBM nephritis	~12	Rare*
	Secondary glomerular diseases	
Henoch-Schönlein purpura	10–15	10–20
Lupus nephritis	<1	None
HUS	13–25	40–50
Diabetic nephropathy	100	<5
Amyloidosis	5–30	Unknown
Wegener granulomatosis	Case reports	Unknown
Essential mixed cryoglobulinemia	50	Unknown
	Nonglomerular disease	
Oxalosis	90–100	Majority
Cystinosis	~10	Rare
Fabry's disease	Rare	Unknown
Sickle cell nephropathy	Rare	Unknown
PSS	Unknown	Unknown
Alport's syndrome	Rare	Rare

FSGS, focal sclerosing glomerulonephritis; MGN, membranous glomerulonephritis; MPGN, membranoproliferative glomerulonephritis; GBM, glomerular basement membrane; HUS, hemolytic-uremic syndrome; PSS, progressive systemic sclerosis.
* As long as anti-GBM antibody has been negative for 6 months prior to transplantation.

tion.[15] Although the cause of FSGS is not known, it is possible that there exists a circulating factor that changes the permeability of the basement membrane and initiates the process of glomerular sclerosis.

Several approaches have been attempted to reduce the rate of recurrent FSGS and to manage the nephrotic syndrome after the disease has recurred. Most have involved treatment in the early posttransplant period. If such treatment is proposed, the planning should be initiated during the evaluation process. Postoperative plasmapheresis has been attempted with some success in a small number of patients.[40,41] Whether pretransplant plasmapheresis is helpful to a recipient before transplantation of an organ from a living related donor has not been established but might be a consideration for patients at high risk in the context of a clinical trial.

After transplantation, the use of angiotensin-converting enzyme (ACE) inhibitors has been useful in controlling proteinuria and may have a theoretic advantage in delaying the progression of renal failure once the disease has recurred.[41,42]

None of the currently available immunosuppressive agents has been found to be effective in reducing the recurrence rate of FSGS or other glomerulopathies. Recurrent FSGS has been described both with cyclosporine and with tacrolimus (Shapiro R, personal communication, 1996).[41,43] It is unclear whether any of the new agents currently under investigation will be more effective in this regard.

Membranous Glomerulonephritis

Recurrent membranous glomerulonephritis (MGN) is relatively uncommon. Most series report a 3–7% incidence,[44,45] but rates of nearly 60% have been described.[46] GN after transplantation may be recurrent or de novo; unfortunately, no histologic findings differentiate between the two entities. The clinical course of de novo disease may be more ominous, with a greater tendency for graft loss. As with most forms of recurrent glomerulonephritis, the rates of graft loss and recurrence vary widely among published reports. In general, however, graft loss is uncommon. HLA-identical living related recipients may be at a high risk for recurrence,[45] and some authors have suggested that HLA-identical transplantation be avoided in this setting.[34]

Membranoproliferative Glomerulonephritis

The recurrence rate for membranoproliferative glomerulonephritis (MPGN) varies depending on the type of disease. Patients with MPGN type I have been found to have recurrence rates of 20–30%,[35,47] although other reports have documented rates of 40–70%.[48] Because the histologic features of transplant glomerulopathy are similar to those of MPGN type I and MPGN related to hepatitis B and other causes, there may be a tendency to overestimate the rate of recurrence. Unlike the situation with the primary disease, depressed serum complement levels are not regularly seen with recurrence.[49] Graft loss occurs in 28–42% of patients with recurrence.

Type II MPGN is a relatively rare disease; however, recurrence is almost universal after transplantation. Reported rates are 50–100%.[15] Loss of grafts because of recurrence has been reported in 10–20% of patients, although graft loss rates approximating 50% also have been reported. Risk factors for graft loss included male sex and rapidly progressive glomerulonephritis in the native kidneys.[50] No therapy has been found to be effective in the management of recurrence of either form of MPGN after transplantation.

Immunoglobulin A Nephropathy (Berger's Disease)

Immunoglobulin A (IgA) nephropathy recurs in approximately 50% of patients, with a range of 20–75%.[46] Patients with transplants from living related donors may have a higher recurrence rate.[51] Patients with B35 and DR4 HLA antigens may also be at greater risk for recurrence.[57] However, graft loss due to recurrence occurs in less than 10% of patients. One report has suggested that use of cyclosporine A may reduce the rate of recurrence from 50 to 16%,[52] but there is little confirmation of this finding.

Anti–Glomerular Basement Membrane Disease

Anti–glomerular basement membrane (GBM) disease recurs in approximately 50% of renal transplants,[15] but clinically evident disease develops in only 25% of the patients with histologic recurrence. Renal transplantation should be delayed in potential recipients until circulating anti–GBM antibodies are undetectable for 6 to 12 months. Transplantation for patients with detectable antibodies may increase the risk of recurrence to between 50% and 80%.

Henoch-Schönlein Purpura

Clinically evident Henoch-Schönlein purpura recurs in less than 10–15% of patients.[34] Histologic recurrence may develop in approximately 30%. Clinical disease develops between 8 and 18 months posttransplant. Recurrence rates are higher in children (75–88%) and recipients of transplants from living related donors. The incidence of graft loss is typically low (10–20%), but may increase to 40–50% if proteinuria, hematuria, or purpura develops.

Lupus Nephritis

Recurrent lupus nephritis in an allograft is rare and may be related to the practice of avoiding renal transplantation for patients with active lupus. Most nephrologists wait until serologic and clinical evidence of lupus has disappeared (so-called burned-out lupus). Cyclosporine has been reported to reduce the systemic manifestations of lupus and possibly stabilize the histologic changes of lupus nephritis in native kidneys.[53] Treatment with cyclosporine and steroids before transplantation has been reported to result in successful transplantation in patients with active lupus,[54] but this practice should be reserved for very unusual situations in which no other renal replacement alternatives are available.

Hemolytic-Uremic Syndrome

Hemolytic-uremic syndrome (HUS) has many causes, each of which can be associated with a different likelihood of recurrence. Analyses of HUS are typically pooled, because it is a relatively uncommon cause of ESRD. When all cases are combined, recurrence is seen in 13–25% of patients.[34] Once HUS recurs, the risk of graft loss is relatively high, approximately 50%. Familial HUS tends to recur at an even higher rate. Patients and their family members have been demonstrated to have decreased or absent factors involved in prostacyclin synthesis.[34] Likewise, patients with HUS recurrent in a prior transplant have a high rate of recurrence after a subsequent transplant. In contrast, patients with other primary renal diseases who experience cyclosporine A–associated HUS have been successfully treated by conversion to tacrolimus.[55]

Diabetic Nephropathy

Diabetic nephropathy is the leading cause of ESRD and the most commonly recurring glomerular disease after transplantation. Histologic recurrence can be seen in as many as 100% of patients.[56] Few patients, however, have clinically evident diabetic nephropathy, and histologic changes are typically limited to thickening of the basement membrane, mesangial expansion, and hyalinization of the afferent and efferent arterioles.[34] The rate of loss of graft function due to recurrence of diabetic nephropathy is less than 5%. Early use of ACE inhibitors after transplantation may have a hypothetical advantage in delaying the progression of renal disease for patients who have persistent hyperglycemia and hyperfiltration. Balanced against this is a greater tendency toward hyperkalemia, because both diabetes and the use of cyclosporine (or tacrolimus) predispose patients to type IV renal tubular acidosis.

Other Glomerular Diseases

There is limited information on several forms of glomerulonephritis. The recurrence rate in patients with amyloidosis has been reported to be 5–30%.[34] Patient survival tends to be less than in the general renal transplant population, and these rates probably underestimate the actual rate of recurrence. Recurrence of Wegener granulomatosis has been described, although the descriptions have been primarily case reports.[57] Treatment with cyclophosphamide and increased doses of prednisone may be beneficial. Recurrent essential mixed cryoglobulinemia has also been reported,[58] and histologic recurrences of multiple myeloma and light chain nephropathy have been reported.[59,60]

Alport's Syndrome

Hereditary nephritis (Alport's syndrome) is an X-linked progressive glomerular disease associated with hearing loss and lenticular abnormalities.[61] Women are carriers and may have hematuria but do not usually develop renal failure. Transmission is from mother to son; no transmission from father to son occurs. Patients with Alport's syndrome have a defect (or absence) of a basement membrane component in the noncollagenous domain of type IV collagen ($\alpha5$ chain) that is X linked and may be due to a mutation of *COL4A5*.[62] The $\alpha5$ chain occurs only in the basement membrane. This defect leads to an absence of $\alpha3$ immunoreactivity. Recurrence of Alport's syndrome after renal transplantation is uncommon[34]; there has been one case report documenting histologic recurrence.[63] Patients with Alport's syndrome may have anti-GBM disease after transplantation.[64] Because patients with Alport's syndrome do not respond to anti-GBM antibody and are missing a normal α3 chain, transplant recipients may develop antibodies to this new antigen in the donor graft and have typical anti-GBM renal disease (crescentic glomerulonephritis).[65] Graft loss is then almost universal. Pulmonary manifestations are absent, because the α5 chain is limited to the kidney.[64] Plasmapheresis and cyclophosphamide treatment should be considered, but there are limited data on the utility of these measures.

Sickle Cell Nephropathy

Sickle cell nephropathy has been reported to be associated with MPGN type I and FSGS. Other histologic findings appear to be due to ischemic injury directly related to the sickling process. Transplantation for patients with sickle cell disease has been marked by graft loss primarily due to thrombosis. In one series only one of eight patients retained graft function for 1 year.[66] Graft loss was attributed directly to sickling of red cells and thrombosis. No individual study has reported on more than 15 cases. Recurrence has been reported in one case report.[67] More optimistic results were presented in a national study of sickle cell disease after renal transplantation in which the 1-year graft survival rate was 67%.[68] Bone marrow transplantation for sickle cell anemia also has had promising results.[69] Whether combined bone marrow and renal transplantation will improve patient and graft survival has yet to be determined.

Nonglomerular Diseases

The nonglomerular causes of renal failure have also been reported to recur. As discussed above, oxalosis has a recurrence rate that approximates 100%. Cystinosis is seen primarily in the pediatric population and is caused by an inborn error of metabolism that leads to deposition of cystine crystals in the renal interstitium. Histologic evidence of recurrence develops in approximately 10% of patients but rarely causes renal failure.[34] Fabry's disease is caused by a hereditary deficiency of α-galactosidase, which leads to accumulation of glycophospholipids and renal failure. It was initially hoped that the transplanted kidney might provide the deficient enzyme, but unfortunately it does not. Early experience with transplantation for these patients was marked by death due to sepsis, pulmonary hemorrhage, and thrombosis.[34] A report by the European Dialysis Transplant Association Pediatric Registry documented a 1-year graft survival rate of 80%.[70] Based upon this encouraging evidence, renal transplantation should be offered to patients with this disease.

Scleroderma Kidney

Scleroderma (progressive systemic sclerosis, PSS) is an uncommon cause of renal failure, and reports are sparse. In one series, two of ten patients developed recurrence.[34] A similar histologic appearance between PSS and vascular rejection makes the confirmation of recurrence difficult. Furthermore, scleroderma with ESRD is usually accompanied by severe extrarenal manifestations, which increases the risk of transplantation. Current recommendations are to offer transplantation only to patients without active disease.

▲ GASTROINTESTINAL EVALUATION

Gastrointestinal complications that develop after transplantation can be life threatening, and patients with a history of gastrointestinal problems should receive a careful evaluation before transplantation. For example, patients with a history of peptic ulcer disease should probably undergo upper gastrointestinal endoscopy before transplantation. The prevalence of peptic ulcer disease may be as high as 25% among potential recipients. Endoscopy is preferable to a barium study, since the latter may miss small ulcerations, gastritis, or fungal overgrowth, and does not allow biopsy of suspicious lesions. Patients with active ulcers or gastritis should be deferred from activation on the waiting list until the problems are resolved.

Posttransplant gastritis or ulcer disease may be related to high doses of steroids. Aggressive antiulcer prophylaxis for all patients will minimize this problem after transplantation. We use a combination of H2 blockers and sucralfate until the daily prednisone dose has been reduced to 10 mg or less a day. Omeprazole occasionally needs to be substituted for the H2 blocker.

With regard to colonic disease, all potential candidates have stool tested for occult blood. All candidates older than 50 years undergo routine flexible sigmoidoscopy. Further evaluation is individualized.

Pancreatitis that develops after transplantation is potentially lethal. The mortality rate after transplantation has been reported to be 70% or greater.[71] As with peptic ulcer disease and gastritis, pancreatitis can be initiated or exacerbated by steroids. Other causes include cytomegalovirus (CMV) infection, mumps, gallstones, and azathioprine. For patients with a history of pancreatitis, it is important to try to minimize the steroid dosage postoperatively if possible.

If gallstones are found during the pretransplant evaluation, the gallbladder should be removed, preferably using laparoscopic techniques. Cholelithiasis not only can cause pancreatitis but also may lead to cholecystitis or cholangitis after transplantation; we have even seen two cases of gallbladder perforation. These conditions can be associated with high morbidity and mortality.

The presence of preexisting liver dysfunction requires close attention during the evaluation. Significant hepatic disease develops in 7–24% of patients in the early postoperative period and is the cause of late death in 8–28% of patients.[72,73] Hepatitis B virus (HBV) and hepatitis C virus (HCV) infections are the leading causes of viral hepatitis after transplantation. The management of patients with prior exposure to these viruses is problematic. Patients who are hepatitis B surface antigen (Hb_sAg)–positive are generally not considered suitable candidates for renal transplantation, although some centers will transplant selected patients with stable liver function who are HBV DNA–negative and who have evidence of quiescent disease. Patients who are HCV-positive currently undergo HCV-RNA and polymerase chain reaction (PCR) testsing; if positive, these patients undergo liver biopsy. Patients with chronic active hepatitis are referred for treatment and are not listed, while patients without clinically significant hepatic disease can be listed.

▲ CARDIAC EVALUATION

The leading cause of death after transplantation is cardiac disease, and it occurs with a relative risk three to ten times that in the general population.[74] Coronary artery disease is the most frequent cause of cardiovascular death among both dialysis and transplant patients. Factors that predict coronary artery disease in patients with ESRD include age 50 years or older, white race, male sex, elevated cholesterol level, myocardial infarction or angina before the initiation of dialysis, abnormal left ventricular wall motion, and diabetes.[75]

As part of the cardiac evaluation for prospective transplant candidates who do not have diabetes, many centers recommend that all patients over 40–50 years of age undergo echocardiography or a gated heart pool scan to determine wall motion and ejection fraction. Patients who do not have diabetes but have a history of myocardial infarction or angina should undergo a pharmacologic thallium stress test and an echocardiogram regardless of age (Table 3–6). Patients with demonstrable cardiac ischemia should undergo coronary angiography.

The precise age at which thallium stress testing should be recommended in asymptomatic patients is not precisely known, but it would be prudent to begin test-

TABLE 3–6 ▲ CARDIAC EVALUATION

Patient Group	Evaluation
All patients over 40–50 years of age	Echocardiagraphy or gated heart pool scan
Patients without diabetes	Stress thallium exercise test or pharmacologic stress test at 50–55 years of age or older
History of CAD	Angiography
Symptomatic CAD	Angiography
Patients with diabetes	
Age ≥45 years	Coronary angiography
Diabetes ≥20–25 years	
Age ≤45 years	Dipyridamole or adenosine stress thallium test and echocardiography

CAD, coronary artery disease.

ing at 50–55 years of age. The presence of multiple risk factors or a history of congestive heart failure or peripheral vascular disease may dictate testing at an earlier age. Thallium exercise stress testing may be less predictive of coronary artery disease in patients with ESRD because of poor exercise tolerance, difficulty interpreting an electrocardiogram (ECG) in the presence of left ventricular hypertrophy or conduction disturbances, and the use of β blocking agents. For these reasons, we perform an adenosine (or dipyridamole) thallium study without attempting an exercise test. Although pharmacologic thallium testing avoids the requirement that patients increase their heart rate by exercise, it is not without hypothetical limitations. One study suggested that dipyridamole thallium studies are less sensitive and specific in ESRD patients than in the general population.[76] Others have found both exercise stress tests and dipyridamole studies to predict perioperative cardiac events for patients without diabetes.[77,78] Finally, dobutamine echocardiography may be a useful substitute for pharmacologic thallium testing and echocardiography.

Cardiac Evaluation for Patients with Diabetes

Premature cardiovascular disease is the leading cause of death in patients with ESRD secondary to diabetes. Approximately 24% of patients with diabetes who begin dialysis do not survive the first year. The 5-year patient survival rate in renal transplant recipients with diabetes is as low as 53% but also as high as 84% in single-center reports.[79,80] The cardiac evaluation for patients with diabetes is subject to variation among centers. It ranges from routine coronary angiography for all adults with diabetes to an exercise stress test only. The cardiac evaluation for patients with diabetes is complicated by the high prevalence of coronary heart disease, which may be associated with silent ischemia, and cardiomyopathy. Many studies have found that exercise stress tests with or without thallium are of limited predictive value in diabetes.[81] Only 45% of patients with diabetes are capable of reaching 70–80% of their maximum predicted heart rate. Reasons for inadequate or false-negative thallium stress tests include use of β blockers at the time of the study, autonomic neuropathy, poor patient motivation, and poor physical conditioning.[82]

Manske et al[83] developed an algorithm in an attempt to identify low-risk diabetic patients who can safely avoid angiography in the pretransplant evaluation. The investigators found an 88% prevalence of coronary artery disease in diabetics older than 45 years of age. They recommended angiography for all patients with diabetes in this age group. In younger patients without a smoking history or ST-T wave changes on an ECG, and in patients with diabetes for less than 25 years, the risk of coronary disease was found to be lower. These patients were advised to undergo a dipyridamole thallium stress test as the initial study. Any abnormality on this study would require angiography, even for the group at low risk. Although this was a relatively small study, this approach probably represents the most useful way to screen patients with diabetes. Once coronary artery disease has been found, the lesions should be bypassed or dilated before transplantation. Coronary revascularization before transplantation in the diabetic clearly has been shown to decrease the frequency of cardiac events and mortality after transplantation.[84]

▲ MALIGNANCY

With the increasing age and complexity of medical problems of potential recipients has come a greater prevalence of preexisting carcinoma and the associated risk of recurrent cancer after transplantation. Immunosuppression is believed to accelerate the growth of preexisting cancers and may be associated with an increased rate of tumor recurrence after excision. In addition, reduced immune surveillance may allow new cancers to develop. These risks make the identification of malignancy before and after transplantation extremely important. Determining an appropriate interval between therapy for pre-existing cancers and transplantation is important, both to minimize the rate of recurrence and to provide appropriate access to transplantation.

The pretransplant evaluation should be structured to identify occult malignancy. We use the American Cancer Society recommendations for early detection of cancer in patients without symptoms as the framework for pretransplant screening and posttransplant follow-up care (Table 3–7).[85] Skin cancers are the leading carcinoma before and after transplantation. The initial physical examination should include a detailed skin examination, including the soles of the feet. The latter is particularly important for African-American patients, since melanomas, although uncommon, can be found on the soles of the feet. All patients over 50 years of age should undergo screening flexible sigmoidoscopy. After two normal annual studies, it should be repeated every 3–5 years. Similarly, a rectal examination and stool guaiac test should be performed on all potential adult recipients and repeated annually for patients aged 40 years and older. A detailed pelvic examination and Papanicolaou (Pap) smear should be performed in women beginning at 20 years of age or when they become sexually active. Cervical dys-

TABLE 3–7 ▲ AMERICAN CANCER SOCIETY RECOMMENDATIONS FOR EARLY DETECTION OF CANCER IN PEOPLE WITHOUT SYMPTOMS

Test	Sex	Age (y)	Frequency
Sigmoidoscopy	M and F	>50	After two normal studies 1 year apart, repeat every 3–5 y
Stool guaiac	M and F	>40	Every year
Digital rectal examination	M and F	>40	Every year
Pap smear and pelvic exam	F	>20, earlier if sexually active	Every year
Mammography	F	35–40	Baseline, then every 2 y
		41–50	Every 1–2 y
		>50	Yearly

(Adapted from Kimball and Miller)

plasia, warts, or other lesions should be treated before transplantation. Although the role of routine mammography is controversial in the general population, all women 35 years and older undergo a baseline study at our center. Studies are repeated according to the patient's age (Table 3–7). Prostate specific antigen (PSA) is measured in men 40 years and older as a screen for prostate cancer, although it is not included in the evaluation by the American Cancer Society.

In general, transplantation and immunosuppression increase the risk for subsequent cancers, although the risk varies according to the type of tumor. Several general observations can be made. Malignant tumors that are common among the general population (carcinoma of the lung, breast, prostate, colon, and invasive uterine or cervical carcinomas) do not occur more frequently in transplant recipients; the prevalence may even be slightly decreased.[86] This decrease may be related to aggressive pretransplant screening for malignancy. Squamous cell carcinoma of the skin occurs at a high rate in transplant patients and is the most common cancer in this population. This is especially true in countries with a high degree of sun exposure, such as Australia. Many cancers are seen more in transplant patients than in the general population; these include lymphoma (20% versus 5%), lip cancer (8% versus 0.3%), Kaposi sarcoma (6% versus near zero), carcinoma of the kidney (5% versus 2%), carcinoma of the vulva and perineum (4% versus 0.6%), hepatobiliary tumors (2.6% versus 1%), and non–Kaposi's sarcomas (1.7% versus 0.5%) (See also Chapter 11.).

Recurrence of Cancer After Transplantation

For most patients with a history of cancer, a 2-year tumor-free interval from the termination of cancer therapy to transplantation is sufficient. In some cases, a shorter or longer waiting time is appropriate. The Transplant Tumor Registry at the University of Cincinnati maintains the largest set of records of transplant patients with malignant disease. The rate of recurrence and the recommended waiting times are shown in Table 3–8).[89] Overall, patients treated 0 to 24 months before transplantation experienced a 53% recurrence rate. Those who received transplants 25–60 months after treatment had a 34% rate of recurrence, and those transplanted over 60 months after completion of treatment experienced only a 13% recurrence rate. Recurrence rates can be predicted by cancer type and have been grouped into low, intermediate, and high. Late recurrences have developed in all three patient groups and have been noted even in the low-recurrence-rate group as long as 12 years after treatment. Thus longer waiting periods decrease but do not eliminate the risk of recurrence. Once cancer recurs, the risk for death is substantial and approaches 100% for some cancers (Table 3–8). Patients with in situ carcinomas, low-grade bladder cancers, basal cell skin carcinoma, and possibly focal malignant lesions (single focus) have very low recurrence rates and can probably undergo transplantation without waiting. Clinical judgment should be exercised even in the treatment of these favorable groups. Similarly, incidentally discovered renal cell carcinomas have not

TABLE 3–8 ▲ RECURRENCE OF CANCER AFTER RENAL TRANSPLANTATION

Tumor	Recurrence rate (%)	Deaths (%)	Recommended Wait (y)
	Low recurrence rate (0–10%)		
Incidental renal cancer	0	0	None
Testicular	3	0	2
Cervix or uterus	3	33.3	2
Thyroid	8	12.5	2
Lymphoma	10	33.3	2
	Intermediate recurrence rate (11–25%)		
Body of uterus	11	100	2
Wilms	16	80	2
Colon	21	62.5	>2
Prostate	24	20	2
Breast	25	81.3	>2
	High recurrence rate (≥26%)		
Bladder	26	36.4	>2
Sarcoma	28	50	2
Melanoma	30	100	>2
Symptomatic renal cell	30	76.5	2
Nonmelanoma skin	62	2	2
Myeloma	88	100	2

Adapted from Penn I: The effect of immunosuppression on pre-existing cancers. *Transplantation* 4:742–747, 1993.

been reported to recur, and these patients can undergo transplantation without delay. Other malignant lesions require longer waiting times; these include melanoma, breast cancer, invasive bladder cancer, and colorectal carcinoma.

▲ THE WAITING LIST

After patients have been accepted as candidates for renal transplantation, they are placed on a waiting list. Organs are allocated according to a computer-driven point system defined by HLA matching, waiting time, and panel reactive antibody (PRA) criteria (Table 3–9). The allocation system is currently administered by the United Network of Organ Sharing (UNOS). In general, the better the match, the more points a patient receives, and the more likely a patient is to receive a given kidney. Patients with a zero-antigen mismatch are mandated to receive the kidney according to UNOS

TABLE 3–9 ▲ UNOS ALOGORITHM FOR ORGAN ALLOCATION

Category	Points
HLA antigen matching	
0 antigen mismatch	mandatory share
0 BDR mismatches	7
1BDR mismatch	5
2 BDR mismatches	2
Panel reactive antibody (PRA)	
>80%	4
<80%	0
Waiting time	
	1 to patient with longest waiting time, others receive fraction of a point based on position on list.
	1.0 per full year on list.
Pediatric candidates	
<11 years of age	3 additional
>11 years of age	2 additional

policy, and these kidneys are shipped to appropriate recipients around the United States. However, zero-antigen mismatch kidneys are relatively uncommon. In 1990, the mean number of mismatches was 3.5 among whites, 4.0 among African-Americans, and 4.2 among other groups. Time spent waiting on the list is given relatively little weight but may play an important role for patients who are equally matched on the basis of HLA. The algorithm also attempts to give priority to patients who are highly sensitized (PRA >80%) and are destined to have extremely long waiting times for an organ. Pediatric patients are assigned additional points when they are placed on the waiting list. These children retain the added points until they reach 18 years of age.

Although not part of the allocation criteria, other factors, such as blood type or race, may affect waiting time (Figure 3–3).[88] Patients with blood type O typically have had the longest waiting time,[89] although in our program, patients with blood type B have been waiting longer.[93] Because type O cadaveric kidneys are universal donors, some of these kidneys were routinely transplanted into non-O recipients. The frequency of this practice decreased from 12% in 1985 to 4% in 1990. The practice is now against UNOS policy, except for zero-antigen mismatch kidneys.

The effect of race on waiting time is a controversial area. In 1991 the Office of the Inspector General of the United States Department of Health and Human Services released a study revealing that African-Americans wait approximately twice as long as their white counterparts (13.9 vs 6.3 months).[10] After publication of this study, many groups examined their results and conducted further studies directed at explaining this phenomenon. When single-center data were examined, some centers found differences in waiting time,[90] but others did not.[91,92] Between 1987 and 1992, the mean waiting time at the University of Pittsburgh was 6.5 ± 9.2 months for whites and

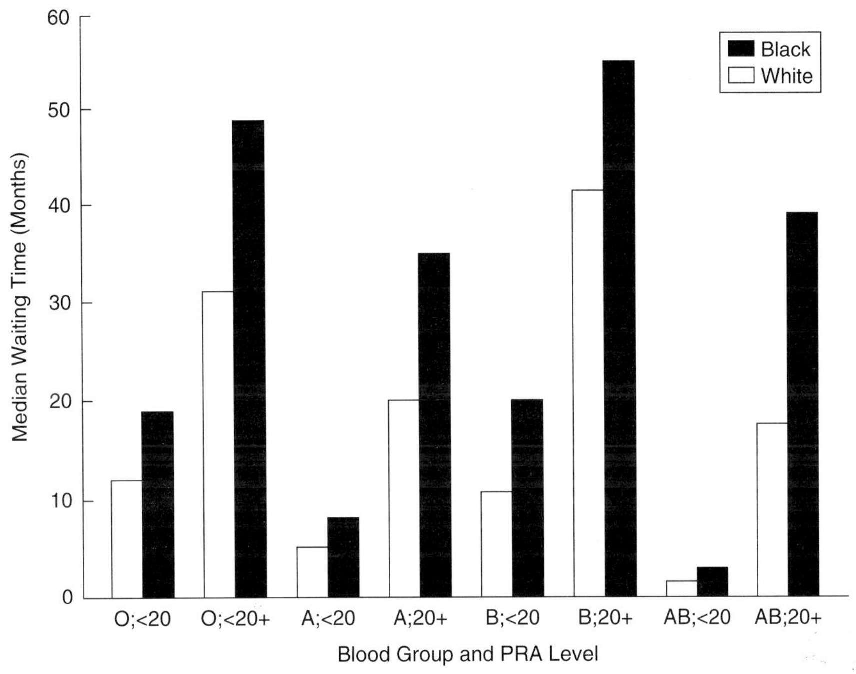

Figure 3–3. Waiting time among renal transplant candidates based on blood group, panel reactive antibody level, and race. (*Data from United Network of Organ Sharing [UNOS] Update, February 1994.*)

7.8 ± 8.9 months for African-Americans, a difference that was not statistically significant.[93] The emphasis on HLA matching may well play a role in the longer waiting times for African-Americans. The donor pool is predominantly white, and African-Americans are less likely to obtain a good match than whites.[90] Other undefined factors also may play a role, since the discrepancy cannot be explained entirely by tissue typing.

Patients on the waiting list must be monitored for new medical problems that might preclude transplantation. Patients with cardiovascular disease should be reevaluated at least annually. Asymptomatic patients with coronary artery disease should undergo stress tests yearly. Any patient who experiences angina or myocardial infarction should undergo coronary angiography and be removed from the waiting list until these problems are corrected. Other problems, such as infections, peptic ulcer disease, or psychiatric illness should prompt removal from the waiting list until the problems are resolved.

The pretransplant recipient evaluation is straightforward in the young, relatively healthy patients with no clinically significant problems other than renal failure. However, an increasing number of older patients and patients with medically complex conditions are being referred for transplantation. It is important to evaluate them carefully to ensure as smooth a postoperative course as possible.

▲ REFERENCES

1. United States Renal Data System: USRDS 1993 Annual Data Report. National Institute of Diabetes and Digestive and Kidney Diseases. Bethesda, National Institutes of Health, 1993: E.13, 18, 50–54, 61, 62.
2. Krakauer H, Grauman JS, McMullan MR, Creede CC: The recent US experience in the treatment of end stage renal disease by dialysis and transplantation. *N Engl J Med* 308: 1558–1563, 1983.
3. Vollmer WM, Wahl PW, Blagg CR: Survival with dialysis and transplantation in patients with end stage renal disease. *N Engl J Med* 308:1553–1558, 1983.
4. United States Renal Data System: USRDS 1991 Annual Data Report. National Institutes of Health, National Institute of Diabetes and Digestive and Kidney Diseases. *Am J Kidney Dis* 18 (Suppl 2):1–127, 1991.
5. Port FK, Wolfe RA, Mauger EA, et al: Comparison of survival probabilities for dialysis patients vs cadaveric renal transplant recipients. *JAMA* 270:1339–1343, 1993.
6. Eggers PW: Effect of transplantation on the Medicare end stage renal disease program. *N Engl J Med* 318:223–229, 1988.
7. Simmons RL, Kjellstrans CM, Buselneier TJ, Najarian JS: Renal transplantation in high risk patients. *Arch Surg* 103:290–298, 1971.
8. Ismail N, Hakim R, Hederman HJ: Renal replacement therapies in the elderly. II. Renal transplantation. *Am J Kidney Dis* 23:1–15, 1994.
9. Cardella CJ, Harding ME, Abraham G, et al: Renal transplantation in older patients on peritoneal dialysis. *Transplant Proc* 21:2022–2023, 1989.
10. Office of the Inspector General: The distribution of organs for transplantation: Expectations and practices. Department of Health and Human Services Publication OE-01-89-00550. Washington, DC, Office of Analysis and Inspections, 1991.
11. Hurley CK: HLA diversity in African Americans. *Transplant Proc* 25:2399, 1993.
12. Opelz G, Wujciak T, Schwarz V, et al: Collaborative transplant study analysis of graft survival in African-Americans. *Transplant Proc* 25:2443–2445, 1993.
13. Pasulka PS, Bistrian BR, Benotti PN, et al: The risk of surgery in obese patients. *Ann Intern Med* 104:540, 1986.
14. Holley JL, Shapiro R, Lopatin WB, et al: Obesity as a risk factor following cadaveric renal transplantation. *Transplantation* 49:387–389, 1990.
15. Gill IS, Hodge EE, Novick AC, et al: Impact of obesity on renal transplantation. *Transplant Proc* 25:1047–1048, 1993.
16. Kjellstrand CM: Giving life-giving death. *Acta Med Scand* (Suppl) 725:1–88, 1988.
17. Tzakis A, Cooper M, Dummer JS, et al: Transplantation in HIV+ patients. *Transplantation* 49:354–358, 1990.
18. Scheinman JI: Primary hyperoxaluria: therapeutic strategies for the 90's. *Kidney Int* 40:389, 1991.
19. Danpure CJ: Metabolic and clinical heterogeneity of primary hyperoxaluria type 1. *Am J Kidney Dis* 17:366, 1991.
20. Morgan SH, Watts RWE: Perspectives in the assessment and management of patients with primary hyperoxaluria type I. *Adv Nephrol* 18:95–106, 1989.
21. Binswanger U, Keusch G, Frei D, et al: Kidney transplantation in primary hyperoxaluria of adult patients. *Transplant Proc* 18:14–15, 1986.
22. Watts RWE, Morgan SH, Purkiss P, et al: Timing of renal transplantation in the management

of pyridoxine resistant type I primary hyperoxaluria. *Transplantation* 45:1143–1145, 1988.
23. Katz A, Kim Y, Scheinman J, et al: Long term outcome of kidney transplantation in children with oxalosis. *Transplant Proc* 21:2033–2035, 1989.
24. Broyer M, Brunner FP, Brynger H, et al: Kidney transplantation in primary oxalosis: data from the EDTA Registry. *Nephrol Dial Transplant* 5:332–336, 1990.
25. Katz A, Mauer SM: Transplantation in primary hyperoxaluria type I. *Am J Med* 92:341–342, 1992.
26. Schurmann G, Scharer K, Wingen AM, et al: Early liver transplantation for primary hyperoxaluria type I in an infant with chronic renal failure. *Nephrol Dial Transplant* 5:825–827, 1990.
27. Cochat P, Scharer K: Should liver transplantation be performed before advanced renal insufficiency in primary hyperoxaluria type I2. *Pediatr Nephrol* 7:212–218, 1993.
28. Morgan SH, Purkiss P, Watts RWE, et al: Oxalate metabolism in end stage renal disease. *Nephrol Dial Transplant.*
29. Watts RWE, Calne RY, Rolles K, et al: Primary hyperoxaluria (type I): attempted treatment of combined hepatic and renal transplantation. *Q J Med* 57:697–703, 1985.
30. DePauw L, Gelin M, Danpure CJ, et al: Combined liver-kidney transplantation in primary hyperoxaluria type 1. *Transplantation* 50:886, 1990.
31. Watts RWE, Morgan SH, Danupure CJ, et al: Combined hepatic and renal transplantation in primary hyperoxaluria type I: clinical reports of nine cases. *Am J Med* 90:179–188, 1991.
32. Watts RWE, Danupure CJ, DePauw L, et al: Combined liver-kidney and isolated liver transplantation for primary hyperoxaluria type 1: European experience. *Nephrol Dial Transplant* 6:502–511, 1991.
33. Fyfe B, Israel DH, Quish A, et al: Reversal of primary hyperoxaluria cardiomyopathy after combined liver and renal transplantation. *Am J Cardiol* 75:210–212, 1995.
34. Ramos E: Recurrent diseases in the renal allograft. *J Am Soc Nephrol* 2:109–121, 1991.
35. Cameron JS: Glomerulonephritis in renal transplants. *Transplantation* 34:237–245, 1982.
36. Cameron JS, Senguttuvan P, Hartley B, et al: Focal segmental glomerulosclerosis in fifty-nine renal allografts from a single center: analysis of risk factors for recurrence. *Transplant Proc* 21:2117, 1989.
37. Tejani A, Stablein DH: Recurrence of focal segmental glomerulosclerosis post-transplantation. *J Am Soc Nephrol* 2 (Suppl 3):S258, 1992.
38. Striegel JE, Sibley RK, Fryd DS, Mauer M: Recurrence of focal segmental sclerosis in children following renal transplantation. *Kidney Int* 30 (Suppl):S44, 1986.
39. Lewis EJ: Recurrent focal sclerosis after renal transplantation. *Kidney Int* 22:315, 1982.
40. Laufer J, Ettenger RB, Ho WG, et al: Plasma exchange for recurrent nephrotic syndrome following renal transplantation. *Transplantation* 46:540, 1988.
41. Artero M, Biava C, Amend W, et al: Recurrent focal glomerulosclerosis: natural history and response to therapy. *Am J Med* 92:375, 1992.
42. Vangelista A, Frasca GM, Martella D, Bonomoni V: Glomerulonephritis in renal transplantation. *Nephrol Dial Transplant* 5(Suppl):1 42–46, 1990.
43. Vincenti F, Biava C, Tomlanovitch S, et al: Inability of cyclosporine to completely prevent the recurrence of focal glomerulosclerosis after kidney transplantation. *Transplantation* 47:595, 1989.
44. Mathew TM: Recurrence of disease after renal transplantation. *Am J Kidney Dis* 12:85–96, 1988.

45. Berger BE, Vincenti F, Biava C, et al: De novo and recurrent membranous glomerulopathy following kidney transplantation. *Transplantation* 35:315–319, 1983.
46. Morzycka M, Croker BP, Seigler HF, Tisher CC: Evaluation of recurrent glomerulonephritis in kidney allografts. *Am J Med* 72:588–598, 1982.
47. O'Meara Y, Green A, Carmody M, et al: Recurrent glomerulonephritis in renal transplants: fourteen years experience. *Nephrol Dial Transplant* 4:730–734, 1989.
48. Habib R, Antignac H, Hinglais N, et al: Glomerular lesions in the transplanted kidney in children. *Am J Kidney Dis* 10:198–207, 1987.
49. Glicklich D, Mata AJ, Sablay LB, et al: Recurrent membranoproliferative glomerulonephritis type I in successive renal transplants. *Am J Nephrol* 7:143–149, 1987.
50. Oberkircher OR, Enama, M, West JC, et al: Regression of recurrent membranoproliferative glomerulonephritis type II in a transplanted kidney after plasmapheresis therapy. *Transplant Proc* 20:418–423, 1988.
51. Bachman U, Biava C, Amend W, et al: The clinical course of IgA nephropathy and Henoch-Schonlein purpura following renal transplantation. *Transplantation* 42:511–515, 1986.
52. Tomlanovich S, Vincenti F, Amend W, et al: Is cyclosporine effective in preventing recurrence of immune-mediated glomerular disease after renal transplantation. *Transplant Proc* 20(Suppl):285–288, 1988.
53. Favre H, Miescher PA, Huang YP, Chatelanat F, Mihatsch MJ: Ciclosporin in the treatment of lupus nephritis. *Am J Nephrol* 9(Suppl 1):57–60, 1989.
54. Cantarovich M, Hiesse C, Lantz O, Charpentier B, Fries D: Renal transplantation and active lupus erythematosus. *Ann Intern Med* 109:254–255, 1988.
55. McCauley J, Shapiro R, Bronsther O, et al: Renal transplantation under FK 506 in patients with previous loss of renal function due to hemolytic uremic syndrome. *Transplant Proc* 23 (6):3068–3070, 1991.
56. Lundgren G, Wilczek H, Tyden G, et al: Recurrent diabetic nephropathy in renal allografts of diabetic patients. *Transplant Proc* 19:2290–2293, 1987.
57. Aunsholt NA, Ahlbom G: Recurrence of Wegener's granulomatosis after kidney transplantation involving the kidney graft. *Clin Transplant* 3:159–161, 1989.
58. Hiesse C, Bastuji-Garin S, Santelli G, et al: Recurrent essential mixed cryoglobulinemia in renal allografts. *Am J Nephrol* 9:150–154, 1989.
59. De Lima JJG, Kourilsky O, Meyrier A, et al: Kidney transplant in multiple myeloma. *Transplantation* 31:223–224, 1981.
60. Gerlag PGG, Koene RAP, Berden JHM: Renal transplantation in light chain nephropathy: case report and review of the literature. *Clin Nephrol* 25:101–104, 1986.
61. Grunfeld JP: The clinical spectrum of hereditary nephritis. *Kidney Int* 27:83, 1985.
62. Reeders ST: Molecular genetics of hereditary nephritis. *Kidney Int* 42:73, 1992.
63. Mathew TH, Mathews DC, Hobbs JB, Kincaid-Smith P: Glomerular lesions after renal transplantation. *Am J Med* 59:177–190, 1975.
64. Shah B, First MR, Mendoza NC, et al: Alport's syndrome: risk of glomerulonephritis induced by anti–glomerular basement membrane antibody after renal transplantation. *Nephron* 50:34–38, 1988.
65. Hudson BG, Kalluri R, Gunwar S, et al: The pathogenesis of Alport's syndrome involves type IV collagen molecules containing the a3 (IV) chain: evidence from anti-GBM nephritis after transplantation. *Kidney Int* 42:179, 1992.
66. Barber WH, Deierhoi MH, Julian BA, et al: Renal transplantation in sickle anemia and sickle cell disease. *Clin Transplant* 1:169–175, 1987.
67. Miner DJ, Jorjasky DK, Perloff LJ, et al: Recurrent sickle cell nephropathy in a transplanted kidney. *Am J Kidney Dis* 10:306–313, 1987.

68. Chatterjee SN: National study on natural history of renal allografts in sickle cell disease or trait. *Nephron* 25:199–201, 1980.
69. Abboud MR, Jackson SM, Barredo J, et al: Bone marrow transplantation for sickle cell anemia. *Am J Pediatr Hematol Oncol* 16:86–89, 1994.
70. Broyer M, Rizzoni G, Brunner H, et al: Combined report on regular dialysis and transplantation of children in Europe, XIV. *Proc Eur Dial Transplant Assoc* 22:55, 1984.
71. Fernandez JA, Rosenberg JC: Post-transplant pancreatitis. *Surg Gynecol Obstet* 143:795, 1976.
72. LaQuaglia MP, Tolkoff-Rubin NE, Dienstag JL, et al: Impact of hepatitis on renal transplantation. *Transplantation* 32:504, 1981.
73. Boyce NW, Holdsworth SR, Hooke D, et al: Non-hepatitis B related liver disease in a renal transplant population. *Am J Kidney Dis* 11:307, 1988.
74. First R: Transplantation for the nephrologist: long term complications after transplantation. *Am J Kidney Dis* 22:477–486, 1993.
75. Rostrand SG, Rutsky EA: Ischemic heart disease in chronic renal failure: management considerations. *Semin Dial* 2:98–101, 1989.
76. Marwick TH, Steinmuller DR, Underwood DA, et al: Ineffectiveness of dipyridamole SPECT thallium imaging as a screening technique for coronary disease in patients with end stage renal failure. *Transplantation* 49:100–103, 1990.
77. Derfler K, Kletter K, Heinz G, et al: Predictive value of thallium-201-dipyridamole myocardial stress scintigraphy in chronic hemodialysis patients and transplant recipients. *Clin Nephrol* 36:192–202, 1991.
78. Cottier C, Pfisterer M, Muller-Brand J, et al: Cardiac evaluation of candidates for kidney transplantation: value of exercise radionuclide angiocardiology. *Eur Heart J* 11:832–838, 1990.
79. United States Renal Data System: 1990 Annual Data Report. National Institute of Diabetes and Digestive and Kidney Diseases, Bethesda, 1990.
80. The United States Renal Data System: 1994 Annual Data Report. National Institute of Diabetes and Digestive and Kidney Diseases, Bethesda, 1994: 107.
81. Morrow CE, Schwartz, Sutherland DER, et al: Predictive value of thallium stress testing for coronary and cardiovascular events in uremic diabetic patients before renal transplantation. *Am J Surg* 146:331–335, 1983.
82. Holley JL, Fenton RA, Arthur RS: Thallium stress testing does not predict cardiovascular risk in diabetics patients with end stage renal disease undergoing cadaveric renal transplantation. *Am J Med* 90:563–570, 1991.
83. Manske CL, Thomas W, Wang Y, Wilson R: Screening diabetic transplant candidates for coronary artery disease: identification of a low risk subgroup. *Kidney Int* 44:617–621, 1993.
84. Manske CL, Wang Y, Rector T, et al: Coronary revascularization in insulin dependent diabetic patients with chronic renal failure. *Lancet* 340:998–1002, 1992.
85. National Cancer Institute: Cancer control objective for the nation: 1985–2000. US Department of Health and Human Services, 1986. DHHS publication no. (NIH) 86–2880. (NCI monograph #2).
86. Penn I: Occurrence of cancers in immunosuppressed organ transplant recipients. *Clin Transpl* 1990.
87. Penn I: The effect of immunosuppression on pre-existing cancers. *Transplantation* 4:742–747, 1993.
88. UNOS Update: 10:(2) 1994.
89. Port FK, Held PJ, Wolfe RA, et al: The impact of non-identical ABO cadaveric renal transplantation on waiting times and graft survival. *Am J Kidney Dis* 17:519–523, 1991.

90. Koyama H, Cecka JM: Race effects. *Clin Transpl* 269–280, 1991.
91. Sommer BG, Sing DE, Henry ML: The influence of recipient race on renal allograft survival: a single institute analysis. *Transplant Proc* 21:3929, 1989.
92. Shapiro R, Tzakis AG, Hakala TR, et al: Renal transplantation in African-American recipients at the University of Pittsburgh. *Transplant Proc* 21:3921, 1989.
93. Shapiro R, McCauley J, Scantlebury V, et al: Effect of recipient race on waiting time for renal transplantation at the University of Pittsburgh. *Transplant Proc* 25:2458–2459, 1993.

4

Cadaveric and Living Donation

Velma P. Scantlebury

The successful results after kidney transplantation have led to the referral for transplant evaluation of increasing numbers of patients with end-stage renal disease (ESRD). Unfortunately, although the number of patients being considered for transplantation has increased steadily, the number of donors has remained relatively stagnant. As of the end of 1995, 31,115 patients in the United States were on the waiting list for kidney transplantation (a number that increases by more than 200 a month), even though 11,810 transplants were performed that year. Twenty-five percent of these transplants were with kidneys from living donors.[1,2] Because organ donation is being outpaced by the increasing number of potential recipients, it is important to utilize all viable donors while at the same time avoiding kidneys that are unlikely to provide good function. This chapter discusses the evaluation, technical issues, and ethical aspects of cadaveric and living donation.

▲ THE CADAVERIC DONOR

Cadaveric organ donation begins with the determination of brain death in a given patient and the recognition that such an individual may be a potential donor. The latter is a responsibility that falls on all health care professionals. A large number of potential donors are lost because of failure of the medical community to identify such candidates.[3] Less than 2% of all people who die fulfill the criteria for organ donation. The success of organ recovery depends on a team effort between health care professionals and personnel from the local organ procurement organization (OPO). The role of the OPO is to coordinate donor identification and obtain consent from the donor's family. The OPO also organizes the process of organ recovery and distribution. OPOs are located throughout the United States and function either as independent not-for-profit organizations that serve one or more transplant centers or as direct affiliates of a specific center, providing services only to that center.

The need to increase organ donation has been the focus of a number of groups, on both the local and national levels. In 1994, however, cadaveric organ donation increased by only 2.5%, demonstrating the continued need for public education and an examination of the factors that contribute to an insufficient number of donors.[2] These factors range from general distrust of the health care system to religious myths and misperceptions regarding consent to donation. Such fears are especially common among some minority groups.[4,5] In a survey conducted by Manninen and Evans[6] 70% of families approached were found to be supportive of organ donation. However, most respondents did not think about donation until they were informed of its possibility. In general, it has become the duty of members of the local OPO to assume the most difficult aspect of the entire process—approaching a newly grieving family to obtain consent for organ donation.

▲ DONOR SELECTION

In general, the diagnosis of brain death precedes any consideration for organ donation. This determination is made independently of the transplantation team. The criteria for brain death are listed in Table 4–1 and have been formally enacted into legislation in all 50 states.

Once a person with irreversible brain injury has been referred, determining the potential donor's suitability is best coordinated by the OPO in consultation with the transplant surgeons. The criteria used to decide whether to use a given organ are reasonably well established, but certain relative contraindications to donation are often weighed differently by different surgeons. When relative contraindications exist, the donor is sometimes described as marginal (Table 4–2). For example, some centers prefer not to use organs from very young donors because of a higher risk of technical complications and reports of decreased graft survival.[7,8] However, such organs can be successfully transplanted into selected recipients (eg, first transplant, low body weight, low panel reactive antibody [PRA] level), and should not be routinely excluded from the donor pool. Several centers have reported good results with pediatric kidneys in adult recipients.[9,10] Similarly, organs from donors older than 60 or even 70 years can often be used; however, older donors may have other medical problems (eg, hypertension, cardiac disease) that may make their organs less suit-

TABLE 4–1 ▲ CRITERIA FOR ESTABLISHING BRAIN DEATH

The presence of
Deep coma without induced hypothermia or the use of depressant drugs
No spontaneous respiratory motion in the absence of muscle relaxants
No spontaneous movements in the absence of decerebration and decorticate posturing
No response to deep painful stimuli
Absent cranial reflexes, ie, fixed and dilated pupils, no corneal reflexes, no oculocephalic reflex (doll's eyes)

TABLE 4–2 ▲ CONTRAINDICATIONS TO CADAVERIC DONATION

Absolute	Relative
Chronic renal disease	Hypertension Diabetes
Malignant tumor (except primary brain tumors)	Bacterial sepsis (treated)
Positive HbsAg test	Anti-HCV positive
Positive HIV test	Age >70 y Age <2 mo
Untreated systemic bacterial, fungal, or viral infections	
Prolonged warm ischemia	Prolonged cold ischemia Donor ATN

HbsAg, hepatitis B surface antigen; HCV, hepatitis C virus; HIV, human immunodeficiency virus; ATN, acute tubular necrosis.

able for transplantation. Although age alone is not a reason to exclude a candidate as a potential donor, routine histologic examination of the recovered kidneys is useful to help determine their suitability for transplantation.[11]

The use of organs from hepatitis C virus (HCV) antibody–positive donors has been controversial. At one extreme, some centers have refused to recover organs from HCV-positive donors; at the other extreme some centers transplant these organs into HCV-negative recipients. A consensus seems to have been reached to transplant these kidneys into HCV-positive recipients (with appropriate informed consent) in view of the lack of associated morbidity.[12–15] Exclusion of these potential donors would lead to a decrease in the donor pool and would unnecessarily waste valuable organs. With the development of newer tests for antibody to HCV using the second-generation enzyme-linked immunosorbent assay (ELISA-2) and recombinant immunoblot assay (RIBA), the rate of false-positive testing should decrease. Many centers are now using reverse transcriptase polymerase chain reaction (PCR) testing to detect HCV-RNA sequences in both donors and recipients. It is also possible to eliminate 99% of the HCV virus load by means of pulsatile preservation; some centers use this technique in an effort to decrease the transmission rate.[16]

In situations in which a patient has profound irreversible neurologic injury but brain death criteria cannot be strictly met, some donors can serve as non–heart beating donors. In these situations, consent is obtained, and the patient is extubated in the operating room; once the heart has ceased beating, the organs are rapidly removed. There are other circumstances in which organs can be recovered from non–heart beating donors when sudden circulatory arrest takes place in an uncontrolled situation.[17–19] Retrieval of organs in these situations is discussed below.

Donor Management

Once the diagnosis of brain death has been established and consent has been obtained for organ donation, the OPO continues to play an important role in coordinating organ recovery and allocation. It is also the responsibility of the OPO to assist the hospital in donor management (in consultation with the transplant surgeon if necessary) and ensure that families are not billed for costs incurred during the process of organ donation.

The goal of donor management is to provide physiologically ideal organs for transplantation. Once brain death has been declared, hospital care givers have a tendency to reduce the premortem intensity of care. It becomes crucial for the OPO coordinator to assist in the care of the donor to ensure that appropriate ventilatory and hemodynamic stability are maintained.[20] Brain death is associated with many pathophysiologic problems, including hypotension, hypothermia, diabetes insipidus, and cardiopulmonary dysfunction. These problems must be avoided or corrected to prevent ischemic injury to any potentially usable organs. Table 4–3 lists the commonly encountered problems and their management.

In the event that cardiac arrest occurs in potential donors with brain death, immediate resuscitation should be initiated to restore effective circulation. If circulation cannot be reestablished within 15 minutes, the resulting warm ischemia may render the organs unusable unless immediate recovery can be performed. The use of the super rapid in situ cold flush technique has allowed successful use of both livers and kidneys in situations in which cardiac arrest has occurred and there is the capability for immediate retrieval of the organs.[21]

Hemodynamic instability can occur simply because replacement of fluid (both insensible and urinary) is inadequate. Aggressive intravenous crystalloid infusion is necessary to keep urine output greater than 1 mL/kg per hour. Excessive urine losses due to diabetes insipidus may warrant the use of vasopressin, although it may sometimes be desirable instead to replace the high urinary output intravenously. Severe hypernatremia and hypokalemia, which can occur in donors with diabetes insipidus, may be avoided by frequent electrolyte monitoring. Persistent untreated hypokalemia may result in ventricular tachycardia and cardiac arrest.

Avoiding infections in potential donors is a necessity. Ongoing antibiotic therapy

TABLE 4–3 ▲ MEDICAL PROBLEMS IN DONOR MANAGEMENT

Problem	Management
Cardiopulmonary dysfunction	Avoidance of atelectasis, use of PEEP, frequent suctioning, correction of electrolyte abnormalities, avoidance of the use of inappropriate pressor agents
Hypotension and dehydration	Intravenous replacement of fluid to maintain CVP within normal limits, use of blood products and inotropic drugs (dopamine) to maintain a normal mean blood pressure
Diabetes insipidus	Replacement of losses with fluids low in sodium with 5% dextrose, potassium replacement, administration of exogenous ADH to reduce urine output to a level compatible with IV fluid replacement
Infection	Use of aseptic technique at all times, especially for catheter insertion, wound care, and tracheobronchial suctioning

PEEP, positive end-expiratory pressure; CVP, Central venous pressure; ADH, antidiuretic hormone.

should be continued even after brain death is declared to control systemic infections. Pulmonary atelectasis and infections must be prevented with the use of positive end-expiratory pressure (PEEP), frequent tracheobronchial suctioning, and chest physiotherapy. Blood, urine, and sputum cultures should be performed daily, and serologic testing should also be performed for hepatitis A, B, and C, cytomegalovirus (CMV), Epstein-Barr virus, herpes, human immunodeficiency virus (HIV), *Toxoplasma gondii* (for cardiac donors), and syphillis (VDRL). Many of these serologic studies should be drawn both before and after transfusion of blood and blood products to avoid missing transfusion-related infections.

The rapid infusion of large volumes of cold fluids, such as crystalloid solutions, blood, or blood products, can aggravate preexisting hypothermia. This can be seen in most donors and is attributed to generalized vasodilatation coupled with the dysfunction of the temperature regulatory system. Intravenous fluids should be warmed and body temperature kept as close to normal as possible if metabolic acidosis and cardiac dysrhythmias are to be avoided.

Management at the Time of Organ Recovery

Continuity of preoperative to intraoperative care is necessary to ensure the recovery of suitable organs for transplantation. Intraoperative monitoring by an anesthesiologist has proved useful; if an anesthesiologist is not available, monitoring can be assumed by a member of the local OPO. All efforts must be directed at maintaining hemodynamic stability by continuous replacement of blood loss and urine output with crystalloid.

Use of α adrenergic agonists should be avoided to minimize peripheral vasoconstriction and reduced renal and hepatic perfusion. Muscle relaxants are usually required to optimize surgical exposure, because spinal reflexes sometimes prevent abdominal relaxation. Full intravenous heparinization (300 U/kg) is performed before cross clamping of the aorta. The need for an anesthesiologist continues until the time of aortic cross clamping and in situ hypothermic perfusion. Retrieval of the organs can then proceed in an expeditious and careful manner.

Techniques of Cadaveric Organ Recovery

With the development of multiple organ recovery techniques,[22–24] coordination and cooperation among the various surgical teams involved are essential for the successful retrieval of transplantable organs. The time to procure each solid organ should be minimized to decrease any unnecessary ischemic injury. Kidney retrieval usually follows removal of the heart, lungs, liver, and pancreas.

Preliminary dissection in the chest is often carried out by the cardiac team to isolate the aorta and superior vena cava before cannulation. The inferior vena cava is also isolated for easy access to allow quick venting of blood once in situ perfusion has been initiated. For adequate perfusion of the liver, intestine, kidneys, and pancreas, the distal aorta is used for cannulation. Preliminary intraabdominal dissection is performed to isolate the aorta, divide the bile duct, and ligate the gastroduodenal artery. If the lungs and/or heart are to be recovered, aortic cross clamping takes place in the abdomen. Some dissection of the supraceliac aorta may be necessary to allow clamping in this location. When the pancreas is not to be used as a solid organ for transplantation, the inferior mesenteric vein is dissected out and cannulated for portal perfusion of the liver, in addition to aortic perfusion. Two liters of University of Wisconsin solution (UW) are used for each cannula. When the aorta alone is used for cannulation, 3 liters of UW solution are infused before organ recovery.

Gerota's fascia can be opened to expose the kidneys for surface cooling. While the heart is being removed and the cold perfusate is being infused, ice slush is placed into the abdominal cavity to provide surface cooling for the liver, kidneys, and pancreas.

Once the heart is removed, and the liver is to be retrieved, careful attention should be given to ensure the following:

1. The aortic cannula is not extended beyond the ostia of the renal arteries. Such placement can result in inadequate flushing of the kidneys, leading to unnecessary warm ischemia.
2. In the event that the superior mesenteric artery (SMA) is not taken along with the celiac artery for the liver, the upper portion of the remaining aorta can be reclamped to allow continued perfusion of the kidneys and cooling while the liver is being removed (Fig. 4–1A). If the SMA is taken with the liver and removed, it may not be possible to place a curved clamp in a tangential manner on the remaining segment of aorta. Although this would allow continued flushing of the kidneys, there is some risk of occluding of the renal artery orifices, especially on the right side (Fig 4–1B).
3. At the time of transection of the vena cava between the liver and the kidneys, care must be taken to avoid injury to the right renal vein or misidentification of the vein as a portion of the vena cava. The right renal vein can often extend superiorly before entering the vena cava and may be inadvertently transected (Fig 4–2A). Because a segment of infrahepatic vena cava is required in liver transplantation, communication is necessary between the liver and kidney retrieval teams to leave a desirable amount of cuff of vena cava to go with the liver and to prevent injury to the right renal vein (Fig. 4–2B).
4. If consent includes retrieval of the pancreas, this procedure is performed before removal of the kidneys. Again, injury to the left renal artery or vein can occur as the dissection of the pancreas is performed. Often the pancreas and occasionally the kidneys are recovered en bloc with the liver and then separated on the back table (see below).

It is unnecessary to perform extensive mobilization of the kidneys prior to their removal, especially in cases of multiple organ recovery. Such retroperitoneal dissection, with mobilization of the small and large intestine to expose the kidneys, can jeopardize the liver by interfering with the venous return through the portal system. In addition, accidental injury or ligation of aberrant renal arteries can occur, leading to incomplete perfusion and warm ischemia of the kidneys.

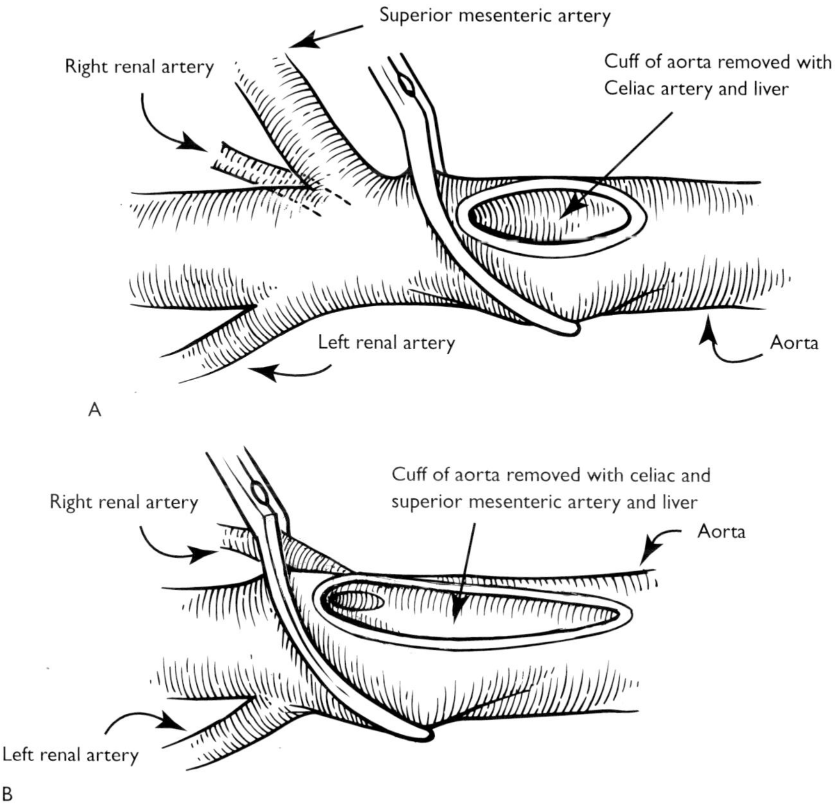

Figure 4–1. A. Reclamping of the aorta after hepatectomy to allow continued perfusion of the kidneys, if the origin of the superior mesenteric artery is not taken with the liver. B. Reclamping not possible because of proximity to orifices of renal artery.

All that is needed to recover the kidneys safely in a multiple organ recovery is appropriate placement of the aortic cannula for the cold in situ flush with UW solution. Once the liver has been removed, the kidneys can be recovered by mobilizing the right and left colon. The ureters are then divided distally as close to the bladder as possible. They are dissected superiorly with adequate amounts of periureteral tissue left in place to avoid interference with the ureteral blood supply. Culturing of the tips of the ureters can be performed at this time. The distal aorta with the cannula in place and the distal vena cava at the level of the bifurcation are both transected and dissected off the vertebral column (Fig. 4–3). This dissection is carried cephalad and kept as far posterior as possible; the line of dissection is maintained at the level of the paraspinal muscles. Gerota's fascia is kept attached to the kidneys. At the superior poles of the kidneys, the adrenal glands are left intact attached to the kidneys. The kidneys are removed en bloc without identification of the hilar structures.

On the back table, any surrounding excess perinephric fat is excised and re-

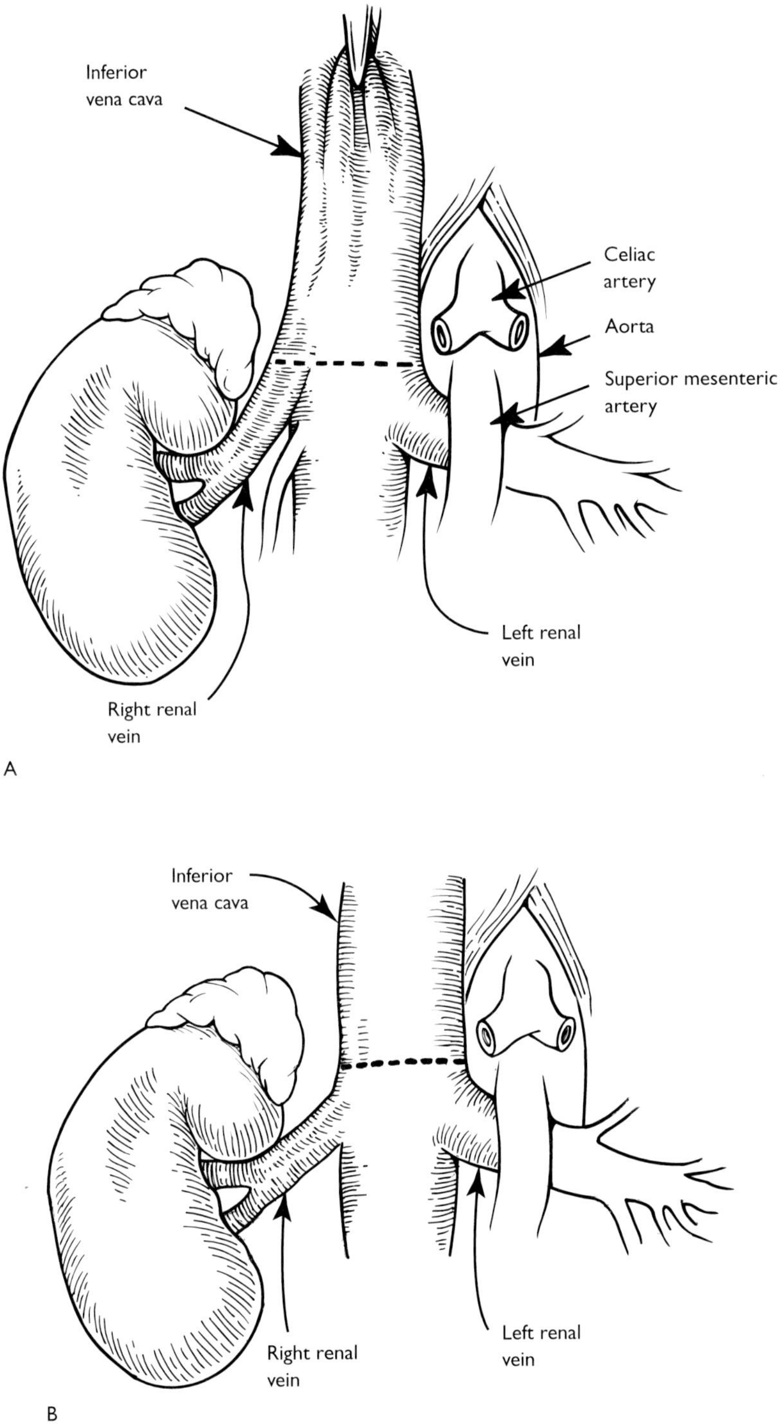

Figure 4–2. A. Inadvertent transection of right renal vein when inferior vena cava is being divided. B. Appropriate level of transection of inferior vena cava.

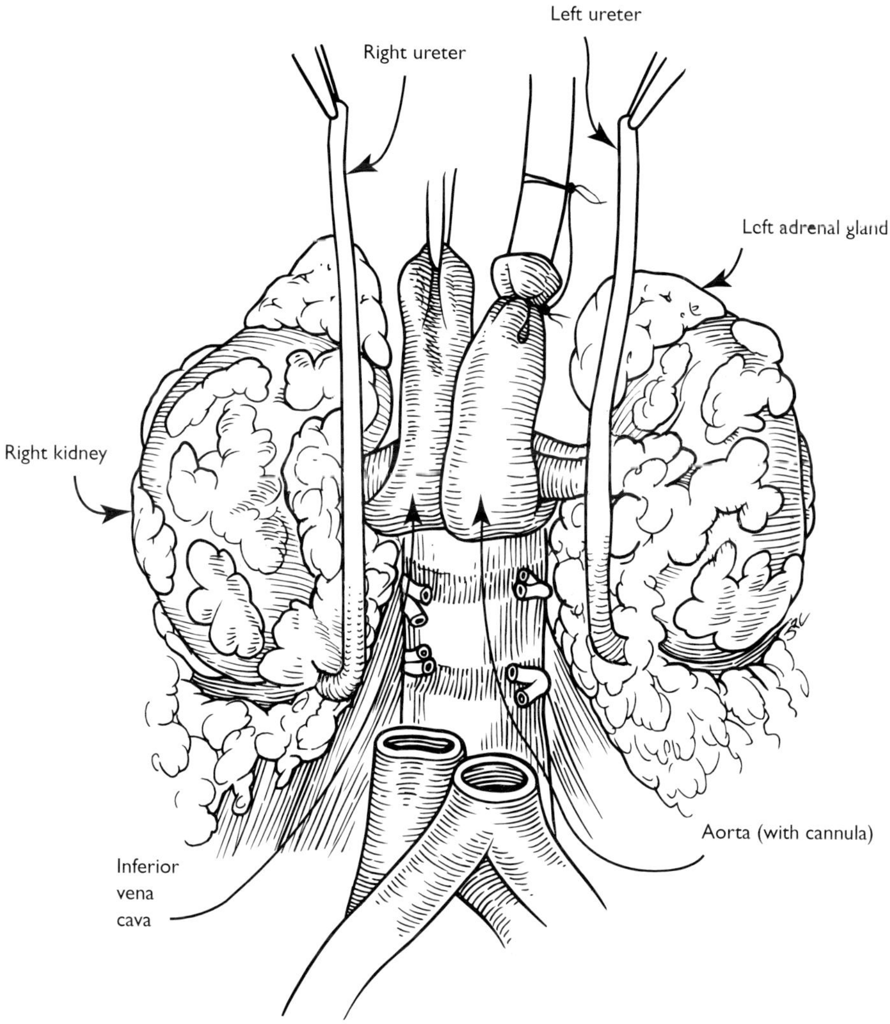

Figure 4–3. En bloc removal of kidneys and ureters.

moved from the lateral aspects of the kidneys to allow for appropriate cooling. The surfaces of the kidneys are inspected for petechiae, anatomic abnormalities, and adequacy of the cold in situ flush. The renal veins are examined, and the left renal vein is transected with a small cuff of vena cava. The entire vena cava is left with the right kidney (Fig 4–4). The aorta is split posteriorly by dividing between the lumbar arteries and then anteriorly down the middle. The ostia of the renal arteries are examined to identify multiple renal arteries and the presence of atherosclerotic occlusion. Care must be taken to identify aberrant renal arteries, which may originate from the iliac arteries or distal aorta. The aortic segment is left intact. The ureters are examined for length, numbers, and size.

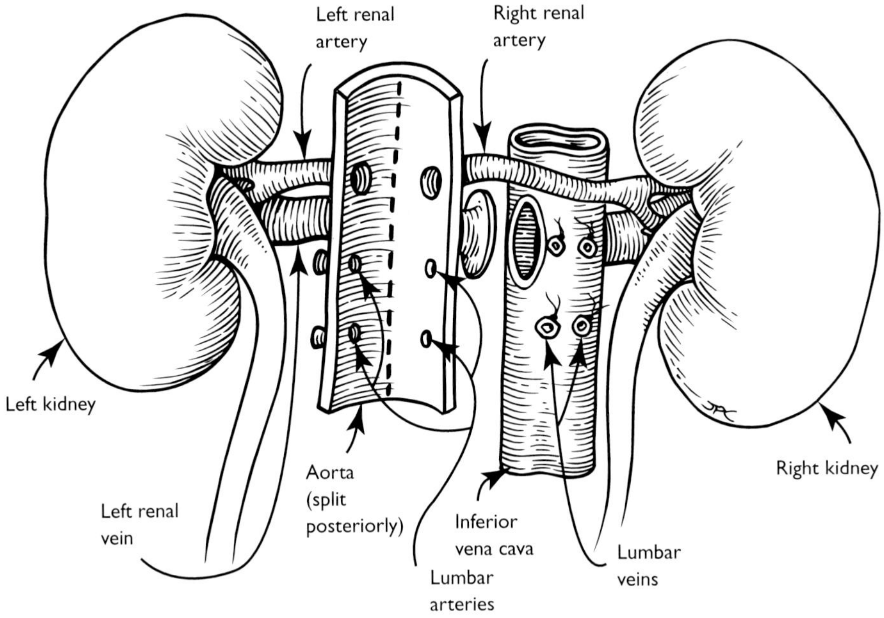

Figure 4–4. Separation of kidneys on the back table.

It is useful to reflush each kidney until the effluent is free of blood before packaging. The organs are packaged separately in a cold solution of the perfusate; the container is wrapped in two sterile plastic bags and stored in a Styrofoam plastic container of crushed ice. The organs can then be transported to any part of the country.

If the *liver is not to be recovered,* dissection of the kidneys can proceed with mobilization of the right colon, exposing the right kidney, the inferior vena cava, and lower aorta. Identification and ligation of the inferior mesenteric artery and vein are performed, and the lesser splanchnic nerves are divided, allowing mobilization of the left mesocolon and exposure of the left kidney. The SMA can then be identified, ligated, and divided. At this point, the upper abdomen is approached and the supraceliac aorta is identified as it exits the diaphragmatic crus. Alternatively, mobilization of the aorta can be performed within the thoracic cavity for better control, if consent includes opening the chest. The celiac axis is identified, ligated, and divided. Mass clamping of the hepatoduodenal ligament can also be performed (Fig 4–5) to minimize flushing of the liver. The ureters are then divided distally and mobilized superiorly; culture of the ureteral tips can be performed at this point.

After heparinization, the kidneys can be flushed via the distal aortic cannula with simultaneous clamping of the upper aorta and venting of the vena cava into the chest, if possible. Removal of the kidneys can then proceed as described above.

If the donor is younger than 3–4 years, the surgeon must make sure the aortic cannula is not occluding the renal artery orifices. Dissection of the kidneys proceeds in a manner similar to that described above, but the kidneys are kept as a pair and

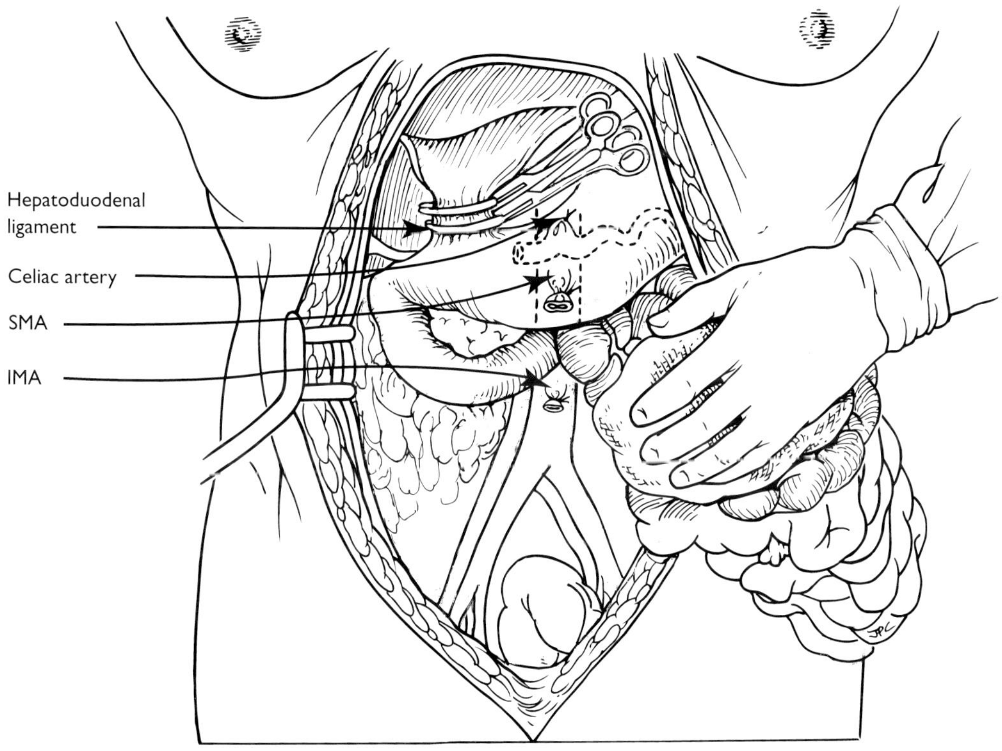

Figure 4–5. Cadaveric nephrectomy without hepatectomy. Ligation of the inferior mesenteric, superior mesenteric, and celiac arteries, with division of the hepatoduodenal ligament.

are not separated. With very small donors, it may be necessary to place the aortic cannula into one of the common iliac arteries so as not to compromise the length of aorta to be used for anastomosis in the recipient. Kidneys from a donor 3–4 years or older can usually be used separately, if they are large enough.

The retrieval of multiple intraabdominal organs by an en bloc total abdominal evisceration technique that prevents prolonged warm ischemia and traction injuries to the vascular tree has been described in the literature.[25] This technique was associated with a lower rate of primary non-function of livers and no statistical difference in the incidence of delayed renal allograft function when compared with conventionally retrieved kidneys. The organs to be used are separated on the back table.

Improving techniques of harvesting organs from non–heart beating donors has allowed the use of organs that otherwise would not be considered for transplantation. Reports of the satisfactory function of organs retrieved in this manner[17,26] have been followed by methods of proposed effective cooling by various aortic infusion techniques.[18,19,27] Such methods of recovery have allowed good organs to be obtained from non–heart beating donors in countries that do not have brain death laws.[28]

The retrieval of organs when cardiac arrest occurs immediately before or during preliminary dissection can best be conducted with simultaneous chest and abdominal exposure. This ensures placement of the aortic cannula for perfusion and immediate cross clamping of the upper thoracic aorta with venting of the vena cava. In rare situations, it is the request of the family that the pronouncement of death be made and witnessed by them before removal of organs. In such circumstances, the donor is placed in a setting near the operating room, and in the presence of family members, the ventilator is disconnected. At the time of cardiac standstill, pronouncement is made, and procurement is initiated after immediate transport to the operating room.

Organ Preservation

Many of the techniques of kidney preservation were pioneered by the late Folkert Belzer. In 1967, Belzer developed hypothermic perfusion preservation at the University of California at San Francisco. His work was based on the concept that exposure to cold decreases oxygen consumption by slowing cellular energy metabolism.[29,30] Soon thereafter, Geoffrey Collins[31] developed a technique of cold storage preservation. He maintained that initial perfusion, followed by simple immersion in a cold (4°C) solution containing large amounts of potassium and glucose, would achieve good results.

These two techniques of organ preservation revolutionized renal transplantation and made cadaveric organs available for transplantation across the country. The Collins solution (or a modified version called Euro-Collins) dominated the field of organ preservation, but was not as effective for the preservation of extrarenal organs (eg, pancreas, liver) as for the preservation of kidneys. In 1987, the University of Wisconsin (UW) solution, developed by Southard and Belzer, was introduced.[32] The UW solution markedly extended the preservation time for both liver and pancreas and proved effective for all intraabdominal organs, both for in situ flushing and for subsequent cold storage.[33] The composition of the UW solution is shown in Table 4–4. The effectiveness of the solution is due mainly to the presence of impermeable molecules, such as lactobionate and raffinose, which prevents hypothermia-induced cell swelling. Expansion of the extracellular space is prevented by hydroxyethyl starch.

The introduction of better preservation of kidneys has allowed organ allocation based on tissue typing and matching (see Chapters 3 and 8). Organs can be shipped from one part of the country to another. Preservation has made kidney transplantation a somewhat more elective procedure; in addition, the use of kidneys once considered marginal (in terms of long ischemia times) has become possible. Within our institution, the average cold ischemia time is 31.4 hours.[34]

Cold ischemia time is defined as the time from aortic cross clamping during organ retrieval to the time of reperfusion of the kidney in the recipient. Warm ischemia time is described as either the initial warm ischemia time at harvesting or the warm

TABLE 4–4 ▲ COMPOSITION OF UNIVERSITY OF WISCONSIN SOLUTION

K^+ Lactobionate	100 mM
KH_2PO_4	25 mMn
$MgSO_4$	5 mM
Raffinose	30 mM
Adenosine	5 mM
Glutathione	3 mM
Insulin	100 U/L
Dexamethasone	8 mg/L
Allopurinol	1 mM
Hydroxyethyl starch	50 g/L
Penicillin	200,000 u/L
PH	7.45
K	120 ± 5 mM
Na	30 ± 5 mM
OsM	320 ± 5 mOsm/L

ischemia time during the recipient operation. It can also be the sum of these two. Warm ischemia time may not be an important factor in the era of in situ perfusion (although it may become an issue if the duration of the donor hepatectomy is excessively long) and with the frequent use of an ice blanket wrapped around the kidney during reimplantation (see Chapter 6). The latter keeps the kidney reasonably cold while the vascular anastomoses are being performed and allows for a more careful, less anxious reimplantation; this is particularly important in a teaching institution.

The use of Euro-Collins solution for the in situ flush during organ procurement, followed by flushing with UW solution on the back table has been advocated by some centers as being less expensive than and as effective as the use of UW solution alone. Belzer specifically advised against this practice, and it is probably detrimental to the extrarenal organs. Our center uses UW solution as the sole flushing solution; Euro-Collins solution can be used to store the kidneys if cost is an issue. Reflushing with UW solution just before reimplantation has little beneficial effect.

Continuous pulsatile preservation is being used by several centers in the United States. This technique was used initially to allow extended preservation time and to provide the kidney with nutrients even in a state of low metabolism. With the adoption of better preservation solutions, this method of preservation has decreased in popularity, although there may be a resurgence of interest. Large series have shown no difference in initial graft non-function rates between perfused and stored kidney grafts.[35–37] However, individual centers have claimed remarkably low rates of delayed graft function with pulsatile preservation; it may be that this is confounded with a low cold ischemia time and better donor management prior to recovery.[38,39] Machine perfusion may be considered for kidneys from non–heart beating donors to decrease the incidence of delayed graft function.[40,41] Injuries to the renal vessels can occur with pulsatile perfusion, and this method is expensive and requires highly trained personnel to operate the machines.

Trials are underway with other preservation solutions, including histidine tryptophan ketoglutarate (HTK), Carolina rinse solution, and a simplified UW-type solution called sodium lactobionate sucrose (SLS) solution.[42–44]

Ethical Issues

The continuing shortage of donor organs has raised several ethical issues. The National Organ Transplant Act of 1984 (HR5586, Title II) explicitly forbids the purchase and sale of human organs for profit. Given the ongoing shortage, however, there has been some discussion regarding compensation to donor families to increase the consent rate.[45] Possible financial incentives have included contribution toward burial costs, cash payment, donations to a charity of the family's choosing, or a small insurance policy or tuition credit for any offspring. These issues have been the subject of considerable debate, without any consensus to date.[46–48]

Although the Uniform Anatomical Gift Act provides a legal basis for such gifts in advance of the death of the donor, it is the family or next of kin who makes the final decision regarding donation. The family has the right to veto the decision of the donor card signer. The ability to do so raises questions about the utility of having a signed donor card. Community education to increase organ donation should focus not only on the need to sign a donor card but also on the need to discuss such issues with family members and friends. Many states have adopted a revision of the Uniform Gift Act that eliminates the necessity for consent from the next of kin for organ donation, if the necessary document agreeing to donation has been given to the donor's physician. This revision also eliminates the previous requirement for the signature of a witness on the donor card. The concept of presumed consent carries this idea a step further and assumes agreement to donation unless refusal is clearly stated. This concept has met with much resistance and has not been adopted in any state for solid organ retrieval, although it has become legally sanctioned practice in several European countries.

Other ethical issues under discussion include allocation of organs to recipients from foreign countries when there are so many U.S. citizens on the waiting list. There is debate about whether foreign nationals should be listed separately to give first priority to U.S. recipients.

The equity of transplant allocation has been debated by many authorities with the goal of balancing justice and medical utility. One modification that has not been adopted would give preference to African-American recipients, who currently have a longer waiting time.[49] The need to ensure that all potential recipients have the resources to benefit from transplantation is perhaps more fundamental an issue, to avoid wastage of organs because of lack of appropriate support systems. These issues remain unresolved.

▲ THE LIVING DONOR

The use of living donors for renal transplantation was critical to the early development of the field and preceded the use of cadaveric donors. The first completely successful kidney transplantation occurred on December 23, 1954, at the Peter Bent Brigham Hospital in Boston. This transplant took place between identical twins after identity was verified by means of cross skin grafting and blood group verification.[50] At present, 20–25% of all kidney transplants performed in the United States are with living donors. Most donors are closely related genetically. In a small but increasing percentage of cases, however, donors are genetically unrelated and include spouses, friends, or other emotionally related individuals. Ethical guidelines mandate that the living donor not be coerced and that there be no evidence of financial profit by the donor. Donation should be considered "a gift of extraordinary value."[51]

The use of living donors has been associated with a higher success rate than that seen with cadaveric donation (see Chapter 1). Given the increase in the number of patients awaiting transplantation and the lack of a parallel increase in the number of available cadaveric organs, living donation allows some patients to avoid long waiting times and occasionally even the need for dialysis (Table 4–5).

Evaluation

It is usually the potential living donor who initiates the discussion about donation, although the recipient or the physician also can raise the issue. The donor then meets with the nephrologist, transplant surgeon, social worker, and transplant nurse coordinator. All donors are informed of the risks and benefits of transplantation compared with dialysis and the risks to themselves of donating a kidney, both short and

TABLE 4–5 ▲ ADVANTAGES OF LIVING DONATION

Better results (both long and short-term)
Consistent early function and easier management
Avoidance of long waiting time for transplantation
Less aggressive immunosuppressive regimens
Emotional gain to donor

long term.[52,53] A 1995 report of U.S. practices found the reported mortality rate for living donors to be 0.03% and the morbidity rate to be 0.23%.[54] It is important to screen any relative of a patient with familial renal disease (polycystic kidney disease, hereditary nephritis) for evidence of occult signs and symptoms; such donors are excluded.[55] On the other hand, kidneys with minor renal abnormalities can be used safely, once it is determined that function of such kidneys will not be impaired after transplantation.[56]

Initial evaluation of all potential donors consists of blood and tissue typing. Those with ABO incompatibility are excluded; compatibility with the Rh factor is unnecessary. All blood group–compatible donors are then tested with a T-lymphocyte cross match. A negative cross match will allow for further consideration for donation. In the case of multiple potential donors, the better the antigen match, the greater is the likelihood of being selected for donation, if all other testing is within normal limits.

In general, as long as the donor and recipient have a negative T-cell cross match, the operation can be carried out. This is true for both related and nonrelated donors who are ABO compatible. The cross match between donor cells and recipient serum is the only immunologic test performed routinely at our institution. Many centers perform a mixed lymphocyte reaction (MLR) as part of the routine evaluation. The importance of this test has decreased with the introduction of better immunosuppression.

Further evaluation for a potential donor consists of a complete history and physical examination, routine laboratory testing, and serologic evaluation for EBV, herpes virus, CMV, HIV, and hepatitis B and C viruses. A urinalysis and culture, along with a 24-hour urine collection for creatinine clearance and protein excretion, are included as part of the routine evaluation. If there is any concern regarding a borderline hypertensive blood pressure reading, the blood pressure should be measured on at least three and as many as ten separate occasions.

Once all laboratory testing has been performed, the next step is renal arteriography with an excretion phase to visualize the collecting system. This eliminates the need for a separate intravenous pyelogram. Such testing can be performed on an outpatient basis. Spiral CT scanning has been used instead of conventional angiography in some centers. The use of magnetic resonance (MR) angiography is still investigational.

Donors are judged unsuitable for a variety of reasons (Table 4–6). Anyone at risk for the development of acquired renal disease should be excluded. This includes individuals with diastolic blood pressures consistently above 90 mm Hg, or who require antihypertensive medications to control their blood pressure. A history of hypertension is not in itself a reason for exclusion if the donor is normotensive and off medication, but the donor should be carefully examined for preexisting renal disease or for the risk for development of renal disease later in life.

Potential donors for siblings with diabetes routinely undergo a 5-hour glucose tolerance test, and the 24-hour urine specimen must be free of proteinuria. Some centers require that the donor be at least 10 years older than the age of the recipient at the time of the diagnosis of diabetes. The measurement of hemoglobin A_{1C} and anti-

TABLE 4–6 ▲ EXCLUSION CRITERIA FOR LIVING DONORS

Absolute
Age <18 years
Hypertension (blood pressure >140/90 mm Hg or necessity for medication)
Diabetes (abnormal glucose tolerance test or Hb A_{Ic})
Proteinuria (>300 mg/24 hours)
Abnormal glomerular filtration rate (creatinine clearance <75 mL/min)
Microscopic hematuria
History of thrombosis or thromboembolism
Medically significant illness (chronic lung disease, recent malignant tumor, heart disease)
History of bilateral kidney stones
Relative
Abnormalities of the donor kidney (urologic, vascular)
Obesity (30% or more above ideal weight)
Psychiatric disorders

islet antibodies also can be included in the evaluation of any potential related donor for a recipient with diabetes.

Unexplained microscopic hematuria may be an indication of underlying renal disease such as glomerulonephritis and as such may not be detected before donation. Finding as few as three red cells per high-power field may appear unimportant at first but may be an indicator of potential future problems.

A history of thromboembolism or thrombophlebitis places a potential donor at increased risk for pulmonary embolism and therefore excludes donation. This also is true of patients with heart disease, or a history of malignant neoplasia. Obesity may be a relative contraindication for any potential donor more than 30% above ideal body weight. These individuals should be advised to lose the excess weight before the transplant is scheduled to decrease the risk of pulmonary embolism or cardiac complications.

Patients with clinically significant psychiatric disorders should be evaluated fully by a psychiatrist to establish that the donor understands and agrees to the proposed procedure. In our center, we tend not to accept such donors.

Once a full evaluation has been performed, if examination of the donor's vascular supply and drainage system reveals an abnormality, it must be decided whether the risks imposed on the donor or the recipient are too great. With regard to vascular abnormalities, we tend not to use donor kidneys with three or more arteries. Abnormalities such as aneurysms, renal artery stenosis, or fibromuscular dysplasia, if limited in size and area, can often be resected and repaired or excised on the back table. Such pathologic conditions should be limited to one kidney, leaving a normal kidney in place. Given these caveats, it may be possible to use such donors.[57,58] Excision and reconstruction of such abnormalities is in a sense a form of treatment for these donors, although care must be taken to avoid leaving either the donor or the recipient with less than a perfect outcome.

Preoperative Management

Once the evaluation has demonstrated that there are no abnormalities serious enough to exclude donation, the donor can be admitted to the hospital after arteriography. Many insurance companies are now restricting admissions to the day of the operation. In such cases, intravenous hydration can be given overnight on an outpatient basis or started on arrival at the hospital. Such hydration is important to help ensure adequate diuresis during the donor operation. Assessment by the anesthesiologist and the pain management team preoperatively can make for a more comfortable postoperative recovery. We use one of two options for postoperative pain management for the donor: epidural catheter placement for narcotic administration or a patient controlled analgesia (PCA) pump.

The donor is instructed preoperatively on the use of the incentive spirometer, and on the use of leg support stockings and the sequential compression device (SCD) system to prevent venous stasis. After entering the operating room but before the incision, the patient should receive a dose of an intravenous antibiotic (1–2 g of a first- or second-generation cephalosporin is sufficient). Although preoperative skin cleaning is recommended, eg, with a Hibicleas shower, hair clipping is avoided until just before the incision.

Perioperative Management

When the donor arrives in the operating room, the epidural catheter (if that option is chosen) is placed and general anesthesia is induced. Positioning of the patient is critical. We prefer to use the left kidney because of the longer vein if the arterial supply to both kidneys is similar. The patient is placed in the right lateral decubitus position with the table flexed maximally and the kidney rest raised under the 12th rib. Once the patient is appropriately positioned and hemodynamic stability is confirmed, it is important to adjust the urinary catheter tubing so that it is draining in a continuous downward flow. It is usually necessary to give additional crystalloid to increase the urine output. Care must be taken not to restrict venous return to the heart by raising the kidney rest excessively and compressing the vena cava.

A slightly curved flank incision is made from the tip of the 12th rib to the lateral border of the rectus muscle at the level of the umbilicus. This type of incision avoids removal of a portion of the rib and results in less postoperative discomfort; the possibility of pneumothorax also is eliminated. The fascial layers are incised and the peritoneum is reflected medially. The ureter is identified, and Gerota's fascia is incised. The kidney is then mobilized from inside Gerota's fascia using electrocautery to minimize blood loss. The ureter is then dissected free proximally.

Once the hilum is approached, care is taken to dissect out the vessels gently to avoid arterial spasm. Papaverine is infiltrated around the renal artery before any dissection is attempted. Renal vein branches are ligated and divided as necessary. Once the renal vein and artery are mobilized, the ureter is mobilized distally and transected at the level of the iliac bifurcation. It is imperative at this point to verify that the contralateral kidney is making adequate amounts of urine.

The renal artery and renal vein are transected immediately after each vessel is clamped with a vascular clamp. Systemic heparinization is unnecessary. The kidney is immediately flushed on the back table with cold Ringer's lactate, to which procaine, 100 mg/L, and heparin, 10,000 U/L, have been added. Once the kidney is adequately flushed and surface cooled, it is transported to the recipient room for implantation. Any necessary vascular repairs are best performed at this time.

The use of an antibiotic-containing solution (1 g cefazolin per liter of saline solution) to irrigate the wound periodically during the operation and meticulous hemostasis before wound closure are important steps in minimizing postoperative complications.

Recent descriptions of laparoscopic techniques to perform the donor nephrectomy and the associated reduced morbidity may have a broad impact; at present, only two centers are using this approach routinely.[60,61]

Postoperative Care

The postoperative care of a living kidney donor is fairly standard. Adequate postoperative analgesia is the key factor in preventing postoperative complications such as atelectasis and pneumonia.[59] Infections should not occur with appropriate prophylaxis. The continuous use of leg stockings and sequential compression devices is essential to prevent deep venous thrombosis of the lower extremities. Most patients are often ambulatory by postoperative day 1 or 2 and tolerating oral feedings by postoperative day 3 or 4. The donor can be discharged by postoperative day 2 to 6. Renal function should be assessed 1 and 6 weeks after the operation, as some patients experience a 25% increase in serum creatinine level; this should return to near baseline by 3 months after the operation. The serum creatinine level should again be measured 6 months and then yearly after discharge.

There are no convincing data to suggest that living donors are at any increased long-term risk as a result of having donated a kidney. Nevertheless, it is not unreasonable to recommend ongoing periodic long-term follow-up evaluation for these patients. This can be performed by the donor's personal physician.

▲ REFERENCES

1. UNOS Update: Waiting list charts by organ by ABO group, age, race and UNOS region. 11:38, Sept 1995.
2. UNOS Update: United States organ transplants increase. 11:39, Feb 1995.
3. Nathan HM, Jarrell BE, et al: Estimation and characterization of the potential renal organ donor pool in Pennsylvania. *Transplantation* 151:142–149, 1991.
4. Norton-Reitz N, Callender C: Organ donation in the African American population: a fresh perspective with a simple solution. *Natl Med Assoc* 85:353, 1993.

5. Davidson MN, Devney P: Attitudinal barriers to organ donation among black Americans. *Transplant Proc* 25:2531–2532, 1991.
6. Manninen DL, Evans RW: Public attitudes and behavior regarding organ donation. *JAMA* 253:311–3115, 1985.
7. Wetzels JFM, Hoitsma AJ, et al: Influence of cadaver donor age on renal graft survival. *Clin Nephrol* 25:256, 1988.
8. Brown MW, Akyol AM, et al: Transplantation of cadaver kidneys from pediatric donors. *Clin Transplant* 2:87, 1988.
9. Ratner LE, Flye MW: Successful transplantation of cadaveric en-bloc paired kidneys into adult recipients. *Transplantation* 51:273, 1991.
10. Darris F, Jordon ML, et al: Transplantation of pediatric en-bloc kidneys under FK506 immunosuppression. *Transplant Proc* 23:3089, 1991.
11. Alexander JW, Vaughn WK: the use of "marginal" donors for organ transplantation: the influence of donor age on outcome. *Transplantation* 51:135, 1991.
12. Brunson ME, Lau J, et al: Non-A, non-B hepatitis and elevated serum aminotransferases in renal transplant patients. *Transplantation* 56:1364, 1993.
13. Kahan BD: Pro/con: Hepatitis C-positive organ donation (letter). *Transplant Immunol* 9:1993.
14. Stempel GA, Lake J, et al: Hepatitis C: its prevalence in end stage renal failure patients and clinical course after transplantation. *Transplantation* 55:273–276, 1993.
15. Morales JM, Campistol JM, et al: Transplantation of kidneys from donors with hepatitis C antibody into recipients with pre-transplantation anti-HCV. *Kidney Int* 47:236–240, 1995.
16. Roth D: Hepatitis C positive individuals are suitable for organ donation (letter). *Transplant Immunology* 9:1993.
17. Ruers TJM, Vroemen JPAM, Kootstra G: Non–heart beating donors: a successful contribution to organ procurement. *Transplant Proc* 18:408, 1986.
18. Yland M, Anaise M, Ishimaru M, Rapaport FT: New pulsatile perfusion method for non–heart-beating cadaveric donor organs: a preliminary report. *Transplant Proc* 25: 3087–3090, 1993.
19. Matsuno M, Kozaki M, Sakurai E, et al: Effect of combination in situ cooling and machine perfusion preservation on non–heart beating donor kidney procurement. *Transplant Proc* 25:1516–1517, 1993.
20. Lavery G: The cadaveric donor. In: McGeown MG (ed), *Clinical Management of Renal Transplantation.* Academic publishers, Dordrecht, Netherlands, Kluwer 1992:135–151.
21. Yanaga K, Kakizoe S, Ikeda T, et al: Procurement of liver allografts from non-heart beating donors. *Transplant Proc* 22:275–278, 1990.
22. Starzl TE, Hakala T, et al: A flexible procedure for multiple cadaveric organ procurement. *Surg Gynecol Obstet* 158:223–230, 1984.
23. Starzl TE, Miller C, Broznick B, et al: Improved technique for multiple organ harvesting. *Surg Gynecol Obstet* 165:343, 1987.
24. Starzl TE, Iwatsuki S, Shaw WB, et al: Orthotopic liver transplantation in 1984. *Transplant Proc* 17:250, 1985
25. Nakazato PZ, Concepcion W, Bry W, et al: Total abdominal evisceration: an en bloc technique for abdominal organ harvesting. *Surgery* 111:37–47, 1992.
26. Casavilla A, Ramirez C, Shapiro R, et al: Experience with liver and kidney allografts from non-heart-beating donors. *Transplantation* 59:197–203, 1995.
27. Anaise D, Smith R, Ishiman M, et al: An approach to organ salvage from non-heart beating cadaver donors under existing legal and ethical requirements for transplantation. *Transplantation* 49:290–294, 1990.

28. Ericzon BG, Lundgren G, Wilczek H, Groth CG: Experience with human liver grafts obtained after donor cardiac standstill. *Transplant Proc* 18:3862–3863, 1987.
29. Belzer FO, Ashby BS, Dumphy JE: 24- and 72-hour preservation of canine kidneys. *Lancet* 3:536, 1967.
30. Belzer FO, Southard JH: Principles of solid organ preservation by cold storage. *Transplantation* 45:673–676, 1988.
31. Collins GH, Bravo-Shugarman MB, Terasaki PI: Kidney preservation for transplantation: initial perfusion and 30 hour ice storage. *Lancet* 2:1219, 1969.
32. Southard JH, Pienaar H, et al: The University of Wisconsin solution for organ preservation. In: *Transplantation Reviews*. Philadelphia, Saunders, 1989:103–130.
33. Cofer JB, Klintmalm GB, Morris CV, et al: A prospective randomized trial between Euro-Collins and University of Wisconsin solutions as the initial flush in hepatic allograft procurement. *Transplantation* 53:995–998, 1992.
34. Shapiro R, Jordan M, Scantlebury V, et al: A prospective randomized trial of FK506 based immunosuppression after renal transplantation. *Transplantation* 59:485–490, 1995.
35. Opelz G, Terasaki PI: Advantage of cold storage over machine perfusion for preservation of cadaver kidneys. *Transplantation* 23:64, 1982.
36. Halloran P, Aprile M: A randomized prospective trial of cold storage versus pulsatile perfusion for cadaveric kidney preservation. *Transplantation* 43:827, 1987.
37. Merion RM, Oh HK, Port FK, et al: A prospective controlled trial of cold-storage versus machine perfusion in cadaveric renal transplantation. *Transplantation* 50:230, 1990.
38. Tesi RJ, Elkhammas EA, Davis EA, et al: Pulsatile kidney perfusion for preservation and evaluation: use of high-risk kidney donors to expand the donor pool. *Transplant Proc* 25:3099–3100, 1993.
39. Heil JE, Canafax DM, Sutherland DER, et al: A controlled comparison of kidney preservation by two methods: machine perfusion and cold storage. *Transplant Proc* 19:20–46, 1987.
40. Manis T, Hong JH, Bronsther OL, et al: Superior results with machine-perfused kidneys in cyclosporine-treated transplant recipients. *Transplant Proc* 17:1483, 1985.
41. Booster MH, Wijnen RMH, Yin M, et al: Enhanced resistance to the effects of normothermic ischemia in kidneys using pulsatile machine perfusion. *Transplant Proc* 25:3006–3011, 1993.
42. Groenewooud AF, Thorogood J, for the HTK Study Group: Current status of Eurotransplant randomized multicenter study comparing kidney graft preservation with histidine-tryptophan-ketoglutarate, University of Wisconsin, and Euro-Collins solutions. *Transplant Proc* 25:1582–1585, 1993.
43. Tokunaga Y, Wicomb WN, Concepcion W, Nakazato P, Collins GM, Esquivel C. Successful 20-hour rat liver preservation with chlorpromazine is sodium lactobionate sucrose solution. *Surgery* 110:80–86, 1991.
44. Nakazato PZ, Itasaka H, Concepcion W, Lim J, Esquivel C, Collins G. Effects of abdominal en bloc procurement and of a high sodium preservation solution in liver transplantation. *Transplant Proc* 25:1604–1606, 1993.
45. Peters TG: Financial incentives for organ recovery: An update. *Dialy Nephrol* 23, 1993.
46. Rothenberg LS: Ethical and legal issues in kidney transplantation. In: *Handbook of Kidney Transplantation* 1992:358–371.
47. Peters TG: Financial incentives in organ donation. *Curr Issues Dialy Transplant* 21:270, 1992.
48. Peters TG: Life or death: the issue of payment in cadaveric organ donation. *JAMA* 265:45–48, 1991.
49. Newman JM: Equity in transplant allocation: A patient's view (letter). *Transplant Immunol* 9:5, 1993.

50. Kuss R, Bourget P: In: *An Illustrated History of Organ Transplantation: The Great Adventure of the Century.* Rueil-Malmaison, France, Sandoz, 1992.
51. Council of the Transplantation Society: Commercialization in transplantation: the problems and some guidelines for practice. *Lancet* 2:715–716, 1985.
52. Levey AS, Milford EL: Donor and recipient selection. In: Brenner BM, Stein JH (eds), *Contemporary Issues in Nephrology: Renal Transplantation.* vol. 19:247–285, 1989.
53. Rosenthal JT, Danovitch GM: Live related and cadaveric kidney donation. In: *Handbook of Kidney Transplantation.* 1992:105–118.
54. Bia MJ, Ramos EL, Danovitch GM, et al: Evaluation of living donors: the current practice of U.S. transplant centers. *Transplantation* 60:322–327, 1995.
55. Spanos PK, Simmons RL, Kjellstrand CM, Buselmeir TJ, Najarian JS: Screening potential related donors for renal disease. *Lancet* 1:645–648, 1984.
56. Spanos PK, Simmons RL, Rattazzi LC, Goldberg ME, Najarian JS: The fate of kidney transplants from donors with minor renal abnormalities. *Surgery* 76:252–258, 1974.
57. Brandina L, Marcos A, Fraga A, et al: Kidney transplantation: the use of abnormal kidneys. *Nephron* 35:78–81, 1983.
58. Waltzer WC, Engen DE, Stanson A, Sterioff S, Zincke H: Use of radiographically abnormal kidneys in living-related donor renal transplantation. *Nephron* 39:302–305, 1985.
59. Eklund B, Eklund P, Lindfors O, Lindstrom BL: Living donor nephrectomy: surgical aspects. *Scand J Urol Nephrol* 64(Suppl):157–161, 1981.
60. Ratner LE, Kavoussi LR, Sroka M, et al: Laparoscopic assisted live donor nephrectomy—a comparison with the open approach. *Transplantation* 63(2):229–233, 1997.
61. Flowers JL, Jacobs SC, Bartlett ST, et al: Comparison of laparoscopic and open live donor nephrectomy. Presented at the American Surgical Association 117th Annual Meeting, April, 1997.

5

Anesthetic Management in Kidney Transplantation

Yoogoo Kang

The anesthetic care of patients undergoing kidney transplantation remains a challenge for anesthesiologists because of the pathophysiologic changes that occur with end-stage renal disease (ESRD) and the presence of coexisting systemic diseases. In addition, there is the need to optimize the physiologic environment for the newly transplanted kidney. The role of the anesthesiologist is thus crucial to the success of the transplant procedure.

▲ PREPARATION FOR THE OPERATION

Because of the general availability of dialysis, patients are usually admitted for transplantation in fairly reasonable condition, and any further interventions to enable the patient to go to the operating room are usually handled by the surgeon and the nephrologist. Immediate preoperative consultation by the anesthesiologist is important, however, so that other medical problems can be evaluated, and any additions to or modifications of anesthetic management can be planned.

As premedication, sodium citrate (30 mL) may be administered to reduce the degree of potential aspiration pneumonitis. Midazolam (0.05–0.1 mg/kg, IM) is given for sedation, and atropine (20 μg/kg, up to 2 mg) is administered for vagolytic action.

▲ INTRAOPERATIVE MONITORING

Intraoperative monitoring is similar to that for patients undergoing any major operation. A five-lead electrocardiogram is placed: lead II shows conduction abnormalities and the precordial lead is used to identify ischemic episodes. A noninvasive blood pressure monitor is used in patients who have no complications, and a radial intraarterial catheter is used for patients with cardiopulmonary dysfunction. Gas exchange is monitored by percutaneous pulse oximetry and capnography or mass spectrometry. Monitoring of central venous pressure (CVP) is a common practice for the precise titration of intravascular volume. A pulmonary artery catheter may be used for patients with cardiovascular dysfunction, because pressure from the right side of the heart may not reflect that of the left side, and determination of cardiac output is helpful in choosing an appropriate treatment mode. For patients with severe cardiovascular dysfunction, a two-dimensional transesophageal echocardiogram may be used to identify preload, wall motion abnormality, pericardial effusion, and valvular dysfunction. A neuromuscular blockade monitor is essential for the titration of muscle relaxants, and body temperature is monitored. The availability of a stat laboratory is mandatory to determine arterial blood gas tensions and acid-base state, hematocrit, and serum levels of electrolytes and glucose. A large-bore intravenous catheter is secured for administration of drugs and fluids. The arteriovenous fistula is protected during the operation: a heating pad is applied, and intravenous and intra-arterial catheters are placed in the contralateral extremity.

▲ ANESTHETIC MANAGEMENT

All major anesthetic techniques can be used for kidney transplantation. The type of anesthesia selected depends on the physiologic condition of the patient and the preference of the anesthesiologist and surgeon. Regional anesthesia (spinal and epidural) has been used successfully[1,2] and has the advantage of avoiding central nervous system depressants and muscle relaxants. Epidural anesthesia is preferred to spinal anesthesia because the sympathetic blockade is less dramatic, the duration of anesthesia can be tailored, and postoperative narcotic analgesia can be combined. However, coagulopathy may rule out the epidural technique because of the risk of epidural hematoma. With general anesthesia, on the other hand, the physiologic state of the patient is easily controllable, particularly for patients with moderate to severe systemic diseases.[3,4]

For *epidural anesthesia,* an epidural catheter is inserted via a Tuohy needle at the L3–4 level. A local anesthetic (commonly 15–20 mL of bupivacaine 0.5%) is administered via the catheter to achieve the sensory level of T6-8. An adequate anesthesia level is maintained by adding one half to two thirds of the original dose about every 2 hours or when the sensory level begins to recede. Hypotension associated with sympathetic blockade should be prevented by the administration of fluids and managed with ephedrine sulfate (5–10 mg increments). Oxygen is supplemented, and it is helpful to reduce anxiety and discomfort with narcotics (fentanyl, 25–50 μg increments) and sedatives (midazolam, 1–2 mg increments). Toward the end of the operation, narcotics (commonly 4–5 mg of preservative-free morphine) are administered through the catheter to provide postoperative analgesia.

General anesthesia begins with preoxygenation. Anesthesia is commonly induced with thiopental (4–6 mg/kg) or etomidate (0.2–0.6 mg/kg) and narcotics (fentanyl, 2–5 μg/kg). The pharmacodynamics of thiopental are similar to those in patients without renal disease. More free drug is available, but the half-life of the drug is close to normal because of increased volume of distribution and clearance.

Endotracheal intubation is facilitated with the use of a depolarizing agent (succinylcholine, 1–2 mg/kg) after a small dose of d-tubocurarine (3 mg) or pancuronium bromide (1 mg) to prevent muscle fasciculation. For patients with a high-normal serum potassium level, a nondepolarizing muscle relaxant (vecuronium, 0.015 mg/kg [priming dose] followed by 0.08 mg/kg) is chosen because muscle fasciculation caused by the depolarizing agent increases the serum potassium level. When a full stomach is a concern, the airway is secured by awake intubation or rapid-sequence induction with cricoid pressure to avoid aspiration pneumonitis. For patients with a difficult airway, awake intubation is preferred.

Anesthesia is frequently maintained with a combination of inhalation and intravenous anesthetics. For inhalation agents, isoflurane is the agent of choice, because it is associated with less myocardial depression, biodegradation, nephrotoxicity, and hepatotoxicity than other agents. Enflurane increases the inorganic fluoride level in the kidney in a dose-dependent manner, and may induce nephropathy in the presence of renal insufficiency. Halothane may be hepatotoxic in the presence of hepatic ischemia or dysfunction. Nitrous oxide may be used, but it may depress the myocardium, distend intestinal loops, and depress the bone marrow. Fentanyl, sufentanil, and alfentanil are commonly used because of their short half-life and ease of titration in patients with limited renal function.

Although complete muscle relaxation is not necessary when the kidney is placed extraperitoneally in the right or left lower quadrant, some muscle relaxation is needed to facilitate the operation. In general, muscle relaxants with the least dependence on renal function for metabolism and excretion are chosen. The dose of muscle relaxant is carefully titrated to avoid prolonged weakness or paralysis after the operation. Most of these agents and their metabolites are eliminated by the kidney.

Succinylcholine, a depolarizing agent used primarily for endotracheal intubation, is quickly metabolized by plasma pseudocholinesterase, although the enzyme level is about half of normal in patients with ESRD. However, succinylmonocholine, the metabolite of succinylcholine with 5% of the potency of the parent drug, is excreted by the kidney and may produce prolonged muscle relaxation.[5] Succinylcholine increases the serum potassium level (0.2–0.5 mmol/L)[6] even when fasciculation is prevented by d-tubocurarine. Succinylcholine may induce arrhythmias because of its hyperkalemic effects and stimulation of nicotinic receptors of sympathetic and parasympathetic ganglia and muscarinic receptors in the sinus node.

d-Tubocurarine and pancuronium bromide are commonly used for muscle relaxation because they are less dependent on renal function compared with other drugs. d-Tubocurarine may decrease the blood pressure by releasing histamine, and pancuronium bromide may increase the heart rate by its vagolytic action.

Vecuronium is a new nondepolarizing muscle relaxant. A large portion of vecuronium (80%) is absorbed by the liver and excreted in bile. The onset, duration, and recovery time after a single vecuronium injection in patients with ESRD are similar to those in healthy people.[7] However, a repeated dose of vecuronium can interfere with recovery from muscle relaxation.

Atracurium, a curare-like molecule, is a short-acting muscle relaxant that is eliminated by Hofmann elimination reaction and ester hydrolysis.[8] Atracurium does not have a cumulative effect, and the prolonged duration of action and recovery time in patients with ESRD are not clinically significant.[9] Atracurium does decrease blood pressure and increase heart rate by releasing histamine. The metabolite of atracurium, laudanosine, is excreted by the kidney and may accumulate in patients with renal disease. Laudanosine can cause seizures in animals, but a toxic level is unlikely to be reached even in anephric patients.[10]

▲ MAINTENANCE OF THE PHYSIOLOGIC STATE

Intraoperative care of the recipient is focused on prevention of complications from underlying systemic diseases and maintenance of optimal perfusion of the grafted kidney. Normal ventilation is used because renal perfusion and glomerular filtration decrease with hypercarbia and hypocarbia.[11,12] Low intravascular volume caused by dialysis is corrected by administration of half normal saline solution on the basis of CVP and other hemodynamic variables to optimize cardiac output and tissue perfusion. Additional fluid is given to replace third-space losses (3–7 mL/kg per/hour). Blood glucose level is monitored for diabetic patients, and either additional glucose in the form of a 5% solution or regular insulin may be necessary to maintain a blood glucose level of 100–200 mg/dL[13] (5.55–11.1 mmol/L). Transfusion of packed red blood cells may be necessary to maintain the hematocrit above 25 mg/dL.

Hypertension is not usually a major concern with anesthesia. However, mild to moderate hypertension is corrected with hydralazine (5-mg increments). Severe hypertension is treated with an infusion of sodium nitroprusside. Thiocyanate, a metabolite of sodium nitroprusside, is excreted by the kidneys, but its toxic effects do not appear to be a clinical problem; in addition, it is readily dialyzable.[14] Hypertension with myocardial ischemia is treated with an infusion of nitroglycerin.

During vascular anastomosis of the renal vessels, preparation is made for reperfusion of the grafted kidney. Patients with a relatively high preload appear to have a better graft outcome with a reduction in the incidence of delayed graft function from 36% to 6%.[15–17] Many other factors, however, enter into this issue, prolonged cold ischemia time being perhaps one of the most important. Increasing the systolic blood pressure to 140 mm Hg appears to be beneficial for the grafted kidney. In some centers, preload is increased to a CVP of 15–17 cm H_2O with crystalloid and, if necessary, hetastarch, albumin, or packed red blood cells. If systolic blood pressure remains low, dopamine (up to 5 μg/kg/min) is administered to increase cardiac contractility and renal perfusion. Dopamine improves graft function after transplantation in animal models, although its beneficial role in clinical kidney transplantation is controversial. It is agreed that dopamine may improve renal function in patients with hypotension or a less than perfect donor kidney. Furosemide (1 mg/kg) can be administered during and after the performance of the vascular anastomoses. Furosemide appears to be protective against acute tubular necrosis by maintaining the renal blood flow and oxygen consumption ratio of the medulla through oxidation of cytochrome a_3. Mannitol (1 g/kg) is given to decrease the incidence of delayed graft function[18] because it increases renal blood flow to a greater degree than changes in plasma volume, cardiac output, and systemic vascular resistance.

Various hemodynamic changes may be seen on reperfusion of the grafted kidney. Hyperkalemia can be caused by the residual hyperkalemic preservation solution that enters the systemic circulation, although this is not usually significant clinically.[19] Symptomatic hyperkalemia, with tall, peaked T waves and ventricular conduction defects on an electrocardiogram, is treated with $CaCl_2$ (300–500 mg) and $NaHCO_3$ (40 mmol). Hypertension may occur when renin is released from the graft, and hypotension may occur with a sudden decrease in preload after unclamping of the iliac artery. Mild to moderate acidosis may be seen with the release of acidic substances from the kidney and the lower extremity. Once the kidney begins to function, CVP gradually decreases to the normal range with diuresis and a decrease in vascular resistance.[20] Urine output is replaced with half-normal saline solution, and electrolyte balance should be maintained in patients with extreme diuresis (>300 mL/h). Intraoperative bleeding is not usually a concern, although two units of packed red blood cells are always available.

At the end of the procedure, the patient is allowed to recover from inhalational anesthesia by ventilation and from intravenous agents by hepatic metabolism. The residual effect of the muscle relaxant is reversed with the combination of an anticholinergic agent (atropine sulfate [15–20 μg/kg]) or glycopyrrolate (10–15 mg) and a reversal agent (edrophonium (0.2–0.4 mg/kg), neostigmine (40–45 μg/kg), or pyridostigmine (0.1–0.16 mg/kg). The patient is extubated and allowed to recover in the postanesthesia care unit with supplemental oxygen. Postoperative analgesia is provided by careful titration of narcotics (fentanyl or morphine).

Hypertension is the most common complication in the immediate postoperative period and is managed initially with calcium channel blockers (nifedipine, 10 mg sublingually); if necessary, vasodilators such as hydralazine and nitroprusside may be required to prevent adverse effects on the graft and the recipient (see Chapter 7).[21] β-Adrenergic blockers (labetalol, esmolol) may be used to treat hypertension and tachycardia, but their use is limited because of their hyperkalemic effect. Other serious cardiovascular complications that may occur in the early postoperative period include arrhythmia in 5–10% of patients, myocardial infarction in 0.5%, and cardiac death in as many as 1% of patients.[21]

▲ REFERENCES

1. Vandam LD, Harrison JH, Murray JE: Anesthetic aspects of renal homotransplantation in man. *Anesthesiology* 23:783–792, 1962.
2. Linke CL, Merin RG: A regional anesthetic approach for renal transplantation. *Anesth Analg* 55:69–73, 1976.
3. Heino A, Orko R, Rosenberg PH: Anaesthesiological complications in renal transplantation: a retrospective study of 500 transplantations. *Acta Anaesthesiol Scand* 30:574–580, 1986.
4. Graybar GB: Choice of anesthesia. In: Graybar GB, Bready LL (eds), *Anesthesia for Renal Transplantation.* Boston, Martinus Nijhoff, 1987:139–155.
5. Bishop MJ, Hornbien TF: Prolonged effect of succinylcholine after neostigmine and pyridostigmine administration in patients with renal failure. *Anesthesiology* 58:384–386, 1983.
6. Koide M, Waud BE: Serum potassium concentrations after succinylcholine in patients with renal failure. *Anesthesiology* 36:142–145, 1972.
7. Fahey MR, Morris RB, Miller RD, Nguyen TL, Upton RA: Pharmacokinetics of Org NC45 (norcuron) in patients with and without renal failure. *Br J Anaesth* 53:1049–1053, 1981.
8. Nigrovic V, Auen M, Wajskol A: Enzymatic hydrolysis of atracurium *in vivo. Anesthesiology* 62:606–609, 1985.
9. Hunter JM, Jones RS, Utting JE: Use of atracurium in patients with no renal function. *Br J Anaesth* 54:1251–1258, 1982.
10. Ingram MD, Scalabassi RJ, Cook DR, Stiller RL, Bennett MH: Cardiovascular and electroencephalographic effects of laudanosine in "nephrectomized" cats. *Br J Anaesth* 58(Suppl 1): 14S–18S, 1986.
11. Dhabuwala CB, Bird M, Salaman JR: Relative importance of warm ischemia, hypotension, and hypercarbia in producing renal vasospasm. *Transplantation* 27:238–241, 1979.
12. Hunter JM, Jones RS, Utting JE: Effect of acute hypocapnoea on renal function in the dog artificially ventilated with nitrous oxide, oxygen and halothane. *Br J Anaesth* 52:197–198, 1980.
13. Drexler AJ: Management of the diabetic patient during surgery. In: Bergmann M (ed), *Principles of Diabetic Management.* New York, Medical Examination, 1987;337–341.
14. Tinker JH, Michenfelder JD: Increased resistance to nitroprusside-induced cyanide toxicity in anuric dogs. *Anesthesiology* 52:40–47, 1980.
15. Diethelm AG, Aldrete JS, Sterling WA, Morgan JM: Large volume diuresis as a mechanism for immediate maximum renal function after transplantation: advantage of fluid load under pulmonary arterial pressure monitoring during surgical period. *Surg Gynecol Obstet* 138:869–874, 1974.
16. Luciani J, Frantz P, Thibault P, et al: Early anuria prevention in human kidney transplantation. *Transplantation* 28:308–312, 1979.
17. Carlier M, Squifflet JP, Pirson Y, Gribomont B, Alexandre GP: Maximal hydration during anesthesia increases pulmonary artery pressures and improves early function of human renal transplants. *Transplantation* 34:201–204, 1982.
18. Weimar W, Geerlings W, Bijnen AB, et al: A controlled study on the effect of mannitol on immediate renal function after cadaver donor kidney transplantation. *Transplantation* 35:99–101, 1983.

19. Hirshman CA, Leon D, Edelstein G, et al: Risk of hyperkalemia in recipients of kidneys preserved with an intracellular electrolyte solution. *Anesth Analg* 59:283–286, 1980.
20. Freilich JD, Waterman PM, Rosenthal JT: Acute hemodynamic changes during renal transplantation. *Anesth Analg* 63:158–160, 1984.
21. Marsland AT, Bradley JP: Anaesthesia for renal transplantation: 5 years' experience. *Anaesth Intensive Care* 11:337–344, 1983.

6

The Transplant Procedure

Ron Shapiro

This chapter discusses the technical details related to the actual performance of a kidney transplant. The first part deals with the immediate preoperative evaluation of the recipient. The bulk of the chapter focuses on the back table preparation and implantation of the kidney. It describes both routine and the less straightforward procedures. In addition, the principles of intraoperative management are discussed.

An uncomplicated kidney transplantation is not a difficult operation to perform; it is, however, unforgiving of technical error. The range of anatomic variability in both donor organs and recipients is sufficiently great that flexibility is required on the part of the surgeon. Most difficulties in renal transplantation can be ascribed to nonsurgical considerations, but this is true only when the achievement of technical perfection has become routine.

▲ THE IMMEDIATE PREOPERATIVE PERIOD

After a recipient has been chosen for a given kidney (see Chapter 3), the patient's nephrologist is called to make sure that there are no acute medical problems that would contraindicate transplantation. The recipient is then called and brought into the hospital.

After being admitted, the patient is seen by the surgeon, nephrologist, and anesthesiologist. Blood is drawn and sent for routine chemistry and hematologic studies. In the absence of other medical problems, the main determinants of whether the patient can go directly to the operating room are the serum potassium level and volume status of the recipient[1–4] and the need for a repeat cross match.[2,5,6]

A potassium level is obtainable within minutes from an intensive care unit (ICU) laboratory. A level of 5.0 mmol/L or less is acceptable; a level greater than 6.0 mmol/L mandates preoperative dialysis.[2–4] A level between 5.0 and 6.0 mmol/L is sometimes treated with a potassium-binding resin enema (Kayexalate, 30–50 g),[1,3] but this can often be ineffective and time consuming and is not always worthwhile. It is perhaps more realistic to accept a level as high as 5.2–5.3 mmol/L and to perform dialysis routinely if the potassium level is higher.

Volume status can be determined by means of physical examination, although a chest radiograph is also obtained and reviewed.[5] Euvolemia and a normal potassium level allow a patient to proceed directly to the operating room.[2,4,5]

For a patient whose negative cross match is with a specimen less than 1 month old and who has not undergone a transfusion in the interim, a repeat cross match probably is unnecessary. However, some centers routinely draw a fresh blood sample for a repeat cross match.[5] Certainly, for a patient with a recent blood transfusion or a patient whose sample is more than 3 months old or who has a high panel reactive antibody (PRA) level, a repeat cross match should be performed. This imposes a 2 1/2–4 hour delay before transplantation can take place.

Preoperative assessment also allows the transplantation team to assess the patient's other medical problems, all of which presumably have been identified during the evaluation process. For patients considered at high cardiac risk, for example, plans may be made to monitor the patient intraoperatively with an arterial line and Swan-Ganz catheter and to take the patient to the ICU postoperatively for observation.

Once the preoperative assessment and interventions, if any, have been made, the patient can be sent to the operating room. Oral immunosuppression can be given with a sip of water; intravenous medications can be given in the operating room.

Back Table Preparation

Cadaveric kidneys are ordinarily recovered en bloc and then separated before being packaged and stored; in some centers, the organs are placed on a pump and perfused (see Chapters 1 and 4).[7–11] In any event, before transplantation, the excess fat, muscle, and connective tissue must be removed from the kidney, and the vessel branches not leading to or from the kidney must be ligated.[3,7] The cuff of the aorta and vena cava are then trimmed appropriately so that vessels can be anastomosed to the recipient vessels without difficulty. This back table preparation ordinarily is straightforward, but there are a variety of circumstances in which more complex reconstruction is necessary.[3,13]

A back table is set up in the operating room with a large shallow basin set on a sterile field. A 1-liter bag of sterile frozen saline solution is crushed with a mallet and placed in the basin. A large, clear, sterile bag is placed around the basin, and a sling is created on which to rest the kidney during dissection and repair (Fig. 6–1). Cold saline or lactated Ringer solution is poured into the basin.

In the case where a left kidney is used, the vessels are placed on slight tension with 4-0 silk sutures through their ends (Fig. 6–2). The left renal vein ordinarily has

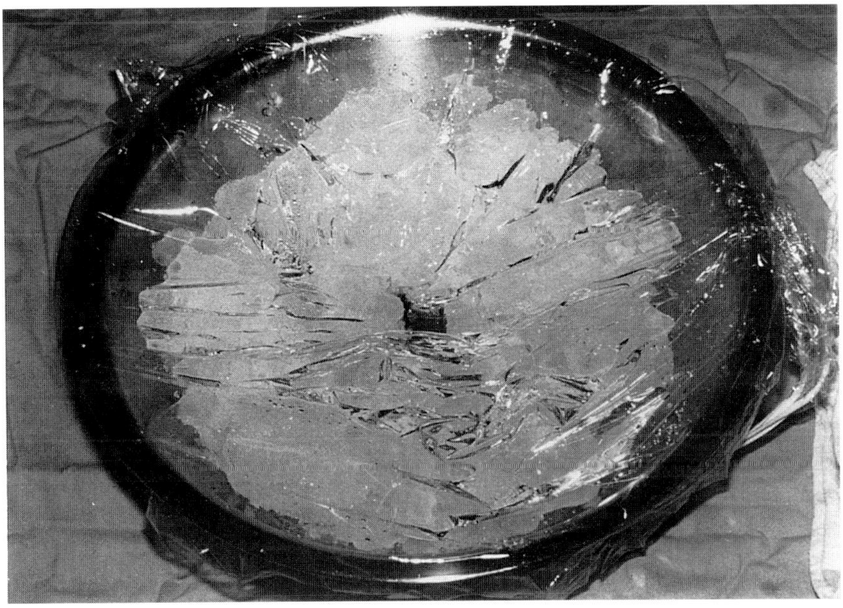

Figure 6–1. Back table basin.

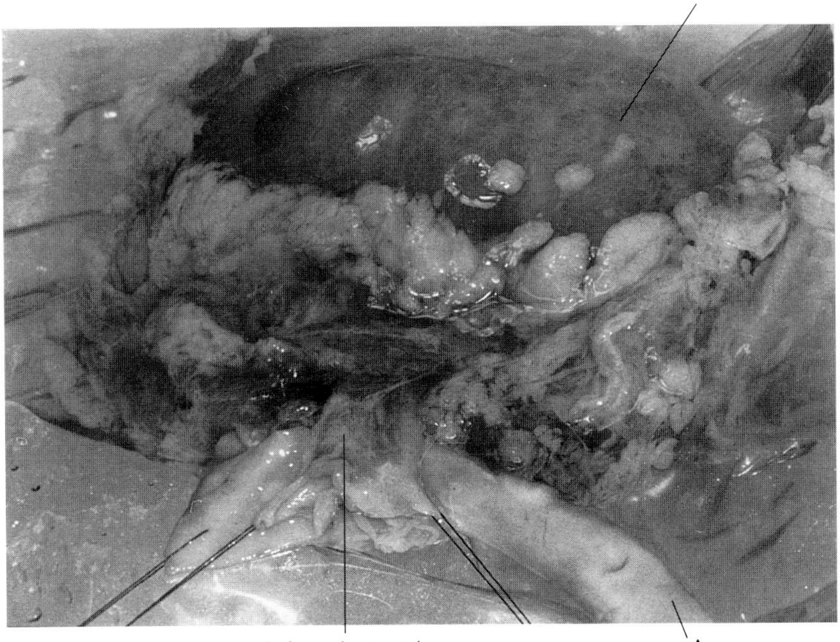

Figure 6–2. Back table preparation of kidney before dissection.

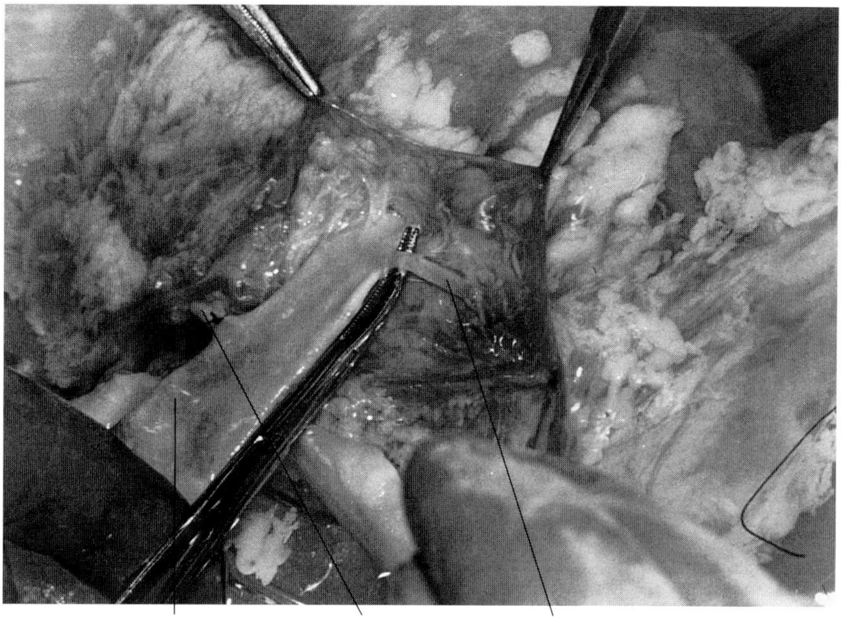

Figure 6–3. Ligation of renal vein branches.

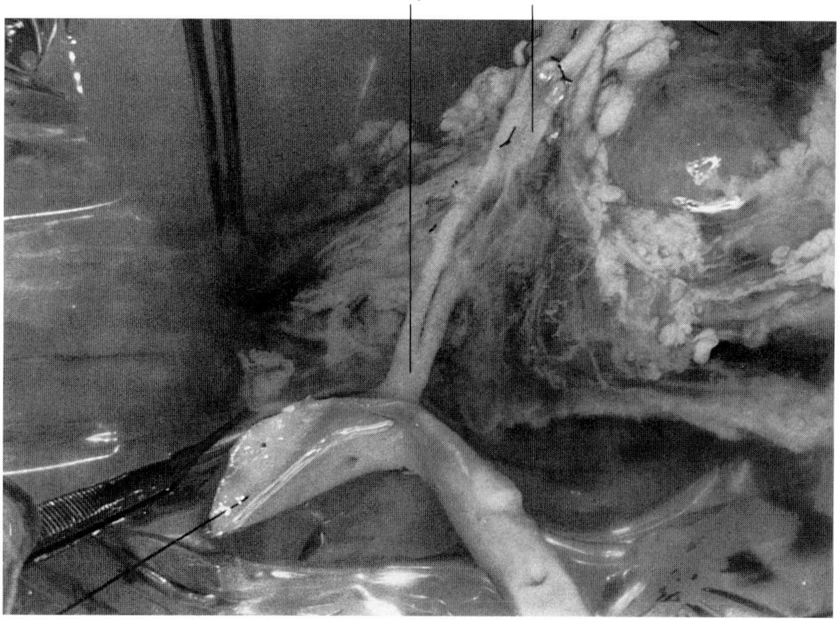

Figure 6–4. Dissection of renal artery.

three vein branches, the adrenal, gonadal, and lumbar (some anatomy books refer to the latter as the inferior phrenic);[14,15] these are ligated and divided with 4-0 silk ties (Fig. 6–3). The vein is dissected free from the surrounding connective tissue to a point close to its exit from the parenchyma. The artery is similarly dissected free, although branches are less common (Fig. 6–4). An adrenal branch, if present, may require ligation, but care needs to be taken to ensure that the branch does not supply the kidney. There is no collateral arterial supply in the kidney, whereas a rich collateral venous supply is almost always present.[16]

Once the vessels have been mobilized, the perinephric fat and adrenal gland are removed (Fig. 6–5). Some surgeons prefer to ligate the fat in the hilum to prevent bleeding. Care is taken not to strip the ureter of its blood supply. Finally, the excess vena cava and aorta are trimmed off to leave a small cuff for anastomosis to the recipient vessels (Fig. 6–6).

When the right kidney is used, there tends to be a discrepancy between the length of the short renal vein and of the long artery,[14,15] which can lead to kinking of the latter. The use of the donor vena cava to extend the vein or an iliac vein graft from the same donor (or another ABO-compatible donor) can correct this potential problem[16] (Fig. 6–7). Many surgeons do not consider this necessary.

Anatomic variations are common, and repair or reconstruction often is necessary. Two or more renal arteries can supply a kidney.[14] Generally they both originate from the aorta, but it is possible to have a lower-pole branch that originates from the

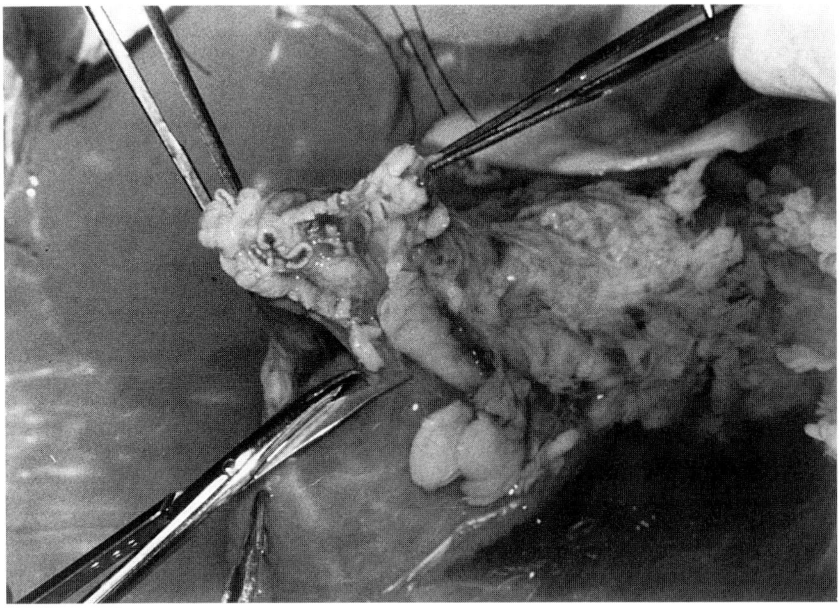

Figure 6–5. Removal of perinephric fat.

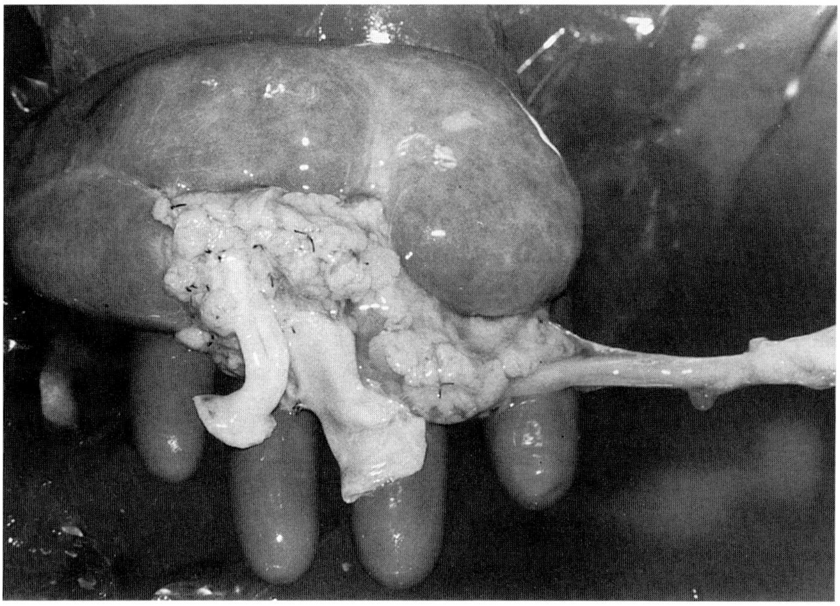

Figure 6–6. Left kidney after completion of back table dissection.

common iliac artery.[14] Arterial branches cannot be sacrificed, and the goal is to devise a solution that enables straightforward implantation. When there are multiple arteries on one continuous patch of aorta, it is a simple matter to retain a long cuff that allows direct anastomosis[3,17] (Fig. 6–8). At times, there may be a considerable gap between vessels, and two separate arterial anastomoses are required (Fig. 6–9). Another way of handling this problem, if the vessels are long enough, is to cut out the intervening segment of aorta and anastomose the vessels closer to each other, to create a shorter, single aortic cuff (Fig. 6–10).

Arterial injuries during organ recovery can be corrected by back table reconstruction.[3,13] Partial transections often can be repaired primarily (Fig. 6–11). If the artery has been completely transected, and the proximal artery and aortic cuff are available, end-to-end anastomosis can be performed (Fig. 6–12). Sometimes this is not possible, and end-to-side anastomosis to the main renal artery is required (Fig. 6–13). In the case of a short stump of artery or multiple injuries (Fig. 6–14), the branches can be implanted separately, partially anastomosed to form a single channel (Fig. 6–15),[31] or reconstructed with an iliac arterial graft from the same donor (or an ABO-compatible donor) (Fig. 6–16).[13] These reconstructions are not difficult but usually require magnification with loupes and the use of 7-0 or 8-0 suture material.

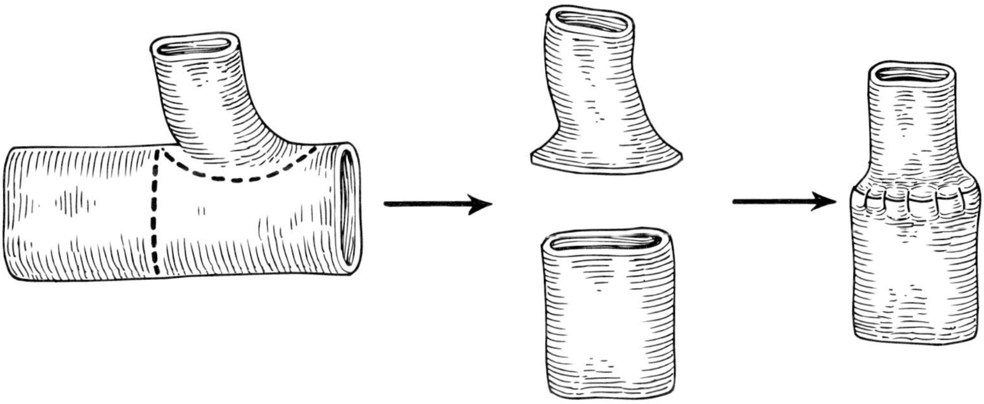

A

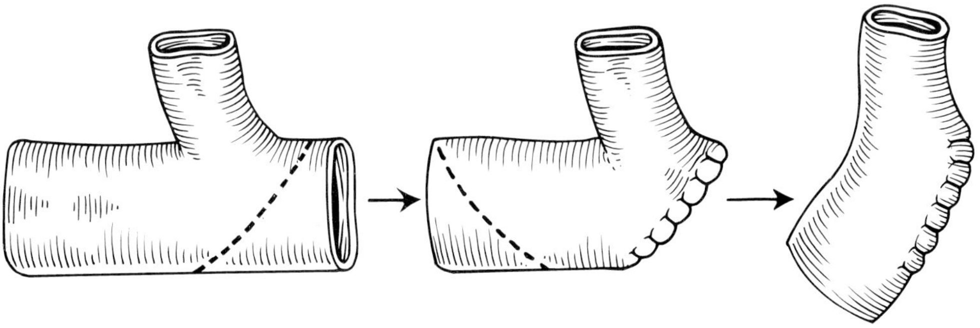

B

Figure 6–7. A,B. Lengthening the right renal vein with donor vena cava.

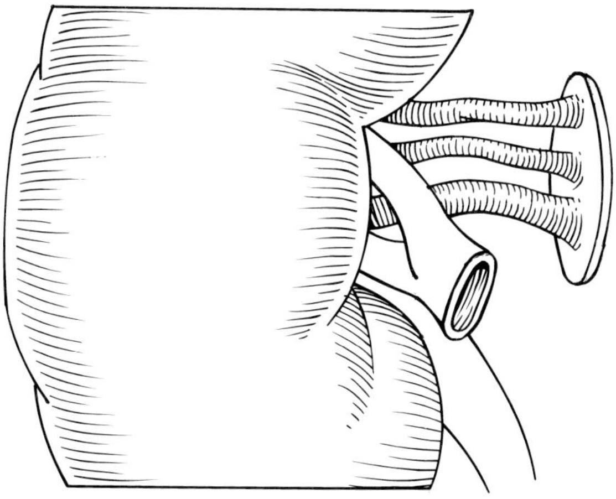

Figure 6–8. Multiple renal arteries on a single cuff of aorta.

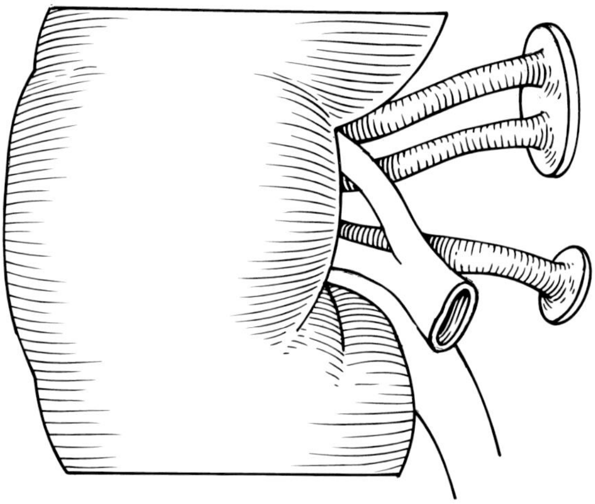

Figure 6–9. Multiple renal arteries on two separate cuffs of aorta.

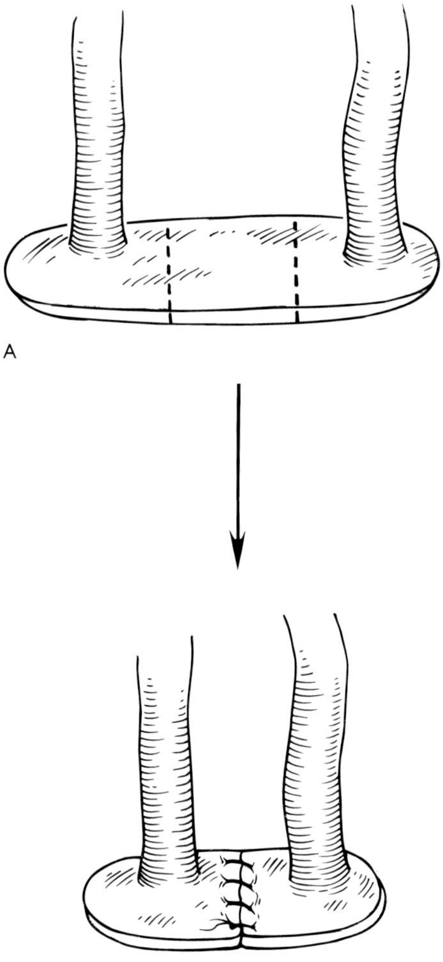

Figure 6–10. A,B. Multiple renal arteries. Construction of single aortic cuff after removal of excess intervening aorta.

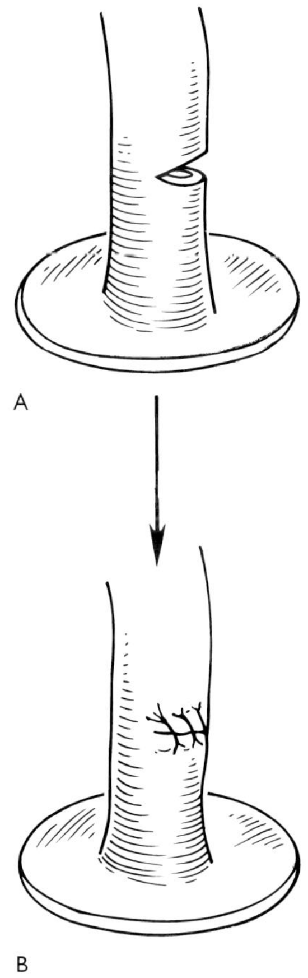

Figure 6–11. A,B. Partial transection and repair of renal artery.

The Vein

The venous system is forgiving in that vein branches can be ligated without serious consequence, as long as the dominant vein is intact.[18] The techniques described to increase the length of the right renal vein can be applied to any short vein. Transection of a vein can be repaired primarily if it is partial (Fig. 6–17); if it is complete, reconstruction with a vein graft can be performed if the remaining stump is too short (Fig. 6–18).

All end-to-end reconstructions, unless they involve an anastomosis of cuffs of larger vessels, are at risk for narrowing because of a pursestring effect. A "growth factor," which involves tying the vascular sutures loosely with up to a one-half diameter excess after completion of the anastomosis, diminishes the likelihood of stenosis but does not result in bleeding if performed correctly (the excess suture material is incorporated into the suture line)[19] (Fig. 6–19). It should only be performed with monofilament suture that will slide, such as polypropylene. (Polybutester, in contrast, does not slide, and a growth factor should not be used with it.)

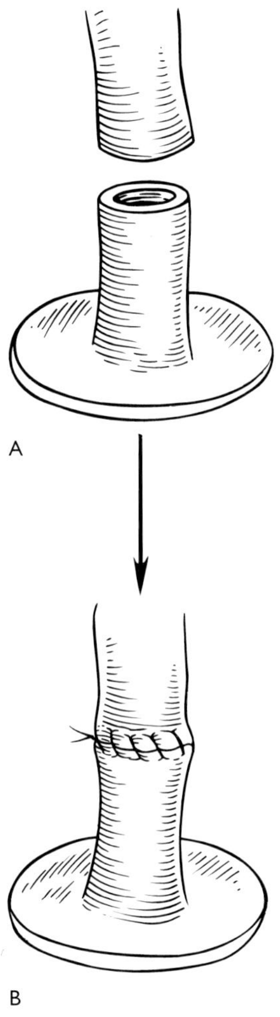

Figure 6–12. A,B. Complete transection and repair of renal artery.

The Ureter

In general, the ureter requires little attention on the back table. Whereas vessels are carefully dissected free of the surrounding connective tissue, it is preferable to manipulate the ureter as little as possible. The ureteral blood supply comes from three sources in life—the kidney, the bladder, and small iliac or gonadal branches.[14,15] The transplanted ureter has only one residual blood supply from the kidney. Excessively close dissection of the ureter may lead to ureteral necrosis after transplantation. Thus the periureteral vessels and fat are best left alone, although the adjacent gonadal vessels can and should be removed.

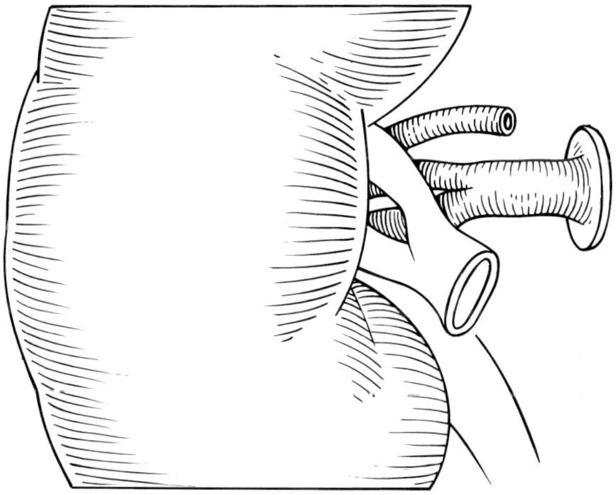

A

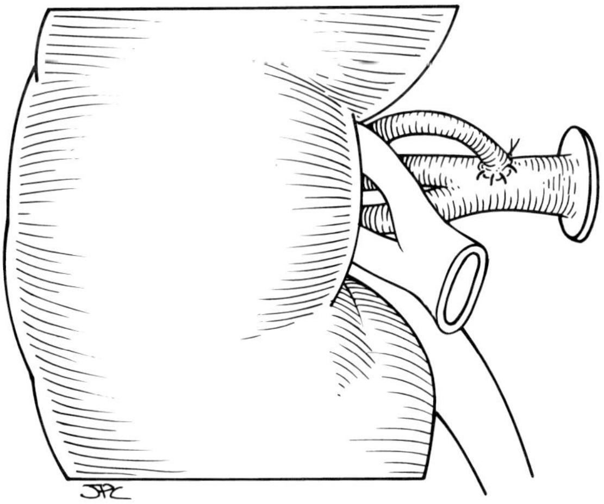

B

Figure 6–13. A,B. Transected polar artery and implantation into main renal artery.

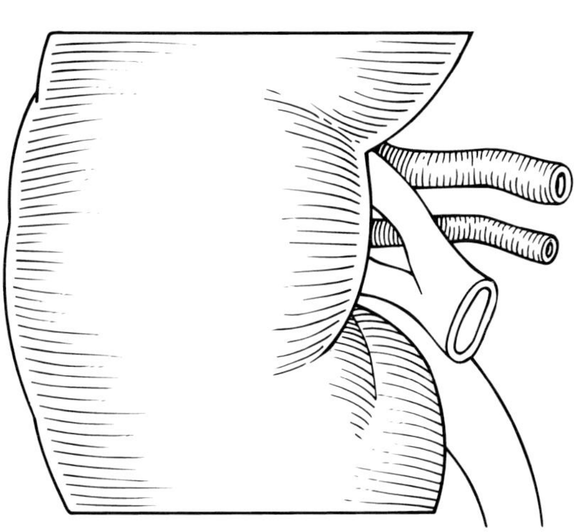

Figure 6–14. Multiple transected renal arteries.

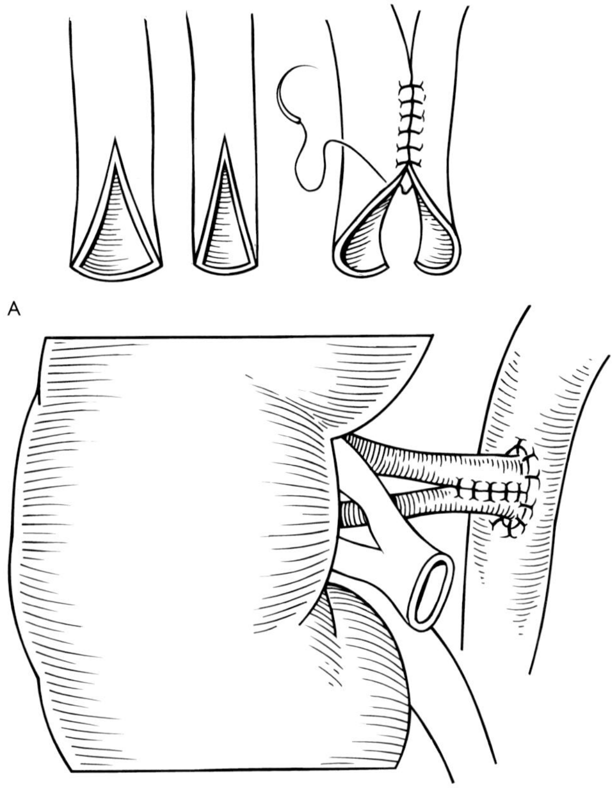

A

B

Figure 6–15. A,B. Reconstruction by means of formation of a single channel.

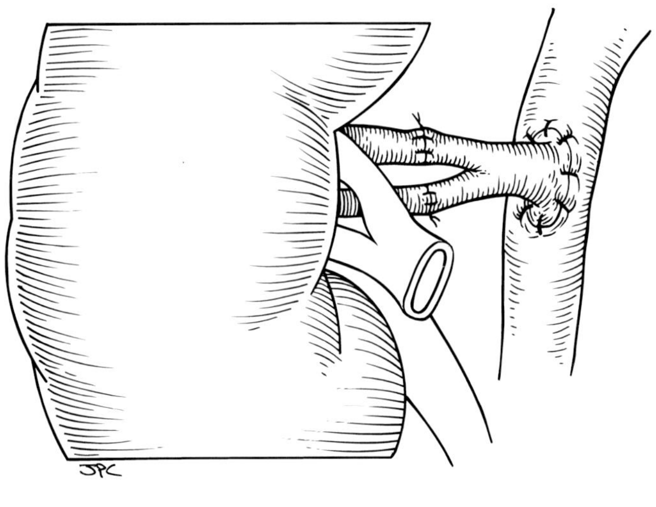

Figure 6–16. Reconstruction with an iliac arterial graft.

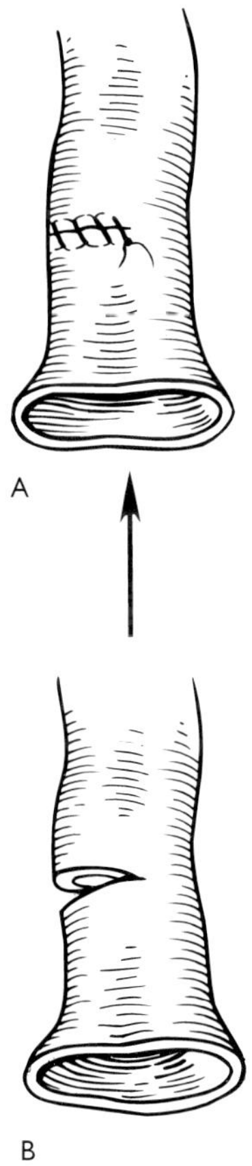

Figure 6–17. A,B. Partial transection and repair of renal vein.

Some authors argue against ureteral dissection above the lower pole of the kidney. However, unless there is a lower-pole artery, there is not a blood supply other than that coming from the hilum. Mobilizing the ureter from the lower pole of the kidney for a short distance, perhaps 2 cm, does not harm the ureter and may simplify the ureteroneocystostomy.

Ureteral anomalies include double ureters and ureters with ureteropelvic junction obstruction.[15] The latter may not have been of functional significance in the life of the donor but may be important as a single kidney in a transplant patient. There is little to be done on the back table about these variations, and they are discussed in more detail in the section on implantation.

Pediatric Donors

From the point of view of back table preparation, kidneys from pediatric donors older than 4–5 years can be handled in a manner similar to that of kidneys from adult donors. Some authors claim that all kidneys from pediatric donors can be handled

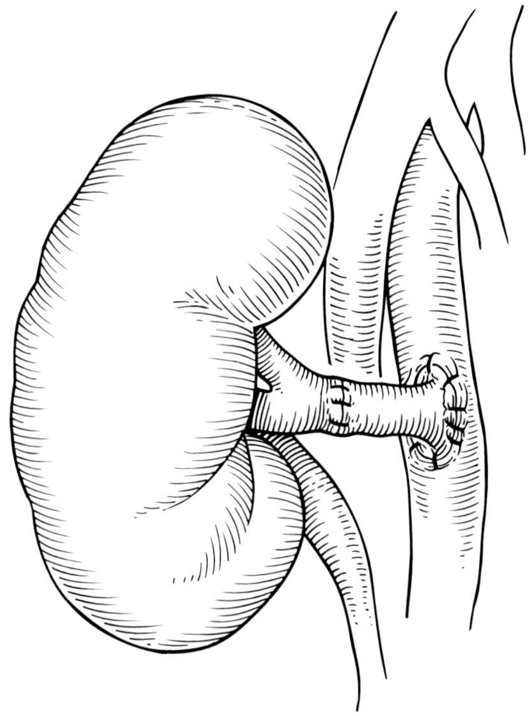

Figure 6–18. Reconstruction of a transected vein with an iliac vein graft.

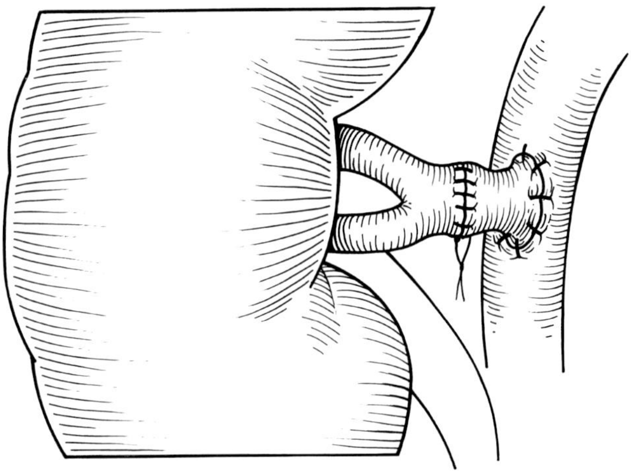

Figure 6–19. Use of a "growth factor" to prevent stenosis after reconstruction with a vein or artery graft.

the same way, although modification of the ureteral reimplantation may be required.[20] However, in the case of donors 3 years of age and younger, there has been considerable experience with the transplantation of both kidneys into a single (usually adult) recipient.[21–26] Whether transplanted singly or en bloc, there is a higher technical complication rate than with adult kidneys. On the other hand, once an individual surgeon has learned how to prepare these kidneys and transplant them safely, the results can be quite acceptable.

The back table preparation of en bloc pediatric kidneys is not difficult but requires attention to detail.[3] The kidneys are placed in the back table basin facing anteriorly (Fig. 6–20). The proximal and distal aorta and inferior vena cava are transfixed with 4-0 silk sutures. The tips of the ureters are clamped with fine tip mosquito clamps. Lumbar and gonadal vein branches entering the inferior vena cava are dissected free and ligated with 4-0 silk ties (Fig. 6–21). The right and left renal vein are then dissected free, with appropriate branch ligation (Fig. 6–22). Lumbar, gonadal, and various unnamed arteries that originate from the aorta are ligated, and the renal arteries are dissected free. The kidneys are then flipped over. Enough dissection will have been done that the excess connective tissue and muscle can be safely divided. This tissue can be dissected off each kidney, as can the perinephric fat. As with adult kidneys, ligation of the remaining fat in the hilum is important to minimize bleeding. The kidneys are flipped over again, so that they are once again anterior, and the re-

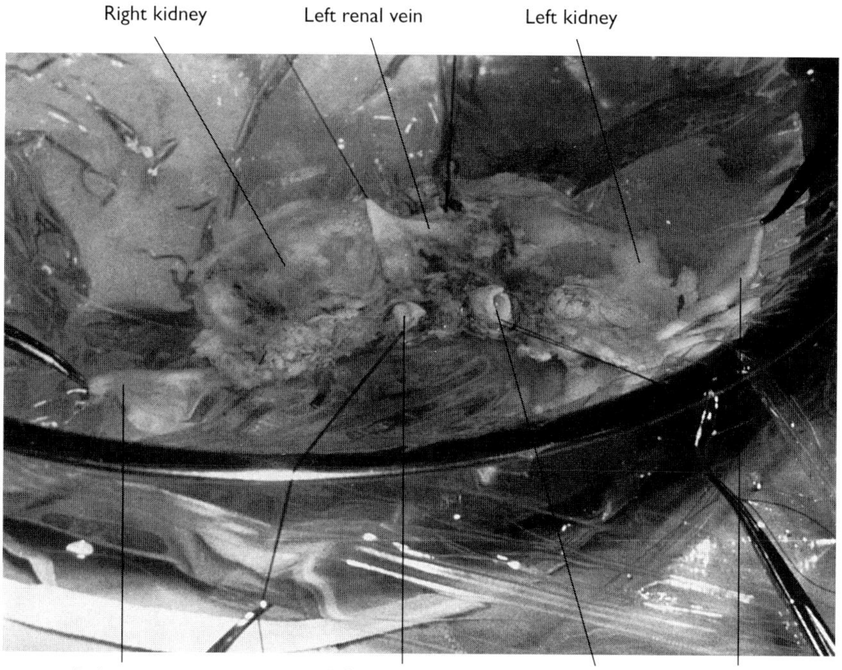

Figure 6–20. Pediatric en bloc kidneys from an 18-month-old donor.

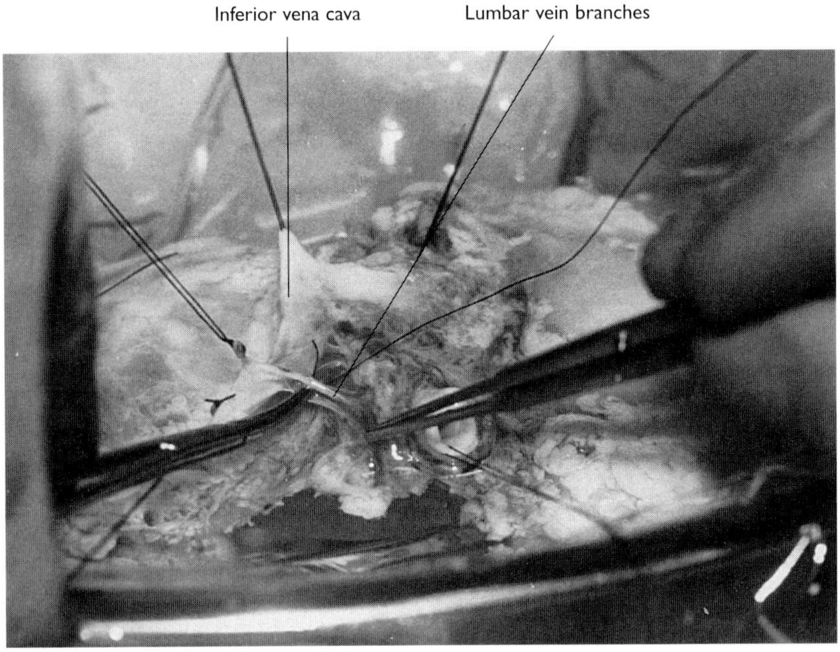

Figure 6–21. Pediatric en bloc kidneys, back table preparation. Ligation of lumbar vein branches of the donor inferior vena cava.

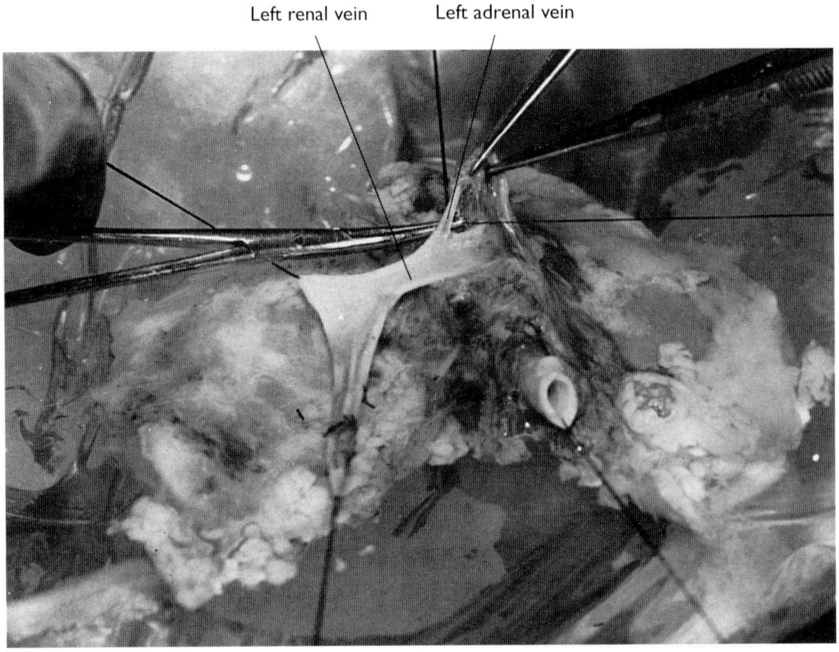

Figure 6–22. Pediatric en bloc kidneys, back table preparation. Ligation of left adrenal vein.

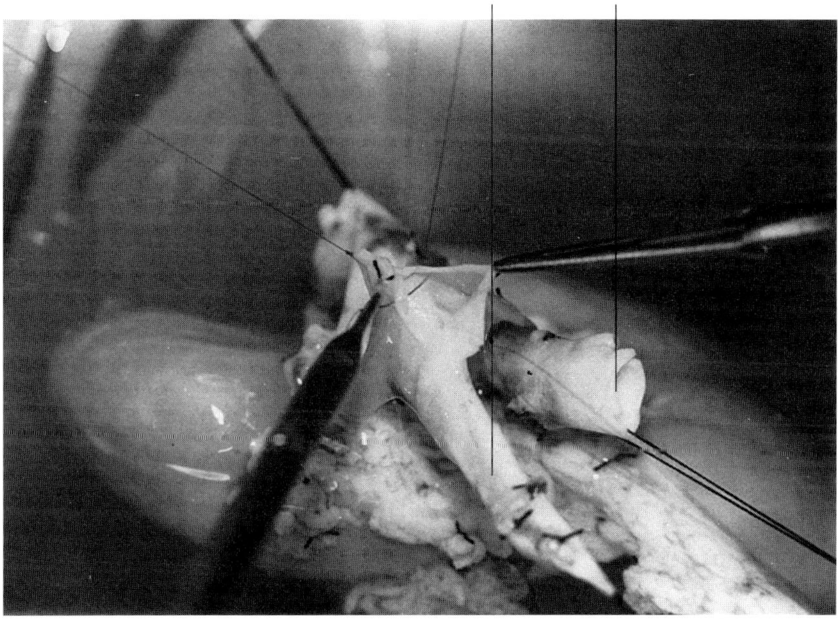

Figure 6–23. Pediatric en bloc kidneys, back table preparation. Closure of suprarenal inferior vena cava.

maining excess tissue is dissected free. Finally, the superior aspects of the inferior vena cava and aorta are closed, usually with running 6-0 polypropylene suture (Fig. 6–23). An anterior-posterior closure may be less likely to compromise the vessel openings if the margin of vessel is small (Fig. 6–24). The inferior aspects of the inferior vena cava and aorta are then appropriately trimmed; care is taken to remove a minimum amount of vessel (Fig. 6–25).

Iatrogenic injuries to en bloc kidneys during organ recovery may render them unusable, but certain injuries can be repaired or reconstructed. If there is insufficient superior inferior vena cava or aorta to close the vessels without compromising the vessel lumens, a cap of ABO compatible (or donor, if available) vessel may be sutured circumferentially (Fig. 6–26). Transected vessels can be reimplanted into the inferior vena cava or aorta, if the length of vessel lost is not excessive (8-0 polypropylene or polybutester is probably the best suture material in this situation).[27] The aorta and inferior vena cava may be too short, and vein and arterial graft extensions may be required. If, however, the main vessels are even 2–3 cm long, that should be sufficient.

Ureteral ischemia is, surprisingly, not a common problem, but insufficient length, particularly of the left ureter, may render the kidneys unusable. When en bloc kidneys are transplanted into the right iliac fossa, the left ureter has the longest reach to the bladder.

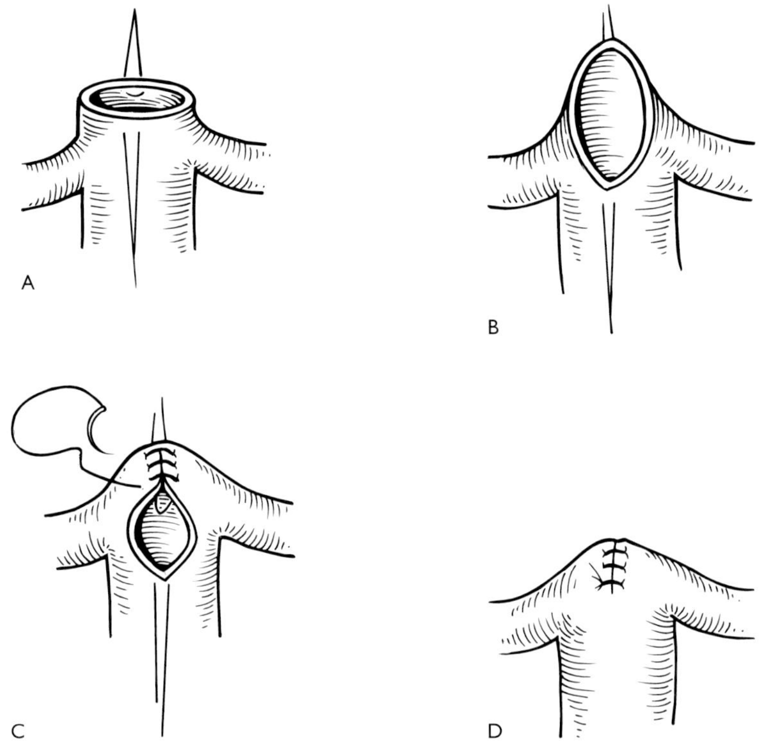

Figure 6–24. A–D. Pediatric en bloc kidneys, back table preparation. Anterior-posterior closure of suprarenal inferior vena cava or aorta.

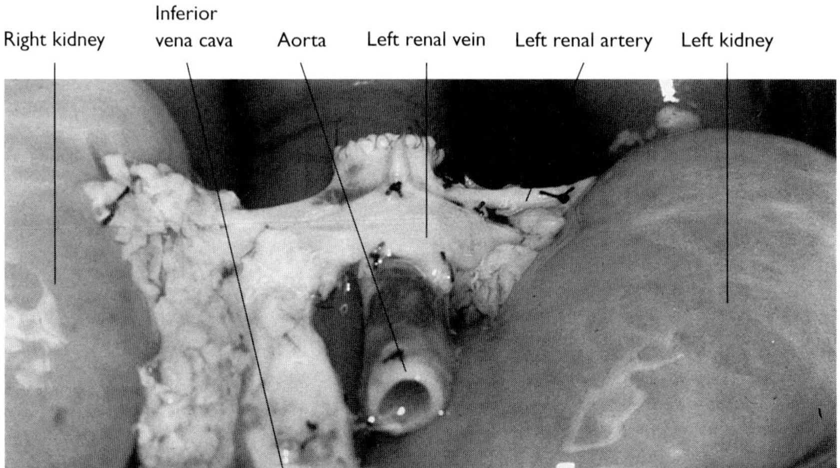

Figure 6–25. Pediatric en bloc kidneys after completion of back table preparation.

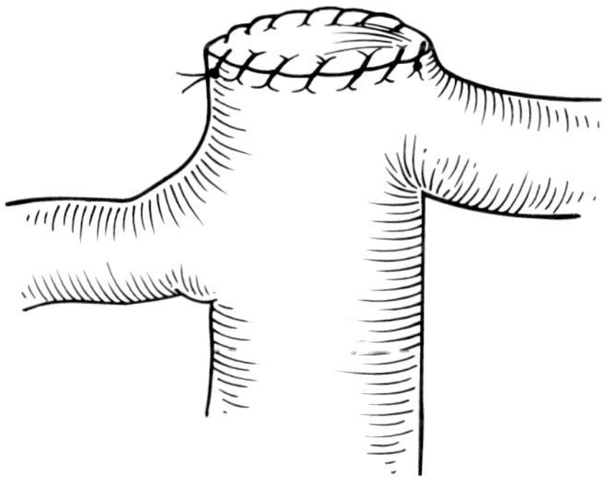

Figure 6–26. Pediatric en bloc kidneys, back table preparation. Closure of the suprarenal vena cava or aorta with a cap of vessel.

Horseshoe Kidney

Horseshoe kidneys are uncommon,[14,15] and donors with horseshoe kidneys are a rarity. Nevertheless, if the renal function is good, it may be possible to separate a horseshoe kidney into two usable kidneys (Fig. 6–27). There will most likely be multiple arteries supplying each kidney, and it is important to dissect the vessels carefully to determine where each vessel goes. Once the blood supply has been separated and the excess perinephric tissue removed, the two kidneys are connected only by a bridge of renal tissue. Occasionally a fibrous plane divides the two parts; usually the kidneys are separated by dividing the parenchyma at its thinnest spot. The transected area of kidney is best oversewn with a long-lasting monofilament absorbable suture (4-0 polyglyconate works well) (Fig. 6–28). If the kidneys are fundamentally sound, it is possible to transplant them successfully.[28]

Living Donor Kidney

Back table preparation for a kidney from a living donor usually is accomplished during the donor nephrectomy. Additional back table separation of the artery and vein occasionally is required. If there are two arteries, individual preference may be to anastomose partially the arteries so as to implant them together; alternatively, they can be kept separate.[29–31]

We have seen two living donors with an asymptomatic, incidentally discovered renal artery aneurysm in a branch vessel.[32] In both cases, the affected kidney was removed, the aneurysm excised and repaired on the back table, and the kidney transplanted uneventfully with an excellent result (Fig. 6–29).

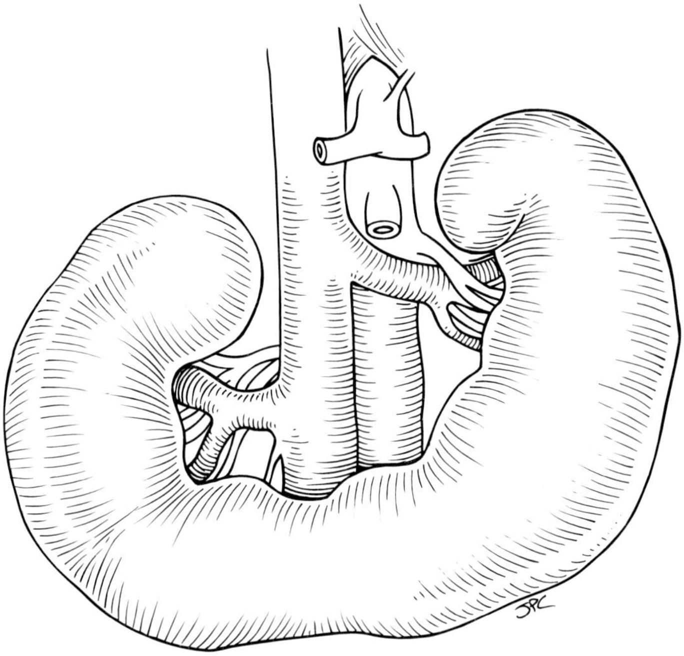

Figure 6–27. Horseshoe kidney.

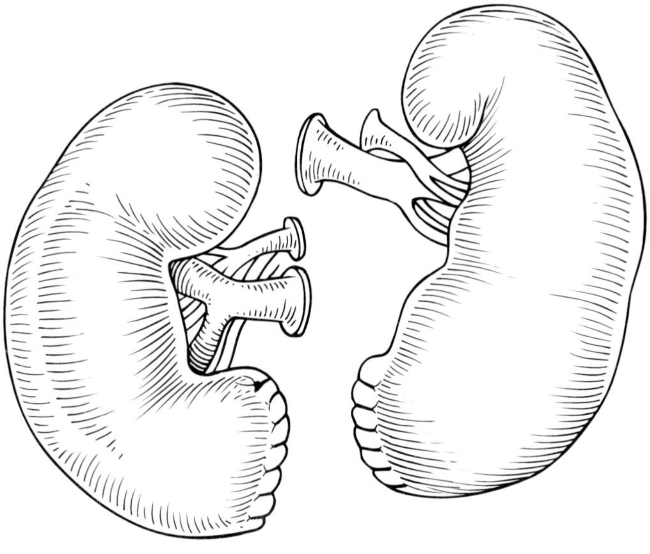

Figure 6–28. Horseshoe kidney after back table preparation and separation into two kidneys.

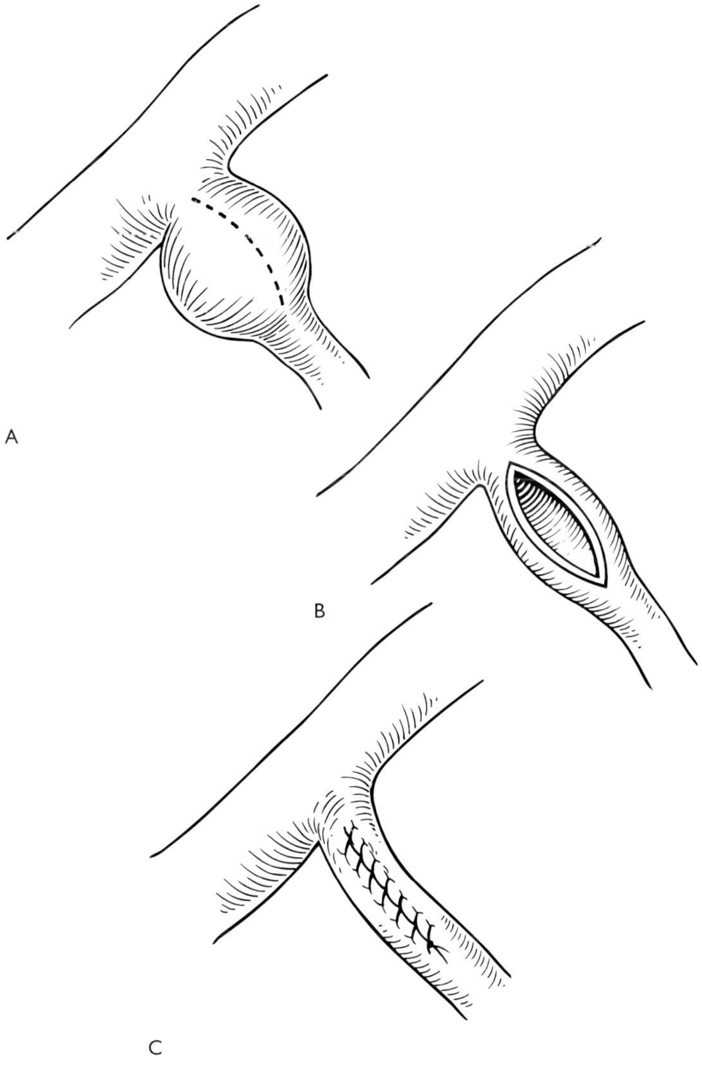

Figure 6–29. A,B,C. Renal artery aneurysm in a living-related-donor kidney. Excision and repair on the back table after nephrectomy and before transplantation.

▲ IMPLANTATION

Preliminary Dissection

Once a recipient is in the operating room and after induction of anesthesia, a Foley catheter is inserted. To facilitate the eventual ureteroneocystostomy, the bladder is distended by the instillation of up to 200 mL of an antibiotic solution (the composition is not critical—0.25% neomycin or 1 mg/mL cefazolin is commonly used).[3,33] The bladder distention is done by gravity only; forcing excess fluid into a small-capacity bladder that may not have been used for years can lead to rupture. The catheter tubing is clamped to keep the bladder distended. If the recipient has a large native urine output, the bladder is emptied before instillation of the antibiotic solution. An alternative approach is to attach the Foley catheter to a 1-liter bag of saline solution. The bag is raised on a pole to allow the bladder to distend and is lowered after the ureteroneocystostomy is performed (Jordan ML, personal communication, 1994).

After appropriate clipping of the pubic and abdominal wall hair, the entire abdomen is prepped and draped. A first-generation cephalosporin is given intravenously just before incision; frequent wound irrigation with a topical antibiotic solution (eg, 1 mg/mL of the first-generation cephalosporin) also is employed during the procedure.

The specific type of incision is based on surgeon preference, but for a first transplantation in an adult, a curving right (or left) lower abdominal incision is usual. The incision extends from the pubic symphysis at the midline to a point 2–3 cm superomedial to the anterior superior iliac spine[34–37] (Fig. 6–30). Some surgeons prefer a paramedian incision with a hockey-stick deviation to the midline inferiorly.[3,38] In any event, the goal is to incise the abdominal wall fascial and muscle layers, leaving the peritoneum intact. The peritoneum is then mobilized medially to expose the external iliac artery and vein. The kidney will reside in this retroperitoneal space. Ligation

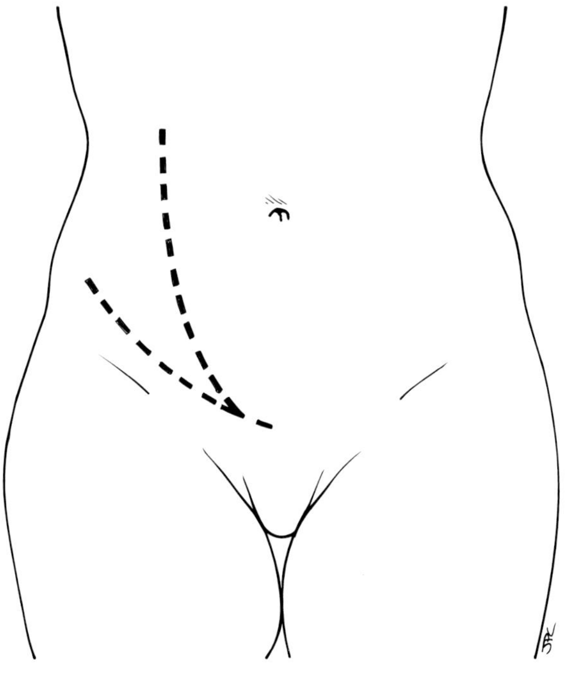

Figure 6–30. Incision for renal transplantation.

and division of the inferior epigastric vessels and, in female patients, of the round ligament, are routinely performed during this phase.[29]

Once the preliminary exposure has been accomplished, any of a number of retraction systems is assembled to maintain the exposure. Examples include the Bookwalter (a personal preference), the Thompson, the Iron Intern, the Turner-Warwick, or the Omni-Trac. A simple Balfour retractor with the bladder blade attachment and a second assistant holding a Harrington or Deaver retractor will also work.

Further mobilization of the vessels is subject to personal preference. Some surgeons (myself included) prefer to mobilize most of the external iliac artery and vein; others clean off only the length needed to perform the vascular anastomoses. The advantage of the former approach is that exposure is maximized, and this is especially useful in a teaching situation. Regardless of whichever style is used, an important principle is that the lymphatic vessels should be divided between ligatures to minimize the risk of lymphocele formation (see Chapter 11).[29,33]

Details of Vascular Anastomosis

There are perhaps as many slightly different techniques of vascular anastomosis as there are transplant surgeons; a few of the more common ones are presented. The simplest approach is to place two sutures, one at each corner of the vessel, and then anastomose each side successively[29] (Fig. 6–31). A popular variation is to place two sutures in the middle to provide traction and minimize inadvertent suture of the back wall[29] (Fig. 6–32). Some surgeons perform one side of the vessel anastomosis from within, borrowing from the techniques of liver transplantation[39] (Fig. 6–33). Still others use a single-stitch technique, particularly for the artery (Fig. 6–34). Familiarity with all these variations is useful, as it may be necessary to use different techniques in certain situations. The goal, of course, is to perform a technically perfect and expeditious vascular anastomosis.

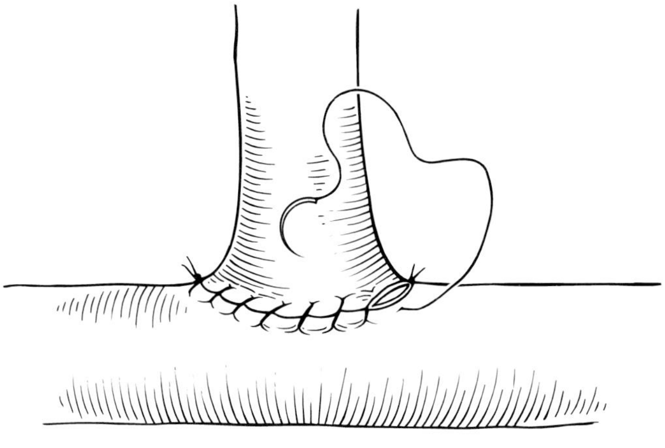

Figure 6–31. Vascular anastomosis. Two-stitch technique.

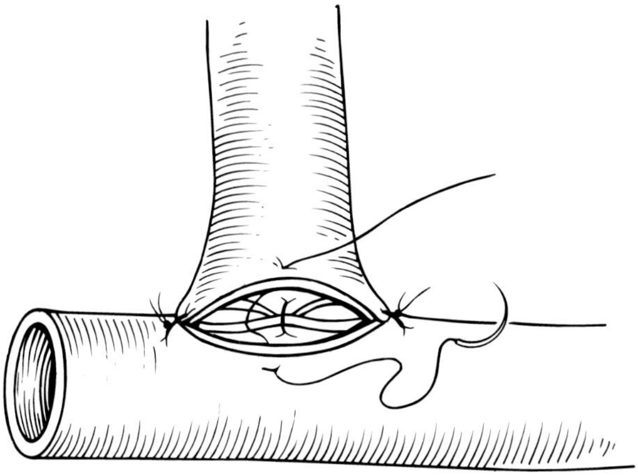

Figure 6–32. Vascular anastomosis. Four-stitch technique.

The vein is customarily anastomosed first, end to side to the external iliac vein.[5,29] Suture of 5-0 or 6-0 polypropylene is commonly used (Fig. 6–35). The artery is sutured usually end to side to the external iliac artery with either 5-0 or 6-0 polypropylene[5,33] (Fig. 6–36). There are several variations with regard to the recipient vessels. Some surgeons prefer an end-to-end anastomosis to the internal iliac artery[35] (Fig. 6–37). This was one of the earliest techniques in renal transplantation.[29,34] Disadvantages include an increased risk of atherosclerosis of the internal iliac artery orifice in an older or diabetic recipient and the risk of inducing impotence in the retransplant setting when both internal iliac arteries have been divided.

In cases of multiple retransplantations, excessive scarring may render exposure

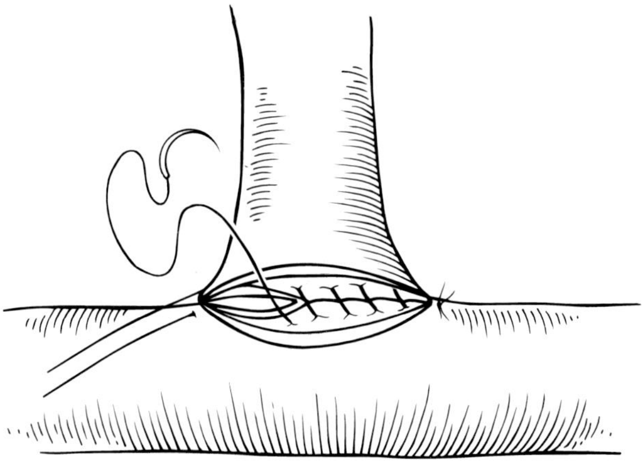

Figure 6–33. Vascular anastomosis. Suturing the back wall from within.

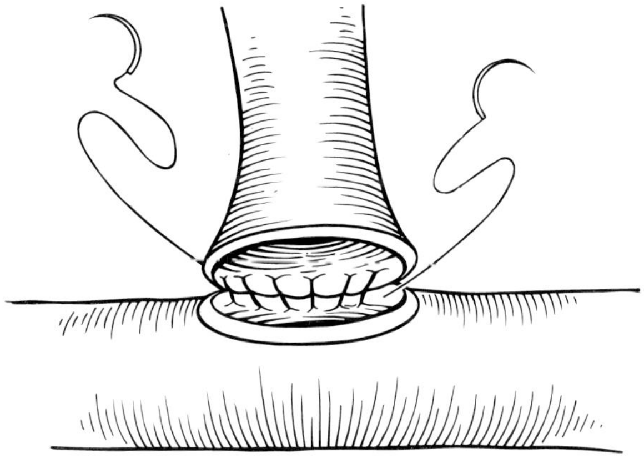

Figure 6–34. Vascular anastomosis. Single-stitch technique.

of the external iliac vessels difficult, and it may be easier to expose the common iliac vessels.[29,33] Some surgeons even place a kidney intraabdominally and anastomose to the inferior vena cava and right common iliac artery or aorta[29,33] (Fig. 6–38). The basic principles of exposure, dissection, and vascular anastomosis remain the same.

In living-donor transplantation, the donor vessels do not have cuffs of aorta and vena cava. It is still possible to perform the vascular anastomoses in an end-to-side

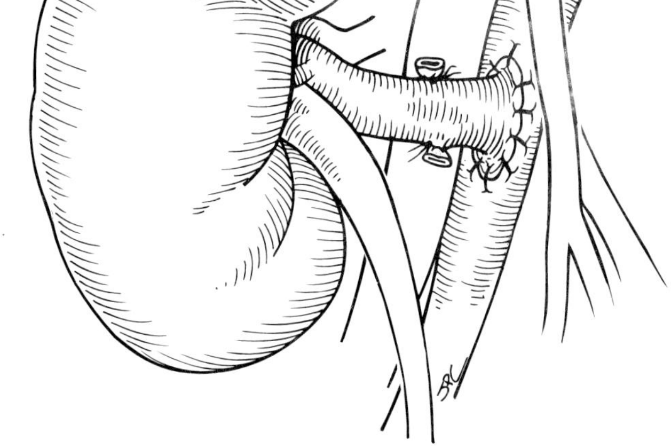

Figure 6–35. Renal vein anastomosis end to side to the external iliac vein.

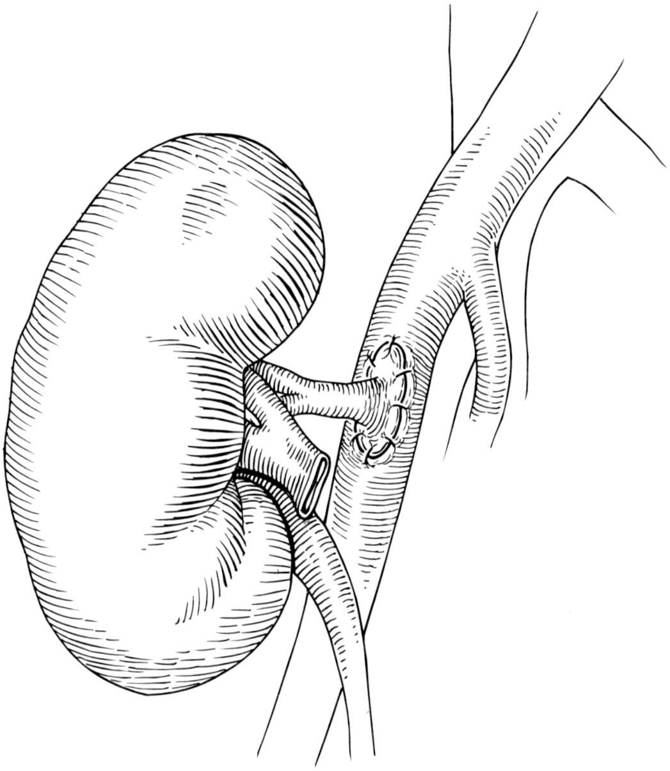

Figure 6–36. Renal artery anastomosis end to side to the external iliac artery.

manner to the external iliac vessels, although many surgeons prefer end-to-end anastomosis to the internal iliac artery.[2,3,29,33] Additional mobilization of the recipient vessels may facilitate implantation in this situation.

Just as there are different styles of vascular anastomosis, so are there variations of adjunctive measures performed while the vessels are being sutured. A popular local maneuver is to wrap the kidney in an ice blanket during the actual performance of the vessel anastomoses (Fig. 6–39). The kidney remains fairly cold until reperfusion, and warm ischemia is reduced. This is particularly useful in a teaching situation. Another useful adjunct is to administer intravenous furosemide, 1 mg/kg, and mannitol 1 g/kg, as the vessels are anastomosed.[4,38] An additional 1 mg/kg of intravenous furosemide is administered over 30 minutes after release of the cross clamp. Some surgeons prefer a systolic blood pressure of 140 mm Hg when the kidney is reperfused;[4,38] others insist on a central venous pressure (CVP) of 11–17 cm H_2O and appropriate volume loading.[40] A few surgeons administer small doses of intraarterial calcium channel blockers (nifedipine) or smooth-muscle relaxants (papaverine) at

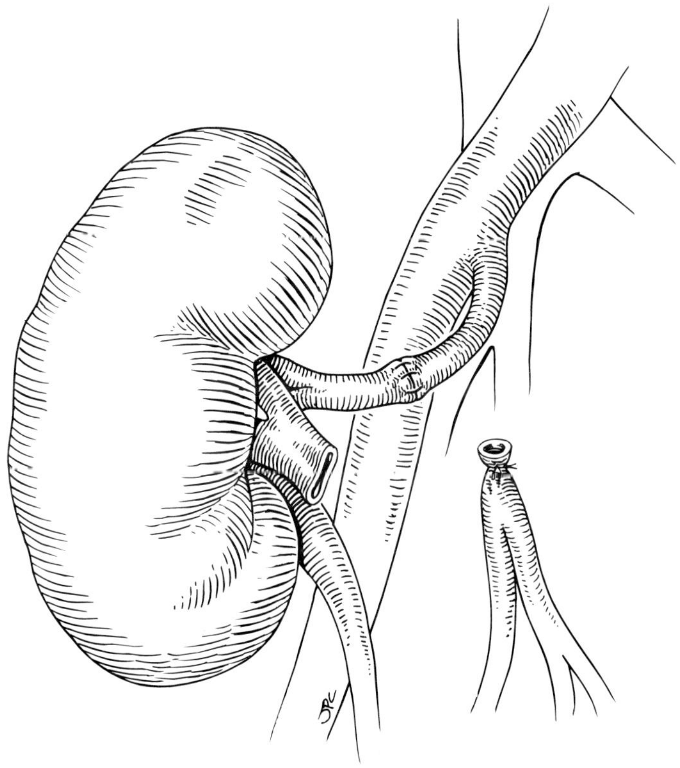

Figure 6–37. Renal artery anastomosis end to end to the internal iliac artery.

the time of cross-clamp release (Light J, personal communication, 1991). The goal of all of these maneuvers is to have the newly reperfused kidney begin to make urine immediately.

Ureteral Reimplantation

The technical aspects of ureteroneocystostomy are subject to more variation than those of vascular anastomosis. The more common variations are discussed. The most common technique is extravesical.[2,3,33,41,42] It involves incision of the bladder wall musculature at the dome for a distance of 2–3 cm to expose the bladder wall mucosa (Fig. 6–40A). A small incision is made in the distal mucosa. The ureter is trimmed to an appropriate length and cut (usually) at an angle; some surgeons prefer to ligate the periureteral vessels. The anastomosis of full-thickness ureter to the bladder mucosa is performed with running or interrupted suture, usually of ab-

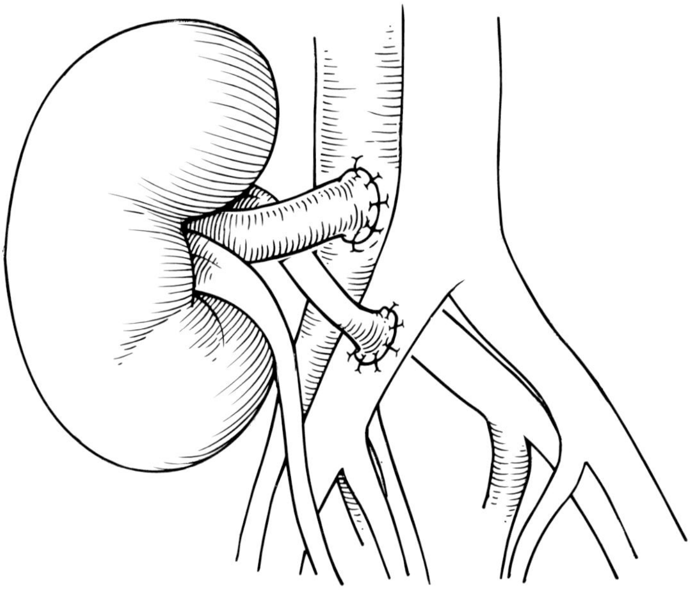

Figure 6–38. Intraabdominal placement of renal allograft with venous anastomosis to the inferior vena cava and arterial anastomosis to the right common iliac artery.

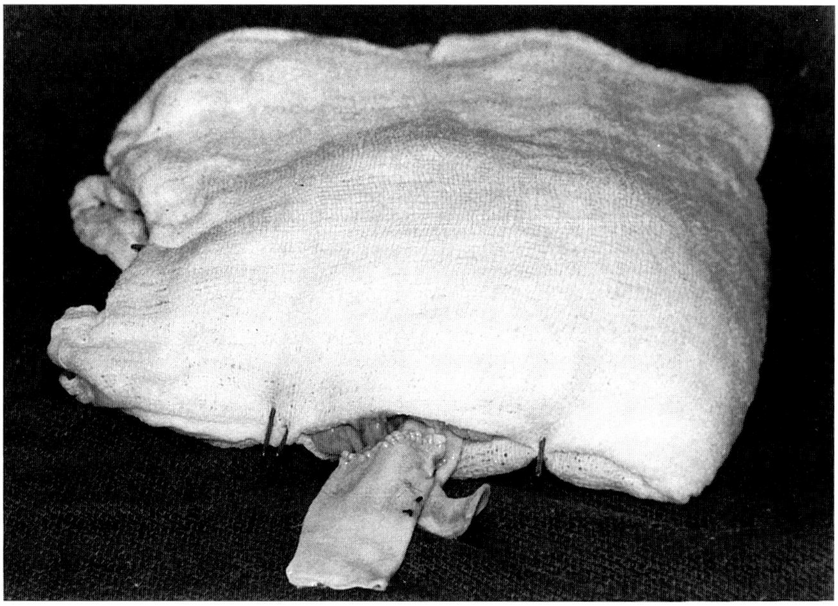

Figure 6–39. Renal allograft wrapped in an ice blanket. (Note: Ice is within the laparotomy pad and is not in direct contact with the kidney.)

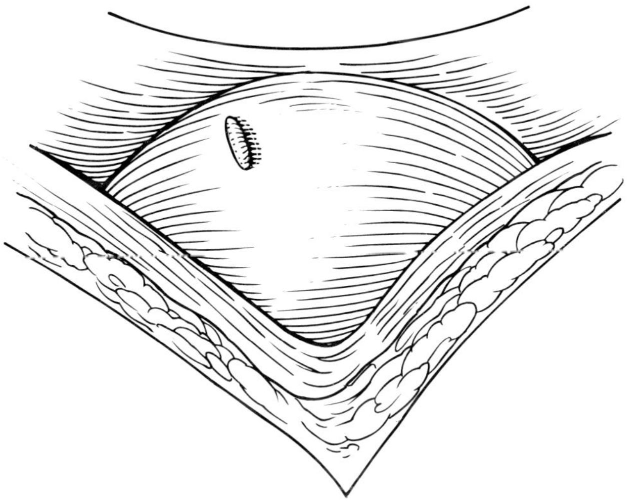

A

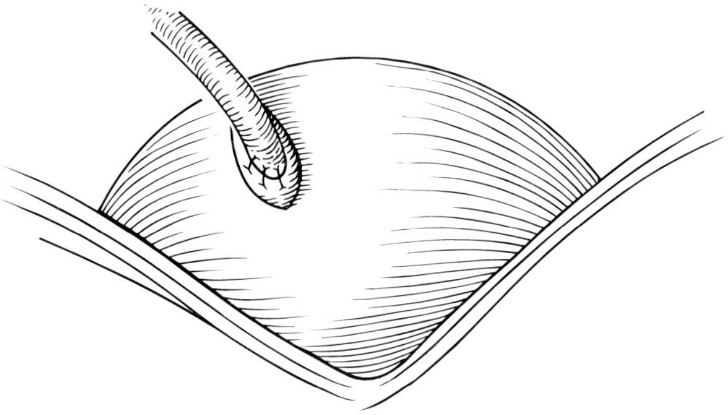

B

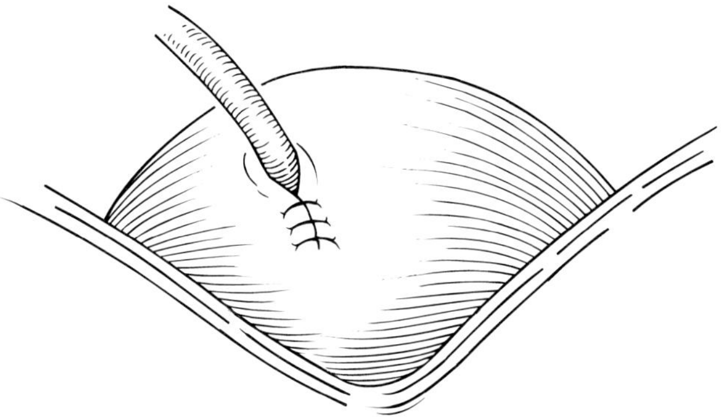

C

Figure 6–40. A. Extravesical ureteroneocystostomy. Exposure of the bladder mucosa. B. Ureteral anastomosis to bladder mucosa. C. Reapproximation of bladder wall musculature to produce a submucosal tunnel.

sorbable material (a personal preference is 6-0 polyglyconate) (Fig 6–40B). The bladder muscle layer is then reapproximated for a short distance, enough to create a submucosal tunnel but not so long as to constrict the ureter (Fig 6–40C). This concept of the submucosal tunnel was adopted from a technique described by Lich et al[41] to correct reflux in children.

Variations of the extravesical technique range from not reapproximating the bladder wall musculature[43] (Fig. 6–41) to using a single suture to telescope the ureter into the bladder before reapproximating the muscle layer. In the latter circumstance, the ureter is not actually sutured to the bladder mucosa[44] (Fig. 6–42).

The original, open technique attributed to Politano and Leadbetter[45,46] involves producing a large opening in the bladder, fashioning a submucosal tunnel, and performing the ureteroneocystostomy from within (Fig. 6–43).

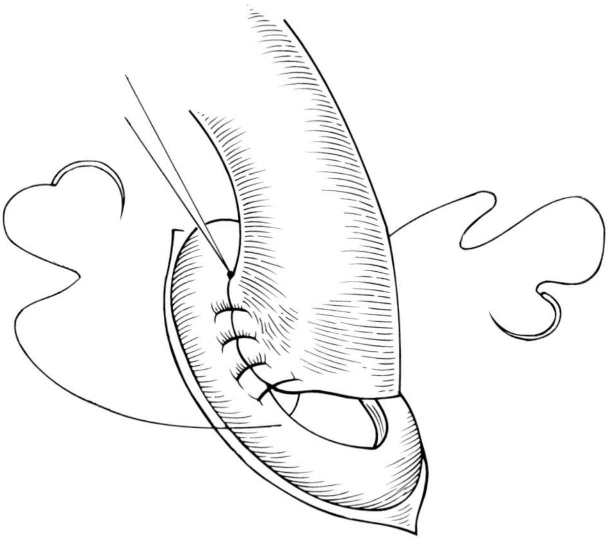

A

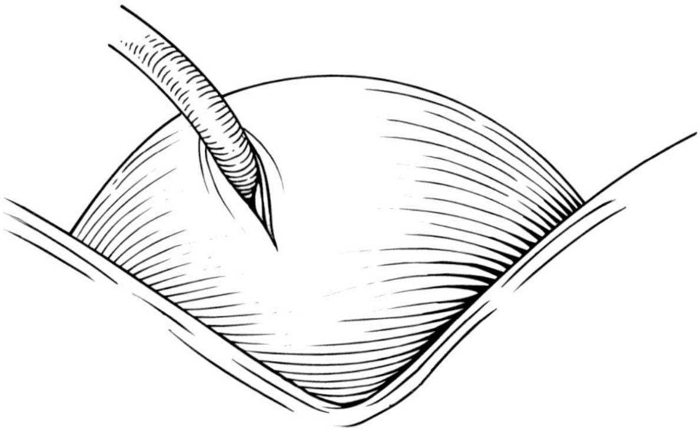

B

Figure 6–41. A,B. Extravesical ureteroneocystomy, variation. Ureteral anastomosis to bladder wall mucosa without reapproximation of muscle layer.

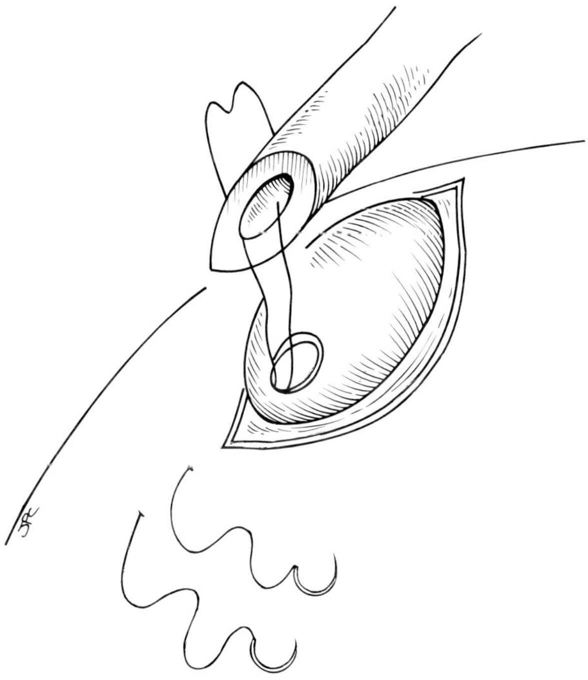

A

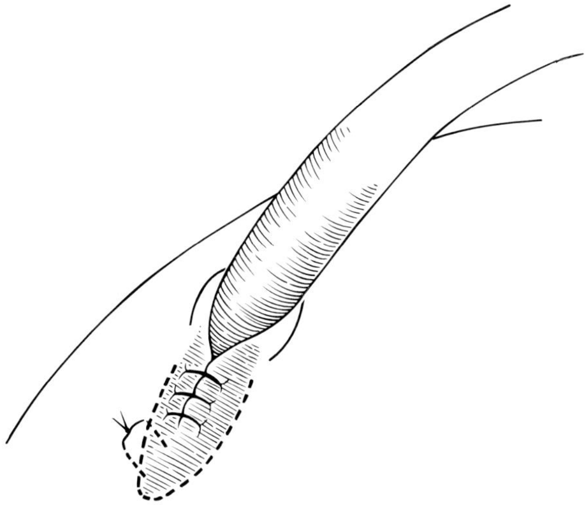

B

Figure 6–42. A,B,C. Extravesical ureteroneocystostomy variation. Telescoping of ureter into bladder followed by closure of bladder wall musculature. Ureteral anastomosis to bladder mucosa is not performed.
(Continued)

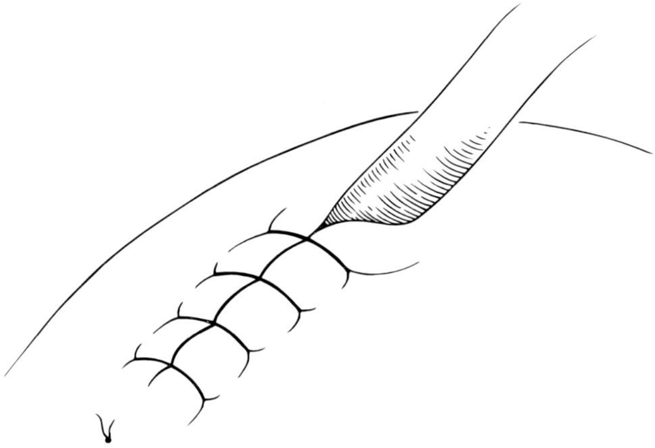

Figure 6–42. *(Continued)*

In the case of a double ureter, there are two options. The ureters can be implanted separately into the bladder (Fig. 6–44A), or they can be partially anastomosed and then implanted as a single unit (Fig. 6–44B). With either variation, it is important to dissect minimally the ends of the ureters so as not to disturb the blood supply.

A ureteropelvic junction obstruction in the transplanted ureter may be of no functional importance. On the other hand, it may result in significant obstruction. Unfortunately, it is not always possible to predict the outcome at the time of transplantation. Furthermore, ureteropelvic junction obstruction may not even be noticed because the ureter has not been dissected proximally enough to uncover it. Options include simple stenting at the time of the transplant, performance of a pyelovesicostomy or a pyeloureterostomy end to side or end to end to the native ureter (Fig. 6–45), or performance of an endopyelotomy through a nephrostomy.[47,48]

There are techniques that avoid the bladder altogether in which the native ureter is used for end-to-end or side-to-end anastomosis to the proximal transplant ureter or pelvis (with or without native nephrectomy)[33,47–49] (Fig. 6–46). This technique is useful if the donor ureter has been stripped and is ischemic.

In the uncommon case of a patient with an ileal loop, a full-thickness, interrupted anastomosis to the diverted intestine is performed[3,33] (Fig. 6–47).

A final issue is whether to stent the ureter; here again there is enormous variation. Ureteroureterostomies or pyeloureterostomies are generally stented, as are implantations into an ileal loop. If they are used, stents are removed cystoscopically 6 weeks after transplantation.

The goal of all of these techniques is to perform a watertight, technically perfect anastomosis and use a healthy, nonischemic donor ureter.

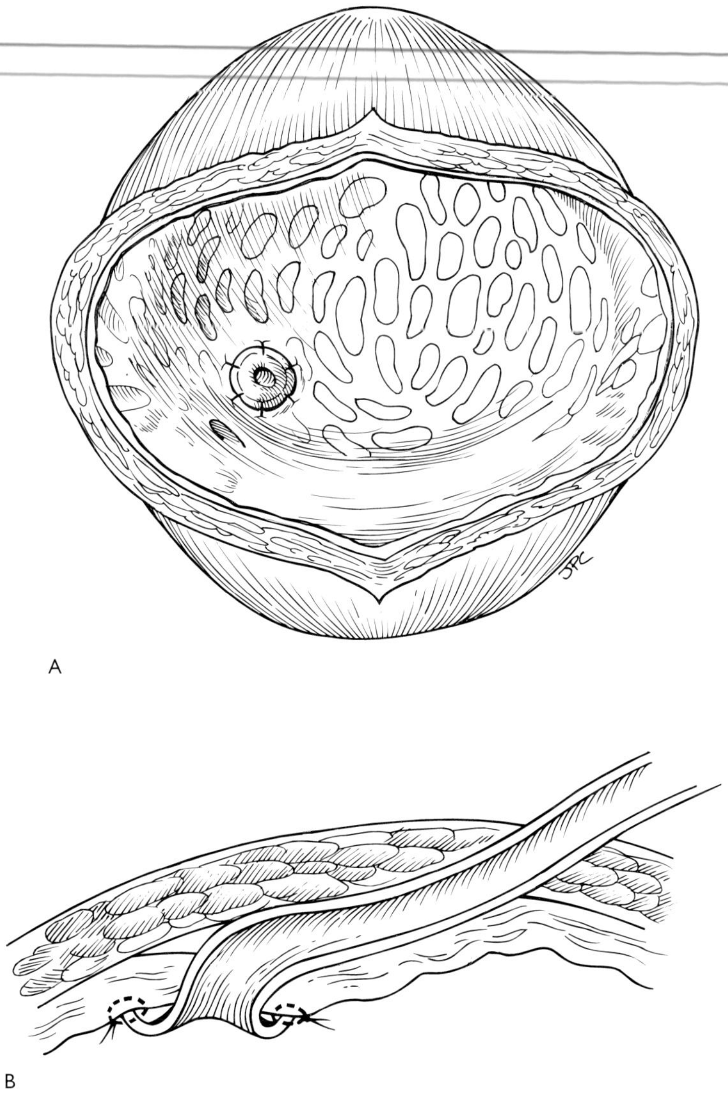

Figure 6–43. A,B. Open ureteroneocystostomy, with ureteral anastomosis performed from within and construction of a submucosal tunnel.

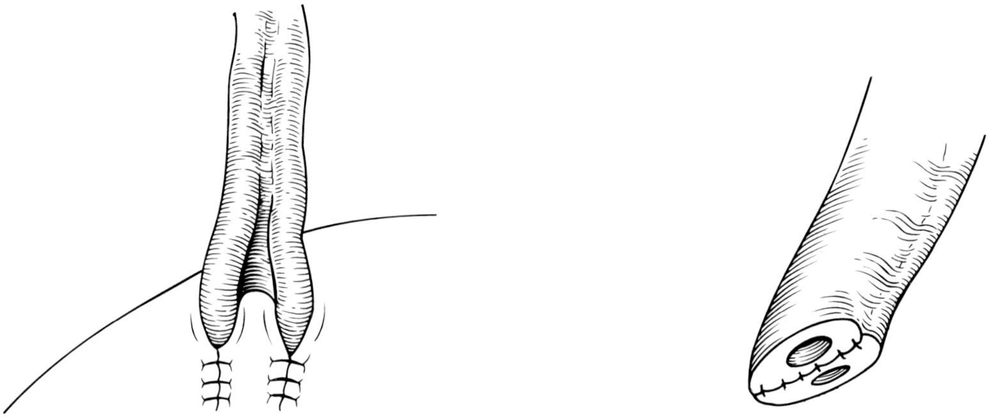

A B

Figure 6–44. A. Double ureter. Separate ureteroneocystostomies. B. Partial anastomosis of the ureters with a single ureteroneocystostomy.

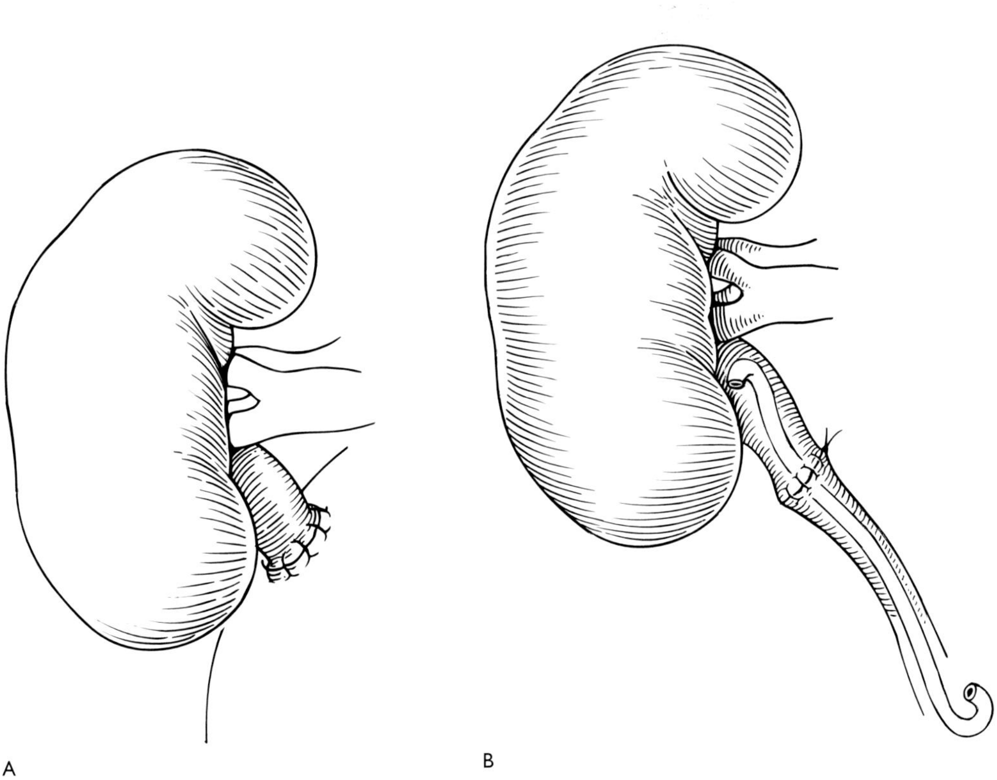

A B

Figure 6–45. A. Pyelovesicostomy. B. Pyeloureterostomy to the native ureter.

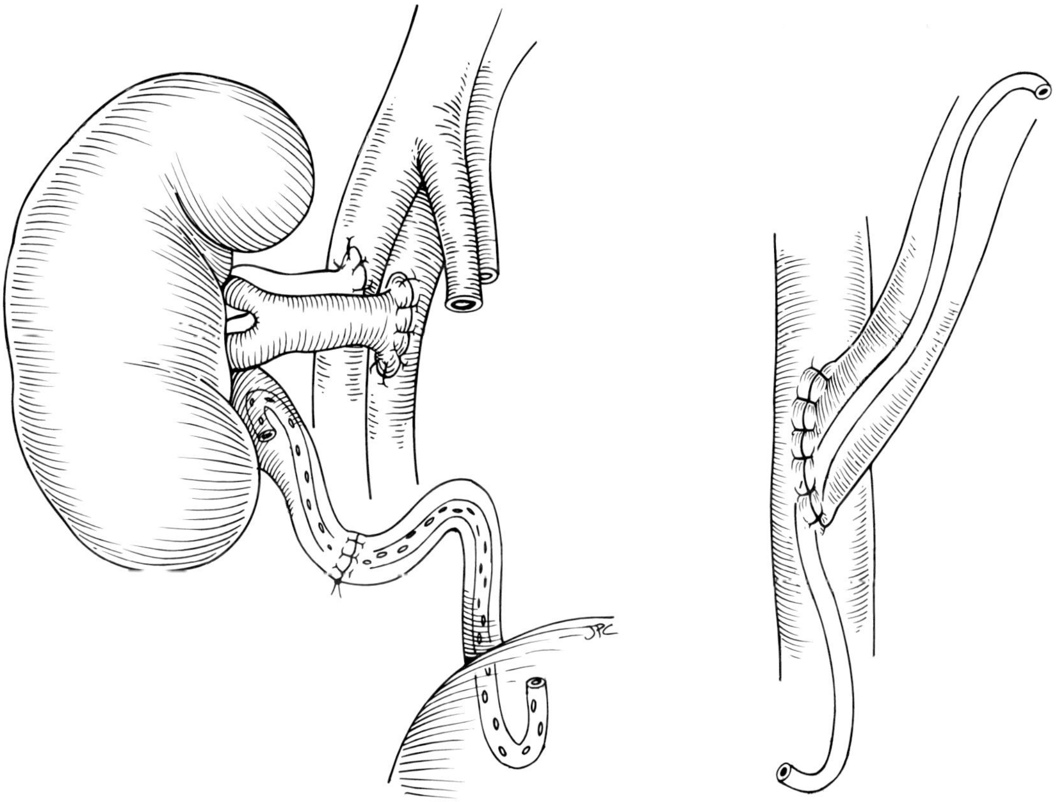

A

B

Figure 6–46. Ureteroureterostomy to the native ureter. A. end-to-end. B. end-to-side.

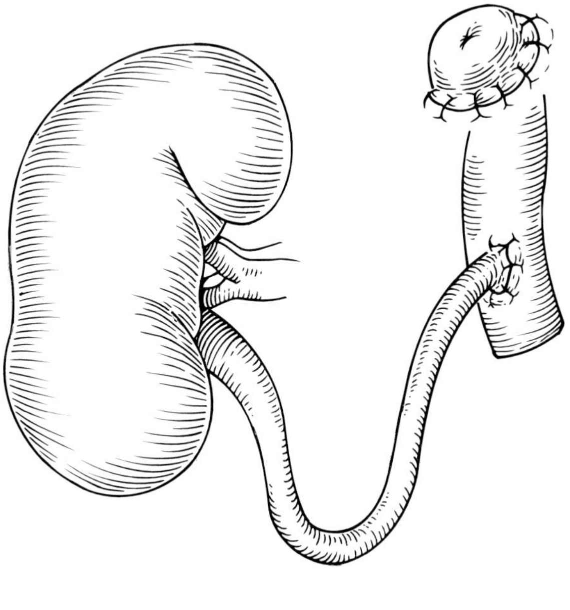

Figure 6–47. Ureteral anastomosis to an ileal loop.

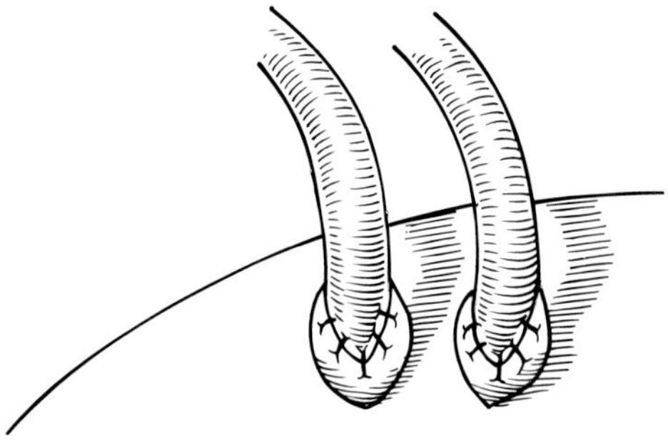

Figure 6–48. Pediatric en bloc kidneys. Two separate ureteroneocystostomies.

En Bloc Kidneys

Implantation of en bloc kidneys is technically more problematic than implantation of single adult kidneys. Vessel anastomosis involves suturing the donor inferior vena cava to the external iliac vein end to side and the donor aorta to the external iliac artery end to side. Wrapping the kidneys in an ice blanket can prevent twisting during implantation.

Ureteral reimplantation can be performed as two separate ureteroneocystostomies (a personal preference) (Fig. 6–48) or as a single anastomosis after partially suturing together the two ureters.[21,22] The ureters are stented at the surgeon's discretion. The length of the left ureter, when the kidneys are implanted on the right side, can be the important limiting factor.

Perhaps the most critical issue is the positioning of the kidneys in the iliac fossa. The kidneys must lie so that they have uncompromised arterial inflow and venous outflow and so that the ureters reach the bladder without excessive tension. Careful placement is needed to find a comfortable and stable location for the kidneys.

▲ REFERENCES

1. Holmes JH: Preparation of recipient for transplantation. In: Starzl TE (ed), *Experience in Renal Transplantation.* Philadelphia, Saunders, 1964:17–29.
2. Rosenthal JT: The transplant operation and its surgical complications. In: Danovitch GM (ed), *Handbook of Kidney Transplantation.* Boston, Little Brown, 1992:135–150.
3. Shapiro R, Simmons RL: Renal transplantation. In: Starzl TE, Shapiro R, Simmons RL (eds), *Atlas of Organ Transplantation.* New York, Gower, 1992:4, 1–21.
4. Shapiro R, Simmons RL: Kidney transplantation. In: Makowka L (ed), *The Handbook of Transplantation Management.* Austin, R.G. Landes 1991:168–191.
5. Kjellstrand CM, Simmons RL, Buselmeier TJ, Najarian JS: Kidney. In: Najarian JS, Simmons RL (eds). Philadelphia, Lea and Febiger, 1972:418–495.
6. Ting A, Welsh K: HLA Matching and crossmatching in renal transplantation. In: Morris PJ (ed), *Kidney Transplantation: Principles & Practice,* ed 4. Philadelphia, Saunders, 1994: 109–126.

7. Yanaga K, Podeta LG, Broznick B, Shapiro R, Stieber A, Makowka L: Multiple organ recovery for transplantation. In: Starzl TE, Shapiro R, Simmons RL (eds), *Atlas of Organ Transplantation.* New York, Gower, 1992:3, 1–49.
8. Schwartz, Podesta L, Morris M, Makowka C, Miller C: Donor management, techniques and procurement. In: Makowka L (ed), *The Handbook of Transplantation Management.* Austin, R.G. Landes 1991:44–71.
9. Rosenthal JT, Danovitch GM: Live related and cadaveric kidney donation. In: Danovitch GM (ed), *Handbook of Kidney Transplantation.* 1992:105–118.
10. Marshall VC, Jablonski P, Scott DF: Renal preservation. In: Morris PJ (ed), *Kidney Transplantation: Principles & Practice,* ed 4. Philadelphia, Saunders, 1994:86–108.
11. Belzer FO, Ashby BS, Dunphy JE: 24-Hour and 72-Hour preservation of canine kidneys. *Lancet* 2:536–539, 1967
12. Claes G, Blohme I: Organ preservation. In: Pegg DE (ed), New York, Churchill-Livingstone, 1973:51–59.
13. Tzakis A, Mazzaferro V, Pan C-E, et al: Renal artery reconstruction for harvesting injuries in kidney transplantation with particular reference to the use of vascular allografts. *Transplant Int* 1:80–85, 1988.
14. Gray H; Pickering Pick T, Howden R (eds): *Gray's Anatomy.* New York, Bounty, 1977.
15. Pansky R: *Review of Gross Anatomy.* New York, Macmillan, 1975.
16. Corry RJ, Kelley ST: Technic for lengthening the right renal vein of cadaver donor kidneys. *Am J Surg* 135:867, 1978.
17. Hume DM: Progress in clinical renal homotransplantation. *Adv Surg* 2:419–498, 1966.
18. Marchioro TL: Donor nephrectomy. In: Starzl TE (ed), *Experience in Renal Transplantation,* 1964:68–83.
19. Starzl TE, Iwatsuki S, Shaw BW Jr: A growth factor in fine vascular anastomoses. *Surg Gynecol Obstet* 159:164–165, 1984.
20. Lippman H, Jacoby K, McFarlin L, et al: Surgical complications in 50 adult renal transplant recipients of single kidneys from cadaveric donors aged 11 to 48 months. *Clin Transplant* 6:350–356, 1992.
21. Jordan ML, Shapiro R, Sundberg R, et al: Transplantation of pediatric en bloc kidneys under FK506 immunosuppression. *Transplant Proc* 23:6:3089–3090, 1991.
22. Nghiem D: En bloc transplantation of kidneys from donors weighing less than 15 kg into adult recipients. *J Urol* 145:14–16, 1991.
23. Kinne DW, Spanos PK, DeShazo MM, Simmons RL, Najarian JS: Double renal transplant from pediatric donors to adult recipients. *Am J Surg* 127(3):292–5, 1974.
24. Lindstrom BL, Ahonen J: The use of both kidneys obtained from pediatric donors as en bloc transplant adult recipients. *Scand J Urol Nephrol* 29:71, 1975.
25. Dreikorn J, Rohl L, Horsch R: The use of double renal transplant from pediatric cadaver donor. *Br J Urol* 49:361, 1977.
26. Najarian JS: Long term success with double pediatric cadaver donor renal transplant. *Ann Surg* 197:439–442, 1983.
27. Shapiro R, Tzakis AG, Starzl TE: Bilateral venous reconstruction of pediatric en bloc kidneys for transplantation. *Transplantation* 50:1055–1056, 1990.
28. Menezes de Goes G, De Campos Freire G, Borelli M, Pompeo ACL, Wrociawski ER: Transplantation of a horseshoe kidney. *J Urol* 126:537, 1981.
29. Starzl TE: Recipient operations. In: Starzl TE (ed), *Experience in Renal Transplantation.* Philadelphia, Saunders, 1964:84–110.
30. Woodruff MFA, Robson JS, Ross JA, Nolan B, Lambie AT: Transplantation of a kidney from an identical twin. *Lancet* 1:1245–1249, 1961.

31. Simmons RL, Talolent MB, Kjellstrand CM, Najarian JS: Kidney transplantation from living donors with bilateral double renal arteries. *Surgery* 69:201–207, 1971.
32. Shapiro R, Scantlebury VP, Zajko AB, Simmons RL: Renal artery aneurysm in a living-related kidney donor: a report of 2 cases. *Clin Transplant* 6:323–324, 1992.
33. Lee HM: Surgical techniques of renal transplantation. In: Morris PJ (ed), *Kidney Transplantation: Principles & Practice,* ed 4. Philadelphia, Saunders, 1994:127–137.
34. Kuss R, Teinturier J, Millienz P: Quelques essais de greffes du rein chez l'homme. *Mem Acad Chir* 77:755, 1951.
35. Murray JE, Harrison JH: Management of 50 patients with kidney transplants including 18 pairs of twins. *Am J Surg* 105:205, 1963.
36. Hume DM, Magee JH, Kauffman HM, Rittenbury MS, Prout GR: Renal homotransplantation in man in modified recipients. *Ann Surg* 158:608, 1963.
37. Starzl TE, Marchioro TL, Dickinson TC, Rifkind D, Stonington OG, Waddell WR: Technique of renal homotransplantation: experience with 42 cases. *Arch Surg* 89:87, 1964.
38. Simmons RL, Najarian JS: Kidney transplantation: In: Simmons RL, Finch MB, Ascher NL, Najarian JS (eds), *Manual of Vascular Access: Organ Donation and Transplantation.* 1984:292–328.
39. Stieber AC, Makowka L, Starzl TE: Orthotopic liver transplantation. In: Starzl TE, Shapiro R, Simmons RL (eds), *Atlas of Organ Transplantation.* New York, Gower, 1992:7, 1–49.
40. Diethelm AG, Aldrete JS, Sterling WA, et al: Large volume diuresis as a mechanism for immediate maximum renal function after transplantation. *Surg Gynecol Obstet* 138:869, 1974.
41. Lich R, Howerton LW, Davis LA: Recurrent urosepsis in children. *J Urol* 86:554–558, 1961.
42. Gregoir W, van Regemorter G: Le reflux vesico-ureteral congential. *Urol Int* 18:122–128, 1964.
43. Starzl TE, Shapiro R, Tzakis A, Hakala TR: A new technique of extravesical ureteroneocystostomy for renal transplantation. *Transplant Proc* 21:3856–3858, 1989.
44. Matas AJ, Tellis VA, Karwa GL, et al: Comparison of posttransplant urologic complications following extravesical ureteroneocystostomy by a "single-stitch" or "mucosal" anastomosis. *Clin Transplant* 1:159–163, 1987.
45. Politano VA, Leadbetter WF: An operative technique for the correction of vesicoureteral reflux. *J Urol* 79:932–941, 1958.
46. Paquin AJ: Ureterovesical anastomosis: the description and evaluation of a technique. *J Urol* 82:573–583, 1959.
47. Leadbetter GW, Monaco AP, Russell PS: A technique for reconstruction of the urinary tract in renal transplantation. *Surg Gynecol Obstet* 123:839–841, 1966.
48. Cranston D: Urologic complications after renal transplantation. In: Morris PJ (ed), *Kidney Transplantation: Principles & Practice,* ed 4. Philadelphia, Saunders, 1994:330–338.
49. Lord RH, Pepera T, Williams G: Ureteroureterostomy and pyeloureterostomy without native nephrectomy in renal transplantation. *Br J Urol* 67:349, 1991.

7

Postoperative Management of the Renal Transplant Recipient

Brian C. Bennett / Carlos A. Vivas

This chapter focuses on the nonimmunosuppressive aspects of the postoperative care of renal transplant patients. The principles are straightforward, and much of the care is not different from that of any other patient undergoing a major surgical procedure. A few important differences, however, must be appreciated, and some potential pitfalls must be avoided to ensure an uncomplicated postoperative recovery. The first section deals with the postoperative management in the recovery room; the second discusses care during the first week after transplantation; and the third deals with the rest of the first postoperative month.

▲ CARE IN THE IMMEDIATE POSTOPERATIVE PERIOD

After the renal transplant has been completed, the patient is routinely admitted to the recovery room. Admission to an intensive care unit (ICU) is not usual and is limited to patients who have complicated prior or perioperative medical problems. The initial concerns are similar to those of any surgical patient, although they are affected by the presence of end-stage renal disease (ESRD). Most renal transplant patients are successfully extubated during the immediate postoperative period and treated thereafter with aggressive pulmonary physiotherapy (although the altered metabolism of particular agents used by anesthesiologists is important to note [see Chapter 5]). A chest radiograph is obtained in the recovery room to assess central venous pressure (CVP) line placement, to rule out pneumothorax, and to look for evidence of pulmonary edema.

Hemodynamic issues can be problematic. Hypertension is common and is related to the patient's underlying renal disease, possible withdrawal from preoperative medications, and intraoperative fluid administration. Review of the anesthetic record is helpful in evaluating intraoperative fluid balance, hemodynamic stability, and possible intraoperative drug administration (ie, antihypertensive agents, diuretics, vasopressor agents). Hypertension may be managed with vasodilating agents such as nitrates and calcium channel blockers. β-Blocking agents should be avoided in the management of acute hypertension because of the increased risk of hyperkalemia, particularly in the setting of delayed graft function (DGF).[1] Hypotension is uncommon and should raise questions about surgical bleeding or a myocardial event. An electrocardiogram (ECG) is routinely obtained in the recovery room for all patients. Cardiac isoenzymes are measured and serial ECGs are obtained for patients with a history of coronary artery disease and for patients who have experienced any intraoperative hemodynamic instability. These two groups of patients are admitted to an ICU immediately after transplantation.

Once the airway, ventilatory, and hemodynamic issues are under control, the two remaining issues to be addressed in the recovery room are serum electrolytes, principally the potassium level, and early function of the allograft. Elevations of the serum potassium level are seen frequently during the immediate postoperative period and require prompt intervention. Treatment options include administration of intravenous calcium gluconate, intravenous sodium bicarbonate, and the use of glucose and insulin (50 mL D50, 10 units regular insulin).[2,3] Kayexalate (sodium polystyrene sulfonate), a potassium exchange resin, may be administered as an enema and can lead to a decrease in total body serum potassium level. A rare complication of colonic necrosis and perforation can occur with early postoperative Kayexalate enema administration, probably related to the sorbitol carrier; therefore, this treatment option should be avoided.[4,5] Patients with oliguria, or those who are unresponsive to conservative management, require immediate dialysis.

Kidneys can function variably after transplantation, diuresing as much as 1000 mL or more an hour or making no urine at all. Intravenous fluid management during the first 24 hours reflects the urine output. Large volumes, >300 mL/h, are replaced 0.8–1.0 mL/mL on an hourly basis for 24–48 hours. Urine outputs <300 mL/h, are replaced 1 mL/1 mL every hour. Replacement is most often with 0.9% or 0.45% saline solution and 5% dextrose. Dextrose 1% may be preferred in the replacement solution of a well-functioning allograft to avoid hyperglycemia and possible osmotic diuresis. Potassium is never included in routine fluid replacement. Hypokalemia is unusual and should be corrected only as needed.

Although not absolutely necessary, a CVP catheter allows accurate measurement of volume status for patients without heart disease. Patients with a history of cardiac disease may be better managed with a Swan-Ganz catheter, and volume status is assessed by measurement of left atrial filling pressures.

For patients with initial anuria or oliguria, volume status, fluid balance, and urethral catheter patency should be assessed. Patients who appear to be hypovolemic should be treated with careful volume replacement; in practice, this is rare. In patients who are euvolemic or hypervolemic, intravenous furosemide (1 mg/kg) may induce diuresis and may have to be given periodically during the first 24–48 hours after transplantation. The term *delayed graft function* is used when early (<48 h) allograft non-function occurs or if dialysis is needed within the first week. A number of variables determine early function. Cold ischemia time plays an important role; long ischemia times are associated with an increased incidence of DGF.[6] Stability of the donor's condition, speed with which the kidneys are removed and later transplanted, and the type of preservation solution all play a role in early allograft function.[6,7] Some centers routinely use pulsatile perfusion and claim remarkably low DGF rates;[8–10] other published reports show no benefit associated with pumping compared with simple cold storage (see Chapters 1 and 4).[11–13] There are instances of immunologically mediated DGF, although it is not always possible to demonstrate this. Research on reperfusion injury has suggested free radical formation as a mediator of early non-function.[14,15] Aggressive efforts to minimize DGF are important, because early function is an important determinant of graft survival. Many studies have demonstrated a 10–20% deterioration in the 1-year graft survival rate in patients with early non-function.[16]

Once patients have recovered from anesthesia, are hemodynamically stable, and have stable electrolytes, they can be safely transferred to the floor.

▲ THE FIRST POSTOPERATIVE WEEK

Although most renal transplant recipients can be treated successfully on a surgical ward, patients with cardiac disease are most appropriately treated in an ICU during the immediate postoperative period. Daily weights and accurate inputs and outputs should be followed closely in all patients. Adjustment of antihypertensive medications is commonly necessary. Metabolic issues are important, such as control of serum potassium and bicarbonate levels and close monitoring of calcium, phosphorous, and magnesium levels. Hypophosphatemia can be seen with the rapid normalization of renal function and may lead to calcium depletion from the bones. Hypomagnesemia may occur, most likely as a side effect of cyclosporine or tacrolimus.

Blood sugar homeostasis can be a problem. A substantial number of transplant patients have diabetes mellitus as the cause of ESRD, and hyperglycemia can occur early in the postoperative course, particularly when large doses of corticosteroids are being administered. An insulin drip occasionally is necessary for the first 1–2 days after transplantation. Both tacrolimus and cyclosporine are diabetogenic[17,18] and occasionally may lead to hyperglycemia in nondiabetic patients when administered in combination with corticosteroids. Blood sugar levels should be checked at least four times a day in patients with diabetes.

With regard to fluid management, after the first 24–48 hours, patients can be given maintenance intravenous fluids until gastrointestinal function has recovered and oral intake is tolerated. The goal is to maintain adequate hydration without overloading the patient, although many renal transplant recipients gain several kilograms during the first few days after transplantation.

The management of the gastrointestinal tract during the first postoperative week is most often uncomplicated. Although the retroperitoneal dissection may be associated with postoperative ileus, most patients can be managed without a nasogastric tube. Patients are slowly advanced to a regular diet once they are passing flatus. However, they may have delayed recovery of bowel function; in its most extreme form, this is called Ogilvie's syndrome, or colonic pseudo-obstruction. Ogilvie's syndrome is characterized by marked dilatation of the colon without mechanical obstruction or appreciable involvement of the small intestine. Massive abdominal distention is the most common physical finding and frequently occurs without pain unless colonic perforation has occurred. Plain abdominal radiography is the most useful diagnostic test in the assessment of acute abdominal distention. A cecal diameter of 10–12 cm in the setting of acute pseudo-obstruction is potentially dangerous and can be associated with perforation.[19] Conservative treatment includes correction of all fluid and electrolyte abnormalities, discontinuation of oral intake, placement of a nasogastric tube, and discontinuation of all narcotics and anticholinergic agents, which may inhibit gastrointestinal mobility. Placement of a rectal catheter may be helpful, but is often ineffective, since the point of dilatation is most often proximal to the splenic flexure. For patients who experience dilatation of the cecum >9 cm, emergent colonoscopic decompression is necessary and can be lifesaving. Successful colonoscopic decompression is achievable in 60–90% of patients.[20] Delay in the diagnosis or management of this entity may result in catastrophic cecal perforation.[21]

Because of the increased risk of peptic ulcer disease and hemorrhage in the setting of high-dose corticosteroid administration,[22] all patients receive gastrointestinal ulcer prophylaxis. Prophylactic use of antacids, sucralfate, and H2 blockers have been effective in the prevention of peptic ulcers in renal transplant patients on high-dose steroids. Occasionally, omeprazole is necessary instead of an H2 blocker.[23] Prophylaxis is continued for several months until the maintenance dose of prednisone is decreased to 10 mg/d or less.

Foley catheter drainage routinely is continued for 2–7 days postoperatively. The length of time of Foley catheter drainage often depends on the individual preference of the transplant surgeon. The catheter may be removed as soon as 48 hours after an uncomplicated renal transplant in patients without evidence of pathologic changes in the bladder wall. Foley catheter drainage should be continued beyond 48 hours after any technically difficult anastomosis and for patients with a small, defunctionalized, or scarred bladder, who may be at increased risk for postoperative complications. For patients who receive pediatric en bloc kidneys, the catheter may be left in for as long as 1 week. The surgeon occasionally may elect to stent the ureter; the stent can be removed cystoscopically 6 weeks after transplantation.

Early postoperative wound management for renal transplant recipients is similar to that of general surgical patients. Because these patients are immunosuppressed, the postoperative risk for wound infection is somewhat higher than for other surgical patients. The most important causes of wound infections stem from operative complications, which include wound hematoma, urinary leak, and lymphocele formation (see Chapter 11).[24] Corticosteroids have been shown to have profound inhibitory effects on the rate of wound healing by decreasing the rate of protein synthesis and inhibiting the normal inflammatory response.[25] Skin staples are thus routinely left in place for 3 weeks postoperatively.

Patient education is an important aspect of care during the first postoperative week before discharge. Learning about and understanding a large number of medications can be difficult for many patients. Before discharge (and, in some centers, prior to transplantation), patients are taught to manage their own medications and must demonstrate proficiency. Physicians and nursing staff must watch for situations in which a lack of understanding (or motivation) may result in noncompliance. If necessary, a family member or caretaker should be asked to learn the medication regimen. The consequences of lack of compliance, such as rejection, infection, peptic ulcer formation, and allograft loss must be understood by the patient. The importance of close follow-up care is emphasized. The patient is instructed to report any episodes of fever, chills, persistent nausea or vomiting, changes in urinary output, peripheral edema, or pain over the allograft.

In general, it is possible to recover surgically after renal transplantation in 1 week or less. If appropriate arrangements are in place for close daily medical follow-up care (eg, laboratory work, evaluation of immunosuppression), patients can be discharged from the hospital. If the patient has delayed graft function, dialysis and even renal biopsies can be performed on an outpatient basis.

▲ EVALUATION OF THE ALLOGRAFT

A Doppler ultrasound examination and in some centers a DTPA or MAG3 nuclear scan are performed on the first postoperative day to confirm vessel patency and to establish the absence of hydronephrosis or perinephric fluid collections (see Chapter 13). These noninvasive studies can usually rule out technical problems.

Lack of allograft function may be secondary to acute tubular necrosis, drug toxicity, or an immunologic injury. In a patient with early allograft nonfunction, an ultrasound-guided biopsy is performed 1 week postoperatively to rule out rejection. For patients with functioning allografts, any early deterioration in function with normal noninvasive studies is an indication for biopsy. With real-time Doppler ultrasound guidance, biopsies can be performed with minimal risk. Coagulation studies and a platelet count are routinely performed before renal transplant biopsy. A transplant kidney biopsy is technically straightforward. The patient is supine, and the area over the allograft is prepped and draped in a sterile manner. The ultrasound probe is covered with a sterile sheath, and the allograft is imaged. A needle guide attachment to the ultrasound probe allows real-time localization of the precise path of the needle. The allograft is then imaged with color Doppler ultrasound, with attention to the location of the hilar and intrarenal vessels, overlying intestine, and perinephric fluid collections. A local anesthetic (8 to 9 mL 1% [or 5 mL 2%] lidocaine without epinephrine, to which 1 to 2 mL of sodium bicarbonate has been added to reduce discomfort) is used, and an 18-gauge spring-loaded biopsy gun is used to obtain a core of renal cortical tissue from the lateral aspect of either the upper or lower pole of the allograft. Rapid examination of the biopsy core under a low-power microscope can confirm that an adequate sample of cortex with glomeruli has been obtained; this can be performed in the ultrasound suite. Manual pressure is placed on the biopsy site for approximately 10–15 minutes after the biopsy. Color flow Doppler ultrasound allows immediate visualization of any clinically significant hemorrhage after the biopsy. The patient remains at bedrest for 4 hours after the biopsy, and vital signs are evaluated frequently. The urine is monitored for gross hematuria, and a serum hematocrit is obtained 4 hours after the biopsy. Although it is preferable not to perform renal biopsies on dialysis days, patients who must undergo dialysis on the day of a biopsy may do so without heparin.

Fine-needle aspiration with cytologic examination of the renal allograft is also an excellent modality to assess early posttransplant abnormalities.[26] This procedure is technically simple and potentially less traumatic than a conventional biopsy.

▲ FIRST MONTH AFTER TRANSPLANTATION

After discharge from the hospital or the daily outpatient follow-up setting, patients are examined two to three times a week during the early postoperative period. An interval history and physical examination are performed during each follow-up visit. Signs of surgical complications, drug toxicity, acute rejection, or overimmunosuppression are carefully assessed. Any changes in blood pressure, weight, or urine output should be precisely documented, and any history of fever requires a thorough evaluation. Urinalysis and, if necessary, urine culture are routinely performed. Laboratory studies include a complete blood count, serum electrolytes, serum blood urea nitrogen and creatinine, fasting blood glucose, liver function tests, calcium, phosphorous, and magnesium levels, uric acid, cholesterol, and a tacrolimus or cyclosporine level. Attention should be focused on abnormalities in renal function, level of immunosuppression, anemia or myelosuppression, hyperkalemia, and hyperglycemia. Any change in renal function should be investigated promptly. The risk for acute rejection is highest during the first 3 months after transplantation.

Most patients need multiple adjustments in their medications in the early posttransplant period. In addition, immunosuppression must be tapered over time, since long-term immunosuppression can be maintained at a much lower level than that required for induction (see Chapter 8).

The postoperative care of a renal transplant recipient is not particularly difficult. It does require careful attention to detail and constant communication among all members of the transplantation team to ensure a smooth postoperative course.

▲ REFERENCES

1. Arthur S, Greenberg A: Hyperkalemia associated with intravenous labetalol therapy for acute hypertension in renal transplant recipients. *Clin Nephrol* 33:269, 1990.
2. Giebisch GH, Thier SO: Potassium: physiologic and clinical importance. In: Siegal L (ed), *Directions in Cardiovascular Medicine.* Hoechst-Roussel, 1977:48.
3. DeFronzo RA, Felig P, Ferrannini E, Wahren J: Effect of graded doses of insulin on splanchnic and peripheral potassium metabolism in man. *A J Physiol* 238:E421, 1980.
4. Lillemoe KD, Romolo JL, Hamilton SR, Pennington LR, Burdick JF, Williams GM: Intestinal necrosis due to sodium polystyrene (Kayexalate) in sorbitol enemas: clinical and experimental support for the hypothesis. *Surgery* 101:267–272, 1987.
5. Scott TR, Graham SM, Schweitzer EJ, Bartlett ST: Colonic necrosis following sodium polystyrene sulfonate (Kayexalate)–sorbitol enema in a renal transplant patient: report of a case and review of the literature. *Dis Colon Rectum* 36:607–609, 1993.
6. McClelland J, Cecka JM: Kidney preservation. In: Terasaki PI (ed), *Clinical Transplants 1987.* UCLA Tissue Typing Laboratory, Los Angeles, 1987:415.
7. Zhou Y, Cecka JM: Preservation. In: Terasaki PI, Cecka JM (eds), *Clinical Transplants 1992.* UCLA Tissue Typing Laboratory, Los Angeles, 1992:383.
8. Heil JE, Canafax DM, Sutherland DER, Simmons RL, Dunning M, Najarian JS: A controlled comparison of kidney preservation by two methods: machine perfusion and cold storage. *Transplant Proc* 19:2046, 1987.
9. Manis T, Hong JH, Bronsther OL, Friedman EA, Butt KMH: Superior results with machine perfused kidneys in cyclosporine-treated transplant recipients. *Transplant Proc* 17: 1483–1484, 1985.
10. Mendez R, Mendez RG, Koussa N, Cats S, Boggaard TP, Khetan U: Preservation effect on oligo-anuria in the cyclosporin era: a prospective trial with 26 paired cadaveris renal allografts. *Transplant Proc* 19:204–2050, 1987.
11. Opelz G, Terasaki PI: Kidney preservation: perfusion versus cold storage 1975. *Transplant Proc* 8:121–125, 1976.
12. Merion RM, Oh HK, Port FK, Toledo-Pereyra LH, Turcotte JG: A prospective controlled trial of cold-storage versus machine-perfusion preservation in cadaveris renal transplantation. *Transplantation* 50:230–233, 1990.
13. Clark EA, Opelz G, Hickey MR, Terasaki PI: Evaluation of Belzer and Collins kidney preservation methods. *Lancet* 2:361–364, 1973.
14. Green CJ, Healing G, Lunec J, Fuller BJ, Simkin S: Evidence of free radical induced damage in rabbit kidneys after single hyperthermic preservation and autotransplantation. *Transplantation* 41:161, 1986.
15. Koyama J, Bulkey GB, Williams GM, Im MJ: The role of oxygen free radicals in mediating the reperfusion injury of cold-preserved ischemic kidneys. *Transplantation* 45:590, 1985.
16. Lim EC, Terasaki PI: Early graft function. In: Terasaki PI (ed), *Clinical Transplants 1991.* UCLA Tissues Typing Laboratory, Los Angeles, 1991:401.
17. Jindal RM, Popescu I, Schwartz ME, Miller CM: Diabetogenicity of FK506 versus cyclosporine in liver transplant recipients. *Transplantation* 58:370, 1994.
18. Scantlebury V, Shapiro R, Fung J: New onset of diabetes in FK506 vs. cyclosporine treated kidney transplant recipients. *Transplant Proc* 23:3169, 1991.
19. Strodel WE, Brothers T: Colonoscopic decompression of pseudo-obstruction and volvulus. *Surg Clin North Am* 69:1327, 1989.

20. Variers VW, Al-Salti M: Acute pseudo-obstruction of the colon (Olgilvie's syndrome): an analysis of 400 cases. *Dis Colon Rectum* 29:203, 1986.
21. Koneru B, Selby R, O'Hair DP, Tzakis AG, Hakala TR, Starzl TE: Nonobstructing colonic dilatation and perforations following renal transplantation. *Arch Surg* 125:610, 1990.
22. Messer J, Reitman D, Sacks HS, et al: Association of adrenocorticosteroid therapy and peptic ulcer disease. *N Engl J Med* 309:21–24, 1983.
23. Tryba M: Prophylaxis of stress ulcer bleeding. *J Clin Gastroenterol* 13:544, 1991.
24. Kyriakides GK, Simmons RL, Najarian JS: Wound infections in the renal transplant patient: pathogenetic and prognostic factors. *Ann Surg* 186:770, 1975.
25. Medows EC, Prudder JF: A study of the influence of adrenal steroids on the strength of healing wounds. *Surgery* 33:841, 1976.
26. Hayry P, von Willebrand E: Transplant aspiration cytology. *Transplantation* 38:7, 1984.

8

Prevention and Management of Rejection: Immunology of the Allograft Rejection Response

Susan A. McCarthy

▲ OVERVIEW

The immune response to foreign tissue and organ transplants is complex. It affords many possible opportunities for therapeutic regulation with immunosuppressive strategies. This section provides a brief overview of the most important elements of the immune response to allografts and emphasizes actual or theoretic points of intervention for prevention of graft rejection. Subsequent sections of this chapter explore immunosuppression in greater detail and focus on immunosuppressive regimens currently in use or under development.

The immune system is composed of two major types of responses, an antigen-specific response and an antigen-nonspecific (or natural) response.[1] The natural response provides a first line of defense against foreign antigens, and is thought to be particularly important for antimicrobial resistance and less important in allograft rejection. The antigen-specific response, on the other hand, is the main immune barrier to allograft transplantation. The antigen-specific immune response normally involves the activation of T and B lymphocytes by foreign antigens that are processed and presented to lymphocytes by antigen-presenting cells (APC). The activated lymphocytes then produce effector molecules that contribute to elimination of the foreign antigens. B lymphocytes produce antibodies, and T lymphocytes produce cytokines and cytotoxic proteins. Although B cells and antibodies are essential to the elimination of many foreign antigens, they are most effective against soluble antigens (toxins) and extracellular pathogens, and generally do not play a major role in allograft rejection. In contrast, T-cell effector mechanisms are effective against cell-associated foreign antigens such as intracellular pathogens (especially viruses) and tissue or organ transplants. T cells are in fact required for transplant rejection. Nude mice, which express all immune cell types except T lymphocytes, do not reject allogeneic or xenogeneic tissue or organ transplants.[2] This overview therefore focuses on the requirements for T-cell activation by allografts.

T cells normally recognize peptides derived from foreign antigens. Peptides are presented in association with "self" proteins encoded by the major histocompatibility complex (MHC) on the surface of antigen-presenting cells.[3] However, T-cell recognition specificity can have cross-reactive specificity for foreign MHC proteins themselves in association with peptides derived from either self or foreign proteins.[4] This cross-reactive recognition of foreign MHC is called *alloreactivity*. T-cell alloreactivity can be a potent component of the strong immune responses typically generated against allografts.

T-cell recognition of MHC on allografts is mediated by antigen-specific T-cell receptor molecules expressed on the T-cell surface. The T-cell receptors are clonally variant, so each T-cell clone has a different fine specificity.[5] In addition to the T-cell receptor complex, several antigen-nonspecific accessory receptor molecules augment the T-cell response to the antigen that binds the T-cell receptor.[6] These coreceptors and accessory receptors recognize ligand structures on the allografts, and serve both to strengthen the interaction between T cell and allograft cell and to provide activation signals to the T cell. The T-cell receptor and accessory signals lead to a series of intracellular gene activation events that result in the differentiation of the T cells to activated effector T cells.[7]

Activated T-cells can be subdivided into two functional types—the helper T lymphocytes and the cytotoxic T lymphocytes. Helper T-cells and cytotoxic T cells are generated from distinct lineages of naive T-cells, express distinct sets of accessory receptors, recognize distinct sets of MHC molecules on allografts, and exhibit distinct effector functions once they are generated. Helper T cells produce soluble cytokines that recruit and activate other components of the immune response to allografts, such as macrophages and cytotoxic T lymphocytes.[8] Cytotoxic T cells kill target cells within the allograft by several distinct mechanisms.[9] Thus the combined helper T-cell and cytotoxic T-cell activation elicited by the allograft leads to its ultimate destruction.

▲ MAJOR HISTOCOMPATIBILITY COMPLEX AND ANTIGEN-PRESENTING CELLS

Recognition of allograft MHC proteins is central to T-cell immunity and graft rejection. There are two subsets of MHC molecules—MHC class I and MHC class II. These classes have genetic and physical homologies and are encoded by linked genetic loci. In humans, the main MHC class I proteins are called HLA-A, -B, and -C. The main MHC class II proteins are called HLA-DR, -DP, and -DQ. The proteins are encoded by genes of the same names. MHC class I proteins are expressed by almost all nucleated cells, whereas MHC class II proteins are normally expressed mainly by cells of the immune system, including macrophages, dendritic cells, and B lymphocytes. Other cell types, such as endothelial cells, can be induced to express MHC class II proteins in response to inflammatory cytokines, such as interferon-γ, during an ongoing immune response, and can therefore acquire stimulatory roles in allograft rejection responses.[10,11]

The MHC genes are codominantly expressed and are polymorphic; there are at least 50 alleles at each of the six loci. Each person is therefore heterozygous at all or most of the six loci and expresses six different MHC class I and six different MHC class II proteins. The high variability of MHC proteins among individuals is an important limiting factor for transplantation, because it virtually ensures that some MHC alleles are expressed by the graft donor but not by the recipient, leading to the potential for T-cell recognition of the transplant as foreign. One potential therapeutic strategy for reducing allograft responses is reducing graft immunogenicity by reducing the number of MHC disparities between the graft donor and recipient.[12] MHC tissue typing of donor and recipients is an important focus of transplant research and is actively used for some, but not all, organ types, as described in a later section of this chapter. A related, still experimental, strategy aimed at reducing graft immunogenicity would be to reduce expression of all of the MHC proteins on the donor graft, rendering it "invisible" to the recipient's T-cell immune response. Studies with MHC "knock-out" mice,[13–16] in which MHC class I or class II expression or both has been genetically eliminated, have been initiated and may lead to analogous strategies in larger animals. This technology would have its application in the form of xenotransplants rather than allotransplants.

Dendritic cells and macrophages, which express both MHC class I and MHC class II antigens, are the primary initial stimulators of T cells.[17] Dendritic cells and macrophages have therefore been called *professional APC* in recognition of this critical role. The initial priming of T cells can occur in the lymph nodes or at the graft site. In the former case, the donor antigen must migrate to the lymph nodes in the form of either donor or recipient APC. In the latter case, the T cells that predominate in the peripheral blood can find the APC within the graft.

The T cells that coordinate and regulate allograft responses are the helper T cells, which respond best to allogeneic MHC class II proteins expressed by the transplant. Cytotoxic lymphocytes, in contrast, respond best to allogeneic MHC class I proteins expressed by the transplant. Because MHC class I is expressed on virtually all cell types, virtually all cell types can be attacked by activated cytotoxic T lymphocytes. However, because cytotoxic T-lymphocyte activation often requires initial signaling from activated helper T cells, professional APC are also critical to the generation of cytotoxic T cells.[18]

▲ T-CELL ANTIGEN RECOGNITION, ACTIVATION, AND EFFECTOR FUNCTION

Most therapeutic strategies attempt to modify the recipient T-cell response to the allograft. These strategies are based on the biochemistry of T-cell recognition of foreign antigen and subsequent T-cell activation.[5–7] T-cell recognition of allogeneic MHC (plus peptide) complexes on transplanted cells is mediated by antigen-specific T-cell receptors on the T cells. The T-cell receptor contains highly variable, clonally distributed α and β chains, both of which contribute to the fine specificity of binding of T-cell receptors of each T cell to a particular allograft MHC protein. The α and β chains of the T-cell receptors are noncovalently associated on the T-cell surface with a nonvariable signal-transducing protein complex, the CD3 complex. In addition, each mature T cell expresses either the CD4 or the CD8 protein on its surface. Almost all helper T cells express CD4, which has some binding affinity for nonpolymorphic portions of MHC class II proteins and so may contribute to T-APC avidity. Reciprocally, amost all cytotoxic T cells express CD8, which has some binding affinity for MHC class I and so may contribute to T-stimulator avidity. When a critical threshold number of T-cell receptor/CD3 complexes, plus either CD4 or CD8, on a T cell are cross-linked by binding to allogeneic MHC proteins on the transplanted tissue or organ, activation signals are initiated in the T cell.

This recognition specificity raises the possibility of another mode of therapeutic intervention to reduce allograft rejection.[19] Antibodies directed at either the T-cell receptor/CD3 complex or the CD4/CD8 molecules can block T-cell activation in vitro by directly interfering with T-cell recognition of donor MHC. In vivo application of this type of strategy has been attempted but is difficult, because unintended polyclonal activation of T cells can occur if the antibodies directly cross link T-cell receptor/CD3 complexes and mimic antigen recognition by the T cells. A related strategy is to use such anti–T-cell antibodies in vivo to eliminate the T cells rather than merely block their activation.

A novel mode of therapeutic intervention has been raised by the observation that in most cases, the intracellular signals initiated by T-cell receptor/CD3 (plus CD4 or CD8) cross linking are not sufficient for full T-cell activation. In fact, T-cell receptor/CD3 signals can instead ultimately lead to cellular inactivation, called *cellular anergy,* if they are not accompanied by additional signals induced in the T cell by other, antigen-nonspecific receptors. This observation is consistent with the idea, originally proposed by Bretscher and Cohn,[20] that each lymphocyte needs two qualitatively different signals for activation. Signal 1 acts by way of the T-cell receptor and is antigen specific, whereas signal 2 acts by way of one of the auxiliary receptors and is not antigen specific but is produced when the T-cell successfully interacts with an appropriate, competent partner cell such as an APC. At present, the best documented signal 2 system is associated with cross linking of CD28 molecules on helper T cells by interaction with members of the B7 protein family on APC. CD28-initiated signals can prevent induction of anergy in T cells and may prolong T-cell survival. Reagents that can block CD28/B7 interactions in vivo have been described and are being tested for therapeutic efficacy.[21] The injection of APC-depleted donor cells before or with the organ transplant could be another means to anergize allograft-specific T cells in the recipient by providing a stimulus for signal 1 in the absence of signal 2.

Some helper T cells appear to use the soluble APC-derived cytokine interleukin-1, which binds to interleukin-1 receptors on the T cell, for generation of signal 2. Signal 2 for at least some cytotoxic T lymphocytes instead appears to be induced by cytokines such as interleukin-2 and interferon-γ produced and secreted by helper T cells. Strategies aimed at blocking these cytokine activities could therefore block T-cell activation in response to allogeneic MHC on the donor graft.

Once a T cell has received a coordinated signal 1 plus signal 2 stimulus, intracellular second-messenger systems such as calcium mobilization and protein kinase activation initiate a cascade that ultimately results in cellular proliferation and the transcription and translation of genes that encode the functional effector proteins of the cell. These proteins are predominantly cytokines in the case of helper T cells.[8] The precise cytokines produced define subsets of helper T cells, the TH1 cells and TH2 cells. TH1 cells produce interleukin-2 and interferon-γ, whereas TH2 cells produce interleukins-4, -5, and -10. This difference in cytokine production leads to important differences in the functional activities of TH1 and TH2 cells. TH1 cytokines activate primarily cytotoxic T lymphocytes and macrophages and therefore promote cell-mediated immunity that is directly relevant to transplant rejection. TH2 cytokines activate primarily B cells and therefore promote humoral immunity.[22]

The cytokines produced and secreted by helper T cells (and by other cells) act by binding to cytokine receptors on the surface of cytotoxic T lymphocytes, B cells, the helper T cells themselves, macrophages, and other cells. Binding of cytokines to cytokine receptors induces activation signals in the target cells that lead to new protein production, cellular proliferation, differentiation, and effector function.

The activation of T cells leading to cytokine production is one of the main immune regulatory points at which immunosuppressive strategies are currently directed.[23] Drugs such as cyclosporine and tacrolimus interrupt the intracellular signaling cascade initiated by T-cell receptor/CD3 cross linking, preventing initiation of immune responses. Similarly, drugs such as sirolimus (rapamycin) block the activity of some cytokines by interrupting the intracellular signaling cascade initiated by the binding of the cytokine to its cytokine receptor. These strategies have the advantage of being quite potent but have the important disadvantage of being antigen-nonspecific, so that immune responses to opportunistic pathogens also are suppressed.

Once helper T cells have become activated and have provided cytotoxic T lymphocytes and macrophages with cytokines to activate or augment the effector mechanisms of those cells, the rejection of an allograft by these effector cell types is possible. The first step in this process is the migration of activated leukocytes to the graft site followed by infiltration of these cells into the graft tissue. Leukocyte migration and tissue entry depend on expression of adhesion molecules on both the leukocytes and the vascular endothelium.[24,25] Critical leukocyte adhesion molecules include LFA-1, VLA-4, and L-selectin; critical vascular endothelial adhesion molecules include ICAM-1, ICAM-2, and VCAM-1. Cell-cell interactions facilitated by these adhesion molecules allow the T cells and macrophages to slow their movement through the bloodstream, adhere to the vascular endothelium at the graft site, and migrate across the endothelial barrier by diapedesis. Once the leukocytes have entered the graft and are in direct contact with donor organ cells, transplant destruction can proceed. Interference with the expression or function of adhesion molecules at the graft site, perhaps by the use of antibodies to these structures, could therefore represent a feasible strategy for modulating the strength of the rejection response.

The effector phase of cytotoxic T-lymphocyte activity has both an immunologically specific antigen-recognition stage and an immunologically nonspecific cytotoxic stage.[26] Recognition of the allogeneic MHC on the graft by the antigen-specific T-cell receptors of the cytotoxic T cells in conjunction with auxiliary nonspecific cytotoxic T-lymphocyte/target adhesion triggers the cytotoxic stage in the cytotoxic T cells, which then can kill graft cells.[9] Activated cytotoxic T lymphocytes are rich in intracellular cytoplasmic granules that contain proteins believed to contribute to the ultimate destruction of the graft target cell. At target-cell recognition, the cytotoxic T-lymphocyte granules are mobilized to the face of the cytotoxic T cell bound to the allogeneic target cell. Some of the granules and their contents are then released into the narrow space between the cytotoxic T cells and the target by a process called *granule exocytosis.* The granule proteins include a protein related to the C9 component of the complement membrane attack complex. This protein, known as *cytolysin* or *perforin,* can insert into the target-cell membrane to produce a pore. The cytotoxic T-lymphocyte granules also contain a number of serine proteases called *granzymes* (granule enzymes) whose function is unclear but may include activation of cytolysin, alteration of target-cell surface structures, or entry into the target cell after it is perforated by cytolysin.

This latter proposed action of the serine proteases may be central to target-cell death. In some, if not all, instances of target-cell killing by cytotoxic T lymphocytes the target cell undergoes programmed cell death, or *apoptosis.* Apoptotic cell death involves many intracellular reactions, most notably the extensive fragmentation of the DNA of the cell by the cell's own nucleases. Serine proteases have been reported to activate apoptosis in membrane-permeabilized cells, and these proteases may therefore function as a mediator of target-cell death by activation of endogenous nucleases. A second apoptosis-inducing mechanism used by cytotoxic T lymphocytes to kill allogeneic target cells involves the engagement of the Fas protein on the target cell by the Fas ligand on the cytotoxic T lymphocyte. Fas is a cell surface protein expressed on many histologically distinct cell types that can initiate the apoptotic pathway when cross linked to its ligand (or by anti-Fas antibodies). After delivery of its lethal hit to the target cell, the cytotoxic T lymphocyte disengages and can seek out and kill another allograft target cell.

This scenario of cytotoxic T-lymphocyte effector function raises several possible means to suppress graft destruction by cytotoxic T lymphocytes. In addition to blocking the initial activation and differentiation of the cytotoxic T lymphocytes as outlined in the discussion of nonspecific T-cell immunosuppression, strategies might be devised to inhibit the cytotoxic machinery of the cytotoxic T cell itself. For example, in an allogeneic transplant setting, antibodies against the Fas ligand on cytotoxic T cells or soluble forms of Fas might be used to protect the graft by interfering with Fas engagement with Fas ligand. In a xenogeneic transplant setting, genetic elimination of Fas expression on the graft would inhibit Fas-induced apoptosis in xenograft cells. Similarly, donor grafts might be genetically modified to express an inactivator of perforin. These strategies are clearly speculative at this time, but they have the advantage of inhibiting only the transplant-specific cytotoxic T lymphocyte activity while sparing the recipient's cytotoxic T-cell immunity against intracellular pathogens.

Macrophages are also important participants in cell-mediated immunity to, and rejection of, allografts. Helper T cells produce and secrete cytokines that attract macrophages to the graft site and then inhibit their escape, thereby increasing the number of effector cells available for graft destruction.[27] Helper T cells also produce and secrete cytokines that activate macrophages to develop cytotoxic activity; interferon-γ is particularly effective in this regard. Interference with cytokine production and action by the immunosuppressive drugs already mentioned may therefore also protect the graft from macrophage-induced damage. The ability of an immunosuppressive strategy to affect several components of the allograft response reflects the highly interrelated nature of the immune components and highlights the central role of the helper T cells in initiating and perpetuating the rejection reaction.

▲ T-CELL TOLERANCE INDUCTION

This overview of allograft responses presumes that T cells specific for MHC antigens expressed on the graft exist in the recipient at the time of transplantation. The immunosuppressive strategies proposed to protect the allograft therefore focus on preventing T-cell activation, differentiation, and effector function. A distinct strategy would be to eliminate allograft-specific T cells from the recipient, producing immunologic tolerance of the graft. Such strategies are being developed for possible clinical use in the not-too-distant future. They usually entail elimination of most or all of the pre-existing mature T cells in the recipient followed by induction of a new wave of T-cell generation in the thymus to provide a new cohort of mature T cells to the periphery. During generation of the new cohort of T cells, donor APC expressing donor MHC alloantigens can be introduced into the recipient thymus so that donor-specific immature T cells are deleted from the thymic T-cell population. The optimal type of donor cell to be used is not yet clear, but a bone marrow–derived hemopoietic stem cell would be most likely to provide a long-lived donor cellular component in the thymus to maintain tolerance to the donor alloantigens.[28] This strategy has the obvious advantage that the recipient's immune system is fully intact and can respond to all foreign antigens with the single exception of those expressed on the donor graft.

Immunologic Monitoring

Adriana Zeevi

Many attempts have been made to develop in vitro procedures that can be used for reliable and accurate assessment of the immunologic status of the allograft. Immunologic monitoring can, in theory, be used to differentiate rejection from other forms of dysfunction, such as infection or primary nonfunction. Furthermore, the ideal tool would allow one to gauge accurately a patient's response to antirejection therapy and might help prevent overimmunosuppression. Immune monitoring also can be important in helping to predict which recipients can have their immunosuppression reduced without increasing the risk for acute and chronic rejection. Although no one immunologic test can accomplish all these tasks, there are a number of tests which can be used together to assess the immunologic status of transplant recipients.

▲ ASSESSMENT OF IMMUNOCOMPETENCE

Increased immunosuppression, which is associated with the development of opportunistic infections, may also affect immune reactivity. Strober et al[29] reported suppression of in vitro proliferative responses and an increase in viral infections in renal transplant recipients as long as 1 year after total lymphoid irradiation. A significant correlation between suppressed helper T-cell function and the incidence of opportunistic infections was reported also in recipients of lung transplants[30] and in pediatric patients with human immunodeficiency virus (HIV) type 1 infections.[31]

Helper T-cell functional status can be assessed in vitro according to the amount of interleukin-2 production or the proliferation of T cells in response to various stimuli, including soluble antigens (influenza or tetanus toxoid, which are recall antigen responses), alloantigens, and mitogens (concanavalin A [ConA] and phytohemagglutinin [PHA]).[30,31] Significant inhibition of helper T function was observed in renal transplant recipients at the time of cytomegalovirus (CMV) infection; after recovery, the helper T responses were fully restored.

▲ MONITORING THE DEVELOPMENT OF ANTI-HLA ANTIBODIES

As discussed in Chapter 1, the currently available immunosuppressive regimens are not routinely effective in the prevention or control of chronic rejection. Anti–human leukocyte antigen (HLA) antibodies may contribute to the development and progression of chronic rejection. Several investigators have shown in kidney and heart transplant recipients that long-term survival is lower in patients who develop anti-HLA antibodies after transplantation than in patients who do not develop these antibodies.[33–35] Suciu-Foca et al[33] identified anti-HLA antibodies in 57% of the sera obtained from patients undergoing chronic rejection of renal allografts compared with only 5% in patients who kept their graft for 4 years.[34] In addition, they showed that long-term graft loss was associated with the presence of immune complexes formed by soluble HLA antigens (released from the injured graft) and the circulating anti-HLA antibodies.[33,34] The rate of chronic graft loss was lower among recipients who developed anti-idiotypic antibodies that blocked the cytotoxic activity of the antigraft HLA antibodies.[33,34]

Lobo et al[35] showed that acute rejection associated with the development of donor-specific anti-HLA antibodies was a poor prognostic factor for kidney graft survival. In addition, the prevalence of anti-HLA antibodies in patients' sera depleted of soluble HLA antigens was significantly increased in kidney and heart transplant recipients with chronic rejection but not in patients without rejection.[33,36]

The evaluation of anti-HLA antibodies in sequential samples of sera thus may be a useful tool for the prediction of graft outcome. Monitoring of anti-HLA antibodies also should be performed on sera depleted of HLA antigens that may mask the presence of anti-HLA antibodies.

▲ ASSESSMENT OF DONOR-SPECIFIC HYPOREACTIVITY

An important goal in the long-term care of transplant recipients is to reduce maintenance immunosuppression to a minimum. In vitro testing for the development of donor-specific hyporeactivity has been studied by several investigators.[37–43] Though both mixed lymphocyte culture (MLC) and cell-mediated lymphocytotoxicity (CML) assays have been used to identify patients who are hyporeactive to donor antigens, it appears that the MLC is a better predictive tool than the CML assay.

The evaluation of donor-specific hyporeactivity is based on MLC assays in which recipient cells are used as responders and the donor splenocytes and control third-party panel cells as stimulators.[32] To determine the degree of donor-specific hyporeactivity, recipients' donor-specific ML responses at various times after transplantation are compared with both recipients' pretransplant MLC and their responses to third-party control cells. Donor-specific hyporeactivity is defined as at least a 70% decrease in posttransplant versus pretransplant donor-specific ML response while reactivity to both third-party control stimulator cells and mitogens is maintained.[32,44] Reinsmoen et al[42,43] used homozygous typing cells (HTCs), cells that are well-characterized with respect to HLA and are homozygous for HLA class II DR antigens. These HTCs were used as stimulators in the MLC to identify possible hyporeactivity of recipients' cells to donor HLA class II antigens.

Improved long-term renal transplant outcome has been associated with the development of in vitro donor-specific hyporeactivity.[43,45] Patients who exhibited donor-specific hyporeactivity had fewer episodes of late acute rejection than the reactive patients and were free of chronic rejection.[43] In one center, donor-specific hyporeactivity in MLC has been used as a criterion for discontinuation of prednisone.[45] Thus stable donor-specific hyporeactivity might be a useful parameter for identification of recipients who may be able to taper immunosuppression.

However, sequential testing is needed for monitoring of the recipient's immune status, particularly if immunosuppression has been modified. We and others have observed in some renal transplant recipients the development of donor-specific hyporeactivity while they were on steroid or triple drug therapy.[32,46] After steroid withdrawal, a few patients became donor reactive and experienced late acute cellular rejection. Thus sequential immunologic monitoring after transplantation was more informative than a single evaluation to help predict the patients' immune status.

▲ QUANTITATION OF DONOR ANTIGEN–REACTIVE HELPER CELLS

Lymphokine-secreting helper T cells have been shown to be an important component of allograft rejection.[47] Acute allograft rejection is associated with increased numbers of donor-reactive helper T lymphocytes in renal and cardiac allografts.[32,48] Furthermore, recent studies in recipients of cardiac transplants showed that long-term graft acceptance was associated with a decrease in donor-reactive helper T lymphocytes.[49] In this study frequencies of helper T lymphocytes were determined using peripheral blood samples before transplantation and 1 month and 1 year after transplantation. Patients with stable graft function had lower frequencies of helper T lymphocytes 1 year after transplantation and were withdrawn from steroids. In contrast, the MLC-reactive recipients who maintained large numbers of donor reactive helper T lymphocytes 1 year after transplantation experienced persistent rejection and required more immunosuppression.[49] Quantitation of donor-specific helper T lymphocytes was done by limiting dilution analysis.[32,48] The minimal frequency of helper T lymphocytes was calculated with a computer program.[48]

We have also found that the frequency of donor-specific helper T cells in bone marrow augmented renal transplant recipients correlated with the donor MLC profile.[4] Increased donor-specific helper T-lymphocyte frequency was associated with a reactive MLC pattern and clinical rejection.[32,44] Finally, increased frequency of host-reactive helper T lymphocytes were found to be predictive of the severity of graft-versus-host disease (GVHD) in recipients of bone marrow transplants.[50] We believe that serial rather than random monitoring of donor-specific helper T lymphocyte frequency could be useful in predicting allograft outcome after changes in immunosuppression.

▲ PROPAGATION OF LYMPHOCYTE CULTURES FROM ALLOGRAFT BIOPSIES

The histologic evaluation of biopsies from rejected organ transplants has shown infiltration of mononuclear cells. In human studies characterization of these cells with immunohistochemical staining demonstrated a preponderance of T cells. Both CD4 (helper) and CD8 (cytotoxic) subsets were present in the graft and expressed interleukin-2 receptors and HLA class II DR antigens, indicating that they were activated T cells. Several studies in all solid organ (heart, liver, lung, and kidney) allografts suggested that in vitro proliferation of lymphocytes infiltrating the allograft identifies activated T cells, which mediate acute cellular rejection. These activated T cells manifest donor-specific alloreactivity.

Lymphocyte growth in cardiac transplant recipients correlated with the histologic grade of rejection, and positive growth from histologically negative biopsy specimens was associated with subsequent biopsy-proven rejection.[51,52] Lymphocyte growth from renal transplant biopsies also correlated with acute cellular rejection, and the production of interleukin-2 by the infiltrating cells was associated with irreversible rejection.[53]

The lymphocyte growth assay is a technically simple assay that may contribute to the clinical management of kidney transplant recipients. Demonstrating lymphocyte growth in certain situations, such as follow-up biopsies after treatment of rejection, may define a high-risk group who require augmented immunosuppression.

▲ INTRAGRAFT EXPRESSION OF CYTOKINE mRNA

Accurate diagnosis of acute cellular rejection is critical to the successful clinical management of renal transplant recipients. Much work has been done in the assessment of intragraft cytokine gene expression in an attempt to improve the diagnostic methods and to promote a better understanding of the mechanisms involved in allograft rejection.[54–56] Lipman et al[57] showed that the detection of cytotoxic T lymphocyte–specific serine protease gene expression was seen almost exclusively in rejecting samples, indicating that cytotoxic T lymphocytes are important effectors of graft dysfunction in the process of allograft rejection. Granzyme B, which belongs to the serine protease family, and perforin, which is the cytolytic pore-forming protein, are expressed in cytolytic granules of activated cytotoxic T cells. Both molecules are expressed in infiltrating lymphocytes during rejection of renal, cardiac, and lung allografts.[58–61] Immune staining with anti–granzyme B and anti-perforin monoclonal antibodies, as well as detection of gene transcripts for these molecules, was significantly associated with allograft rejection.[61,62] In addition, their absence coincided with stable function. These results suggest that granzyme B and perforin expression could constitute an effective modality for monitoring transplant recipients as long as appropriate tissue specimens are available. Recently, Xu et al[63] found that intragraft interleukin-10 messenger RNA (mRNA) expression was associated with renal allograft rejection.[31,33] Although the expression of interleukin-2 mRNA was also increased in rejecting kidneys, the sensitivity of interleukin-2 mRNA expression during acute rejection was much lower than that observed for interleukin-10 mRNA.[63] These results are intriguing in light of the immunosuppressive property of interleukin-10 that is believed to dampen the immune response by inhibiting the release of proinflammatory cytokines.[64] However, under some conditions, interleukin-10 may function in vivo as an immunostimulatory polypeptide.[65] Detection of cytokine gene expression in allograft biopsies may shed new light on intragraft events during different processes, but it is not a simple or straightforward method for prospective monitoring of allograft rejection.

Mechanisms of Action of Immunosuppressive Agents

Angus W. Thomson

Immunosuppressive agents are widely used in both solid organ and bone marrow transplantation. Over the past 25 years, the development of more powerful and more selective immunosuppressive drugs has revolutionized the field of transplantation. These agents, which have diverse modes of action (Table 8–1), also provide powerful tools for the investigation of the molecular mechanisms underlying immune responses. There have been several recent reviews[66–71] of immunosuppressive and antiinflammatory drugs, to which the reader is referred for more detailed information.

▲ ADRENAL CORTICOSTEROIDS

Adrenal corticosteroids are the immunosuppressive agents most commonly used in clinical practice.[72,73] The many diverse antiinflammatory actions of glucocorticoids make them potent immunosuppressants. Within the first 6 hours of steroid administration, a profound decrease occurs in the blood lymphocyte count. In humans, this decrease reflects a redistribution of lymphocytes from the intravascular space into lymphoid tissues. Recirculating lymphocytes (approximately two thirds of all lymphocytes) are mainly T cells, which travel back and forth between the intravascular compartment and lymphoid tissues such as the spleen, bone marrow, thoracic duct, and lymph nodes. Sessile lymphocytes, including some T and most B cells, stay within the lymphoid compartment. Glucocorticoids cause emigration of the recirculating T cells from the intravascular compartment to the lymphoid tissues with less effect on the distribution of B cells. The mechanism of lymphocyte distribution is probably an alteration in cell surface phenotype that promotes adhesion to the vascular endothelium.

An important property of steroids appears to be their ability to inhibit cytokine (interleukins-1 and -6, tumor necrosis factor [TNF]) gene transcription and secre-

TABLE 8–1 ▲ MODES OF ACTION IMMUNOSUPPRESSIVE DRUGS

Alteration of gene expression
Cyclosporine
Tacrolimus (FK 506)
Inhibition of cytokine action
Sirolimus (rapamycin)
Inhibition of DNA synthesis
Blockade of purine biosynthesis
Mizoribine
Mycophenolate mofetil
Blockade of pyrimidine biosynthesis
Brequinar
Inhibition of cell maturation
Deoxyspergualin

tion by macrophages. Steroids also suppress the production and effects of T-cell cytokines, which amplify the responses of lymphocytes and macrophages. Thus interleukin-2 production and the binding of interleukin-2 to its receptor is inhibited by glucocorticoids. Moreover, steroids block the ability of macrophages to respond to lymphocyte-derived signals such as migration inhibition factor and macrophage activation factor. These effects may underlie the marked inhibition of delayed-type hypersensitivity reactions observed with these agents. Steroids, however, have little net effect on antibody production. An additional effect of steroids is the suppression of prostaglandin synthesis.

Some of the molecular mechanisms by which glucocorticoids exert their effects have been recently elucidated. Much of the steroid action is initiated at the subcellular level by means of hormone receptors. Unlike polypeptide mediators with receptors on the cell surface, steroids move freely through the cell membrane and bind to receptors in the cytoplasm, producing steroid-receptor complexes. These complexes then move into the nucleus, where they attach to DNA. They act on gene promoters either to depress or to activate part of the genome and influence the transcription of specific messenger RNAs. Thus protein synthesis may be differentially down- or up-regulated.

Specific cytoplasmic receptors for glucocorticoids have been identified in normal human lymphocytes, monocytes, neutrophils, and eosinophils. In addition, varying degrees of receptor density have been demonstrated in different lymphoid cell subpopulations. The sensitivity of a particular subpopulation of lymphocytes is presumed to relate to the relative density of the intracytoplasmic steroid receptors. These messengers can act to inhibit DNA, RNA, and protein synthesis. Glucose and amino acid transport also may be affected.

The effectiveness of cortisone in suppressing allograft rejection was first recognized more than 40 years ago when it was found to prolong skin graft survival in rabbits. In organ transplantation, steroids are not effective by themselves but are valuable when used in combination with other agents. In high doses, steroids are especially useful in reversing ongoing graft rejection, but their prolonged use leads to unacceptable side effects, including hypertension, weight gain, hyperglycemia, peptic ulceration, and gastrointestinal bleeding. Increased susceptibility to pyogenic and opportunistic infections is a direct result of the suppression by steroids of microbial killing by macrophages and neutrophils. The outcome of clinical organ transplantation will improve when more specific means of immunosuppression are developed for routine use and existing steroid dosages can be reduced substantially or eliminated.

▲ ANTIPROLIFERATIVE AGENTS

Antiproliferative agents inhibit immune responses by preventing differentiation and division of immunocompetent lymphocytes after their encounter with antigen.[74] They either resemble essential metabolites in structure or combine with certain cellular components to interfere with cellular function. Their effects are exerted late in the cell cycle compared with other immunosuppressive agents (Table 8–2).

Methotrexate

Methotrexate, a folic acid antagonist, inhibits the enzyme dihydrofolate reductase. It prevents conversion of folic acid to tetrahydrofolic acid, which is necessary for the synthesis of DNA, RNA, and certain coenzymes. The low therapeutic ratio of immunosuppression to toxicity has precluded the use of methotrexate in most clinical settings outside of bone marrow transplantation.

Cyclophosphamide

Cyclophosphamide belongs to the class of alkylating agents. These drugs have highly reactive rings that combine with electron-rich nucleophilic groups, such as the tertiary nitrogens in purines and pyrimidines. The alkylating agents combine with these constituents to form stable covalent bonds. Alkylation of DNA strands, if not repaired, results in faulty chromosomal replication. Cyclophosphamide acts on both humoral and cellular immune responses. B lymphocytes appear to be more susceptible than T cells. The drug is a potent inhibitor of antibody formation. However, the usefulness of cyclophosphamide is limited by its toxicity.

Azathioprine

Azathioprine (Imuran, Burroughs Wellcome, Research Triangle Park, NC) was the most widely used immunosuppressive drug until the introduction of cyclosporine

TABLE 8–2 ▲ DIFFERENTIAL EFFECTS OF IMMUNOSUPPRESSIVE AGENTS ON CELL SIGNALING IN THE REJECTION RESPONSE

		Phase of Cell Cycle Affected				
Agent	**APC Function**	G_0	G_1 *(Early)*	G_1 *(Late)*	*S*	**Immune Amplification**
OKT3		+				
Antilymphocyle globulin		+				
Anti-ICAM		+				
Anti-CD28		+				
Cyclosporine	(+)		+			(+)
Tacrolimus			+			(+)
Sirolimus	(+)			+		
Anti–interleukin-2R				+		
Antisense nucleotides				+		
Azathioprine					+	
Mycophenolate mofetil					+	
Mizoribine					+	
Brequinar					+	

APC, antigen presenting cell; + principal effect; (+), secondary effect, often dose dependent.
Modified from Thomson AW, and Starzl TE (eds), *Immunosuppressive Drugs.* Boston, Little, Brown, 1994:63–81.

into widespread clinical use in 1983. Azathioprine interferes with DNA synthesis. Several other agents have since been developed that interfere selectively with DNA synthesis in lymphocytes. Azathioprine is cleaved to 6-mercaptopurine principally by erythrocyte glutathione. 6-Mercaptopurine is then converted into a series of mercaptopurine-containing nucleotides that interfere with the synthesis of DNA and polyadenylate-containing RNA. The synthesis and action of coenzymes are disrupted, and chromosomal breaks occur. By interfering with mitosis, azathioprine affects the division of both T and B lymphocytes. Unfortunately, the antiproliferative activity of azathioprine is not limited to lymphocytes; this accounts for the toxicity of the drug.

Mycophenolate Mofetil

Mycophenolate mofetil (CellCept, Roche Laboratories, Nutley, NJ) formerly known as RS-61443, is a semisynthetic derivative of the fungal antibiotic mycophenolic acid. It has recently been approved for use in renal transplantation. Mycophenolate mofetil inhibits inosine monophosphate dehydrogenase (IMPDH), the rate-limiting enzyme in guanosine monophosphate (GMP) synthesis.[75,76] Lymphocyte proliferation depends on de novo purine biosynthesis. Specifically, adequate levels of guanosine and deoxyguanosine nucleotides are required for lymphocyte proliferation, wheras an excess of adenosine or deoxyadenosine nucleotides inhibits proliferation. This is mediated by allosteric inhibition of ribonucleotide reductase. By inhibiting IMPDH, guanosine nucleotides are depleted. Lymphocytes do not contain the enzymes of the salvage pathway to compensate for this depletion. With subsequent reduction of ribonucleotide reductase activity, DNA synthesis is suppressed. Mycophenolate mofetil has advantages over nucleoside analogues that inhibit DNA repair enzymes and produce chromosomal breaks, both of which are mutagenic effects. Because mycophenolate mofetil inhibits an enzyme involved in purine biosynthesis, it has no direct effects on DNA.

Mycophenolate mofetil does not inhibit gene expression or signal transduction. Mycophenolate mofetil–mediated depletion of guanosine triphosphate (GTP) inhibits the transfer of fucose and mannose to glycoproteins, some of which are adhesion molecules.[76] By this mechanism, cell-cell interactions can be affected. Some glycoproteins may be sensitive to GTP depletion. This mechanism may account for the near complete inhibition of B-cell antibody formation by mycophenolate mofetil. Antibody formation by polyclonally activated human B lymphocytes is almost completely inhibited by mycophenolate mofetil. Secondary responses of human spleen cells to tetanus toxoid are similarly affected. Mycophenolate mofetil does not deplete GTP in neutrophils and consequently does not affect the growth or responses of these cells to chemoattractants or their ability to produce superoxide and kill bacteria.

Mizoribine

Mizoribine (Bredinin) is an antibiotic substance isolated from culture filtrates of *Eupenicillium brefeldianum.* Mizoribine exerts strong suppressive activity on lymphocyte growth.[77,78] Mizoribine is metabolized into an active form, mizoribine 5′-monophosphate (MZ-5-P) by adenosine kinase. This product inhibits GMP synthesis from inosine monophosphate (IMP). IMPDH, and to a lesser extent GMP synthase, are targeted by MZ-5-P, resulting in almost complete inhibition of guanosine nucleotide synthesis and subsequent DNA synthesis. MZ-5-P is dephosphorylated intracellularly and leaves cells when the extracellular concentration falls. The action of mizoribine depends on its continued presence within the cell. Mizoribine inhibits the passage of cells from the G_1 to the S phase of the cell cycle. T and B lymphocyte proliferation is suppressed, although the effects of mizoribine are not limited to these cells. In addition, MZ-5-P can inhibit DNA repair mechanisms, which explains the presence of chromosome breaks in cells treated with mizoribine. The agent exhibits considerable synergism with cyclosporine and tacrolimus and greater safety than azathioprine.[77]

Brequinar Sodium

Brequinar sodium was developed originally as an antimetabolite for cancer chemotherapy. It acts by its ability to inhibit noncompetitively the activity of the enzyme dihydro-orotate dehydrogenase.[79,80] This enzyme catalyzes the conversion of dihydro-orotate to orotate in the de novo pyrimidine synthesis pathway. As with the purine pathway, lymphocytes cannot use the salvage pathway for pyrimidine biosynthesis. In the presence of brequinar, the nucleotide precursors uridine triphosphate (UTP) and cytidine triphosphate (CTP) are depleted, and DNA and RNA synthesis are inhibited. It has been recently noticed that brequinar may inhibit cytidine deaminase,[80] which converts cytidine to uridine. Cytidine, when combined with brequinar complements the antimetabolic effects of the drug.[80] Cells are most sensitive to brequinar during the active, proliferative phase of an immune response, when DNA and RNA synthesis are at high levels. Brequinar inhibits interleukin-6–induced differentiation of human B cells into IgM-secreting plasma cells.[81] Like mizoribine and mycophenolate mofetil, brequinar exhibits additive immunosuppressive activity with cyclosporine. It carries some toxicity, as its effects are not limited to lymphocytes (see below).[79]

▲ T-CELL–DIRECTED IMMUNOSUPPRESSIVE AGENTS

Cyclosporine

The discovery in 1972 by Borel et al of the immunosuppressive properties of the cyclic peptide cyclosporine, (Sandimmune, Sandoz Pharmaceutical Corp, East Hanover, NJ), a fungal metabolite extracted from *Tolypocladium inflatum Gams,* contributed enormously to the rapid and successful growth of the field of clinical organ transplantation, especially of livers and hearts.[82] When introduced into the clinic in 1978 as an experimental agent for the prophylaxis of allograft rejection and GVHD, cyclosporine represented a completely new class of immunosuppressive agents. The selective, suppressive effects of the drug on T cells appear to be related to its selective inhibition of T cell receptor–mediated activation events. Cyclosporine inhibits cytokine production by $CD4^+$ helper T cells in vitro and blocks the development of mature $CD4^+$ and $CD8^+$ T cells in the thymus. Absence of myelosuppression is an important advantage over the antiproliferative immunosuppressive agents.[69,70,82,83]

Analyses of the effect of cyclosporine on T lymphocytes have shown (1) inhibition of both interleukin-2–producing T lymphocytes and cytotoxic T lymphocytes, (2) inhibition of interleukin-2 gene expression by activated T lymphocytes, (3) no inhibition of activated T lymphocytes in response to exogenous interleukin-2, (4) inhibition of resting T-cell activation in response to alloantigen and exogenous cytokine, (5) inhibition of interleukin-1 production, and (6) inhibition of mitogen (conA) activation of interleukin-2–producing T lymphocytes.

A number of kidney and other solid organ transplantation trials showed that cyclosporine induced potent immunosuppression without myelosuppression. The introduction of cyclosporine into widespread clinical use in 1983 led to substantial improvement in the outcome of cadaveric renal transplantation and allowed the widespread practice of heart and liver replacement.

In addition to nephrotoxicity, the potential adverse effects of cyclosporine include hypertension, hyperkalemia, hirsutism, gingival hyperplasia, tremor and other neurotoxicities, diabetogenicity, and hepatotoxicity. As with other immunosuppressive agents, cyclosporine therapy increases the risk of infection and malignancy but, by reducing steroid requirements, generally decreases infection rates.

Tacrolimus

Tacrolimus (Prograf, Fujisawa USA, Inc, Deerfield, IL [formerly known as FK 506]) is a potent new immunosuppressive agent with a mechanism of action similar but not identical to that of cyclosporine. The agent was isolated in 1984 in Japan from the soil fungus *Streptomyces tsukubaensis*. It is a macrocyclic lactone with a molecular weight of 822 daltons and is structurally distinct from cyclosporine. Both cyclosporine and tacrolimus are now regarded as *prodrugs*. Their antilymphocytic effects result from the formation of active complexes between the drug and its respective intracellular binding protein or *immunophilin*[70] (cyclophilin or FK 506–binding protein [FKBP]). The drug-immunophilin complex blocks the phosphatase activity of calcineurin, a molecule that is important in the regulation of interleukin-2 gene transcription.[69,70] The activity of tacrolimus in vitro, however, is approximately 100 times greater than that of cyclosporine. Like cyclosporine, tacrolimus functions to inhibit (1) interleukin-2 gene expression and interleukin-2 production, (2) T-lymphocyte proliferation in mixed lymphocyte culture, (3) generation of cytotoxic T cells, and (4) the appearance of interleukin-2R on human lymphocytes. In vivo, tacrolimus has been shown to prolong the survival of MHC-disparate skin, cardiac, renal, hepatic, and small-intestinal allografts. Tacrolimus was approved in 1994 for liver transplant recipients. The side effects of cyclosporine and tacrolimus are similar, although tacrolimus does not cause hirsutism or gum hypertrophy.

Sirolimus

Like tacrolimus, the experimental immunosuppressant sirolimus (rapamycin, Rapamune, Wyeth-Ayerst Research, Princeton, NJ) is a macrolide antibiotic. It is a close structural analogue of tacrolimus and binds to the same cytoplasmic receptor (FKBP). Unlike tacrolimus or cyclosporine, however, sirolimus does not block T-cell cytokine gene expression but instead inhibits the transduction of signals from interleukin-2R to the nucleus.[69,70,84] Binding of sirolimus to FKBP inhibits P70S6 protein kinase activity, which is essential for ribosomal phosphorylation and cell cycle progression. Sirolimus potently inhibits experimental allograft rejection. Two additional important properties of this drug are that it acts synergistically with cyclosporine and prevents chronic graft vessel disease in rat transplant models.[84] The combination of sirolimus with low-dose cyclosporine and the use of sirolimus for prevention of chronic rejection and atheromatous disease are important future clinical considerations. However, promiscuity of the inhibitory action of the drug on the response of hematopoietic cells to growth factors and poor oral bioavailability are considered potential clinical limitations.

▲ EICOSANOIDS

Eicosanoids are the largest class of lipid mediators. They are produced by all human cells except lymphocytes and possess a wide variety of biologic activities. The term includes the oxygenation products of long-chain polyunsaturated fatty acids, such as arachidonic acid and linolenic acid, essential fatty acids, and the compounds such as prostaglandins into which they are incorporated for synthesis. The immunomodulatory effects of the eicosanoids are mediated by direct actions on cells and also by indirect influences on the release of platelet-activating factor, cytokines, and other substances.[72] The antirejection eicosanoids (prostaglandin [PG] E_2 and PGD_2) inhibit T-cell proliferation by inhibition of interleukins-1 and -2 and MHC class II antigen expression on macrophages. Other prorejection eicosanoids (thromboxane A_2, leukotrienes B_4, [C_4 and D_4]) enhance T-cell proliferation. Investigations are preliminary but promising, and potential clinical applications to control or prevent rejection by manipulating these agents await further study.

▲ LYMPHOCYTE-DEPLETING AGENTS

Several clinically important immunosuppressive agents are effective because they deplete the host of lymphocytes. As the mechanism of action of these agents becomes understood, a more sophisticated classification system may evolve. For the present, antilymphocyte globulin (ALG) and monoclonal antibody (mAb) therapy appear to act by relatively nonselective lymphocyte depletion or inactivation.[72,85]

Antilymphocyte Globulin

ALGs are produced when lymphocytes are injected into animals of a different species. Rabbit, goat, and horse antisera are commonly used.[72] The action of ALG appears to be directed mainly against T cells; the use of thymocytes for immunization therefore results in the most potent sera. As would be expected, ALG administration interferes most with the cell-mediated reactions—allograft rejection, tuberculin sensitivity, and the graft versus host reaction. ALG can abolish pre-existing delayed hypersensitivity reactions, and larger doses prolong the survival of some xenografts. ALG has a definite, but lesser effect on T-cell–dependent antibody production. Lymphocytes coated with ALG are either lysed or cleared from the blood by reticuloendothelial cells in the liver and spleen. ALG may be administered prophylactically during the early posttransplant period, or it may be used to reverse ongoing rejection. Favorable results depend on the potency of the specific ALG preparation and on prolonged administration rather than a single dose. The use of ALG is not confined to renal transplantation; beneficial results have been reported in other solid organ and in bone marrow transplantation.

The toxicity of any heterologous serum prepared against human tissue depends on two factors: (1) its cross reactivity with other tissue antigens and (2) the ability of the patient to make antibodies against the foreign protein. Anemia and thrombocytopenia can occur and are presumably caused by a reaction between the ALG and host erythrocytes and platelets. Although prior absorption with human platelets and red cell stroma reduces the severity of these side effects, some cross reactivity with these cells persists in all ALG preparations.

Monoclonal Antibody

Monoclonal antibodies have been produced that react with T cells in general (OKT3, anti-CD3) and various T-cell subsets (OKT4, anti-CD4; OKT8, anti-CD8). OKT3 (muromonab-CD3, Orthoclone OKT3, Ortho, Raritan, NJ), first used clinically in 1980, has become the most useful therapeutic mAb. It is used to treat established episodes of acute kidney, liver, heart, or heart-lung rejection. The prophylactic potency of regimens that include OKT3 in renal transplantation has also been demonstrated. OKT3 binds to a site associated with the T-cell receptor (CD3) and functions to modulate the receptor and inactivate T-cell function.[86,87]

By engaging the T-cell receptor complex, OKT3 blocks not only the function of naive T cells but also the function of established cytotoxic T cells, blocking cell-mediated cytotoxicity. OKT3 has been shown to block the T-cell effector functions involved in allograft rejection. After intravenous administration, OKT3 opsonizes or binds to T cells. These are then removed by the reticuloendothelial cells that reside in liver and spleen. The number of circulating T cells decreases abruptly (30–60 minutes) after the first injection of OKT3. Once administration of OKT3 is stopped, $CD3^+$ cells rapidly return to normal levels.[87]

▲ DEOXYSPERGUALIN: INTERFERENCE WITH CELL MATURATION AND DIFFERENTIATION

The drugs reviewed thus far act at the molecular level by altering gene activation, signal transduction, or DNA synthesis and repair. The mechanism of action of 15-deoxyspergualin (DSG; Spanidin, Nippon Kayaku Co, Ltd, Tokyo, Japan), a synthetic analogue of the antitumor antibiotic spergualin, is not so clearly defined. DSG appears to exert a cytostatic effect on precursor cells, preventing cell differentiation. It also impairs antigen processing and presentation.[88,89] Multiple substances are targeted by DSG. It inhibits the enzymes spermine synthase, spermidine synthase, polyamine oxidase, spermidine-spermine N′-acetyltransferase, and ornithine decarboxylase. The resulting depletion of polyamides prevents synthesis of cellular macromolecules necessary for normal differentiation and function.

DSG binds to Hsc 70, a constitutively expressed member of the heat shock protein (hsp) 70 family.[90,91] Heat shock proteins may be involved in numerous cellular functions. They contain peptide-binding grooves similar to those of MHC molecules, and may play a role in binding and intracellular transport of antigenic peptides in

APCs. This may account for the impairment of antigen presentation to T cells by monocytes exposed to DSG. Heat shock protein 70 and hsp90 form complexes with steroid receptors and possibly cyclophilins and are involved in translocation of proteins to the nucleus. Interference with the normal function of these substances may account for the additional effects of this agent.

DSG inhibits proliferation and differentiation of cytotoxic T lymphocytes, probably by preventing interleukin-2R expression.[90] Helper T-cell functions are not affected. DSG does not affect mitogen responses or the early stage of the MLC. Release of interleukin-2 from T lymphocytes, and release of interleukin-1 from macrophages are not impaired.[89,90] The drug inhibits the mitogenic stage of B cells. Primary and secondary antibody responses are inhibited, as is production of xenophile antibodies. DSG suppresses differentiation of human B cells into plasma cells. It suppresses the production of macrophage activating factor by murine cells stimulated with antigens. DSG impairs superoxide production in cells of the monocyte/macrophage lineage and decreases MHC class II expression and interleukin-1 production in these cells. Antigen presentation by monocytes is inhibited. DSG inhibits lymphokine-activated killer (LAK) cell activity and induces lymphocytopenia, granulocytopenia, and anemia.

▲ NEW DIRECTIONS IN DEVELOPMENT OF ANTIREJECTION THERAPIES

The most important goals in the development of new immunosuppressive modalities for the prevention or treatment of allograft rejection are (1) to narrow the target cell population and (2) to induce donor antigen-specific tolerance in the host. Monoclonal antibodies are uniquely suited for the realization of both these goals because of their remarkable specificity.[91,92] After transplantation of an allograft, only a small fraction of the entire T-lymphocyte pool is activated. The ideal mAb would select only this activated subpopulation for either elimination or modulation. This would result in tolerance by the induction of clone-specific anergy. To date, the emphasis in improving the selectivity of mAb therapy has been on identification of suitable molecular targets expressed on the surface of the graft recipient's responding T cells. Anti–interleukin-2R mAbs are excellent examples of this type of approach. By blocking these receptors, the mAbs interfere directly with the ability of activated T cells to respond to normal growth and differentiation signals.

Anti–Interleukin-2R Monoclonal Antibodies

Interleukin-2R is a complex of several transmembrane polypeptide chains. Two interleukin-2 binding chains, α (CD25; p55) and β (p70) have been characterized. Noncovalent association of these chains form the high-affinity binding site for interleukin-2. The α chain is present only on activated T cells and a subset of activated B cells and APC. Thus anti-CD25 mAb treatment targets a small population of cells enriched for antigen-activated T cells. Several anti-CD25 mAbs have been shown to prolong allograft survival in rodents and nonhuman primates.

In an effort to reduce the immunogenicity of rodent mAbs that results in rapid development of neutralizing human anti-mouse antibodies (HAMA), humanized mAbs have been produced. Anti–Tac-H is the best characterized of these. The immunogenicity of this molecule, as measured by in vivo circulating half-life and by the appearance of circulating anti–Tac-H antibodies, is less than that of murine anti-Tac. Although certain limitations have been encountered with the function of humanized mAbs, these should be overcome by further customization (genetic remodeling) of the molecules.

Anti–Adhesion Molecule Monoclonal Antibodies

Another potentially useful group of mAbs are those that block T-cell adhesion molecules, such as lymphocyte function–associated antigen 1 (LFA-1) or very late-appearing antigen 4 (VLA-4), or their endothelial cell ligands, such as intercellular adhesion molecule-1 (ICAM-1) and vascular cell adhesion molecule-1 (VCAM-1). These mAbs have the ability to prevent T cells from homing to the allograft. ICAM-1 is constitutively expressed on about 20% of blood mononuclear cells and on vascular endothelium. It is readily induced on many cell types, including endothelial and epithelial cells by cytokine-induced activation. ICAM-1 functions as a ligand for LFA-1 that is expressed constitutively on T cells. The LFA-1–ICAM-1 interaction provides a costimulatory signal for T-cell activation that is synergistic to the signal delivered via the T-cell receptor–CD3 complex.

Anti–T-Cell Subset Molecule Monoclonal Antibodies

The CD4 and CD8 molecules are expressed on reciprocal subsets of $CD3^+$, $\alpha\ \beta$ T-cell $receptor^+$ T cells that are classified functionally as helper T cells ($CD4^+$) or cytotoxic or suppressor T cells ($CD8^+$). CD4 and CD8 facilitate intercellular adhesion between T cells and APCs bearing class II and class I MHC-associated antigens, respectively. Both CD4 and CD8 have a role in T-cell receptor–CD3-mediated signal transduction by means of interaction with intracellular protein tyrosine kinase. Anti-CD4 mAbs have demonstrated the ability to prolong allograft survival in rodents and nonhuman primates.

Other Target Molecules

Attempts are being made at the experimental level to induce specific T-cell clonal anergy by preventing T cells from receiving the appropriate costimulatory signals from APCs during their initial encounter with graft alloantigens. Potential targets include CD28 and its homologue cytotoxic T-lymphocyte antigen-4 (CTLA-4) on the T-cell surface. These molecules are involved, because of their interaction with B7 family proteins on APCs, with the delivery of the crucial second signal (in addition to antigen) that is essential for T-cell activation. A soluble form of CTLA-4, the recombinant fusion protein CTLA-4-Ig, has been administered to rodents to prevent the interaction of graft cell B7 molecules with host T-cell CD28 and prevent allograft rejection.[93] There is evidence that under these conditions, the T-cell interleukin-2 gene is not expressed, and the cells become specifically unresponsive to donor alloantigens.

Immunotoxins

Immunotoxins are chemical conjugates between mAbs and either toxin moities (eg, ricin A chain) or radionuclides (eg, yttrium-90 or bismuth-120) that selectively deliver a lethal package to specific target cells. These molecules are under development for use in the treatment of cancer, autoimmune disease, or rejection of solid organ allografts. Anti–pan-T cell (CD5) ricin A chain immunotoxin has already been shown to be effective in steroid-resistant acute GVHD. Yttrium-90–labeled murine anti-Tac (CD25) is more effective than nonlabeled anti-Tac in prolonging primate xenografts, presumably because of highly effective killing of interleukin-2R$^+$ cells.

Fusion Proteins and Immunoligands

Unlike an immunotoxin, which is the product of biochemical fusion of payload toxin to mAb, a fusion protein is the translational product of fusion of the genes that encode the two protein elements. For example, various toxins are being genetically appended to antigen-binding domains of preexisting mAbs. An example is the recombinant immunotoxin anti-Tac (Fv)–PE40, in which the antibody variable domains of the anti-Tac mAb are linked to *Pseudomonas* exotoxin. A second type of mAb fusion protein is one in which the antigen-binding domains of the antibody are replaced with another targeting protein. An example is the bivalent molecule interleukin-2/Fc that possesses functional activity of both the incorporated human proteins. In principle, interleukin-2 directs specific binding of the construct to interleukin-2R–bearing cells while the Fc portion directs cytopathic immune effector functions against the target cells. Such immunoligands offer several potential advantages over antireceptor mAbs, including much greater target specificity and affinity.

Anticytokine Monoclonal Antibodies

Other targets for mAb therapy are the leukocyte-derived cytokines that play important roles in intercellular signaling. Already there is evidence that anti-TNFα and anti-TNFβ enhance cardiac allograft survival in rodents. Other potential cytokine targets include interleukins -1, -2, and -6 and interferon-γ. For further discussion of this topic, the reader is referred to the recent literature.[94]

Antisense Oligonucleotides

A new experimental approach to immunosuppressive therapy is selective gene-targeted treatment. The use of antisense technology has been used to prolong organ allograft survival in mice. ICAM-1 antisense oligonucleotides inhibited rejection of murine cardiac allografts and in combination with anti–LFA-1 mAb induced donor specific tolerance.[95] The oligonucleotides exhibited no toxic side effects and did not elicit an immune response.

Gene Transfer Techniques

This novel molecular approach to the therapy of organ allograft rejection offers the potential for induced expression of immunologically relevant molecules within allografts that impair immunity while avoiding the systemic side effects of conventional immunosuppression. A recent report details the transfer of genes that encode transforming growth factor (TGF)–β1 or viral interleukin-10 (immunosuppressive cytokines) in a mouse cardiac allograft model.[96]

Histocompatibility Testing and Cross Matching

Yuichi Iwaki

Histocompatibility (HLA testing) and cross matching are critical aspects of renal transplantation. This section describes the clinical significance of HLA testing and cross matching.

▲ HISTOCOMPATIBILITY TESTING

The human histocompatibility antigen, called *HLA* (human leukocyte antigen), is a group of cell-surface antigens that immunologically define a given individual. The HLA complex is located on the short arm of chromosome 6 and plays an important role in human organ transplantation.

▲ POLYMORPHISM AND NOMENCLATURE OF HLA

HLA antigens are divided into class I and class II; the distinction is based on structural differences and cell distribution. HLA class I and class II antigens are highly polymorphic. The difference between the two antigens is in antigen processing. Class I molecules present peptide from endogenous protein, and class II molecules present peptides from exogenous protein.

Over the past three decades, a number of researchers have spent a great deal of time and effort identifying these polymorphic antigens by exchanging antisera (and recently DNA probes) through an extensive series of international workshops. Although HLA-A, -B, and -C loci are the class I antigens and HLA DR, DP, and DQ are the class II antigens, the HLA-A, -B, and -DR loci are considered the most clinically important. Table 8–3, which includes 21 HLA-A locus antigens, 52 HLA-B locus antigens, and 20 HLA-DR locus antigens, presents the most recent nomenclature.[97]

TABLE 8–3 ▲ NOMENCLATURE OF HLA ANTIGENS

A	B	B (cont'd)	C	DR
A1	B5	Bw50 (21)	Cw1	DR1
A2	B7	B51 (5)	Cw2	DR2
A3	B8	Bw52 (5)	Cw3	DR3
A11	B12	Bw53	Cw4	DR4
A23 (9)	B13	Bw54 (w22)	Cw5	DR5
A24 (9)	B14	Bw55 (w22)	Cw6	DRw6
A25 (10)	B15	Bw56 (w22)	Cw7	DR7
A26 (10)	B16	Bw57 (17)	Cw8	DRw8
A28	B17	Bw58 (17)	Cw9 (w3)	DR9
A29 (w19)	B18	Bw59	Cw10 (w3)	DRw10
A30 (w19)	B21	Bw60 (w40)	Cw11	DRw11 (5)
A31 (w19)	Bw22	Bw61 (w40)		DRw12
A32 (w19)	B27	Bw62 (15)		DRw13 (w6)
Aw33 (w19)	B35	BW63 (15)		DRw14 (w6)
Aw34 (10)	B37	Bw64 (14)		DRw15 (2)
Aw36	B38 (16)	Bw65 (14)		DRw16 (2)
Aw43	B39 (16)	Bw67		DRw17 (3)
Aw66 (10)	B40	Bw70		DRw18 (3)
Aw68 (10)	Bw41	Bw71 (w70)		DRw52
Aw69 (28)	Bw42	Bw72 (w70)		DRw53
Aw74	B44 (12)	Bw73		
	B45 (12)	Bw75 (15)		
	Bw46	Bw76 (15)		
	Bw47	Bw77 (15)		
	Bw48	Bw4		
	Bw49 (21)	Bw6		

▲ EFFECT OF HLA ANTIGENS IN CLINICAL RENAL TRANSPLANTATION

Although there is no doubt about the existence of an HLA matching effect, there exists controversy about the magnitude and importance of the effect relative to other factors (see Chapter 1). The graft survival rates of living and cadaveric donor transplants reveal both the impact and the limitations of HLA matching. United Network for Organ Sharing (UNOS) data show that 1-year graft survival rates in patients with a two haplotype–matched living-related transplant are 95%–96%, which is higher than that in patients with a one haplotype–matched transplant from a living-related donor, in whom the 1-year graft survival rate ranges from 89% to 93%. However, the results with zero haplotype–matched siblings and living-unrelated donors are not terribly different from those with one haplotype–matched living donors; the survival rate ranges from 87% to 96%. All of these recipients of organs from living donors have generally better outcomes than recipients of transplants from cadavers. The 1-year graft survival rate for first cadaver kidneys averages 84%. Longer-term graft survival rates also tend to split between living and cadaveric donors, spousal donors behaving as one haplotype–matched parents. These data cause one to call into question the dogma that matching is the most important determinant of graft survival.

There is an HLA matching effect in cadaveric renal transplant recipients. The most unequivocal finding is the significantly better outcome in zero antigen–mismatched kidneys relative to recipients of other cadaveric kidneys. There are also data to suggest that there is a stepwise decrement in graft survival rates according to the magnitude of HLA matching. Each mismatched antigen supposedly is responsible for a 1%–2% decrease in the 5-year graft survival rate, although recent data suggest that the magnitude of these differences is decreasing. In addition, there are single-center data demonstrating overall results that are superior to the best outcomes in the various registries.[98] Thus, although matching may have some influence on outcome after renal transplantation, the presence of other factors can overshadow its impact. These include the center effect, recipient age, sex, ischemic time (both cold and warm), type of immunosuppression, cause of end-stage renal disease, transplant number, and the presence of preformed anti-HLA antibody (see Chapter 1).

▲ CROSS MATCHING

The cross match is the most important preoperative immunologic test in renal transplantation. Hyperacute or accelerated rejection can occur if a recipient possesses a preformed antibody to the donor HLA antigen, ie, a positive cross match. After the initial observations made by Patel and Terasaki in 1969,[99] cross matching before renal transplantation became mandatory and led to the virtual disappearance of hyperacute rejection by the mid 1970s.

Cross matching has evolved over the past 10–20 years. With the advent of more (perhaps overly) sensitive procedures in the mid 1970s, more false-positive cross matches were reported. During the 1980s, there were attempts to differentiate cytotoxic antibodies from noncytotoxic antibodies or even beneficial antibodies by means of temperature,[100] antiglobulin tests,[101] and, more recently, flow cytometric cross matching.[102] The current consensus regarding cross matching suggests that transplants should be avoided only if the potential recipient possesses a donor-specific IgG antibody to HLA antigens.[103]

The most common National Institutes of Health (NIH) cross-matching procedure is summarized in Tables 8–4 through 8–6. Donor lymphocytes are isolated by various procedures and reacted against recipient sera for 30 minutes at 37°C. Rabbit com-

TABLE 8–4 ▲ LYMPHOCYTE ISOLATION PROCEDURE FOR CROSS MATCHING

1. Centrifuge blood tubes in table-top centrifuge for 15 min at 1800 rpm. *Do not use brake.*
2. Remove buffy coat from all tubes and place in 15-mL screw-cap tube.
   Add an equal amount of McCoy medium and mix well.
3. Place approximately 2 mL of Lymphoprep in each of several 5 mL plastic test tubes.
   Carefully layer approximately 1.5 mL of buffy coat mixture on top of the Lymphoprep (*gently* so as not to disturb the layers).
4. Centrifuge in table-top certrifuge for 15 min at 3000 rpm with brake off.
5. Remove interface-containing lymphocytes and place in Fisher tubes (red blood cells and polymorphonuclear leukocytes are in the precipitate).
   Wash several times with Hanks balanced salt solution (HBSS) to remove platelets and adjust cell count.

TABLE 8–5 ▲ T AND B LYMPHOCYTE ISOLATION PROCEDURE

1. Isolate whole lymphocytes (see Table 8–4).
2. Spin 5–10 × 10^6 cells at 1000*g* for 1 min in Fisher centrifuge.
   Remove supernatant.
3. Add 1 mL 1% ox red blood cells and mix well.
4. Spin in Fisher centrifuge for 5 min at 500*g*.
5. Incubate at room temperature for an additional 10 min.
6. Remove supernatant and add 1 mL 75% Percoll.
   Gently resuspend.
   Add 1 drop of mixture to hemacytometer and check rosette formation.
7. Divide into two 1-mL Fisher tubes.
   Layer approximately 0.2 mL of 0.5% McCoy medium on top of Percoll.
8. Spin at 2000–2500*g* for 2 min; take up speed gradually.
9. Remove interface and place in two tubes marked *T cells*.
   Wash and adjust cell count for cross matching.
10. Remove remaining supernatant and discard.
11. Resuspend pellet containing rosetted B cells in 10% McCoy medium.
    Add one drop of mixture to hemacytometer.
12. Count number of rosettes and nonrosetted cells.
    Calculate percentage of B cells.
13. Spin B-cell rosettes for 2 min at 3500*g*; discard supernatant.
14. Resuspend in ammonium chloride (using two tubes if necessary).
    Incubate in 37°C heat block (to lyse red cells) for 2–4 min.
15. Spin 1 min at 1000*g*.
    Discard supernatant and resuspend in 10% McCoy medium.
    Adjust cell count for cross matching.

TABLE 8–6 ▲ SHORT, B-37, T-37 CROSS MATCH PROCEDURE

1. Short Cross Match
Add whole lymphocytes to patient's serum.
Incubate at 20–25°C for 30 min.
Add 5 μL of ABC complement.
Incubate at 20–25°C for 1 hr.
Stop with 10 μL Stain-fix or Quench.
2. B-37 Cross Match
Add B cells to patient's serum.
Incubate at 37°C for 30 min.
Add 5 μL of rabbit complement.
Incubate at 20–25°C for 2 h.
Stop with 10 μL Stain-fix or Quench
3. T-37 Long Cross Match
Add T cells to patient's serum.
Incubate at 37°C for 30 min.
Add 5 μL of ABC complement.
Incubate at 25°C for 2 h.
Stop with 10 μL Stain-fix or Quench.

plement is then added and incubated for an additional 2 hours at room temperature. Eosin or trypan blue is added to stain, fix, and evaluate the dead cells under an inverse phase microscope.

▲ CHARACTERIZATION OF ANTIBODY

In most instances, positive cross matches reveal an IgG anti-HLA antibody. Caution should be exercised, however, if a patient has an autoimmune disease such as systemic lupus erythematosus (SLE) or is older, because these patients may have an IgM antibody,[104] which is not a contraindication to kidney transplantation.[103] Dithiothreitol (DTT) cleaves the disulfate bond of IgM and eliminates the false positivity associated with IgM; thus only IgG-related cytotoxicity is observed after treatment with DTT.[105] DTT treatment has been well accepted because of its convenience and accuracy (Table 8–7). All the serum can be treated with DTT at the time of cross matching, or it can be treated with DTT and then stored at −80°C until needed.

Antiglobulin tests and flow cytometric cross matching are recommended to identify low levels of IgG antibodies. These tests essentially pick up only recipient IgG antibody, because the secondary antibody used in these procedures is anti-human IgG. In most instances, a combination of these two procedures (conventional dye exclusion complement-dependent cytotoxicity testing with DTT treatment and

TABLE 8–7 ▲ PROCEDURE FOR TREATING DTT SERUM

1. Prepare 10 mL of 1 mol/L DTT.
   Weigh out 1.54g and dilute to 10 mL with normal phosphate-buffered saline solution.
   Store in freezer.
2. Dilute 1 mL of 1 mol/L DTT solution with 19 mL normal phosphate-buffered saline solution (makes 20 mL of 50 mmol/L DTT solution).
   Adjust pH to 7.0–7.5.
3. To treat serum:
   Mix 1 part 50 mmol/L DTT (30 μl) solution to 9 parts (270 μL) serum.
   Mix and incubate in 37°C heat block for 30 min.
4. Centrifuge and use supernatant to set up cross match parallel with untreated serum.

antiglobulin or flow cytometric crossmatching) should be adequate to provide conclusive results.

▲ PANEL REACTIVE ANTIBODY

Once a recipient is placed on the renal transplant waiting list, his or her serum is screened for the presence of anti-HLA antibodies. Sera are tested against lymphocytes, usually from a panel of 30–70 individuals, which represent most HLA antigens, to determine HLA specificities. Results are usually represented as percentage cytotoxicity and are referred to as panel reactive antibody (PRA). PRA screening is important not only for identification of HLA specificities but also to determine the probability of a patient's having a negative cross match at the time a possible donor is located.

For a potential recipient with a history of blood transfusions, pregnancies, or previous transplants, it is likely that the lymphocytotoxic antibodies are IgG in nature; however, without such a history, a positive antiglobulin or flow cytometric cross match may be falsely positive. The higher a patient's PRA level, the lower are his or her chances of receiving a kidney, so when a highly sensitized patient (PRA level greater than 80%) has a negative cross match with a potential donor, the allocation of additional points by the UNOS point system usually ensures that the sensitized patient will receive the organ (see Chapter 3).

Patients awaiting transplantation should have PRA evaluations at regular intervals. This applies particularly to patients receiving blood transfusions or suffering from a systemic infection, even a viral upper respiratory infection, which can stimulate the immune system.

Conventional Immunosuppressive Agents

John J. Fung

Clinical transplantation has been built on the foundation of using drug therapy for nonspecific suppression of the recipient immune response. The goal is both to prevent rejection and also to avoid opportunistic infections and malignancy and to minimize the other toxicities associated with these agents. In this section, the conventional immunosuppressive agents used clinically are described, focusing on their role in current immunosuppressive regimens in renal transplantation and their commonly observed toxicities.

▲ CORTICOSTEROIDS

The approach to manipulation of the immune response with chemical agents actually began in 1951, when locally applied cortisone was used to prolong skin allograft survival.[106] Since then, corticosteroids have been used extensively in clinical immunosuppressive protocols for both induction and maintenance therapy and for the treatment of rejection. Four principal glucocorticosteroid compounds are used in transplantation: hydrocortisone, prednisone, prednisolone, and methylprednisolone. Because hydrocortisone has the greatest mineralocorticoid properties per unit of glucocorticoid activity, its routine application in transplantation has been relatively limited. The latter three agents have more glucocorticoid activity in proportion to their mineralocorticoid activity. Prednisone has an oral bioavailability of about 80% and is metabolized in the liver to its active form, prednisolone. Oral prednisolone has a bioavailability of 100%. The serum half-life of both prednisone and methylprednisolone is about 2–3 hours.[107] However, suppression of cytokine production persists for 24 hours more.

There is no universally accepted fixed dosing regimen. Rather, the dose is often dictated by local protocol. Tornatore et al[107] reported a threefold variation in methylprednisolone clearance and a twofold range in the volume of distribution in recipients of transplants during the early posttransplant period. This suggests that anything short of pharmacokinetic guidance for corticosteroid dosing is essentially empiric. A perioperative dose of 250–1000 mg usually is given followed by a gradual taper over a period of 1–10 weeks. The usual maintenance corticosteroid doses range between 0.1 and 0.2 mg/kg a day. The drug is usually given as a single morning dose in an attempt to minimize interference with the diurnal cortisol rhythm.

Acute rejection may be managed with one to three bolus doses of 250 mg to 1 g intravenous methylprednisolone and/or by a tapering regimen that returns to baseline maintenance corticosteroid doses over 3–21 days. There is evidence to suggest that lower doses than those traditionally used can be equally effective.

Unfortunately, the side effects of corticosteroids are numerous and cause considerable morbidity. Some are related to the total dose and duration of administration. An increased incidence of serious infections has been well documented. Impaired fibroblast growth and collagen synthesis contribute to poor wound healing. Thus surgical wounds and anastomoses are at increased risk, and gastrointestinal ulcerations tend to heal slowly with an increased risk of perforation and rebleeding. Sodium retention, edema, hypertension, potassium loss, and hypokalemic alkalosis can occur with prolonged use. Suppression of the pituitary-adrenal axis can occur with chronic glucocorticoid use but is variable.[107] Although rare, acute adrenal insufficiency can develop if the patient is physiologically stressed. Gastrointestinal ulceration occurs in approximately 2% of patients taking steroids. Decompensation of glucose tolerance can be dramatic. Generalized protein catabolism and bone demineralization can produce a debilitated state. Atherosclerosis may be accelerated, in part because of the abnormal lipid profile associated with chronic corticosteroid use. The risk of cataract formation and increased intraocular pressure (glaucoma) has been well documented. Central nervous system (CNS) effects such as euphoria and mood swings have been described. Soft-tissue and dermatologic changes such as fat redistribution, skin atrophy, and striae produce the characteristic cushingoid appearance. Growth retardation is a serious problem in children.

▲ AZATHIOPRINE

In 1960, Calne used azathioprine, developed earlier by Schwartz and Dameshek,[108] in attempts to obtain success in canine renal transplantation.[109] Azathioprine has been used in numerous maintenance immunosuppressive regimens. Before the availability of cyclosporine, azathioprine was used in conjunction with corticosteroids for maintenance immunosuppression.[110] With the advent of cyclosporine, azathioprine has been relegated to an adjunctive role, generally in three-agent combinations. The addition of azathioprine to cyclosporine-based regimens may allow for dosage reduction of the latter agent and result in fewer side effects.

Azathioprine is well absorbed from the gastrointestinal tract. The metabolism of azathioprine is complex. The parent drug is inactive but is rapidly converted to several metabolites. Thio-inosinic acid is an inhibitor of purine synthesis. The 6-thioguanine nucleotides (TGN) are known to incorporate into DNA. TGN have a very long tissue half-life, about 13 days. On this basis, once-daily dosage is logical. The final inactive end metabolite is 6-thiouric acid, which is excreted by the kidneys. With congenital deficiency of the enzyme thiopurine methyltransferase (1 in 300 patients) or with renal failure, accumulation of TGN can cause increased toxicity.

The drug is usually given orally but also exists in an intravenous formulation. The usual starting dose is between 3 and 5 mg/kg as a single daily dose. Typical maintenance oral dosages after transplantation are between 1 and 2 mg/kg daily but are highly dependent on the use of other immunosuppressive agents and associated toxicities of azathioprine, such as myelosuppression. Dose-limiting myelosuppression usually occurs several weeks into therapy. Pancytopenia and thrombocytopenia with megaloblastic anemia are the most commonly seen side effects. White blood cell (WBC) counts below 3000 cells/mm^3 mandate discontinuation or dosage reduction of azathioprine. As with other antiproliferative drugs, nausea, vomiting, and hair loss may occur. Hepatic injury can occur in two patterns: a reversible hepatitis and a rare but serious hepatic venoocclusive disease that can cause irreparable damage. Azathioprine therapy has been associated with an increased risk of pancreatitis believed to be secondary to a hypersensitivity reaction. The role of azathioprine, however, has been questioned in these instances.[111,112]

Allopurinol inhibits xanthine oxidase, one of the enzymes involved in the degradation of azathioprine metabolites, and can increase azathioprine toxicity. Thus the concomitant use of allopurinol, for the treatment or prevention of gout, with azathioprine mandates dosage reduction of azathioprine and close monitoring of WBC count. It has been suggested that in this situation, the azathioprine dose should be empirically reduced by one half to one fourth.[113] Deaths due to bone marrow suppression have been reported.[114]

▲ CYCLOPHOSPHAMIDE

Cyclophosphamide has been used in place of azathioprine,[115] particularly when there is suspected azathioprine-associated hepatitis, and can reach high hepatic concentrations without hepatotoxicity.[116] It has been stated that cyclophosphamide may have a more selective toxicity toward B cells than T cells, although the data have been scant.[117,118] The drug has been used in immunosuppressive protocols and has been utilized in sensitized patients.[119]

Oral cyclophosphamide is well absorbed (87–96%); peak concentrations are reached in 1 hour.[120] Cyclophosphamide is activated by metabolism in the liver, several metabolites being generated. The active metabolite, phosphoramide mustard, is eliminated by spontaneous hydrolysis with an intracellular half-life of 40–50 minutes. Blood half-life is about 5–7 hours. Cyclophosphamide is removed by hemodialysis. Cyclophosphamide used in transplant regimens is administered at low doses (1–5 mg/kg a day), considerably less than the doses used in most chemotherapeutic regimens (40–100 mg/kg a day).

Side effects of cyclophosphamide administration include gastrointestinal side effects, leukopenia, thrombocytopenia, anemia, interstitial pulmonary fibrosis, and hair loss. As many as 15% of patients experience clinically significant cardiac dysfunction. Infertility also has been infrequently associated with use of cyclophosphamide. Hemorrhagic cystitis is a well-known side effect of cyclophosphamide, but the reported incidence is extremely variable (0.5–40%). This effect can be limited by use of mesna (sodium 2-mercaptoethanesulphonate [Mesnex, Mead Johnson, Evansville, IN])[121] or apparently equally well by aggressive hydration.

▲ CYCLOSPORINE: A CYTOKINE SUPPRESSIVE AGENT

Before the introduction of cyclosporine, immunosuppressive protocols relied heavily on steroids and antimetabolite drugs. These regimens had the disadvantage of nonspecificity and of producing broad suppression of the immune and inflammatory cascades. In 1970, Sandoz Ltd isolated a strain of *Fungi Imperfecti* (*Beauveria nivea*), that was suitable for large-scale cyclosporine production. Borel et al[122] first described the potent immunosuppressive qualities of cyclosporine, and the drug was introduced into clinical trials by Calne et al[123] and Starzl et al.[124] Cyclosporine ushered in a new era of immunosuppression with potent, relatively specific, noncytotoxic suppression of T-cell activation. With the introduction of cyclosporine into clinical transplantation, survival rates for patients and grafts improved dramatically.

Cyclosporine is a cyclic polypeptide with 11 amino acids and a molecular weight of 1202. The drug is insoluble in water and thus must be dissolved in an organic solvent. There currently exist two formulations of cyclosporine—Sandimmune (Sandoz, East Hanover, NJ) and Neoral (Sandoz, East Hanover, NJ). For both healthy volunteers and a variety of patient populations, absorption of the Neoral formulation of cyclosporine is substantially greater than that of the Sandimmune formulation. The overall time to reach peak cyclosporine concentration (t_{max}) is shorter, peak cyclosporine concentrations (C_{max}) are higher, and the area under the curve is greater with Neoral than with Sandimmune. The relative bioavailability of Neoral, compared with Sandimmune, is increased between 74% and 139%.[125] The total area under the curve is increased by 30%.[126,127] The greater variability of bioavailability for Sandimmune is due to its lipophilic nature. Optimal Sandimmune absorption requires adequate pancreatic, biliary, and small-intestinal function, in addition to appropriate gastrointestinal motility and absorptive capacity. Intestinal absorption decreases with small-intestinal dysfunction or reduced bile flow.[128] These requirements appear to be less important with Neoral because of its innovative microemulsion formulation.[129] Intrasubject variability, expressed as the percentage coefficient of variation, varies between 17% and 30% for Neoral and 16% and 38% for Sandimmune. Although proprietary, the microemulsion technology is apparently based on the combination of a lipophilic solvent, a hydrophilic solvent, and a surfactant with the active ingredient, cyclosporine.

The volume of distribution of cyclosporine is large and variable and is similar for both formulations. The steady-state volume of distribution during intravenous dosing ranges from 3 to 5 L/kg of body weight.[130] In the blood compartment, approximately 41%–58% of cyclosporine is bound to red blood cells, 4%–9% is bound to lymphocytes, 5%–12% is bound to granulocytes, and 33%–47% is found in the plasma fraction; more than 90% of the cyclosporine in this latter compartment is bound to plasma proteins (primarily lipoproteins).[131]

The liver is the main site of cyclosporine metabolism by the cytochrome P450 IIIA system, although both the kidneys and small intestine also contribute to cyclosporine metabolism. The drug is excreted through the bile in both native and metabolized forms (95% of excretion) and only in a small amount by the kidney (<5%). The mean half-life of cyclosporine when liver function is normal is 8.4 hours (range 5–18 hours).[128] At least 25 metabolites have been identified, and a few are immunosuppressive, although with considerably less potency than the parent compound.[132] As one might predict, the half-life of cyclosporine increases with hepatic dysfunction.

Monitoring cyclosporine levels is not without problems. Measuring cyclosporine in whole blood or plasma with radioimmunoassay, high-pressure liquid chromatography (HPLC), or fluorescence polarization immunoassay (TdX, Abbott, Abbott Park, IL) gives different results. No method is clearly superior; thus there is no universally accepted blood level. It has been stated that parent compound–specific assays produce results that better correlate with clinical events.[133] HPLC is very specific for both the parent compound and metabolite monitoring, but it is cumbersome and expensive. Both the TdX and radioimmunoassay can be used to detect the parent compound with relative specificity using a monoclonal antibody (mAb-S), or more broadly the parent compound along with its metabolites using a polyclonal antibody. Thus target levels may vary widely from center to center. Table 8–8 shows the ranges for radioimmunoassay, TdX, and HPLC. Higher levels are required during the early posttransplant period and lower levels for maintenance therapy.

Coadministration of a large number of drugs can cause increased or decreased cyclosporine levels because of competitive inhibition or induction of P450 enzymes (Table 8–9). For these reasons, it is essential that levels be monitored regularly and the dosage adjusted accordingly if these agents must be used. It is assumed that both the Sandimmune and Neoral formulations behave similarly. Phenytoin (Dilantin, Parke-Davis, Morris Plains, NJ) phenobarbital, carbamazepine, rifampin, and ticlopidine can induce P-450 microsomal enzymes, increasing cyclosporine metabolic clearance and resulting in a corresponding decrease in blood levels.[134,135] Ketoconazole, erythromycin, chloroquine, and diltiazem increase cyclosporine levels because of a competitive interference with cyclosporine metabolism by these agents.[136–139] Agents that increase cyclosporine levels, as well as those that are inherently nephrotoxic, may potentiate the development of renal dysfunction (Table 8–10).

Some centers attempt to avoid use of any cyclosporine immediately after kidney transplantation, instead using antilymphocyte induction therapy. At centers that use cyclosporine in the perioperative period, cyclosporine may be administered 12–24 hours prior to renal transplantation. For most recipients of renal transplants, it is possible to continue cyclosporine in the posttransplant period by oral administra-

TABLE 8–8 ▲ TARGET RANGES FOR 12-HOUR CYCLOSPORINE TROUGH LEVELS (ng/mL) IN KIDNEY TRANSPLANT RECIPIENTS

Assay	Specificity	Whole Blood	Serum/Plasma
HPLC	Cyclosporine	125–350	50–125
FPIA (TdX)	Cyclosporine and metabolites	300–800	150–400
RIA-mAb-S	Cyclosporine	150–400	75–150
RIA-Poly	Cyclosporine and metabolites	300–800	150–400

HPLC, high-pressure liquid chromatography; FPIA, fluorescence polarization immunoassay; RIA-mAb-S, radioimmunoassay–specific monoclonal antibody; RIA-Poly, Radioimmunoassay–polyclonal antibody.

tion. Patients who cannot take oral cyclosporine can be given cyclosporine intravenously at a dose of 3–4 mg/kg a day. This amount can be given in two divided doses each over 2–6 hours. Some centers prefer to use a slow, continuous infusion over 24 hours. The change to oral dosing usually requires a dose three times higher than the intravenous dose (about 9–12 mg/kg a day usually divided into two daily doses). Because Sandimmune and Neoral are not bioequivalent, lower doses (in the range of 7%–16% less for renal transplant patients) of Neoral have been recommended.[140]

Several adverse effects occur with the administration of cyclosporine. Acute nephrotoxicity, probably resulting from vasoconstrictive effects on the afferent arterioles of the kidney,[141] is a serious problem. This nephrotoxicity is transient and reversible with a decrease in dosage or discontinuation of the drug.[142] The incidence of nephrotoxicity is approximately 25%, 32%, and 38% among kidney, heart, and liver

TABLE 8–9 ▲ DRUGS THAT ALTER CYCLOSPORINE CONCENTRATIONS

Increase	Decrease
Diltiazem	Rifampin
Nicardipine	Carbamazepine
Verapamil	Phenobarbital
Fluconazole	Phenytoin
Itraconazole	Ticlopidine
Ketoconazole	Nafcillin
Clarithromycin	Octreotide
Erythromycin	Isoniazide
Tacrolimus	
Methylprednisolone (high-dose)	
Bromocriptine	
Danazol	

TABLE 8–10 ▲ DRUGS THAT MAY POTENTIATE THE NEPHROTOXICITY OF CYCLOSPORINE

Antibiotics
Gentamicin
Tobramycin
Vancomycin
Trimethoprim-sulfamethoxazole
Antifungals
Amphotericin B
Ketoconazole
Anti-inflammatories
Acetylsalicyclic Acid
Ibuprofen
Diclofenac
Antineoplastics
Melphalan
Antiacids
Cimetidine
Ranitidine
Immunosuppressives
Tacrolimus

transplant patients, respectively.[143] Hypertension occurs frequently within weeks of beginning therapy. The prevalence varies widely among different patient populations and ranges from 10% to 80%.[144] It is hypothesized that hypertension is caused by a vasoconstrictive effect of cyclosporine in both the renal and systemic circulations[145] perhaps caused by antagonism of endothelium-derived relaxation factors or increased synthesis of endothelin, a vasoconstrictor. The hypertension is physiologically responsive to sodium restriction. Therapies that incorporate diuretics or calcium channel blockers have been advocated.[144] Minor neurotoxicity (tremor) is common (10%–55%) and many improve over time without a change in therapy.

Severe symptoms, such as seizures and encephalopathy, have been associated with the use of cyclosporine, but it is not clear whether the association is causal (see Chapter 11).[146] Several reports detail a rare syndrome of confusion and cortical blindness among recipients of liver or bone marrow transplants.[141] Hypomagnesemia and hypocholesterolemia are believed to be risk factors for cyclosporine neurotoxicity.[141] Cyclosporine is diabetogenic, although analysis of this effect is confounded by the frequent concomitant use of steroids with cyclosporine.[141] Other metabolic effects include hypochloremic alkalosis and changes in serum potassium, magnesium, prolactin, and testosterone levels.[147] Hepatotoxicity, manifested by an increased cholestatic tendency, may be quite common,[141] but a reduction in dosage often improves this effect, and it does not appear to be a serious problem. Connective tissue side effects of cyclosporine are common and can be distressing to the patient. These include hirsutism, which occurs over 2–4 weeks in 20%–45% of patients, gingival hyperplasia in 4%–16%, and coarsening of facial features.[148] Cardiac toxicity has been reported as a rare manifestation of cyclosporine toxicity.[149]

Long-term administration of cyclosporine has been associated with nonreversible nephrotoxicity. The incidence is estimated at 15%–40%.[150] The pathologic lesion resembles nephrosclerosis.[141,151]

▲ ANTILYMPHOCYTE ANTIBODIES (POLYCLONAL AND MONOCLONAL)

Antilymphocyte therapy began with the description of heterologous antisera to purified lymphoid cells that were shown to prolong skin graft survival.[152] Soon thereafter, antilymphocyte therapy was introduced for the prevention and treatment of acute rejection in solid organ transplantation.[153–156] Polyclonal antilymphocyte antibodies are heterologous antibody preparations. Animals (including rabbits, goats, and horses) are immunized against human lymphoid cells (which have included thymocytes, lymphoblasts, peripheral T cells, or Jurkat T lymphocytes), and antisera are collected. The resultant antisera, which cross react with other preformed cellular components in human blood, are adsorbed extensively with human red blood cells. The serum fraction can be used (antilymphocyte serum [ALS]), but to reduce the possibility of serum sickness, a more purified γ-globulin fraction is used clinically (antilymphocyte globulin [ALG] or antithymocyte globulin [ATG]). Because of variability among immunized animals, substantial amounts of ALG/ATG are pooled to produce more immunologically homogeneous preparations. The only preparation approved by the U.S. Food and Drug Administration (FDA) is ATGAM (Upjohn, Kalamazoo, MI) although many programs used MALG (University of Minnesota) in the past, and a number of ATG preparations are used in Europe (Merieux horse and rabbit ATG and Fresenius rabbit ATG).

Several inherent properties of conventional ALG prevented its full exploitation.[157,158] Many of the limitations of the ALS and ALG/ATG preparations are related to variability in potency; reactivity to formed blood elements leading to leukopenia, thrombocytopenia, or anemia; and serum sickness to the heterologous proteins. This is due in part to the high level (>90%) of contaminating protein (eg, irrelevant antibodies), contained in these polyclonal antibody preparations.

Each polyclonal ALG/ATG and ALS preparation varies in its constituent antibody specificities, in part because of the variations in the immunogen used, and the species of animals in which the polyclonal antilymphocyte antibody is being raised. Characterization of the antigen specificity of these antibody preparations suggests that multiple cell surface molecules are recognized by the polyclonal antilymphocyte preparations and that the varying specificities may account for the variations in reported clinical efficacy.[159] Bourdage and Hamlin[160] reported the results of antibody specificities of various polyclonal preparations that have been most commonly used. As summarized in Table 8–11, although representative antibodies are directed to the main T-cell surface molecules (eg, CD2, CD3, CD4, CD8, CD28, and the T-cell receptor), there are often antibody specificities to other leukocyte specificities (eg, CD20 and CD40 found on B cells; CD16 found on natural killer (NK) cells and macrophages; LFA-1, and LFA-3, which are common adhesion molecules) and ubiquitous cell surface antigens (eg, MHC class I and class II antigens).[161,162]

Avoidance of the disadvantage of variability in potency became possible with the development of mAb preparations with defined specificities using the hybridoma technology developed by Kohler and Milstein.[163] With mAb preparations, the potent therapeutic qualities of ALG can be retained while the dangers of irrelevant foreign protein administration are reduced. Kung et al[164] were able to produce mouse mAb directed against varying T-cell surface antigens. One such mAb, OKT3, was found to have defined specificity to the CD3 receptor, which is associated with the T cell receptor. OKT3 has been demonstrated to have profound in vivo immunosuppressive qualities and has been shown to be effective in clinical immunosuppressive regimens.[165–168]

TABLE 8–11 ▲ RELATIVE STRENGTHS AND SPECIFICITIES OF VARIOUS CLINICALLY USED POLYCLONAL ANTILYMPHOCYTE ANTIBODY PREPARATIONS TOWARD DEFINED LYMPHOCYTE ANTIGENS[a]

Source	CD2	CD3	CD4	CD5	CD8	CD11	CD18	CD28	CD45	TCR
ATGAM	++	+++	++	+++	++	+++	+++	++++	++	+++
Merieux (rabbit)	–	++	++	–	–	++	+++	+++	+	++
Merieux (horse)	+	+++	++	+	+	++	+++	+++	++	+++
Fresenius	++	++++	++++	+	+++	+++	++++	+++	++	++++
MALG	+++	+++	+++	++	++	+++	+++	++++	++	+++
MALG[b]	NR	+	NR	+++	NR	+++	++++	NR	++	NR
RATG (Carolina)[c]	++	+	++	+	++	++	+++	+++	++	+

+, weakest; ++++, strongest; NR, not reported.

[a] Determination made by inhibition of binding of specific monoclonal antibody binding by the test polyclonal antibody sample.

[b] Data from Bonnefoy-Berard N, et al: Antibodies against functional leukocyte surface molecules in polyclonal antilymphocyte and antithymocyte globulins. *Transplantation* 51:669–673, 1991.

[c] Determined by monoclonal antibody inhibition and immunoprecipitation/gel electrophoresis. Data from Rebellato LM, et al: A comprehensive definition of the major antibody specificities in polyclonal rabbit antithymocyte globulin. *Transplantation* 57:685–694, 1992.

Modified from Bourdage JS, Hamlin DM: Comparative polyclonal antithymocyte globulin and antilymphocyte/lymphoblast globulin anti-CD antigen analysis by flow cytometry. *Transplantation* 59:1194–1200, 1995.

The place of antilymphocyte therapy in immunosuppressive regimens is in a state of flux. Both polyclonal and monoclonal antilymphocyte preparations have been used for the treatment of rejection (generally those considered to be steroid-resistant). These preparations also have been used immediately after transplantation in a strategy of induction therapy. This practice is based on the concept that early incapacitation of the immune system may reduce the propensity for subsequent rejection. The claimed benefits are a delay in time to onset of acute rejection, fewer episodes of rejection, and no increase in infectious complications. The related concept of "sequential" therapy was introduced in response to the renal toxicity of cyclosporine in liver, heart, and kidney transplantation. The practice is to use antibody therapy in the first 1–2 weeks after transplantation in lieu of cyclosporine. It is during this period that renal injury secondary to problems such as donor instability, prolonged ischemia times, or excessive vasopressor use is most likely to become manifest. Administration of cyclosporine is begun after adequate renal function is achieved. Proponents cite a reduced incidence of early renal dysfunction.[169–171] The impact of this strategy on long-term renal function is less clear.

This early intensification of immunosuppression is not universally accepted. Some authors voice concern over the well-known associations of antilymphocyte antibody therapy and immunosuppression in general with infection and malignancy.[172,173] Others describe no benefit, greater expense,[174] or the successful use of regimens that avoid induction altogether.[175] Compromise strategies involve use of prophylaxis to treat only patients at high risk[176] or use of OKT3 (muromonab-CD3) followed by early evaluation of renal function, and discontinuation unless delayed graft function is observed.[177]

A very small number of patients may be sensitized to heterologous proteins from earlier exposure (eg, equine hyperimmune tetanus immune globulin). To avoid an anaphylactic reaction, a test dose of ALS/ALG/ATG, usually diluted 1:1000, is given subcutaneously. Even if no reactions are encountered, it is not unusual for these preparations to cause febrile reactions and chills with the first few doses. Antihistamines, antipyretics, and sometimes steroids (hydrocortisone 1 g) are given as premedication. ATGAM is usually given in the dosage range of 10–15 mg/kg in a single daily dose, although doses up to 30 mg/kg a day have been used. Doses are given either intramuscularly or intravenously (and via central vein catheter). Therapy for acute rejection is usually continued for 14 days. Because the antibodies react with other blood cells, leukopenia (about 14%) and thrombocytopenia (about 30%) can occur. Anaphylaxis occurs in less than 1% of patients. Nonetheless, a skin test before use is recommended. Skin rash is a fairly frequent occurrence (10%–30%). Myalgia, arthralgia, anaphylactoid reactions, and serum sickness are related to the heterologous nature of the administered proteins.

OKT3 is by far the most extensively studied of the mAb. With the first one or two doses, there is a large intravascular release of cytokines by lymphocytes. This first-dose effect frequently causes fever, chills, tachycardia, gastrointestinal disturbances, bronchospasm, and elevation or depression of blood pressure.[178] These effects can be blocked to a large extent by pretreatment with a 1-g intravenous bolus of hydrocortisone with diphenhydramine and acetaminophen, 15–60 minutes before OKT3 infusion. It is important to minimize circulatory overload, which may exacerbate the first-dose effect; patients may need to be dialyzed prior to the first dose. Other side effects of OKT3 include neurologic complications, including aseptic meningitis, psychosis, and seizures. These side effects are selflimited, and it is not necessary to stop therapy with OKT3.

The recommended dose of OKT3 is 2.5 mg a day for pediatric patients who weigh less than 30 kg and 5.0 mg a day for patients who weigh more than 30 kg. The usual length of treatment for acute rejection is 10–14 days, whereas that for induction therapy is 5–7 days. The pharmacokinetics of OKT3 administration are complex, in part because of its large molecular weight (150 kd), the varying levels of its target (CD3 antigen), and an important mechanism of elimination by development of immune complexes.

With the first doses of OKT3, a large circulating and lymphoid-based pool of CD3-positive T cells binds free OKT3 quickly, resulting in a drop in OKT3 levels to 60% to 80% of peak levels within 6 hours.[179] After 3–4 days, trough levels of OKT3 are usually maintained between 250 and 1500 ng/mL.[180] This situation may be markedly different toward the end of OKT3 therapy, or when OKT3 is being reused. Because OKT3 is a murine protein, humans may produce antibodies to the mAb, also known as human anti-mouse antibody, or HAMA. Individuals vary in the amount of HAMA formed, but it may interfere with the effect of OKT3, especially toward the end of mAb therapy. HAMA antibody production can be decreased by continuing the other immunosuppressive agents during the administration of mAb. Retreatment often can succeed if higher doses of antibody are used for subsequent administration. The very highest antibody responders, probably about 5%–20% of patients, form high-titer antibodies, and therapy fails even with increased doses of OKT3. Some advocate following CD3 cell counts with flow cytometry for patients receiving OKT3.[181] If the CD3 count reaches 10%, it is recommended that OKT3 be either increased in dosage (to as much as 15 mg a day) or discontinued. Others suggest monitoring anti-OKT3 antibody titers.[182,183]

The potent suppression of T-lymphocyte populations is known to be associated with an increased incidence of viral infection and lymphoproliferative disorders. It is not clear whether antibody therapy is any worse than other immunosuppressive agents in producing these complications. Some evidence suggests that these problems arise because antibodies are used for too long a time [170] or too late in the course of resistant rejection when the immunosuppressive burden is already high.[184]

▲ LIMITATION OF CURRENT IMMUNOSUPPRESSION

There are two principal limitations of the current immunosuppressive agents. The first is the imperfect effectiveness of these agents, either alone or in combination with one another in preventing rejection. The other is the side effects associated with the agents. Although each immunosuppressive agent is associated with specific side effects, a host of infectious and malignant complications arise from the use of multiple nonspecific immunosuppressive agents (see Chapter 11). Certain types of nonlymphoid, epithelial cancers have an increased incidence in patients on long-term immunosuppression. The use of azathioprine is associated with a fourfold increase in the incidence of skin cancers. Kaposi's sarcoma is associated with long-term cyclosporine immunosuppression. Posttransplant lymphoproliferative disorder (PTLD) is an abnormality of lymphocyte proliferation in an immunosuppressed patient, and its incidence has markedly increased with the use of cyclosporine, as one would expect given its selective inhibition on T cells. The incidence of PTLD in the cyclosporine era is generally estimated to be between 2% and 4%. Most (90%) PTLDs are B cell in origin, and most are associated with integration of Epstein-Barr virus (EBV) DNA into the genome of the B cell.

Current day immunosuppression has led to increasing success in a number of clinical transplant settings. Nevertheless, limitations of the efficacy of these agents exist, and complications of drug toxicity and the consequences of long-term immunosuppression continue to be a problem. These shortcomings have led to the search for new immunosuppressive agents, which are discussed in the next section.

Clinical Experience with New Immunosuppressive Agents in Renal Transplant Recipients

Ron Shapiro

Many new immunosuppressive agents have been studied in a number of clinical trials. This section summarizes the data presented thus far.

▲ TACROLIMUS

Tacrolimus was approved in April 1994 by the FDA for use as an immunosuppressive agent after liver transplantation.[185–188] A great deal of experience in clinical renal transplantation also has been acquired. Although the Pittsburgh group has had the most experience, a number of centers in the United States, Japan, and Europe also have used the drug.

The early Pittsburgh experience included a pilot series, a small randomized trial, and a trial with a larger group of nonrandomized patients ineligible to enter the other trial.[189–191] Patient and graft survival rates were equivalent to those in cyclosporine-treated patients.[191] However, an ability to withdraw steroids in 44% of the patients, a lower need for antihypertension medications, and a lower serum cholesterol level were found in the tacrolimus-treated patients.[191] On the basis of these findings, a second randomized trial was begun in which two tacrolimus-based regimens, with and without azathioprine, were compared.[192–197] The results of this study of 397 transplants demonstrated overall 1- and 3-year actuarial patient survival rates of 95% and 92%, and 1- and 3-year actuarial graft survival rates of 89% and 80%.[196,197] Sixty-nine percent of the patients who underwent successful transplantation were able to discontinue steroids. The benefit of azathioprine was limited to a slightly decreased incidence of rejection, from 55% to 45%, but no improvement in patient survival rate and, in fact, a worse overall graft survival rate (76%, vs 84% for the double-therapy group at 3 years). In a separate, nonrandomized experience with 69 pediatric renal transplants treated with tacrolimus, 100% and 95% 1- and 4-year actuarial patient survival rates and 99% and 85% 1- and 4-year actuarial graft survival rates were seen.[198] Seventy-three percent of the patients who underwent successful transplantation discontinued steriods, with dramatic gains in growth, particularly among the preadolescent patients. Finally, the Pittsburgh group reported a 71% to 74% success rate in "rescuing" patients, most of whom had received transplants outside Pittsburgh and for whom conventional immunosuppressive and antirejection therapies had failed.[199–201]

Side effects of tacrolimus include nephrotoxicity,[202–206] neurotoxicity,[203,207] and diabetogenicity,[203,208] and, children, a trend in the earlier cases toward more viral infections.[209,210] In general, these toxicities are comparable with those that occur with cyclosporine. The overall impression of the Pittsburgh group has been that tacrolimus is an extremely effective immunosuppressive agent in renal transplant patients and that it is more efficacious than cyclosporine.

Experience in Japan to date has included early and late phase II multicenter trials and a phase III trial with historical controls.[211–215] In the phase II trials, which involved 104 patients, 70 of whom received kidneys from living-related donors, the overall 2-year patient and graft survival rates were 97% and 92%, and the incidence of rejection was 44%.[213,214] In the phase III trial, comparable 1-year patient and graft survival rates were seen in cyclosporine and tacrolimus-treated patients.[213,215] The range of side effects was similar to that reported by the Pittsburgh group, and the conclusion was that tacrolimus was "at least as effective" as cyclosporine for renal transplant recipients. There is also a Japanese rescue experience with tacrolimus. Ninety-two patients had an attempt at tacrolimus rescue with a success rate of 68.5%.[213]

In the United States, the results of a multicenter phase II dose-finding trial, in which three different dosages of tacrolimus were compared with one cyclosporine control group, were reported.[216] One hundred twenty patients were entered into the study. One-year patient and graft survival rates in the tacrolimus-treated patients were 98% and 93%; in the cyclosporine-treated patients, the rates were 92% and 89%. Less rejection occurred in the tacrolimus-treated patients. The incidence and range of toxicities were similar to those previously reported.

Several U.S. centers have reported experiences with tacrolimus rescue. The University of Miami, in collaboration with the Pittsburgh group, reported a 95% initial success rate[217] and a 91% 1-year and 88% 2-year actuarial graft survival rate[218] with tacrolimus rescue. The University of Chicago reported an initial success rate of 100% and 9-month actuarial patient and graft survival rates of 92% and 84% with tacrolimus rescue.[219] Finally, a multicenter rescue trial in which 75 patients participated showed a 98.3% initial success rate and a 75% 1–year success rate.[220a]

Gjertson et al[221] looked at the projected half-life with tacrolimus-based immunosuppression in 544 recipients of first cadaver renal transplants at 24 different U.S. centers between 1988 and 1994. When the results were compared with those for 35,147 patients treated with cyclosporine, the projected half-life for the tacrolimus-treated patients was significantly higher than for the cyclosporine-treated patients, 13.8 versus 8.8 years (see Fig. 8–1).

Two phase III multicenter trials, one in the United States and one in Europe, have been performed to compare tacrolimus- and cyclosporine-based therapies. Entry into these trials has been completed, and additional follow-up data are being accumulated. The U.S. trial showed comparable patient and graft survival rates, but less rejection in the tacrolimus group (30.7% versus 46.9%), less steroid-resistant rejection in the tacrolimus group (11% versus 26%), and more crossover from cyclosporine to tacrolimus for refractory rejection,[222,222a] all differences that were statistically significant. The most important adverse event associated with use of tacrolimus was a higher incidence of posttransplant diabetes mellitus.

The phase III European trial also showed less rejection in the tacrolimus-treated patients, but more initial toxicity, probably related to relative inexperience with the drug.[223,223a] Finally, two reports of tacrolimus rescue, from England[224] and Scandinavia,[225] demonstrated 100% and 50% success, respectively.

Taken together, results from these trials confirm the utility of tacrolimus as an important immunosuppressive agent and suggest that it is a superior agent for use in renal transplant recipients.

▲ MYCOPHENOLATE MOFETIL

The first clinical trials of mycophenolate mofetil (CellCept, Roche Laboratories, Nutley, NJ) included a phase I dosing trial and an early rescue experience.[226] In the phase I trial, in which mycophenolate mofetil was used as an azathioprine substitute in a sequential four-drug regimen, a range of dosages, from 100 to 3500 mg a day, were studied in 48 patients. Less rejection was seen at the 2000–3000 mg a day dose range, and a 94% 3-year graft survival rate was obtained. The early rescue experience was with 75 patients, and a 69% success rate was reported.

On the basis of these encouraging early results, three prospective, randomized, double-blind multicenter trials in the United States, Canada, Europe, and Australia were begun. Mycophenolate mofetil was compared with either azathioprine or with placebo in the context of either induction or no induction antilymphocyte therapy.[227–229] Fifteen hundred patients were entered in these trials. The patient survival rate was 96%–97%, and the graft survival rate was 96% for the mycophenolate mofetil groups and 92% for the control groups. In general, there was a 15%–20% lower incidence of rejection among the mycophenolate mofetil–treated patients and a decrease in both the severity of rejection episodes and the need for antilymphocyte therapy (Fig. 8–2.)[227–229] In a randomized trial of mycophenolate mofetil in the treatment of refractory rejection, a somewhat higher graft salvage rate was found among the mycophenolate mofetil group, 86% versus 74%.[230,231] In addition, less subsequent rejection was seen in the mycophenolate mofetil group.

The side effects of mycophenolate mofetil are primarily gastrointestinal and

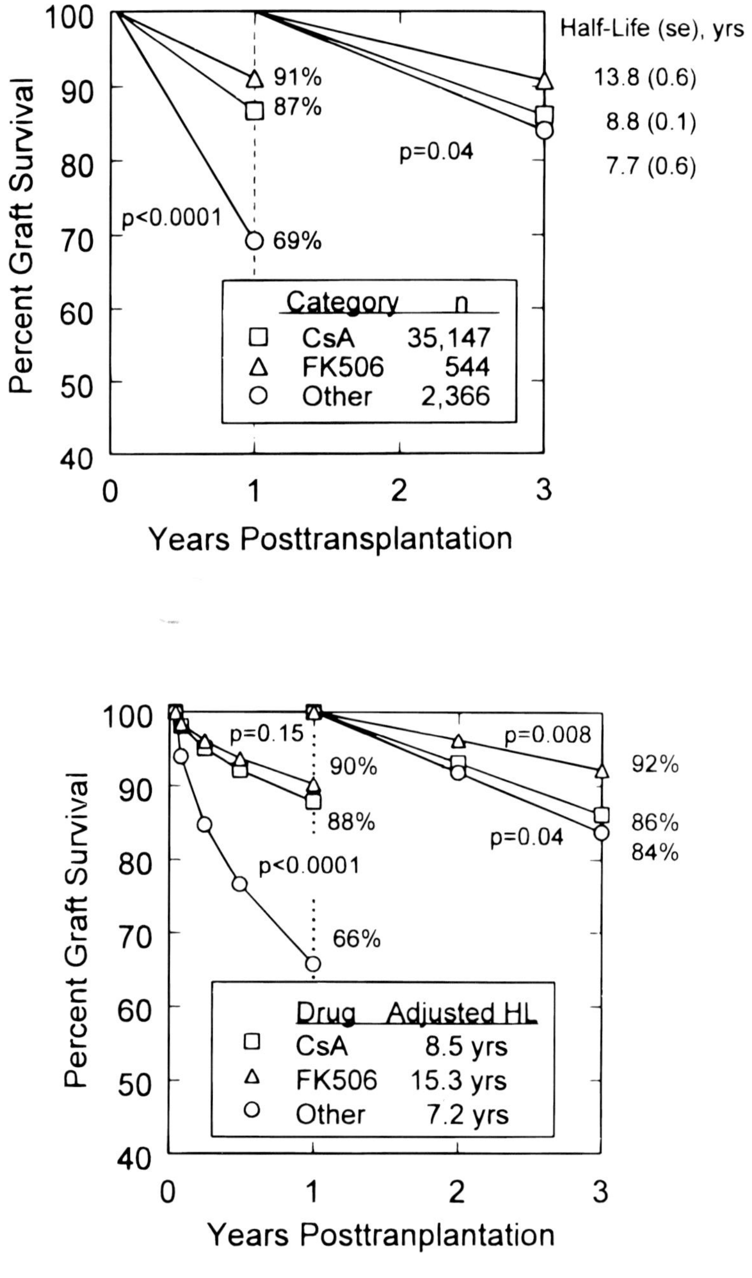

Figure 8–1. A. Graft survival rate and projected half-life among recipients of first cadaveric kidney according to immunosuppressive agent. B. Graft survival rate and projected half-life among recipients of first cadaveric kidneys according to immunosuppressive agent, adjusted for center effect and 19 other variables. *(From Gjertson DW, et al: The relative effects of FK-506 and cyclosporine on short- and long-term kidney graft survival.* Transplantation *60:1388, 1995.)*

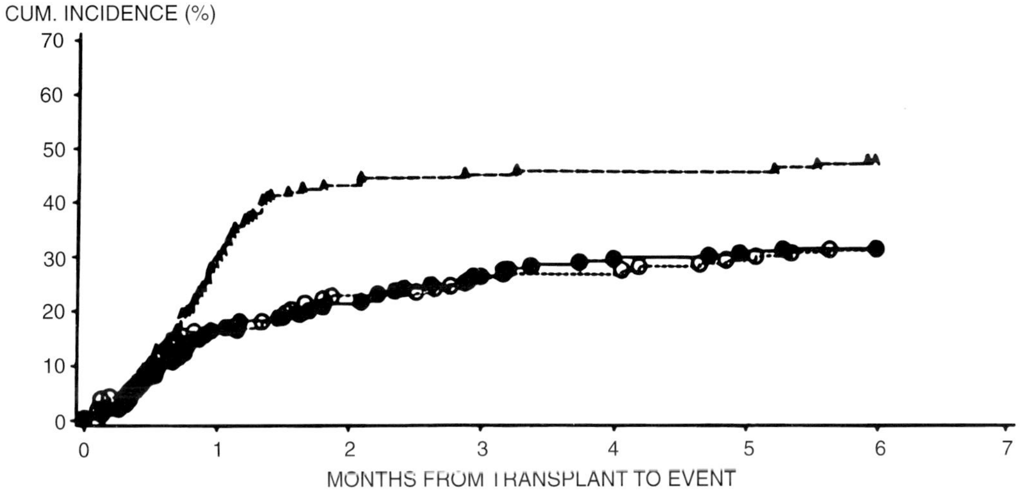

Figure 8–2. Kaplan-Meier estimate of cumulative incidence of rejection or treatment failure according to immunosuppressive agent. ▲, azathioprine; ○, mycophenolate mofetil 2 g a day; ●, mycophenolate mofetil 3 g a day. *(From Sollinger H for the U.S. Renal Transplant Mycophenolate Mofetil Study Group: Mycophenolate mofetil for the prevention of acute rejection in primary cadaveric renal allograft recipients.* Transplantation *60:229, 1995.)*

hematologic; nausea, vomiting, abdominal pain, gastritis, diarrhea, leukopenia, and anemia occur in a dose-dependent manner. The side effects seem to respond to a decrease in dosage.[226–231]

On the basis of these encouraging studies, it seems likely that mycophenolate mofetil will replace azathioprine as a third agent and will be used in combination with cyclosporine and prednisone. Whether mycophenolate mofetil will be effective with tacrolimus is just beginning to be evaluated,[231a] and as yet there are no published data.

▲ SIROLIMUS

Clinical trials with sirolimus (rapamycin, Wyeth-Ayerst Research, Princeton, NJ) began with phase I toxicity studies in dialysis patients with high PRA levels and renal transplant patients.[232, 233] Elevations in triglyceride levels and liver function tests were found. Nephrotoxicity was not observed, and there were no effects on hypertension or cyclosporine pharmacokinetics. High doses of sirolimus were associated with a decrease in the platelet count in recipients of kidneys who received sirolimus as primary immunosuppression (with cyclosporine). Less acute rejection was seen in a small number of patients who received 0.5 mg/m^2, and a complete absence of rejection was seen in patients who received 1–2 mg/m^2.[232,233] However, elevations in serum cholesterol level were seen with the higher doses. A multicenter phase II trial is in progress, and a phase III trial has just started; preliminary (6-month) data from the phase II trial have suggested considerably less rejection in patients receiving sirolimus.[234] A reversible elevation of cholesterol and triglyceride levels and a reduction in platelet counts have been the principal side effects.[234] In recipients of transplants from living donors, sirolimus allowed routine early (1 or 6 month) steroid withdrawal in many patients.[235] If these encouraging early reports are confirmed, sirolimus may well become an important immunosuppressive agent in renal transplant patients.

▲ MIZORIBINE

Mizoribine, also known as Bredinin, has been used as an azathioprine substitute in Japan since the 1980s.[236–242] Mizoribine has been shown to be somewhat more effective and less toxic than azathioprine but has not really been studied outside Japan. Because the mechanism of action is similar to that of mycophenolate mofetil and because the dosage must be adjusted for renal dysfunction, it is unclear whether mizoribine will become an important immunosuppressive agent outside Japan.

▲ 15-DEOXYSPERGUALIN

Because 15-deoxyspergualin is not available in an oral formulation, clinical trials have been limited to rescue and induction therapy.[243–250] Most of these experiences have been in Japan, although small numbers of patients have been treated in Europe and the United States. 15-Deoxyspergualin seems to be effective as a rescue agent. Excellent or good outcomes were obtained in 66% of 270 patients. The success rate was 92% when the drug was used with steroids.[243–245,249] 15-Deoxyspergualin also has been used as a primary agent for induction, again mainly in Japan, with reasonably good outcomes.[247–249] Its side effects include leukopenia, thrombocytopenia, and facial numbness, but are not considered of great importance. However, the lack of availability of an oral formulation will make it difficult to use this drug as a maintenance agent.

▲ BREQUINAR

Early clinical studies with 32 patients treated with brequinar demonstrated excellent patient and graft survival with only one graft loss and a 20% reduction in the rate of rejection.[232,233] Thrombocytopenia was the main adverse side effect and was dose related. Unfortunately, a phase II multicenter trial was stopped in April 1995 because of adverse event–related problems. The pharmaceutical company responsible for brequinar has halted development of this agent for use in transplantation.

▲ LEFLUNOMIDE

Brief mention is made of leflunomide, whose mechanism of action may be similar to that of rapamycin, if only because analogues of leflunomide may one day enter into clinical trials for use in transplant patients. In spite of promising animal studies and other experimental models suggesting that leflunomide might be an effective immunosuppressive agent,[251,252] the pharmaceutical company responsible for the drug has refused for now to develop it further for transplantation.

▲ MONOCLONAL ANTIBODIES

In addition to the aforementioned pharmacologic agents, a large number of mAbs have been studied in clinical trials, either as induction agents or for the management of rejection. They are described by class.

Anti–T Cell

T10B9.1A31

T10B9.1A31 is perhaps the most promising new mAb.[253] It seems to be equivalent to muromonab-CD3 (OKT3) in terms of efficacy, but has none of the side effects associated with the cytokine release syndrome. Although further evaluation is necessary before FDA approval is granted, T10B9.1A31 is likely to become an important alternative to or even replacement for OKT3.

BMA 031

Clinical trials of BMA 031 suggest that it is associated with less early rejection and less graft loss related to rejection. This agent may be a useful agent in clinical practice, although there is little evidence to suggest that it is any better than muromonab-CD3.[254]

WT 32

WT 32 is another agent similar to OKT3 in terms of efficacy and side effects. It appears to offer no advantage over OKT3.[255]

Anti-CD4

There are a number of anti-CD4 mAbs—OKT4a, OKTCDR4a, MT151, BL4, MT412, 16H5, BF5, and an additional unnamed antibody. Although conceptually attractive because of their ability to target selectively a subset of lymphocytes, the clinical potential of these antibodies is still in question. OKT4a, MT151, and BL4 have been disappointing in early trials,[254,256] although a report about OKT4a was encouraging.[257] MT412, a humanized mAb, and 16H5 both have shown promise in thoracic[258] and renal[259] allograft recipients, respectively. There may be a role for some of these anti-CD4 mAbs in the future.

Anti-CD25

A number of anti–interleukin-2 receptor monoclonal antibodies have been developed—anti-Tac, BT563, Campath-6 (YTH906), LO-Tact-1, 33B3.1, humanized anti-tac (Zenapax™), and basiliximab (Simulect™). Two reports of the use of BT563 for steroid-resistant rejection or induction have been promising,[260,261] and both LO-Tact-1[262] and 33B3.1[263] have shown to be comparable in efficacy to ALG. Neither anti-Tac[264] nor Campath-6[265] has been found to be particularly useful. Four recent reports, two on the humanized anti-tac (Zenapax™)[265A,B] and two on basiliximab (Simulect™)[265C,D], have demonstrated significant reductions in the incidence of acute rejection in prospective, randomized double-blind trials, when used as induction agents. Thus, there may well be a role for this class of antibodies.

Anti-CD52

Campath-1H is the humanized form of the rat anti-CD52 monoclonal Campath 1G. Both have been used in pilot clinical trials to manage rejection occurring after kidney transplantation.[266] Campath-1H successfully reversed rejection in 6 of 6 patients, although three of the patients had viral infections, one of them fatal. Antibodies to Campath-1H were not found, although they occurred in 7 of 15 patients treated with Campath-1G. Evaluation of Campath-1H is continuing, using less than half of the original dose.

Anti–Adhesion Molecule

Anti-CD11A mAbs bind to the α chain of LFA-1, an adhesion molecule that binds to ICAM-1. 25-3, an anti–LFA-1 mAb, was used to manage renal allograft rejection and was found to be ineffective in early trials but as effective as ATG in more recent trials.[267,268] Anti-CD54 mAbs target ICAM-1. BIRR-1, an anti-ICAM1 mAb, was studied in a phase I trial of renal transplantation that focused on recipients at increased risk for initial nonfunction. Better outcomes and less delayed function were found among the BIRR-1–treated patients.[269] A prospective, randomized, double-blind trial of BIRR-1 was started following this initial encouraging report.

Anti-CD7

SDZCH380, a human-mouse chimeric anti-CD7 mAb, has the ability to inhibit T-cell proliferation in the MLR. It was used as an induction agent in a small randomized trial of 20 recipients of first cadaveric renal transplants. Half the patients received SDZCH380 and half received OKT3.[270,271] Excellent (90%) allograft survival for more than 4 years was observed in the SDZCH380 group without evidence of chronic rejection. It is likely that further studies will be forthcoming in light of these favorable results.

Anti-CD2

BTI-322 (LO-CD2a) is a rat anti-CD2 monoclonal antibody that blocks the MLR. It has been used to manage acute rejection, both as a first-line agent and for steroid and/or OKT3-resistant rejection.[272,273] In both settings, it has been extremely effective. The mechanism of action is unknown, and further studies will be required to assess the role of this agent in renal transplantation.

▲ CONCLUSIONS

A large number of pharmacologic agents and mAbs are at various stages of clinical development. Sorting out the most effective agents or combinations will likely occupy the next 10 or more years. It is clear, however, that there are or will soon be a number of potential new options for the prevention or treatment of rejection in renal transplant patients.

▲ REFERENCES

Immunology of the Allograft Rejection Response

1. Janeway CA Jr, Travers P: *Immunobiology: The Immune System in Health and Disease.* New York, Garland, 1994.
2. Manning DD, Reed ND, Schaffer CF: Maintenance of skin xenografts of widely divergent phylogenetic origin on congenitally athymic (nude) mice. *J Exp Med* 138:488, 1973.
3. Neefjies JJ, Mombourg F: Cell biology of antigen presentation. *Curr Opin Immunol* 5:27, 1993.
4. Sherman LA, Chattopadhyay S: The molecular basis of allorecognition. *Annu Rev Immunol* 11:385, 1993.
5. Meuer SC, Fitzgerald KA, Hussey RE, Hodgdon JC, Schlossman SF, Reinharz EL: Clonotypic structures involved in antigen-specific human T-cell function: relationship to the T3 molecular complex. *J Immunol* 129:2293, 1982.
6. Janeway CA Jr: The T-cell receptor as a multicomponent signalling machine: CD4/CD8 coreceptors and CD45 in T-cell activation. *Annu Rev Immunol* 10:645, 1992.
7. Weiss A: T cell antigen receptor signal transduction: a tale of tails and cytoplasmic protein-tyrosine kinases. *Cell* 73:209, 1993.
8. Arai K, Lee F, Miyajima A, Arai N, Yokota T: Cytokines: coordinators of immune and inflammatory responses. *Annu Rev Biochem* 59:783, 1990.
9. Kagi D, Vignaux F, Ledermann B, et al: Fas and perforin pathways as major mechanisms of T cell–mediated cytotoxicity. *Science* 265:528, 1994.

10. David-Watine B, Isreal A, Trowsdale J: The regulation and expression of MHC class I genes. *Immunol Today* 11:286, 1990.
11. Glimcher LH, Cara CJ: Sequences and factors: a guide to MHC class II transcription. *Annu Rev Immunol* 10:13, 1992.
12. Ayoub G, Terasaki P: HLA-DR matching in multicenter, single-typing laboratory data. *Transplantation* 33:515, 1982.
13. Zijlstra M, Bix M, Simister NE, Loring JM, Raulet DH, Jaenisch R: β2-micro-globulin deficient mice lack $CD4^{-}8^{+}$ cytolytic T cells. *Nature* 344:742, 1990.
14. Koller BH, Marrack P, Kappler JW, Smithies O: Normal development of mice deficient in β2M, MHC class I proteins, and $CD8^{+}$ T cells. *Science* 248:1227, 1990.
15. Gosgrove D, Gray D, Dierich A, et al: Mice lacking MHC class II molecules. *Cell* 66:1051, 1991.
16. Grusby MJ, Johnson RS, Papaioannou VE, Glimcher LH: Depletion of $CD4^{+}$ T cells in major histocompatibility complex class II–deficient mice. *Science* 253:1417, 1991.
17. Steinman RM: The dendritic cell and its role in immunogenicity. *Annu Rev Immunol* 9:271, 1993.
18. Guerder S, Matzinger P: Activation versus tolerance: a decision made by T helper cells. *Cold Spring Harbor Symp Quant Biol* 54:799, 1989.
19. Waldmann H, Cobbold S: The use of monoclonal antibodies to achieve immunological tolerance. *Immunol Today* 14:247, 1993.
20. Bretscher P, Cohn M: A theory of self-nonself discrimination. *Science* 169:1042, 1970.
21. Lenschow DJ, Zeng Y, Thistlethwaite JR, et al: Long-term survival of xenogeneic pancreatic islet cell grafts induced by CTLA-4Ig. *Science* 257:789, 1992.
22. Mosmann TR, Coffman RL: Th1 and Th2 cells: different pattern of lymphokine secretion lead to different functional properties. *Annu Rev Immunol* 7:145, 1993.
23. Schreiber SL: Chemistry and biology of the immunophilins and their immunosuppressive ligands. *Science* 251:283, 1991.
24. MacKay CR, Marston W, Dudler L: Altered patterns of T-cell migration through lymph nodes and skin following antigen challenge. *Eur J Immunol* 22:2205, 1992.
25. Picker LJ, Butcher EC: Physiological and molecular mechanisms of lymphocyte homing. *Annu Rev Immunol* 10:561, 1992.
26. Kuppers RC, Henney CS: Studies on the mechanism of lymphocyte-mediated cytolysis. IX. Relationships between antigen recognition and lytic expression in killer T cells. *J Immunol* 118:71, 1977.
27. Paulnock DM: Macrophage activation by T cells. *Curr Opin Immunol* 4:344, 1992.
28. Kappler JW, Roehm N, Marrack P: T cell tolerance by clonal elimination in the thymus. *Cell* 49:273, 1987.

Immunologic Monitoring

29. Strober S, Dhillon M, Schubert M, et al: Acquired immune tolerance to cadaveric renal allografts. *N Engl J Med* 321:28, 1989.
30. Keenan RJ, Uknis ME, Pham S, et al: Mitogen responses of lymphocytes from lung transplant recipients: correlation with rejection and infection. *Transplantation* 54:241, 1992.
31. Roilides E, Clerici M, DePalma L, Rubin M, Pizzo P, Shearer GM: Helper T immunosuppressed cell responses in children infected with human immunodeficiency virus type 1. *J. Pediatr* 118:274, 1991.
32. Zeevi A, Pavlick M, Lombardozzi S, et al: Immune status of recipients following bone marrow-augmented solid organ transplantation. *Transplantation* 59:616, 1995.

33. Suciu- Foca N, Reed E, D'Agati VD, et al: Soluble HLA antigens, anti-HLA antibodies and anti-idiotypic antibodies in the circulation of renal transplant recipients. *Transplantation* 51:594, 1991.
34. Reed E, Hardy M, Benvenisty A: Effect of anti-idiotypic antibodies to HLA on graft survival in renal allograft recipients. *N Engl J Med* 316:1450, 1987.
35. Lobo PI, Spencer CE, Stevenson WC, Pruett TL: Evidence demonstrating poor kidney graft survival when acute rejections are associated with IgG donor-specific lymphocytotoxin. *Transplantation* 59:367, 1995.
36. Suciu-Foca N, Reed E, Marboe C, et al: Role of anti-HLA antibodies in heart transplantation. *Transplantation* 51:716, 1991.
37. Goulmy E, Stijnen T, Groenewoud AF, et al: Renal transplant patients monitored by the cell-mediated lympholysis assay. *Transplantation* 48:559, 1989.
38. Cohen DJ, Lee HM, Mohanakumar T: Mechanisms of CML hyporesponsiveness in long-term renal allograft recipients. *Hum Immunol* 14:279, 1985.
39. Thomas J, Johns C, Hoffmann S, Thomas F, Lee HM: Suppressor cells inhibiting the generation of cytotoxic T lymphocytes in long-term human transplant recipients. *Dial Transplant Forum* 7:87, 1978.
40. Pfeffer PF, Hirschberg H, Thorsby E: Donor-specific decreased primary and secondary cell-mediated immune responses in patients with well-functioning grafts. *Transplant Proc* 13:1604, 1981.
41. Charpentier BM, Lang P, Martin B, Fries D: Specific recipient-donor unresponsiveness mediated by a suppressor cell system in human kidney allograft tolerance. *Transplantation* 33:470, 1982.
42. Reinsmoen NL, Matas AJ, Kaufman D, Sutherland D, Najarian JS, Bach FH: Acquired donor-specific hyporesponsiveness in long-term kidney allograft recipients. *Transplant Proc* 23:141, 1991.
43. Reinsmoen NL, Matas AJ: Evidence that improved late renal transplant outcome correlates with the development of in vitro donor antigen-specific hyporeactivity. *Transplantation* 55:1017, 1993.
44. Zeevi A, Pavlick M, Lombardozzi S, et al: Serial evaluation of immune profiles of simultaneous bone marrow and whole organ transplant recipients. *Transplant Proc* 27:213, 1995.
45. Kahan BD, Derman RH, Van Buren CT, Flechner SM, Golden DL, Lewis RM: Clinical outcome in 36 patients after at least one and up to 5 years of steroid withdrawal based upon specific mixed lymphocyte reaction hyporesponsiveness toward the living related donor. *Transplant Proc* 21:1579, 1989.
46. Ingulli E, Shama V, Singh A, Suthanthiran M, Tejani A: Steroid withdrawal, rejection and mixed lymphocyte reaction in children after renal transplantation. *Kidney Int* 43:S-36, 1993.
47. Bishop DK, Shelby J, Eichwald EJ: Mobilization of T lymphocytes following cardiac transplantation: evidence that CD4-positive cells are required for cytotoxic T lymphocyte activation, inflammatory endothelial development, graft infiltration, and acute allograft rejection. *Transplantation* 53:849, 1993.
48. DeBruyne LA, Ensley RD, Olsen SL, et al: Increased frequency of alloantigen-reactive helper T lymphocytes is associated with human cardiac allograft rejection. *Transplantation* 56:722, 1993.
49. DeBruyne LA, Renlund DG, Bishop DK: Evidence that human cardiac allograft acceptance is associated with a decrease in donor-reactive helper T lymphocytes. *Transplantation* 59:778, 1995.
50. Theobald M, Nierle T, Bunjes D, Arnold R, Heinpel H: Host-specific interleukin-2 secret-

ing donor T cell precursors are predictors of acute graft-versus-host disease in bone marrow transplantation between HLA identical siblings. *N Engl J Med* 327:330, 1992.
51. Zeevi A, Fung J, Zerbe T, et al: Allospecificity of activated T cells grown from endomyocardial biopsies from heart transplant patients. *Transplantation* 41:620, 1986.
52. Weber T, Zerbe TR, Kaufman C, et al: Propagation of alloreactive lymphocytes from histologically negative endomyocardial biopsies from heart transplant patients. *Transplantation* 48:430, 1989.
53. Kirk AD, Ibrahim MA, Bollinger RR, Dawson DV, Finn OJ: Renal allograft-infiltrating lymphocytes: a prospective analysis of in vitro growth characteristics and clinical relevance. *Transplantation* 53:329, 1992.
54. Dallman MJ, Andrew CGP, Larsen CP, Morris PJ: Lymphokine production in allografts: analysis of RNA by Northern blotting. *Transplant Proc* 21:296, 1989.
55. O'Connell PJ, Pacheco-Silva A, Bastos M, et al: Sequential analysis of polymerase chain reaction of mononuclear leukocyte activation-associated transcription in pancreatic islet cell allograft rejection. *Transplant Proc* 23:811, 1991.
56. Dallmann MJ, Larsen CP, Morris PH: Cytokine gene transcription in vascularized grafts: analysis using semi-quantitative polymerase chain reaction. *J Exp Med* 174:493, 1991.
57. Lipman ML, Stevens AC, Bleackley RC, et al: The strong correlation of cytotoxic T lymphocyte-specific serine protease gene transcripts with renal allograft rejection. *Transplantation* 53:73, 1992.
58. Clement MV, Haddad P, Ring GH, Pruna A, Sasportes M: Granzyme B gene expression: a marker of human lymphocytes "activated" in vitro or in renal allografts. *Hum Immunol* 28:159, 1990.
59. Griffiths GM, Manikawa R, Mueller C, et al: Granzyme A and perforin as markers for rejection in cardiac transplantation. *Eur J Immunol* 21:687, 1991.
60. Clement MV, Haddad P, Soulie A, et al: Perforin and granzyme B as markers for acute rejection in heart transplantation. *Int Immunol* 3:1175, 1991.
61. Clement MV, Legros-Maida S, Israel-Biet D, et al: Perforin and granzyme B expression is associated with severe acute rejection. *Transplantation* 57:322, 1994.
62. Kataoka K, Naomoto Y, Shiozake S, et al: Infiltration of perforin-positive mononuclear cells into the rejected kidney allograft. *Transplantation* 53:240, 1991.
63. Xu GP, Sharma VJ, Li B, et al: Intragraft expression of IL-10 messenger RNA: a novel correlate of renal allograft rejection. *Kidney Int* 48:1504, 1995.
64. Fiorentino DF, Zlotni K, Vieira P, et al: IL-10 acts on the antigen-presenting cells to inhibit cytokine production by Th1 cells. *J Immunol* 146:3444, 1991.
65. Chen WF, Zlotnik A: Interleukin 10: a novel cytotoxic T cell differentiation factor. *J Immunol* 147:528, 1991.

Mechanisms of Action of Immunosuppressive Agents

66. Thomas AW, Starzl TE: New immunosuppressive drugs: mechanistic insights and therapeutic advances. *Immunol Rev* 136:71–98, 1993.
67. Allison AC, Lafferty KJ, Fliri H: Immunosuppressive and anti-inflammatory drugs. *Ann N Y Acad Sci* 696:1–419, 1993.
68. Kahan BD: New immunosuppressive drugs: pharmacologic approaches to alter immunoregulation. *Ther Immunol* 1:33–44, 1994.
69. Thomson AW, Starzl TE (eds): *Immunosuppressive Drugs: Developments in Anti-rejection Therapy.* Boston, Little, Brown, 1994.

70. Sigal NH, Dumont FJ: Cyclosporin A, FK-506, and rapamycin: pharmacologic probes of lymphocyte signal transduction. *Annu Rev Immunol* 10:519–60, 1992.
71. Kupiec-Weglinski JW (ed): *New Immunosuppressive Modalities and Anti-Rejection Approaches in Organ Transplantation.* Austin, Texas, Landes, 1994.
72. Foker JE, Simmons RL, Najarian JS: Allograft rejection. In: Najarian JS, Simmons RL (eds), *Transplantation.* Philadelphia, Lea & Febiger, 1972:63–145.
73. Gruber SA, Chan GLC, Canafax DM, Matas AJ: Immunosuppression in renal transplantation. II. Corticosteroids, antilymphocyte globulin, and OKT3. *Clin Transplant* 5:219, 1991.
74. Marino IR, Doyle HR: Conventional immunosuppressive agents. In: Thomson AW, Starzl TE (eds), *Immunosuppressive Drugs: Developments in Anti-rejection Therapy.* Boston, Little, Brown, 1994:1–14.
75. Allison AC, Eugui EM: Immunosuppressive and other effects of mycophenolic acid and an ester prodrug, mycophenolate mofetil. *Immunol Rev* 136:5–28, 1993.
76. Allison AC, Eugui EM: Mycophenolate mofetil (RS-61443): mode of action and effects on graft rejection. In: Thomson AW, Starzl TE (eds), *Immunosuppressive Drugs: Developments in Anti-rejection Therapy.* Boston, Little, Brown, 1994:141–159.
77. Amemiya H, Itoh H: Mizoribine (Bredinin): mode of action and effects on graft rejection. In: Thomson AW, Starzl TE (eds), *Immunosuppressive Drugs: Developments in Anti-rejection Therapy.* Boston, Little, Brown, 1994:161–176.
78. Dayton JS, Turka LA: Mizoribine. In: Kupiec-Weglinski JW (ed), *Medical Intelligence Unit: New Immunosuppressive Modalities and Anti-rejection Approaches in Organ Transplantation.* Austin, Texas, Landes, 1994:31–42.
79. Makowka L, Cramer DV: Brequinar sodium: mode of action and effects on graft rejection. In: Thomson AW, Starzl TE (eds), *Immunosuppressive Drugs: Developments in Anti-rejection Therapy.* Boston, Little, Brown, 1994:177–186.
80. Woo J, Lemster B, Tamura K, Starzl TE, Thomson AW: The antilymphocytic activity of brequinar sodium and its potentiation by cytidine: effects on lymphocyte proliferation and cytokine production. *Transplantation* 56:374–81, 1993.
81. Tamura K, Woo J, Bakri MT, Thomson AW: Brequinar sodium inhibits interleukin-6-induced differentiation of a human B-cell line into IgM-secreting plasma cells. *Immunology* 79:487–493, 1993.
82. Kahan BD: Cyclosporine. *N Engl J Med* 321:1725, 1989.
83. Gruber SA, Chan GLC, Canafax DM, Matas AJ: Immunosuppression in renal transplantation. I. Cyclosporine and azathioprine. *Clin Transplant* 5:65, 1991.
84. Boyle MJ, Kahan BD: Immunosuppressive role of rapamycin in allograft rejection. In: Thomson AW, Starzl TE (eds), *Immunosuppressive Drugs: Developments in Anti-rejection Therapy.* Boston, Little, Brown, 1994:129–140.
85. Bach FH, Sachs DH: Transplantation immunology. *N Engl J Med* 317:489, 1987.
86. Demattos AM, Norma DJ: OKT3 for treatment of rejection in renal transplantation. *Clin Transplant* 7:374, 1993.
87. Goldstein G: Overview of the development of orthoclone OKT3: monoclonal antibody for therapeutic use in transplantation. *Transplant Proc* 19:1, 1987.
88. Amemiya H: 15-Deoxyspergualin. In: Kupiec-Weglinski JW (ed), *Medical Intelligence Unit: New Immunosuppressive Modalities and Anti-rejection Approaches in Organ Transplantation.* Austin, Texas, Landes, 1994:75–91.
89. Suzuki S: Deoxyspergualin: mode of action and effects on graft rejection. In: Thomson AW, Starzl TE (eds), *Immunosuppressive Drugs: Developments in Anti-rejection Therapy.* Boston, Little, Brown, 1994:187–202.
90. Tepper MA: Deoxyspergualin: mechanism of action studies of a novel immunosuppressive drug. *Ann NY Acad Sci* 696:123–132, 1993.

91. Masroor S, Schroeder TJ, Michler RE, Alexander JW, First MR: Monoclonal antibodies in organ transplantation: an overview. *Transplant Immunol* 2:176, 1994.
92. Waldmann H: Manipulation of T-cell responses with monoclonal antibodies. *Ann Rev Immunol* 7:407, 1989.
93. Lin H, Bolling SF, Linsley PS, et al: Long-term acceptance of major histocompatibility complex mismatched cardiac allografts induced by CTLA4Ig plus donor-specific transfusion. *J Exp Med* 178:1801–1806, 1993.
94. Pugh-Humphreys RGP, Thomson AW: Cytokines and their receptors as therapeutic targets. In: Thomson AW (ed), *The Cytokine Handbook,* ed 2. Boston, Academic Press, 1994:525–566.
95. Stepkowski SM, Tu Y, Condor TP, Bennett CF: Blocking of heart allograft rejection by intercellular adhesion molecule-1 antisense oligonucleotides alone or in combination with other immunosuppressive modalities. *J Immunol* 153:5336, 1994.
96. Qin L, Chavin KD, Ding Y, et al: Multiple vectors effectively achieve gene transfer in a murine cardiac transplantation model. *Transplantation* 59:809–816, 1995.

Histocompatibility Testing and Cross Matching

97. Bodmer JG, Marsh SE, Albert EK, et al: Nomenclature for factors of the HLA system. *Hum Immunol* 43:149–153, 1995.
98. Mickey MR: Center variability. In: Terasaki PI (ed), *Clinical Transplants 1989.* UCLA Tissue Typing Laboratory, Los Angeles, 1989:435–445.
99. Patel R, Terasaki PI: Significance of the positive crossmatch test in kidney transplantation. *N Engl J Med* 280:735–739, 1969.
100. Iwaki Y, Terasaki PI, Park MS, Billing R: Enhancement of human kidney allografts and B cold lymphocyte cytotoxins. *Lancet* 2:1228–1229, 1978.
101. Fuller TC, Cosimi AB, Russell PS: Use of an antiglobulin ATG reagent for detection of low levels of alloantibody—improvement of allograft survival in presensitized patients. *Transplant Proc* 10:463–466,
102. Iwaki Y, Cook D, Terasaki PI, et al: Flow cytometry crossmatching in human cadaver kidney transplantation. *Transplant Proc* 19:746–766, 1987.
103. Iwaki Y, Lau M, Terasaki PI: Successful transplants across T-warm IgM positive crossmatches. *Clin Transplant* 2:81–84, 1988.
104. Ozturk G, Terasaki PI: Non-HLA lymphocyte cytotoxins in various diseases. *Tissue Antigens* 14:52–58, 1979.
105. Chapman JR, Taylor CJ, Ting A, Morris PJ: Immunoglobulin class and specificity of antibodies causing positive T-cell crossmatches: relationship to renal transplant outcome. *Transplantation* 42:608–613, 1986.

Conventional Immunosuppressive Agents

106. Billingham RE, Krohn PL, Medawar PB: Effect of locally applied cortisone acetate on survival of skin homografts in rabbits. *Br Med J* 2:1049–1053, 1951.
107. Tornatore KM, Reed KA, Venuto RC: Methylprednisolone and cortisol metabolism during the early post-renal transplant period. *Clin Transplant* 9:427–432, 1995.
108. Schwartz R, Dameshek W: The effects of 6-mercaptopurine on homograft reactions. *J Clin Invest* 39:952–958, 1960.
109. Calne RY, Murray JE: Inhibition of the rejection of renal homografts in dogs by Burroughs Wellcome 57-222. *Surg Forum* 12:118, 1961.

110. Starzl TE, Marchioro TL, Waddell WR: The reversal of rejection in human renal homografts with subsequent development of homograft tolerance. *Surg Gynecol Obstet* 117:385, 1963.
111. Lia-no F, Moreno A, Matesanz R, et al: Veno-occlusive hepatic disease of the liver in renal transplantation: is azathioprine the cause? *Nephron* 51:509–516, 1989.
112. Frick TW, Fryd DS, Goodale RL, et al: Lack of association between azathioprine and acute pancreatitis in renal transplant patients. *Lancet* 337:251–252, 1991.
113. Bach JF: *The Mode of Action of Immunosuppressive Agents.* Amsterdam, North-Holland, 1975.
114. Kirkman RL, Strom TB, Weir MR, Tilney NL: Late mortality and morbidity in recipients of long-term renal allografts. *Transplantation* 34:347–351, 1982.
115. Starzl TE, Putnam CS, Halgrimson CG, et al: Cyclophosphamide and whole organ transplantation in human beings. *Surg Gynecol Obstet* 133:981–991, 1971.
116. Floersheim GL: Pharmacologic immunosuppressive agents. *Transplant Proc* 12:315–319, 1980.
117. Kumararatne DS, Gagnon RF, Smart Y: Selective loss of large lymphocytes from the marginal zone of the white pulp in rat spleens following a single dose of cycloposphamide. *Immunology* 40:123–131, 1980.
118. Lagrange PH, Mackaness GB, Miller TE: Potentiation of T-cell mediated immunity by selective suppression of antibody formation with cyclophosphamide. *J Exp Med* 139:1529–1539, 1974.
119. Taube DH, Williams DG, Cameron JS, et al: Renal transplantation after removal and prevention of resynthesis of HLA antibodies. *Lancet* 1:824–828, 1984.
120. Moore MJ: Clinical pharmacokinetics of cyclophosphamide. *Clin Parmacokinet* 20:194–208, 1991.
121. Andriole GL, Sandlund JT, Miser JS, et al: The efficacy of Mesna (2-mercaptoethane sodium sulfonate) as a uroprotectant in patients with hemorrhagic cystitis receiving further oxazaphosphorine chemotherapy. *J Clin Oncol* 5:799–803, 1987.
122. Borel JF, Feurer C, Gubler HU, Stahelin H: Biological effects of cyclosporin A: a new antilymphocytic agent. *Agents Actions* 6:468, 1976.
123. Calne RY, Rolles K, White DJG, et al: Cyclosporin A initially as the only immunosuppressant in 34 recipients of cadaveric organs: 32 kidneys, 2 pancreas, and 2 livers. *Lancet* 2:1022, 1979.
124. Starzl TE, Weil R, Iwatsuki S, et al: The use of cyclosporin A and prednisone in cadaveric kidney transplantation. *Surg Gynecol Obstet* 151:17, 1980.
125. Levy G, Grant D: Potential for CsA-Neoral in organ transplantation. *Transplant Proc* 26:2932–2934, 1994.
126. Kovarik JM, Mueller EA, van Bree JB, et al: Cyclosporine pharmacokinetics and variability from a microemulsion formulation: a multicenter investigation in kidney transplant patients. *Transplantation* 58:658–663, 1994.
127. Sketris IS, Lawen JG, Beauregard-Zollinger L, et al: Comparison of the pharmacokinetics of cyclosporine Sandimmune and Sandimmune Neoral in stable renal transplant patients. *Transplant Proc* 26:2961–2963, 1994.
128. Lindholm A: Factors influencing the pharmacokinetics of cyclosporine in man. Ther Drug Monit 13:465–477, 1991.
129. Vonderscher J, Meinzer A: Rationale for the development of Sandimmune Neoral. *Transplant Proc* 26:2925–2927, 1994.
130. Follath F, Wenk M, Vozeh S, et al: Intravenous cyclosporine kinetics in renal failure. *Clin Pharmacol Ther* 34:638–643, 1983.

131. Wood AJ, Maurer G, Niederberger W, et al: Cyclosporine: pharmacokinetics, metabolism, and drug interactions. *Transplant Proc* 15(Suppl):2409–2412, 1983.
132. Yee GC, Salomon DR: Cyclosporine. In: Evans WE, Schentag JJ, Jusko WJ (eds), *Applied Pharmacokinetics: Principles of Therapeutic Drug Monitoring,* 3d ed. Vancouver, Applied Therapeutics, 1992: 28.1–28.40.
133. Shaw LM, Yatscoff RW, Bowers LD, et al: Canadian consensus meeting on cyclosporine monitoring: report of the consensus panel. *Clin Chem* 36:1841–1846, 1990.
134. Ptachcinski RJ, Burckart GJ, Venkataramanan R: Cyclosporine. *Drug Intell Clin Pharm* 19:90–100, 1985.
135. Yee GC, McGuire TR: Pharmacokinetic drug interactions with cyclosporine. I. *Clin Pharmacokinet* 190:319–322, 1990.
136. Morgenstern GR, Powles R, Robinson B, et al: Cyclosporine interaction with keoconazole and melphalan. *Lancet* 2:1342, 1982.
137. Murray BM, Edwards L, Morse GD, et al: Clinically important interaction of cyclosporine and erythromycin. *Transplantation* 43:602–604, 1987.
138. Nampoory MRN, Nessim F, Gupta RK, et al: Drug interaction of chloroquine with cyclosporin. *Nephron* 62:108–109, 1992.
139. Wagner K, Henkel M, Heinemeyer G, et al: Interaction of calcium blockers and cyclosporine. *Transplant Proc* 20(Suppl 2):561–568, 1988.
140. Frei U, Taesch S, Niese D for the International Sandimmun Neoral Study Group: Use of Sandimmun Neoral in renal transplant patients. *Transplant Proc* 26:2928–2931, 1994.
141. Remuzzi G, Bertani T: Renal vascular and thrombotic effects of cyclosporine. *Am J Kidney Dis* 13:261–272, 1989.
142. Keown PA, Stiller CR, Wallace AC: Effect of cyclosporine on the kidney. *J Pediatr* 111:1029–1033, 1987.
143. American Hospital Formulary Service: *AHFS Drug Information 91.* ed 33. Bethesda, MD, American Society of Hospital Pharmacists, 1991.
144. Luke RG: Mechanism of cyclosporine-induced hypertension. *Am J Hypertens* 4:468–471, 1991.
145. Mason J: The pathophysiology of Sandimmune (cyclosporine) in man and animals. *Pediatr Nephrol* 4:554–574, 1990.
146. Mason J: The pathophysiology of Sandimmune (cyclosporine) in man and animals. *Pediatr Nephrol* 4:686–704, 1990.
147. Scott JP, Higgenbottam TW: Adverse reactions and interactions of cyclosporin. *Med Toxicol Adverse Drug Exp* 3:107–127, 1988.
148. Reznick VM, Lyons Jones K, Curham BL, et al: Changes in facial appearance during cyclosporine treatment. *Lancet* 1:1405–1407, 1987.
149. Karch SB, Billingham ME: Cyclosporine induced myocardial fibrosis: a unique controlled case report. *J Heart Transplant* 5:210–212, 1985.
150. Lorber MI: Cyclosporine: lessons learned—future strategies. *Clin Transplant* 5:505–516, 1991.
151. Kopp JB, Klotman PE: Cellular and molecular mechanisms of cyclosporin nephrotoxicity. *J Am Soc Nephrol* 1:162–179, 1990.
152. Woodreff MFA, Anderson NA: Effect of lymphocyte depletion by thoracic duct fistula and administration of antilymphocyte serum on the survival of skin homograft in rat. *Nature* 200:702, 1963.
153. Najarian J, Simmons R, Condie R, et al: Seven years experience with antilymphoblast globulin for renal transplants from cadaver donors. *Ann Surg* 184:352–368, 1976.
154. Starzl TE, Marchioro TL, Porter KA, Iwasaki T, Cerilli GJ: The use of heterologous anti-

lymphoid agents in canine renal and liver homotransplantation and in human renal homotransplantation. *Surg Gynecol Obstet* 24:301, 1967.
155. Griepp R, Stinson E, Dong E, et al: The use of antithymocyte globulin in human heart transplantation. *Circulation* 45(Suppl):147–153, 1972.
156. Glass N, Miller D, Sollinger H, et al: A comparative study of steroid and heterologous antiserum in the treatment of acute renal allograft rejection. *Transplant Proc* 15:617–621, 1983.
157. Starzl TE: *Experience in Hepatic Transplantation*. Philadelphia, Saunders, 1969: 193–241.
158. Starzl TE: *Experience in Hepatic Transplantation*. Philadelphia, Saunders, 1969: 242–276.
159. Lum CT, Umen AJ, Kasiske B, et al: Clinical impact of replacing Minnesota antilymphocyte globulin with ATGAM. *Transplantation* 59:371–376, 1995.
160. Bourdage JS, Hamlin DM: Comparative polyclonal antithymocyte globulin and antilymphocyte/antilymphoblast globulin anti-CD antigen analysis by flow cytometry. *Transplanation* 59:1194–1200, 1995.
161. Bonnefoy-Berard N, Vincent C, Revillard JP: Antibodies against functional leukocyte surface molecules in polyclonal antilymphocyte and antithymocyte globulins. *Transplantation* 51:669–673, 1991.
162. Rebellato LM, Gross U, Verbanac KM, Thomas JM: A comprehensive definition of the major antibody specificities in polyclonal rabbit antithymocyte globulin. *Transplanation* 57:685–694, 1994.
163. Kohler G, Milstein C: Continuous cultures of fused cells secreting antibody of predefined specificity. *Nature* 256:495–497, 1975.
164. Kung P, Goldstein G, Reinherz E, et al: Monoclonal antibodies defining distinctive human T cell surface antigens. *Science* 206:347–349, 1979.
165. Cosimi A, Colvin R, Burton R, et al: Use of monoclonal antibodies to T cell subsets for immunologic monitoring and treatment in recipients of renal allografts. *N Engl J Med* 305:308–314, 1981.
166. Cosimi A, Burton R, Colvin R, et al: Treatment of acute allograft rejection with OKT3 monoclonal antibody. *Transplantation* 32:535–539, 1981.
167. Fung JJ, Demetris AJ, Porter KA, et al: Use of OKT3 with cyclosporin and steroids for reversal of acute kidney and liver allograft rejection. *Nephron* 46(Suppl 1):19–33, 1987.
168. Norman D, Shield C, Barry J, et al: Therapeutic use of OKT3 monoclonal antibody for acute renal allograft rejection. *Nephron* 46(Suppl 1):41–47, 1987.
169. Millis J, McDiarmid S, Hiatt J, et al: Randomized prospective trial of OKT3 for early prophylaxis of rejection after liver transplantation. *Transplantation* 47:82–88, 1989.
170. Stratta RJ, D'Alessandro AM, Armbrust MJ, et al: Sequential antilymphocyte globulin/cyclosporine immunosuppression in cadaveric renal transplantation: effect of duration of ALG therapy. *Transplantation* 47:96–102, 1989.
171. Benvenisty AI, Cohen D, Stegall MD, et al: Improved results using OKT3 as induction immunosuppression in renal allograft recipients with delayed graft function. *Transplantation* 40:321–327, 1990.
172. Cockfield SM, Preiksaitis J, Harvey E, et al: In sequential use of ALG and OKT3 in renal transplants associated with an increased incidence of fulminant posttransplant lymphoproliferative disorder? *Transplant Proc* 23:1106–1107, 1991.
173. Taylor RM: Monoclonal and polyclonal antibodies: clinical aspects. *Immunol Lett* 29:113–116, 1991.
174. Barr ML, Sanchez JA, Seche LA, et al: Anti-CD3 monoclonal antibody induction therapy: immunological equivalency with triple-drug therapy in heart transplantation. *Circulation* 82:IV291–IV294, 1990.

175. Menkis AH, McKenzie FN, Thomson D, et al: Benefits of avoidance of induction immunosuppression in heart transplantation. *J Heart Transplant* 8:311–314, 1989.
176. Macris MP, Van Buren CT, Sweeney MS, et al: Selective use of OKT3 in heart transplan tation with the use of risk factor analysis. *J Heart Transplant* 8:296–302, 1989.
177. Thistlethwaite JR, Heffron TG, Stuart JK, et al: Selective use of OKT3 induction therapy in adult cadaveric-donor renal transplant recipients. *Am J Kidney Dis* 8:296–302, 1989.
178. Chatenoud L, Gerran C, Legendre C, et al: In vivo cell activation following OKT3 administration. *Transplantation* 49:697–702, 1990.
179. Goldstein G, Norman DJ, Henell KR, Smith IL: Pharmacokinetic study of Orthoclone OKT3 serum levels during treatment of acute renal allograft rejection. *Transplantation* 46:587, 1988.
180. Chatenoud L, Baudrihaaye MF, Chkoff N, Kreis H, Goldstein G, Bach JF: Restriction of the human in vivo immune response against the mouse monoclonal antibody OKT3. *J Immunol* 137:830, 1986.
181. Kreis H, Legendre C, Chatenoud L: OKT3 in organ transplantation. *Transplant Rev* 5:181–199, 1991.
182. Prieto M, Lake KD, Pritzker MR, et al: OKT3 induction and steroid-free maintenance immunosuppression for treatment of high-risk heart transplant recipients. *J Heart Lung Transplant* 10:901–911, 1991.
183. Schroeder T, First M, Mansour M, et al: Antimurine antibody formation following OKT3 therapy. *Transplantation* 49:48–51, 1990.
184. D'Alessandro AM, Pirsch JD, Stratta RJ, et al: OKT3 salvage therapy in a quadruple immunosuppressive protocol in cadaveric renal transplantation. *Transplantation* 47:297–300, 1989.

Clinical Experience with New Immunosuppressive Agents in Renal Transplant Recipients

185. Todo S, Fung JJ, Starzl TE: Liver, kidney, and thoracic organ transplantation under FK506. *Ann Surg* 212:295, 1990.
186. Fung JJ, Abu-Elmagd K, Jain A, et al: A randomized trial of FK506 vs. cyclosporine. *Transplant Proc* 23:2977, 1991.
187. Klintmalm G and the U.S. Multicenter FK506 Liver Study Group: A comparison of tacrolinus (FK506) and cyclosporine for immunosuppression after liver transplantation. *N Engl J Med* 331:1110, 1994.
188. Todo S, Fung JJ, Starzl TE, et al: Single-center experience with primary orthotopic liver transplantation under FK506 immunosuppression. *Ann Surg* 222:270–280, 1995.
189. Starzl TE, Fung JJ, Jordan M, et al: Kidney transplantation under FK506. *Transplant Proc* 23:920, 1993.
190. Shapiro R, Todo S, Starzl TE: Kidney transplantation under FK506 immunosuppression. *Transplant Proc* 23:920, 1991.
191. Shapiro R, Jordan ML, Scantlebury V, et al: FK506 in clinical kidney transplantation. *Transplant Proc* 23:3065, 1991.
192. Shapiro R, Jordan M, Scantlebury V, et al: Randomized trial of FK506/prednisone vs. FK506/azathioprine/prednisone after renal transplantation: preliminary report. *Transplant Proc* 25:669, 1993.
193. Shapiro R, Jordan M, Scantlebury V, et al: A prospective, randomized trial of FK506 in renal transplantation: a comparison between double and triple drug therapy. *Clin Transplant* 8:508, 1994.
194. Shapiro R, Jordan ML, Scantlebury VP, et al: A prospective, randomized trial of FK506-based immunosuppression after renal transplantation. *Transplantation* 59:485–490, 1995.

195. Shapiro R, Jordan ML, Scantlebury VP, et al: A prospective, randomized trial of FK506/prednisone vs. FK506/azathioprine/prednisone in renal transplant patients. *Transplant Proc* 27:1:814–817, 1995.
196. Shapiro R, Jordan ML, Scantlebury VP, et al: The superiority of tacrolimus in renal transplant recipients: the Pittsburgh experience. In: Terasaki PI, Cecka JM (eds), *Clinical Transplants 1995.* UCLA Tissue Typing Laboratory, Los Angeles, 1996:199–205.
197. Shapiro R, Jordan ML, Scantlebury VP, et al: Tacrolimus in renal transplantation. *Transplant Proc*, 28(4):2117–2118, 1996.
198. Shapiro R, Jordan ML, Scantlebury VP, et al: Tacrolimus in pediatric renal transplantation. Transplantation 62:1752–1758, 1996.
199. Shapiro R, Jordan ML, Scantlebury VP, et al: FK506 in pediatric kidney transplantation—primary and rescue experience. *Pediatr Nephr* 9:S43–S48, 1995.
200. Jordan ML, Shapiro R, Vivas CA, et al: FK506 salvage of renal allografts with ongoing rejection failing cyclosporine immunosuppression. *Transplant Proc* 25:1:638–640, 1993.
201. Jordan M, Shapiro R, Vivas C, et al: FK506 rescue for resistant rejection of renal allograft under primary cyclosporine immunosuppression. *Transplantation* 57:6:860–865, 1994.
202. McCauley J, Takaya S, Fung J, et al: The question of FK506 nephrotoxicity after liver transplantation. *Transplant Proc* 23:1444, 1991.
203. Starzl TE, Abu-Elmagd K, Tzakis A, Fung JJ, Porter KA, Todo S: Selected topics on FK506, with special references to rescue of extrahepatic whole organ grafts, transplantation of "forbidden organs," side effects, mechanisms, and practical pharmacokinetics. *Transplant Proc* 23:914, 1991.
204. Starzl TE: FK506 versus cyclosporine. *Transplant Proc* 25:511, 1993.
205. Demetris AJ, Banner B, Fung JJ, Shapiro R, Jordan M, Starzl TE: Histopathology of human renal allograft function under FK506: a comparison with cyclosporine. *Transplant Proc* 23:944, 1991.
206. Randhawa PS, Shapiro R, Jordan ML, Starzl TE, Demetris AJ: The histopathological changes associated with allograft rejection and drug toxicity in renal transplant recipients maintained on FK506: clinical significance and comparison with cyclosporine. *Am J Surg Pathol* 17:60, 1993.
207. Shapiro R, Fung JJ, Jain AB, Parks P, Todo S, Starzl TE: The side effects of FK506 in humans. *Transplant Proc* 22:1:35, 1990.
208. Scantlebury V, Shapiro R, Fung JJ, et al: New onset of diabetes in FK506 vs. cyclosporine-treated kidney transplant recipients. *Transplant Proc* 23:3169, 1991.
209. Scantlebury V, Shapiro R, Tzakis A, et al: Pediatric kidney transplantation at the University of Pittsburgh. *Transplant Proc* 26:1:46–47, 1994.
210. Ellis D, Shapiro R, Jordan ML, et al: Comparison of FK506 and cyclosporine regimens in pediatric renal transplantation. *Pediatr Nephrol* 8:193–200, 1994.
211. Japanese FK506 Study Group: Japanese study of FK506 on kidney transplantation: the benefit of monitoring the whole blood FK506 concentration. *Transplant Proc* 23:3085, 1991.
212. Japanese FK506 Study Group: Japanese study of FK506 on kidney transplantation: results of late phase II study. *Transplant Proc* 25:649, 1993.
213. Ochiai T, Ishibashi M, Fukao K, et al, and the Japanese FK506 Study Group: Japanese multicenter studies of FK506 in renal transplantation. *Transplant Proc* 22:1:50, 1995.
214: Japanese FK506 Study Group, Yokoyama I, Uchida K, Fukao K, et al: FK506: long-term study in kidney transplantation. *Transplant Proc* 22:818, 1995.
215. Japanese FK506 Study Group, Ochiai K, Fukao K, Takahashi K, et al: Phase III study of FK506 in kidney transplantation. *Transplant Proc* 22:829, 1995.

216. Laskow DA, Vincenti F, Neylan J, Mendez R, Matas A: Phase II FK506 multicenter concentration control study: one-year follow-up. *Transplant Proc* 22:809, 1995.
217. Ciancio G, Roth D, Burke G, et al: Renal transplantation in a new immunosuppressive era. *Transplant Proc* 27:812–813, 1995.
218. Roth D, Shapiro R, Scantlebury V, et al: Long-term follow-up kidney recipients converted from cyclosporine to FK506 for severe rejection. Presented at the 14th Annual Meeting of the Society of Transplant Physicians, May 14–17, 1995, Chicago.
219. Woodle ES, Haas M, Josephson MA, et al: Role of protocol biopsies in the treatment of refractory renal allograft rejection with FK506. *Transplant Proc* 28:1008–1009, 1996.
220. Woodle ES, Thistlethwaite JR, Gordon JH, for the FK506 Kidney Transplant Rescue Study Group: A multicenter trial of FK506 (tacrolimus) rescue therapy in renal transplantation (abstract). *J Am Soc Nephrol* 6:1122, 1995.
220a. Woodle ES, Thistlethwaite JR, Gordon JH: A prospective, multicenter trial of FK506 (tacrolimus) therapy for refractory acute renal allograft rejection. Presented at the 16th International Congress of the Transplantation Society, August 25–30, 1996, Barcelona.
221. Gjertson DW, Cecka JM, Terasaki PI: The relative effects of FK506 and cyclosporine on short- and long-term kidney graft survival. *Transplantation* 60:1384–1388, 1995.
222. Pirsch JD, Miller J, Deierhoi MH, et al: A comparison of tacrolimus (FK506) and cyclosporine for immunosuppression after cadaveric renal transplantation. *Transplantation* 63:977–983, 1997.
222a. Miller J, Pirsch JD, Deierhoi R: FK506 in kidney transplantation: results of the U.S.A. Randomized Comparative Phase III Study. *Transplant Proc* 29:304–305, 1997.
223. Schleibner S, Krauss M, Wagner K, et al: FK506 versus cyclosporin in the prevention of renal allograft rejection: European pilot study—six-week results. *Transplant Int* 8:86–90, 1995.
223a. vanHooff J, Buchholz B, Eigler F, et al: The European multicentre prospective randomized trial comparing tacrolimus and cyclosporine in the prevention of renal allograft rejection. Presented at the 16th International Congress of the Transplantation Society, August 25–30, 1996, Barcelona.
224. Mathew A, Talbot D, Minford EJ, et al: Reversal of steroid-resistant rejection in renal allograft recipients using FK506. *Transplantation* 60:1182–1184, 1995.
225. Felldin M, Backman L, Brattstrom C, et al: Rescue therapy with tacrolimus (FK506) in renal transplant recipients: A multicenter analysis. *Transplant Proc* 27:3425, 1995.
226. Sollinger HW, Deierhoi MH, Belzer FO, Diethelm AG, Kauffman RS: RS-61443-A phase I clinical trial and pilot rescue study. *Transplantation* 53:428, 1992.
227. Sollinger HW: RS-61443 (mycophenolate mofetil). Plenary Address, XVth World of Congress of the Transplantation Society, August 29, 1994, Kyoto, Japan.
228. Sollinger HW for the U.S. Renal Transplant Mycophenolate Mofetil Study Group: Mycophenolate mofetil for the prevention of acute rejection in primary cadaveric renal allograft recipients. *Transplantation* 60:225–232, 1995.
229. Tricontinental Mycophenolate Mofetil Renal Transplantation Study Group: A blinded, randomized clinical trial of mycophenolate mofetil for the prevention of acute rejection in cadaveric renal transplantation. *Transplantation* 61:1029–1037, 1996.
230. Tomlanovich S, Danovitch G, Rosenthal J, et al: Comparison of mycophenolate mofetil versus intravenous corticosteroids for treatment of refractory renal allograft rejection. Presented at XVth World of Congress of the Transplantation Society, September 1, 1994, Kyoto, Japan.
231. Mycophenolate Mofetil Renal Transplantation Study Group: Mycophenolate mofetil for

the treatment of refractory, acute cellular renal transplant rejection. *Transplantation* 61:722–729, 1996.
232. Kahan BD: Concentration-controlled immunosuppressive regimens using cyclosporine with sirolimus or brequinar in human renal transplantation. *Transplant Proc* 27:1:33–38, 1995.
233. Kahan BD: Brequinar and rapamycin trials. Presented at the ASTP/ASTS Joint Symposium, May, 1994, Chicago.
234. Kahan BD, Pescovitz M, Julian B, Chan G, Vanrcterghcm Y, and the Sirolimus Multi-Center Study Group: Multi-center phase II trial of sirolimus in renal transplantation: six-month results. Presented at the ASTP/ASTS Joint Symposium, May, 1996, Dallas.
235. Kahan BD, Katz SM, Jordan S, Van Buren CT: Sirolimus permits rapid corticosteroid withdrawal from a cyclosporine-based regimen in renal transplantation. Presented at the 15th Annual Meeting of the ASTP, May, 1996, Dallas.
236. Tajima A, Hata M, Ohta N, Ohtawara Y, Kazuo S, Aso Y: Bredinin treatment in clinical kidney allografting. *Transplantation* 38:116–118, 1984.
237. Aso K, Uchida H, Sato K, et al: Immunosuppression with low-dose cyclosporine com bined with bredinin and prednisolone. *Transplant Proc* 19:1955–1958, 1987.
238. Marumo F, Okubo M, Yokota K, et al: A clinical study of renal transplant patients receiving triple-drug therapy: cyclosporine A, mizorbine and prednisolone. *Transplant Proc* 20:1:406–409, 1988.
239. Takahara S, Fukunishi T, Kokado Y, et al: Combined immunosuppression with low-dose cyclosporine, mizorbine, and prednisolone. *Transplant Proc* 20:3:147–151, 1988.
240. Kokado Y, Ishibashi M, Jiang H, Takahara S, Sonoda T: A new triple-drug induction therapy with low dose cyclosporine, mizoribine, and prednisolone in renal transplantation. *Transplant Proc* 21:1575–1578, 1989.
241. Mita K, Akiyama N, Nagao T, et al: Advantages of mizoribine over azathioprine in combination therapy with cyclosporine for renal transplantation. *Transplant Proc* 22: 1679–1681, 1990.
242. Takada K, Asada S, Ichikawa Y, et al: Pharmacokinetics of bredinin in renal transplant patients. *Eur J Clin Pharmacol* 24:457–461, 1983.
243. Ameniya H, Suzuki S, Kazuo O, et al: A novel rescue drug, 15-deoxyspergualin. *Transplantation* 49:337–343, 1990.
244. Takahashi K, Ota K, Tanabe K, et al: Effect of a novel immunosuppressive agent, deoxyspergualin, on rejection in kidney transplant recipients. *Transplant Proc* 22:1606–1612, 1990.
245. Suzuki S, Hayashi R, Kenmochi T, Shimatani K, Fukuoka T, Amemiya H: Clinical application of 15-deoxyspergualin for treatment of acute graft rejection following renal transplantation. *Transplant Proc* 22:1615–1617, 1990.
246. Amemiya H, Dohi K, Otsubo O, et al: Markedly enhanced therapeutic effect of deoxyspergualin on acute rejection when combined with methylprednisolone in kidney recipients. *Transplant Proc* 23:1087–1089, 1991.
247. Takahashi K, Tanabe K, Ooba S, et al: Prophylactic use of a new immunosuppressive agent, deoxyspergualin, in patients with kidney transplantation from ABO-incompatible or preformed antibody-positive donors. *Transplantation* 23:1078–1082, 1991.
248. Okazaki H, Sato T, Jimbo M, Senga S, Amada N, Oguma S: Prophylactic use of deoxyspergualin in living related renal transplantation. *Transplant Proc* 23:1094–1095, 1991.
249. Koyama I, Amemiya H, Taguchi Y, et al: Prophylactic use of deoxyspergualin in a quadru-

ple immunosuppressive protocol in renal transplantation. *Transplant Proc* 23:1096–1098, 1991.
250. Groth CG, Ohlman S, Ericzon BG, Barkholt L, Reinhold FP: Deoxyspergualin for liver graft rejection (letter). *Lancet* 336:626, 1990.
251. Chong AS-F, Gebel H, Finnegan A, et al: Leflunomide, a novel immunomodulatory agent: in vitro analyses of the mechanism of immunosuppression. *Transplant Proc* 25:747, 1993.
252. Morris RE, Huang X, Cao W, Zheng B, Shorthouse RA: Leflunomide (HWA 486) and its analog suppress T- and B-cell proliferation in vitro, acute rejection, ongoing rejection, and antidonor antibody synthesis in mouse, rat, and cynomolgus monkey transplant recipients as well as arterial intimal thickening after balloon catheter injury. *Transplant Proc* 27:445–447, 1995.
253. Waid TH, Lucas BA, Thompson JS, et al: Treatment of acute cellular rejection with T10B9.1A-31 or OKT3 in renal allograft recipients. *Transplantation* 53:80–86, 1992.
254. Cosimi AB: Future of monoclonal antibodies in solid organ transplantation. *Dig Dis Sci,* 40(1):65–72, 1995.
255. Frenken LAM, Hoitsma AJ, Tax WJM, Koene RAP: Prophylactic use of anti-CD3 monoclonal antibody WT32 in kidney transplantation. *Transplant Proc* 23:1072–1073, 1991.
256. Land W: Monoclonal antibodies in 1991: new potential options in clinical immunosuppressive therapy. *Clin Transplant* 5:495–500, 1991.
257. Cooperative Clinical Trials in Transplantation (CCTT) Research Group: Murine OKT4A immunosuppression in cadaver donor renal allograft recipients: a cooperative pilot study. *Transplant Proc* 27:863, 1995.
258. Meiser BM, Reiter CH, Reichenspurner H, et al: Chimeric monoclonal CD4 antibody—a novel immunosuppressant for heart clinical transplantation. *Transplantation,* 58(4): 419–23, 1994.
259. Sablinski T, Hancock WW, Tilney NL, Kupiec-Weglinski JW: CD4 monoclonal antibodies in organ transplantation: a review of progress. *Transplantation* 52:579–589, 1991.
260. Carl S, Wiesel M, Daniel V, Staehler G: Effect of anti-IL-2-receptor monoclonal antibody BT 563 in treatment of acute interstitial renal rejection. *Transplant Proc* 27:854–855, 1995.
261. Vaessen LMB, Balk AHMM, Yzemans JNM, Weinar W: Peripheral blood monitoring during and after rejection-prophylaxis with a monoclonal anti-interleukin-2-receptor antibody in kidney and heart transplant recipients. *Transplant Proc* 27:858, 1995.
262. Kriaa F, Hiesse C, Alard P, et al: Prophylactic use of the anti IL-2 receptor monoclonal antibody LO-Tact-1 in cadaveric renal transplantation: results of a randomized study. *Transplant Proc*, 25:817–19, 1993.
263. Soulillou J-P, Cantarovich D, Le Mauff B, et al: Randomized controlled trial of a monoclonal antibody against the interleukin-2 receptor (33B3.1) as compared with rabbit antithymocyte globulin for prophylaxis against rejection of renal allografts. *N Engl J Med* 322:1175–1182, 1990.
264. Kirkman RL, Shapiro ME, Carpenter CB, et al: A randomized prospective trial of anti-TAC monoclonal antibody in human renal transplantation. *Transplantation* 51:107–113, 1991.
265. Friend PJ, Waldmann H, Cobbold S, et al: The anti-IL-2 receptor monoclonal antibody YTH-906 in liver transplantation. *Transplant Proc* 23:1390–1392, 1991.
265a. Vincenti F, and Bi-Continental Triple Therapy HAT Study Group: A phase III multi-center study of humanized anti-tac (HAT) for the prevention of rejection in primary cadaveric renal allograft recipients. Presented at the 23rd Annual Scientific Meeting of the American Society of Transplant Surgeons, May, 1997.
265b. Kirkman RL, Vincenti F, Pescovitz MD, et al: A phase I/II randomized, double blind,

placebo controlled study of zenapax in combination with cellcept, neoral, and steroids. Presented at the 23rd Annual Scientific Meeting of the American Society of Transplant Surgeons, May, 1997.
265c. Kanar BD, Rajagopalan PR, Hall ML, et al: Reduction of acute cellular rejection in renal allograft patients with basiliximab (Simulect™). Presented at the 23rd Annual Scientific Meeting of the American Society of Transplant Surgeons, May, 1997.
265d. Nashan B, Moore R, Schmidt AG, et al: Reduction of acute cellular rejection by basiliximab (SIMULECT™), in renal allograft recipients. Presented at the 23rd Annual Scientific Meeting of the American Society of Transplant Surgeons, May, 1997.
266. Friend PJ, Rebello P, Oliveria D, et al: Successful treatment of renal allograft rejection with a humanized antilymphocyte monoclonal antibody. *Transplant Proc* 27:860–870, 1995.
267. Hourmant M, Bedrossian J, Durand D, et al: Multicenter comparative study of an anti-LFA-1 adhesion molecule monoclonal antibody and antihymocyte globulin in prophylaxis of acute rejection in kidney transplantation. *Transplant Proc* 27:864, 1995.
268. LeMauff B, Hourmant M, Le Meur Y, et al: Anti-LFA-1 adhesion molecule monoclonal antibody in prophylaxis of human kidney allograft rejection. *Transplant Proc* 27:865, 1995.
269. Haug CE, Colvin RB, Delmonico FL, et al: A phase I trial of immunosuppression with anti-ICAM-1 (CD54) mAb in renal allograft recipients. *Transplantation* 55:766–773, 1993.
270. Lazarovits AI, Rochon J, Banks L, et al: Human mouse chimeric CD7 monoclonal antibody (SDZCHH380) for the prophylaxis of kidney transplant rejection. *J Immunol* 150:5163–5174, 1993.
271. Sharma L, Muirhead N, Lazarovits AI: Human mouse chimeric CD7 monoclonal antibody for the prophylaxis of kidney transplant losses and absence of chronic rejection at 4 years. Presented at the 15th Annual Meeting of the American Society of Transplant Physicians, Dallas May, 1996.
272. Latinne D, Cornet A, Bazin H, et al: BTI-322/LO-CD2a for acute rejection after renal transplant: Immunologic monitoring of treated patients. Presented at the 15th Annual Meeting of the American Society of Transplant Physicians, May, 1996.
273. Squifflet JP, Besse T, Latinne D, et al: BTI-322 for acute rejection after renal transplantation LO-CD2A. Presented at the 15th Annual Meeting of the American Society of Transplant Physicians, Dallas May, 1996.

9

Chimerism After Whole Organ Transplantation: An Explanation of Renal and Other Organ Acceptance

Thomas E. Starzl / Anthony J. Demetris / Massimo Trucco / Noriko Murase / Angus W. Thomson / Abdul S. Rao

Chapter 2 described the evolution of a generic therapeutic principle on which the clinical fields of renal and other kinds of whole organ transplantation are based. In kidney recipients who were treated with azathioprine and prednisone in 1962 and 1963, a characteristic cycle was recognized in which rejection in the first postoperative days or weeks could be reversed with increased doses of steroids.[1] Following this critical period, in successful instances it was frequently possible to reduce (Fig. 9–1) or rarely, as it turned out much later, even to stop immunosuppression.

The reproducibility of these events after renal and subsequently other kinds of organ transplantation led to the therapeutic practice that can be observed in every transplantation clinic today. It calls for daily baseline treatment with a maintenance drug (or drugs) plus trial and error intervention with the highly dose-maneuverable adrenocortical steroids to whatever level is required to maintain stable graft function. This can be accomplished without (double-drug therapy) or with the adjuvant use of antilymphoid or other agents in triple or quadruple drug cocktails. Throughout the years, this framework of treatment has accommodated increasingly potent new agents[2-9]. The most commonly used drugs are summarized in Table 9–1.

A great appeal of this empirical therapeutic approach was its simplicity and the consequent ease with which it could be taught or modified. Anyone with reasonable clinical judgment could become an expert after experience with a few patients. Of equal practical importance, the algorithmic steps were not drug specific except for the use of prednisone as a common constituent. Although the other individual drugs

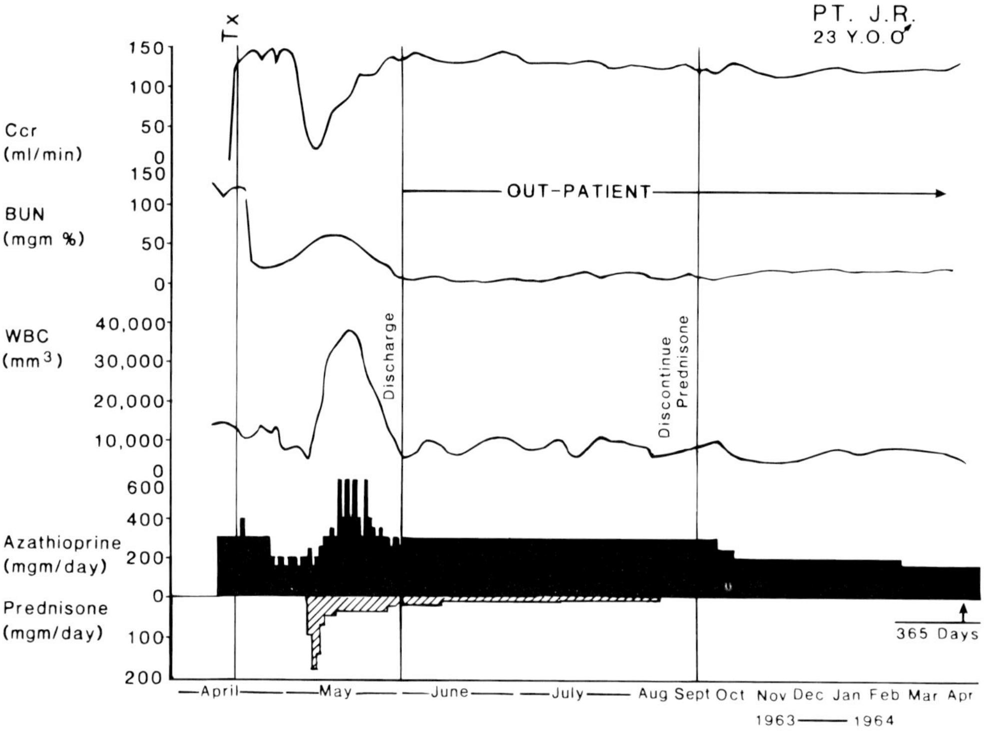

Figure 9–1. The characteristic cycle of immunologic confrontation and recovery after organ transplantation (in this case a kidney) that has dictated the use of immunosuppressive drugs for the last 30 years. After a period of good postoperative renal function, rejection 2 1/2 weeks after transplantation (Tx) was correlated with a fall in creatinine clearance (Ccr), a rise in blood urea nitrogen (BUN), and an increase in circulating white blood cells (WBC). The adverse findings were reversed with prednisone, which was later discontinued along with a reduction of maintenance azathioprine. The kidney allograft in this 23-year-old man functioned continuously from April 1963 until 1990, when the patient died of myocardial infarction. *(From Starzl TE, et al: Donor cell chimerism permitted by immunosuppressive drugs: a new view of organ transplantation.* Immunol Today *14:326–332, 1993.)*

in these cocktails were increasingly characterized in terms of their cellular or molecular site of disruption of the alloactivated T-cell response,[10,11] the cycle of post-transplant recovery was always much the same, differing only in the ease and reliability with which it could be negotiated.

The events of convalescence suggested all along that the drugs or other treatment modalities were affecting a common pathway by facilitating some kind of natural immunologic change in the host, the graft, or both.[12,13] This concept was consistent with a number of early experimental observations in our laboratory. In 1962–1964, drug-free dogs that had survived with kidney or liver allografts for prolonged periods or permanently after a 4-month course of azathioprine had inexplicable waxing and self-resolving rejections.[12,13] In discussing the altered immunologic

TABLE 9–1 ▲ DRUG COCKTAILS WITH EMPHASIS ON DOSE MANEUVERABILITY OF ADRENAL CORTICAL STEROIDS[a]

Agents	Year Described and Reported	Place	Deficiencies	Reference
Azathioprine, steroids	1963	Denver	Suboptimal	1
Antilymphocyte globulin (ALG) as adjunct[b]	1966	Denver	Suboptimal	2
Cyclophosphamide substitute for azathioprine	1970	Denver	No advantage except for patients with azathioprine toxicity	3
Total lymphoid irradiation	1979	Palo Alto, Minneapolis	Dangerous, extensive preparation, not quickly reversible	4, 5
Cyclosporine alone or with cytotoxic drugs[c]	1978–1979	Cambridge, England	Suboptimal	6
Cyclosporine, steroids[d]	1980	Denver	Nephrotoxicity; rejection not always controlled	7
FK 506, steroids[d]	1989	Pittsburgh	Nephrotoxicity; rejection not always controlled	8

[a]Until 1966, these cocktails were developed for kidney transplantation and applied to liver transplantation. From 1966 onward, the liver increasingly became a dominant test organ.
[b]Original ALGs were polyclonal; monoclonal ALG (OKT_3) introduced in 1981.[9]
[c]Steroids were given to some of these patients, but the therapeutic objective was avoidance of steroids.
[d]Compatible with azathioprine or antilymphoid drugs as third or third and fourth agents.

environment following transplantation in 1964, it was suggested, as it turned out correctly, that:

> Prevention of rejection is not entirely dependent upon immunosuppressive agents; a key factor involves a dynamic biologic process in which the immunologic relationship between the host and graft changes rapidly. . . . Through pharmacologic or other means it may become possible to augment the biologic changes. . . . An example of this last possibility is the current research in many laboratories which is directed toward achieving enhancement by inoculating the recipient with [donor] spleen, liver or peripheral white cells. . . .[12]

This strategy, in which bone marrow was the ideal source of augmenting donor antigen, was to become the dominant theme for more than two decades in Monaco's research laboratories[14–16] and elsewhere. However, it was assumed that survival of these cells was limited to a few weeks.

It was soon learned that the postulated "dynamic biologic process" sometimes occurred without immunosuppression, as was demonstrated after liver transplantation in pigs by Garnier et al,[17] Peacock and Terblanche,[18] Calne et al[19] and us.[20] Porter,[21] who had access to tissues from the different research groups, summarized the histopathologic proof that these "non-rejecting" pig recipients were actually going through subclinical rejection and spontaneous remission. Corry et al[22] and Russell et al[23] showed the same thing after heart and kidney transplantation between certain strains of mouse recipients.

Hypotheses to explain graft acceptance under immunosuppression or sometimes without it invoked multiple mechanisms, including graft adaptation, clonal deletion, antibody enhancement, defective macrophage function, and the development of suppressor or veto cells.[12,13,24–29] However, we suggested that the proposed elements of these "concatenation" hypotheses are epiphenomena of the key events of cell migration, repopulation, and systemic chimerism[30–36] on which the ultimate acceptance of kidney and other whole organ grafts depends. In this context, the immunosuppressive drugs used clinically are facilitators that allow the bidirectional host-graft leukocyte migration that leads in successful cases to mixed chimerism in the recipient as well as the transplanted organ (Fig. 9–2). In addition to explaining how allografts are accepted, this concept can be used to improve future therapeutic strategies.

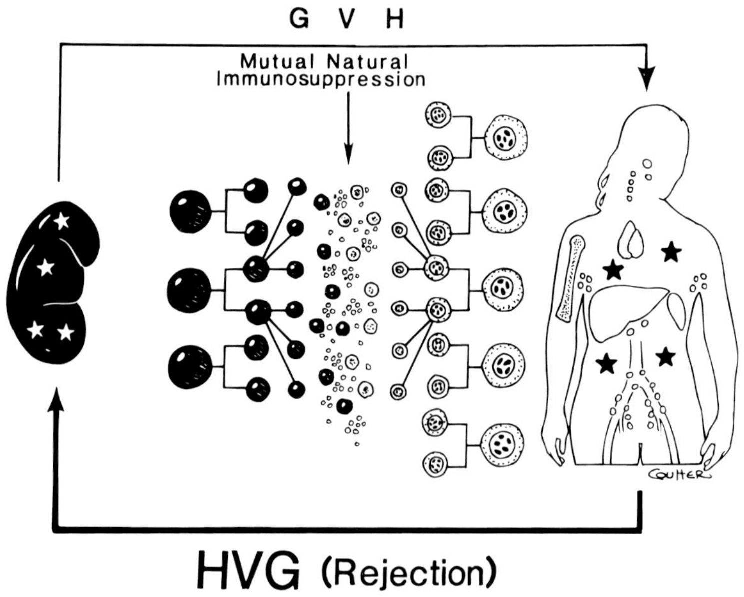

Figure 9–2. The mutual engagement of migratory immunocytes from the graft and the recipient after organ transplantation under potent pharmacologic immunosuppression. The stars represent the migrated cells. Ubiquitous chimerism was inferred from the more extensive studies in recipients of liver, kidneys, and other organs. GVH, graft versus host; HVG, host versus graft.

▲ CHIMERISM IN KIDNEY RECIPIENTS

Historical Neglected Clues

Graft Adaptation

A much discussed hypothesis in the early 1960s was that kidney grafts underwent a diminution in allogenicity after transplantation. Such a change had been noted a decade before by Woodruff in thyroid tissue during a period of privileged sanctuary in the anterior chamber of the guinea pig eye. When Woodruff's "conditioned" endocrine grafts were retransplanted to a subcutaneous location in the same recipient, they were not rejected as normally would have occurred.[37,38] The inability to explain logically how genetically proscribed transplant antigens could change their character caused this "graft adaptation" concept to lose favor. Later, it was shown in skin graft experiments that the antigenicity change was due to depletion of the donor interstitial leukocytes in the graft and their replacement with a recipient population.[39] The kidney transplants became genetic composites.[33,40]

Adoptive Transfer

The results of exhaustive skin test studies (tuberculin, histoplasmin, blastomycin, coccidioidin, mumps, *Candida,* and *Trichophyton)* in our early Colorado kidney recipients and their donors provided an additional lead[41] but one that was not considered plausible at the time. Seventy-seven percent of the skin reactions that were positive preoperatively in the donors but not in the patients crossed over to the previously negative recipients in successful cases, along with the transplanted kidney (Fig. 9–3). Wilson and Kirkpatrick, the immunology fellows who performed these studies under the supervision of David Talmage, speculated that the secondary acquisition of the positive skin tests was "caused by adoptive transfer of donor cellular immunity by leukocytes in the renal graft vasculature and hilar lymphoid tissue."[41]

The implication that cells from the graft had migrated into recipient tissues was considered untenable nearly 30 years ago because the kidney then was thought to be a leukocyte-poor organ. Instead, the transfer factor of Lawrence[42] was suggested as an alternative explanation. Ironically, several of these original patients were actually found to have chimerism nearly three decades later.[33]

Modern Technology of Chimerism Detection

The search in April–July 1992 for chimeric cells in transplanted kidney and other kinds of whole organs and in recipients was made feasible by the distinctive features of two chromosomes.[30–35] In female recipients of organs from male donors, the presence of cells with the Y chromosome in recipient tissues (or blood) was considered unequivocal evidence of systemic chimerism. Alternatively, probes were used that detected human leukocyte antigen (HLA) alleles of chromosome 6. For study of ei-

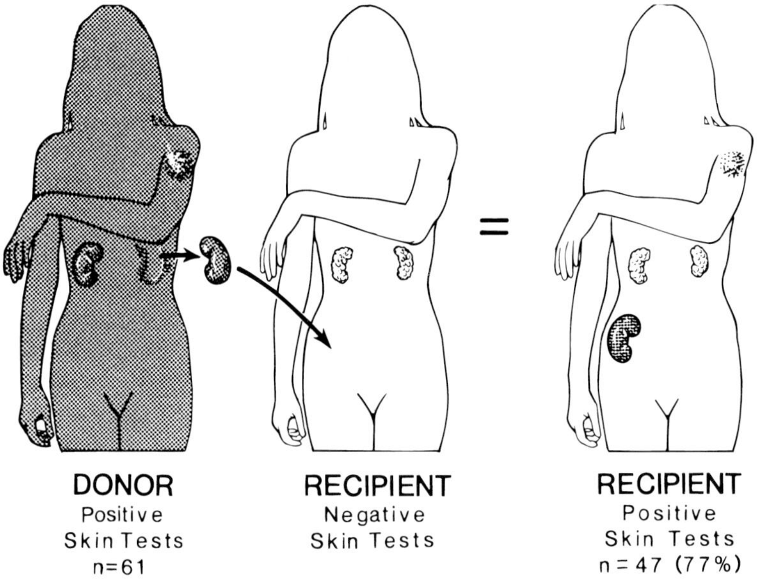

Figure 9–3. Transfer of positive skin test results from kidney donors to recipients at the University of Colorado from 1962 to 1964.[41] Although inexplicable at the time, these observations reflected adoptive transfer after cell migration, repopulation, and chimerism. *(From Starzl TE, et al: Cell migration and chimerism after whole organ transplantation: the basis of graft acceptance.* Hepatology *17:1127–1152, 1993.)*

ther the Y chromosome or chromosome 6, one or the other of two techniques, and usually both, were used. Cytostaining allows the location and morphologic characterization of phenotypically distinct donor and recipient cells. The polymerase chain reaction (PCR) is used to differentiate donor from recipient DNA.

Cytostaining

Staining for the Y probe was performed with a fluorescence method after in situ hybridization. Immunostaining for the HLA markers was with monoclonal antibodies to class I and class II antigen phenotypes present in the donor but not the recipient. Staining with irrelevant anti-HLA antibodies and omission of the primary antibody provided negative controls (See Color Insert, Part C). Tissues with known HLA antigens along with the allograft biopsy and skin sections of the recipient stained with matching anti-HLA monoclonal antibodies were used as positive specificity controls.

Polymerase Chain Reaction

In the PCR search for the Y chromosome, oligonucleotides specific for the satellite region of the Y chromosome centromere Y-A[43] and for the sex-determining region of the Y chromosome[44] were used as primers to determine the presence of male DNA in the female recipient tissues.[31] After Southern blotting, the amplified material was hybridized to radioactively labeled Y-specific probes. PCR tests for donor- and recipient-specific HLA alleles of chromosome 6 were performed according to the reference protocol of the XIth International Histocompatibility Workshop.[45] With this protocol, preliminary generic amplification of the DRB gene is performed followed by allele-specific amplification and testing.

Direct Evidence of Chimerism

One of the five kidney recipients who were studied 27–29 years after transplantation had stopped immunosuppression 12 years earlier. The others were still taking azathioprine with or without prednisone. These five patients were selected for the chimerism study[33] in preference to other surviving kidney recipients from the 1963 era for three reasons. First, four of the five donors still were alive, allowing HLA retyping and use of their lymphocytes for studies of immunologic competence of the recipient. Second, known HLA incompatibilities between these four donors (three parents, one aunt) and their recipients allowed immunocytochemical and PCR differentiation of donor from recipient cells in the biopsy tissues, as described in the preceding section. In the fifth case, in which the donor in a father-to-daughter transplantation had died, chimerism in tissues could be determined by sex typing.

In each of four kidney recipients whose donor was alive, leukocytes with the appearance of dendritic cells that had migrated from the renal allografts were found in recipient skin and lymph node biopsies. Although they were few in number, these HLA mismatched donor cells were unmistakable with the immunostaining techniques (See Color Insert, Part B). Chimerism was confirmed with PCR in the recipient tissues of all four of these patients and in the blood of two of them (Fig. 9–4). In the fifth patient, the woman who had been given her now-deceased father's kidney 29 years previously, cells with the Y chromosome were found in her skin with fluorescent in situ hybridization studies and confirmed with PCR.

In all five cases, biopsies of the kidney showed that the vascular endothelial cells remained donor. The tubular epithelial cells, which did not express HLA antigens well, were proved to be donor with sex karyotyping. In contrast, the leukocytes departing the allograft had been replaced by similar cells from the recipient (See Color Insert, Part A). Thus in addition to showing systemic chimerism, it was established that the kidney grafts were chimeras—composed of cells with two different genomes[33] (Fig. 9–2).

Two of the four recipients of kidneys from the still-living donors had no donor-specific reactivity by mixed lymphocyte reaction (MLR), whereas the other two had greatly reduced antidonor reactivity. With cell-mediated lymphocytotoxicity testing, all four were nonresponsive to donor lymphocytes. Three of the four patients were otherwise fully immunocompetent with responsiveness to third-party lymphocytes and mitogens.[33]

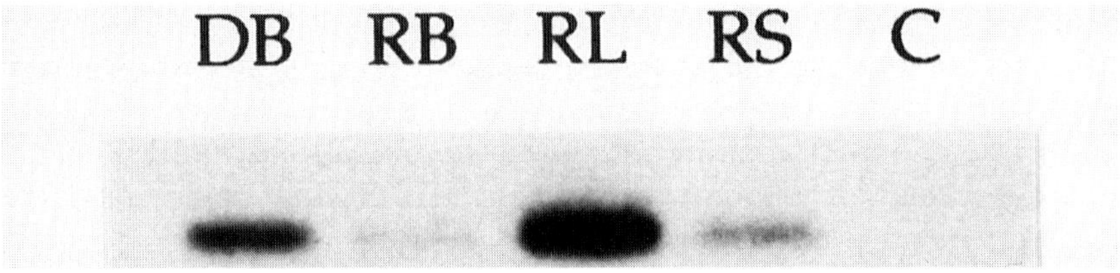

Figure 9–4. LD 90:PCR demonstration with Southern blot technique of chimerism in blood (RB), lymph node (RL), and skin (RS) of the recipient as detected with DR7 (donor) specific oligonucleotide probes. DB, donor blood DNA diluted 100 times to avoid overwhelming the other bands. *(From Starzl TE, et al: Chimerism and donor specific nonreactivity 27 to 29 years after kidney allotransplantation.* Transplantation *55:1272–1277, 1993.)*

▲ LIVER AND OTHER ORGANS

Graft Chimerism

Another underappreciated clue to cell migration was the demonstration in 1969 that the Kupffer cells and other interstitial monocytes and macrophages of a transplanted human liver were replaced within 100 days by cells of recipient phenotype.[46] A composite (chimeric) structure was shown in 1991 also to be a feature of long-surviving transplanted intestine in rats[47] and humans.[48] The suspicion that this process must be generic in all successfully engrafted organs soon was confirmed.[35]

Systemic Chimerism

Like the kidney recipients, most of a cohort of 25 liver recipients studied for chimerism were clinically well and fully immunocompetent according to conventional in vitro testing 2–22 years after transplantation under azathioprine- or cyclosporine-based immunosuppression.[35] Donor cell chimerism was found with cytochemical or PCR techniques in all 25 patients in locations that included skin, lymph nodes, heart, lungs, spleen, intestine, kidneys, bone marrow, and thymus. Chimeric cells were present in larger numbers at any given site than in the contemporaneously studied long-surviving kidney recipients.

▲ CELL TRAFFIC AND SITES OF DONOR-RECIPIENT IMMUNOLOGIC INTERACTIONS

The early events leading to the chimeric state have been studied in rats[36] and mice,[49] including the pathways of passenger leukocyte dissemination. Within minutes or hours, these cells leave the graft and home to the central lymphoid organs (spleen, lymph nodes, thymus, and probably bone marrow), and are destroyed by rejection in most animals except mice. However, with temporary immunosuppression in rats (2 weeks of daily FK 506), these mononuclear cells pause for about 2 weeks in the lymphoid organs but then break out and move secondarily to all recipient tissues[36] (Fig. 9–5). Rat liver recipients treated this way (LEW to ACI) survive indefinitely without further treatment and retain their graft and systemic chimerism.

Interestingly, cell migration and chimerism, with permanent survival of the engrafted livers, occur without any immunosuppression in some rat strain combinations (Brown Norway to Lewis for example), and occur without treatment in virtually all mouse strain combinations. The liver recipients in either species can accept skin, kidney, or a heart from the original donor strain but no other (donor-specific nonreactivity).[36,49] This kind of evidence has indicated that the heavy endowment of the liver with potentially migratory white cells is the basis for the well-known but previously inexplicable phenomenon of "hepatic tolerogenicity." This term has been used to define the ability of the liver to induce its own acceptance or that of companion organs more readily than other kinds of allografts and in some experimental models without immunosuppression.[13,17–20,47,50–53]

By the end of 1992, it was appreciated that all whole organs undergo the same process of potential tolerance induction as the kidney and liver,[34,35] the dynamics being particularly easy to study with the leukocyte-rich intestine.[54,55] The same

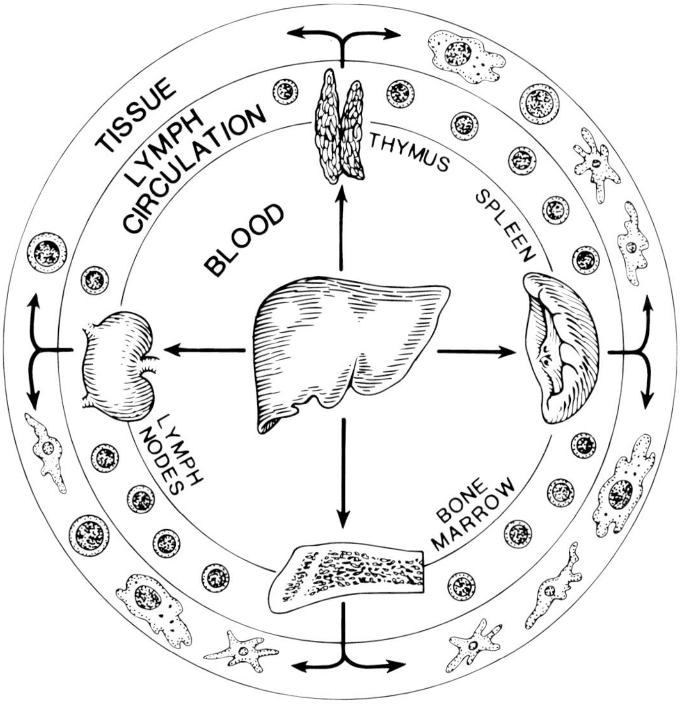

Figure 9–5. The dissemination of passenger leukocytes from the graft (rat liver in these experiments) to the central lymphoid organs and then ubiquitously after a brief pause. The events are similar to those after successful bone marrow transplantation.[36]

kind of traffic in the context of alloactivation and rejection rather than tolerization had been well worked out earlier with the so-called lymphoid-poor organs, including the kidney. Studies with untreated animals have shown that the alloreaction starts in two general sites, peripherally in the graft and centrally in the recipient lymphoid tissues.

In a remarkably complete study in 1981 of untreated rat kidney recipients, Nemlander et al[56] demonstrated the same kind of leukocyte migration as we noted with rat liver allografts 12 years later.[36] If Nemlander et al had given one or two doses of cyclosporine to their recipient animals (an "easy" strain combination) and had followed them further, they almost certainly would have uncovered the events of cell migration and repopulation that awaited another 12 years for exposure with the liver.[36] Larsen et al[57] found that donor dendritic cells from heterotopic cardiac allografts are released into the circulation, where they eventually home into the T-cell areas of the recipient spleen. In the spleen, the donor cells initiate proliferation of recipient cells and vice versa.[56–60] This reaction might be considered to be an in vivo MLR and epitomizes central allosensitization.

Allosensitization (and tolerization) presumably also occur within the graft. Forbes et al[59] were the first to show that clustering of recipient lymphocytes occurs around donor dendritic cells in the interstitium of cardiac grafts within a few days after transplantation. The recipient lymphoid cells undergo blastogenesis and proliferate within these clusters. We have described analogous events in the rejection of rat livers.[58]

In human recipients of kidney grafts under cyclosporine-prednisone immunosuppression, Hayry and Willebrand[61,62] noted what appeared to be a bidirectional MLR in needle aspiration biopsies. When studied with the *Staphylococcus aureus* assay and alloantibodies to nonshared donor and recipient allelic specificities, most of the collected blast cells in some cases were derived from the donor or else the response was split, "resembling a bidirectional mixed lymphocyte reaction in vitro."[61]

▲ FUNCTIONAL CONSEQUENCES OF MICROCHIMERISM

Cause and Effect?

Questions have continued to be raised whether the low-level chimerism found in our long-surviving patients and experimental animals[30–35] was an irrelevant histopathologic curiosity or a condition with immunologic significance. This has been surprising in view of Russell's elegant formal proof of the association of chimerism with acquired tolerance as well as runt disease.[63] The skepticism arose because the chimeric donor cells were so sparse in recipient tissues of the patients and the animals of our studies. The term *microchimerism* (as opposed to *macrochimerism*) to describe a small proportion of chimeric cells in recipient blood was introduced by Liegeois et al[64] in 1974 in a report of experiments with the mouse model used earlier by Monaco et al.[65] Far from being insignificant, there is much evidence that the cumulative effect of these microchimeric cells is substantial, especially after liver transplantation, in which they are most easily demonstrated.

Metabolic Implications

The small population of chimeric cells has been shown to affect total body metabolism in patients treated with liver transplantation for the enzyme deficiencies of type 4 glycogen storage disease and Gaucher's disease in which the consequences of the missing enzymes are widespread storage of amylopectin and B glucocerebroside, respectively.[32] These disorders were thought to be treatable only by bone marrow transplantation because the enzyme deficiency is of all cells. Two to 8 years after liver replacement, however, there was a dramatic resorption of both kinds of storage material from host tissues. As an explanation for the metabolic amelioration, chimeric donor cells were found ubiquitously in recipient tissues, including heart, lymph nodes, bone marrow, intestine, and skin. There apparently had been a coculture effect of a small number of chimeric donor cells on the contiguous overwhelming numbers of enzyme-deficient recipient cells.[32]

If, as we have concluded,[30–36] chimerism differing only in degree with different kinds of organ allografts is an integral feature of all successful engraftments, any such procedure can result in such a gain of systemic metabolic function, as suggested for different reasons by Groth et al[66] in 1979. Although the chimerism in our long-surviving kidney recipients was only one fifth or less of that in the liver recipients, this may have been enough to explain an enigmatic observation made in 1972 by Desnick et al.[67] After successful renal allotransplantation, this group at the University of Minnesota described recovery of function in the patient's diseased kidneys, which had been shut down by the glycosphingolipid accumulations of Fabry's storage disease. A reasonable hypothesis is that donor chimeric cells had settled there (Fig. 9–6).

The Immunologic Interface

The foregoing metabolic observations raise important questions about potential analogous cell-to-cell effects of other molecules directly involved in immunologic processes, including those subserving tolerance induction. Much needs to be learned about how the chimeric donor cells, many of which resemble dendritic cells, are perpetuated for as long as three decades after transplantation. The dendritic and other leukocytes could be spawned by small numbers of pluripotent progenitor cells coming from the allograft interstitium. Dendritic cell precursors have been grown from mouse blood, bone marrow, or whole organs by means of granulocyte-macrophage colony-stimulating factor (GM-CSF)–enriched media.[68] Alternatively, tissue leukocytes in the organ may not have reached terminal differentiation as previously assumed. We have suggested that subsequent survival and renewal of these cells depends on chronic mutual stimulation of the donor and recipient cell populations[34,36] in a process of tolerization that has many of the cellular characteristics associated with immunity.[69] However, there has been no direct way to test how this small population of donor dendritic and other cells can have an impact far exceeding its numbers.

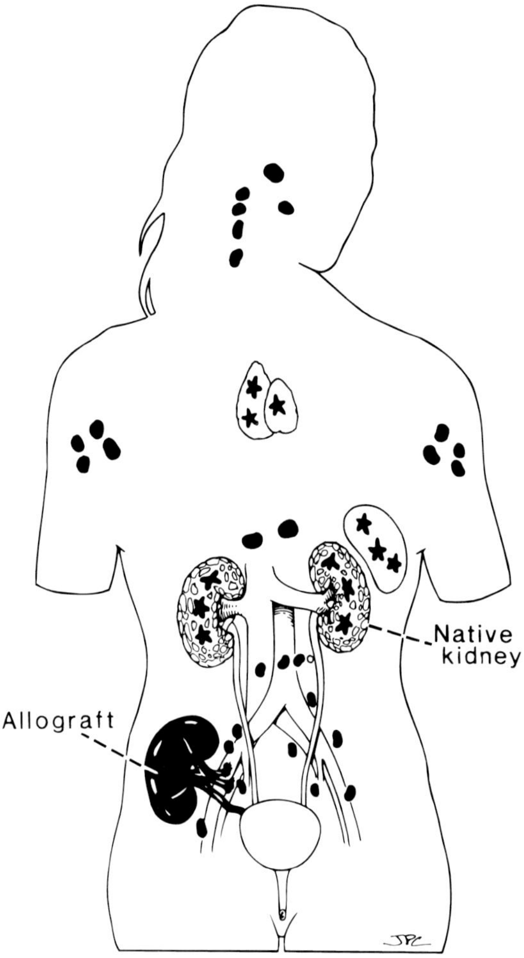

Figure 9–6. Explanation for 1972 observation by Desnick et al[67] of recovery of native kidneys after successful renal transplantation for Fabry disease. The migration of passenger leukocytes from the allograft to the host kidneys and elsewhere is shown with black stars.

Changed Host and Graft Interactions

There are many indications that the coexisting immunocyte populations in successful transplantations come to regard each other in a revised light. The evidence on one hand is the fading of the threat of clinical rejection concomitant with development of decreasing donor-specific reactivity in spite of lightened treatment and on the other the waning specter of graft versus host disease (GVHD). It is quite natural to expect that the threat of GVHD would decline at the same time as the threat of rejection, because both of the cell populations are receiving the same protective immunosuppression in an organ recipient. Appreciation of the intercellular relationship and the need *not* to alter it by ablating one side or other was the crucial conceptual advance allowing the successful engraftment of leukocyte-rich organs such as the liver, intestine, both together, or all of the intra-abdominal organs (multivisceral transplantation).[70] Once it was proved that low-level mixed allogenic chimerism invariably was found after successful whole organ transplantation, the reason seemed clear why GVHD was not common among recipients of liver, intestinal, or multivisceral transplants. The explanation was that mixed chimerism was being produced in the same way as in the classic GVHD-free mouse bone marrow mixed chimerism models of Slavin et al[71] and Ildstad and Sachs.[72]

The Critical Dendritic Cell

Generation of an immune response that leads under normal circumstances to graft destruction or GVHD requires effective antigen presentation and recognition in the initial phase followed by a second costimulatory signal and the response of T cells to the combined signal.[73] Both of these signals are normally delivered to T cells by professional antigen-presenting cells (APC). Of these APCs, the dendritic cell[74,75] (the most prominent chimeric cell according to morphologic criteria) is critical because it can modify the expression of cell interaction, major histocompatibility (MHC) locus, and adhesion molecules, all of which determine how antigen signals are heeded by T cells.[76] Thus the dendritic leukocyte is the prime candidate in this tolerogenicity scenario, even though other lineages may also be essential for the successful outcome of such an immunologic transaction.

Impact on Tissue Matching

In the directions of both host versus graft (rejection) and graft versus host, cellular interactions resulting in "mutual natural immunosuppression" are envisioned as occurring on a sliding scale with each further level of histoincompatibility (Fig. 9–7). With protection by modern-day immunosuppression, the alloreactions caused by the mutual cell engagement usually can be mitigated enough to allow the tolerogenic changes to occur and a rapprochement to be reached between the coexisting immunocytes. The anticipated histocompatibility influence on both rejection and the severity of GVHD are then expected to dwindle. We have postulated that this explains the poor correlation of HLA matching with outcome after cadaveric transplantation of whole organs, including the kidney.[30,34,35]

▲ RELATION OF CELL MIGRATION TO TOLERANCE

The inadequacy of thymic clonal deletion to explain acquired transplantation tolerance has been emphasized in recent reviews.[77] Although a discussion of the meaning

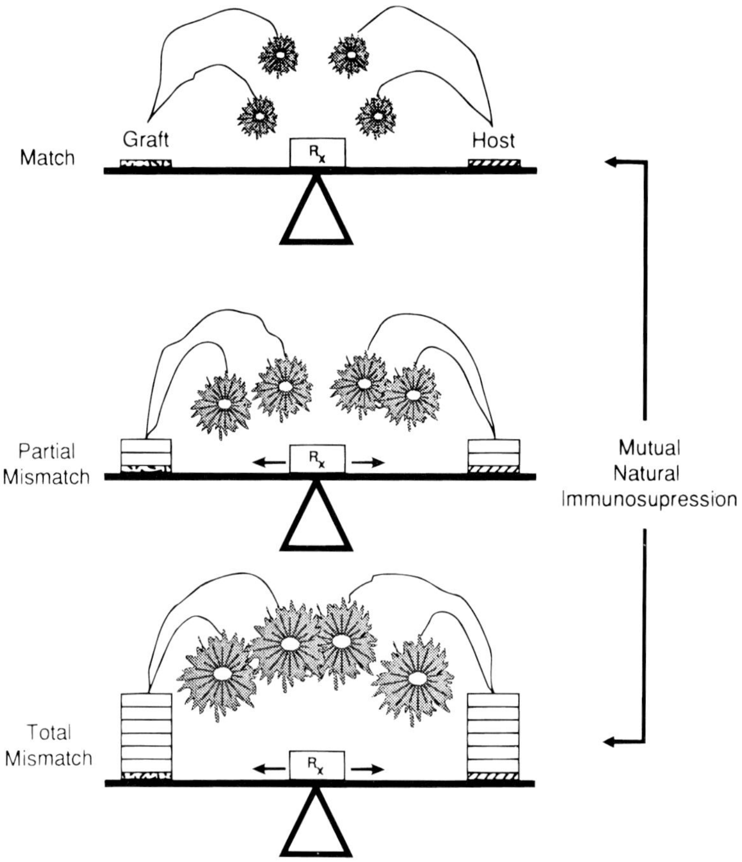

Figure 9–7. The donor-recipient leukocyte interaction is a buffer against rejection on one hand and graft versus host disease on the other. Veto and suppressor cells are postulated to be the result of the interaction shown at the cell population interface. R_x, iatrogenic immunosuppression. *(From Starzl TE, et al: Donor cell chimerism permitted by immunosuppressive drugs: a new view of organ transplantation.* Immunol Today *14:326-332, 1993.)*

of tolerance is beyond our intention, it should be noted that all of the hypotheses to explain clonal "silencing," including peripheral clonal deletion and anergy, could mesh with the discovery of the enduring graft-host intimacy that is inherent with chimerism.

The evidence of long-term vitality and turnover of donor leukocytes in recipient tissues is particularly supportive of the opinions of Coutinho et al[69,78] and Cohen,[79] who defined *acquired tolerance* as a high (not anergic) level of sustained immune activity in networks. These networks presumably interact in a more complex way than the idiotype systems originally postulated by Jerne.[80] Suppressor or veto cells or both could be epiphenomena of this kind of activity.

Such a hypothesis would explain why cell migration and chimerism are a common mechanism of donor-specific nonreactivity no matter what the site of action of immunosuppressive drugs or in some experimental models without drugs. It has been proposed from observations in drug-free models of tolerance induction that T-cell receptor occupancy leads to production of negative regulators of interleukin-2 (IL-2) production (anergy proteins).[73,81] According to this hypothesis, during the course of a normal T-cell response (to alloantigens) these negative regulators of IL-2 production have an inconsequential effect because they are diluted out by vigorous cell replication driven by IL-2. However, these negative regulators would accumulate with consequent anergy if clonal expansion were prevented at any level (Fig. 9–8), for instance, by the absence of a costimulatory signal in drug-free models.[73]

The same effect could be induced iatrogenically by pharmacologic interdiction of IL-2 gene transcription (cyclosporine and FK 506) or administration of a DNA syn-

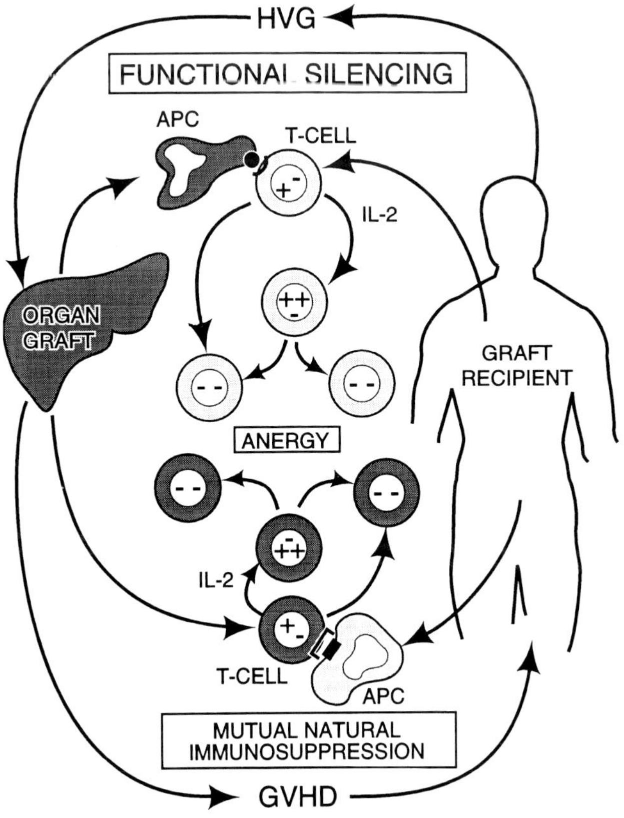

Figure 9–8. Model of dendritic cell (APC)–T_{HI}–cell interaction shows the production within the nucleus of positive (+) and negative (−) regulators (anergy proteins) of interleukin-2 (IL-2) gene transcription. In this model, anergy relates only to the IL-2 gene, and other cytokines (eg, interferon-γ) may be secreted, albeit at suboptimal levels. In the absence of persistent costimulatory signals (or under the umbrella of immunosuppressive drugs), cell division does not proceed, and negative nuclear regulators accumulate, resulting in T-cell anergy. In addition to the action of immunosuppressive agents, chronic antigen stimulation is also envisioned as promoting anergy. In some instances, tolerance can be broken, as by administration of exogenous IL-2. HVG, host versus graft response (allograft rejection); GVHD, graft versus host disease. *(From Thomson AW, Starzl TE (eds):* Immunosuppressive Drugs: *London, Edward Arnold, 1993.)*

thesis inhibitor (azathioprine, cyclophosphamide, and numerous others). The use of non–T-cell depleting monoclonal antibodies, such as those directed against the cell surface CD4 antigen or monoclonal antibodies against adhesion molecules, including ICAM-1 and LFA-1,[82] can also be envisioned.

However it occurs, the reciprocal educational process of donor and recipient leukocytes and its perpetuation resembles in either the direction of rejection or GVHD (Fig. 9–8) the "infectious" transplantation tolerance that can be passed on to naive lymphocytes and be self sustaining in some circumstances.[83] It is postulated that in fully successful transplantations, the mini-immune system of the graft is incorporated into the existing recipient immunologic network,[34,36] compatible with the hypothesis of Coutinho.[78]

▲ UNSTABLE MIXED CHIMERISM

Cell migration conceptually reunites bone marrow transplantation with transplantation of whole organs. Far from involving different mechanisms for successful engraftment, we believe that these two seemingly disparate fields merely reflect contrasting treatment dogmas. For bone marrow transplantation, the conventional treatment strategy of recipient cytoablation eliminates mutual immunocyte engagement and thus necessitates heavy reliance on HLA matching to prevent GVHD in the unbalanced system. The treatment for solid organ transplantation encourages, or at least allows, these consequences of mutual cell engagement, thereby liberating the patient from the restrictions of HLA matching and an overwhelming threat of GVHD.

Failure of clinical organ transplantation implies the inability to achieve mixed allogeneic chimerism despite the best available immunosuppression—almost invariably after kidney transplantation because of an imbalance that leads to rejection. However, because an incipient GVH reaction is a necessary condition for success (this is our fundamental premise), clinical GVHD is a possibility after every transplantation, although the threat varies from organ to organ. We now know that about 5% of all liver recipients experience a bout of clinical GVHD, which in the past usually was attributed to an allergic skin reaction.[35] The incidence after kidney transplantation is not known because it is not considered.

▲ CLINICAL TRIALS OF BONE MARROW AUGMENTATION

The concept developed in this chapter is that the content (and perhaps the specific lineages) of migratory cells that are particularly numerous in the liver confer potential immunologic advantages. These passenger leukocytes, which are of bone marrow origin, have been considered an immunologic liability for transplantation.[84] Under the appropriate conditions, however, they may be tolerogenic, as exemplified by the liver. A corollary, therefore, is that organs, such as the kidney and heart, with a smaller leukocyte component must have similar inherent, although less tolerogenic, potential. The frequently advanced strategy of intravenous infusion of donor bone marrow, donor blood (donor-specific transfusion), or other hematolymphoid cells at the same time or soon after transplantation of whole organs[14–16,64,65,71,72,85–87] is merely an augmentation of the normal posttransplant cell migration. To mimic the natural process, these cells should be given perioperatively, not before or after the operation, as usually has been done with the so-called Monaco model.

This strategy is currently under clinical evaluation, using bone marrow for the leukocyte augmentation. Since December 1992, over 70 patients with end-stage renal disease have received a simultaneous kidney–bone marrow allograft from the same cadaveric donor at our center. Additional renal transplant patients with diabetes (Type I) also have received a pancreas or pancreatic islets from their kidney–bone marrow donor. As a precaution, autologous bone marrow was harvested from the first 10 recipients immediately before kidney transplantation and cryopreserved for potential future use in case of GVHD.[88]

The donor bone marrow was obtained from vertebral bodies at the end of multiorgan procurement: 3–5 $\times$ 10^8 untreated bone marrow cells/kg were administered by means of intravenous infusion immediately after the kidney transplant. The patients with diabetes received the pancreas or pancreatic islets; the latter were infused intraportally. Intravenous bone marrow infusion was performed at the conclusion of the procedure. All patients were treated with FK 506 and steroids. Chimerism was assessed in the recipients by flow cytometry, PCR, and immunostaining from peripheral blood lymphocytes. Immunologic monitoring was by MLR and cell-mediated lympholysis.

Detectable levels of donor cells were present in the peripheral blood lymphocytes of 90% of the recipients. Donor cells were also detected in two patients who underwent lymph node biopsy 2 and 4 months after transplantation. One-year actuarial patient and graft survival have been 100% and 98%, respectively.

None of the recipients manifested GVHD. The only example we observed of such a potential bone marrow–related complication was in a patient who underwent 550 cGy total lymphoid irradiation before a combined liver–bone marrow allograft.[88] The unwise decision to produce an iatrogenic imbalance in the donor-recipient interface by means of total lymphoid irradiation was based on the dogma that "making space" would facilitate engraftment of the marrow. This concept has been eroded with direct experimentation.[89,90]

Further evaluation of passenger leukocyte augmentation (with bone marrow and other leukocyte sources) will be of particular interest for pancreatic islet transplantation. This means of treating diabetes has consistently failed because of the high rate of rejection.[91] If it is possible to increase islet allograft survival with minimum ultimate immunosuppression by concomitant donor bone marrow infusion, this will be an approach opposite to the numerous attempts to reduce islet immunogenicity by selective destruction of the bone marrow–derived antigen presenting cells that are normally contained in islet preparations.[92] Then donor bone marrow would become a dose-maneuverable component of any organ or cellular transplantation for facilitation of graft acceptance and induction of donor-specific nonreactivity.

As discussed earlier, liver transplantation can be envisioned as a mini–bone marrow engraftment. Among a group of 44 human liver recipients who had survived 11–23 years, six (14%) had stopped all immunosuppression 1–11 years postoperatively with subsequent, clinically stable, drug-free intervals of 5–13 years. Another 15 patients with shorter follow-up periods all were drug-free and in stable condition.[35,93] The most extreme example of early successful drug discontinuation in a liver recipient was after 6 months, with a subsequent follow-up period of 3 years. A trial of drug weaning has been started in liver recipients with a rejection-free course exceeding 5 years. Liver graft rejection (if it occurs) can be so effectively treated with FK 506[8] that the benefits of discontinuation of drugs appear to outweigh the risks for selected patients.

The liver experience in which the hepatic graft brings its own intrinsic quota of bone marrow–derived leukocytes should provide insight about what can be achieved with use of bone marrow augmentation for recipients of other organs or cells such as the kidney or pancreatic islets. Even if this strategy to obtain drug independence is successful, there is no way to know when a drug-free state has arrived. It seems clear that if the clinical experience with the tolerogenic livers is taken seriously, renal or heart transplantation with bone marrow augmentation also will require protracted immunosuppression before this treatment can be stopped altogether and then only with precautions. Such conclusions also have been reached by Barber et al[86] using delayed supplementary bone marrow for cadaveric kidney transplantation as advocated by Monaco.

Aided by Research Grants from the Veterans Administration and Project Grant No. DK 29961 from the National Institutes of Health, Bethesda, Maryland.

Although this chapter was written in the spring and early summer of 1993, further work in our laboratories and elsewhere have strengthened the hypothesis it contains. The work and progress of the last 3 years has been summarized in the following three recent reviews:

Thomson AW, Lu L, Murase N, Demetris AJ, Rao AS, Starzl TE: Microchimerism, dendritic cell progenitors and transplantation tolerance. *Stem Cells* 13:622–639, 1995.
Starzl TE, Demetris AJ: Transplantation milestones: Viewed with one- and two-way paradigms of tolerance. *JAMA* 273:876–879, 1995.
Starzl TE, Demetris AJ, Murase N, Trucco M, Thomson AW, Rao AS: The lost chord: Microchimerism and allograft survival. *Immunol Today*, 17(12):577–84, 1996.

▲ REFERENCES

1. Starzl TE, Marchioro TL, Waddell WR: The reversal of rejection in human renal homografts with subsequent development of homograft tolerance. *Surg Gynecol Obstet* 117:385–395, 1963.
2. Starzl TE, Marchioro TL, Porter KA, Iwasaki Y, Cerilli GJ: The use of heterologous antilymphoid agents in canine renal and liver homotransplantation and in human renal homotransplantation. *Surg Gynecol Obstet* 124:301–318, 1967.

3. Starzl TE, Putnam CW, Halgrimson CG, et al: Cyclophosphamide and whole organ transplantation in humans. *Surg Gynecol Obstet* 133:981–991, 1971.
4. Strober S, Slavin S, Fuks Z, et al: Transplantation tolerance after total lymphoid irradiation. *Transplant Proc* 11:1032–1038, 1979.
5. Najarian JS, Ferguson RM, Sutherland DER, et al: Fractional total lymphoid irradiation (TL1) as preparative immunosuppression on high risk renal transplantation. *Ann Surg* 196:442–452, 1982.
6. Calne RY, Rolles K, White DJG, et al: Cyclosporin A initially as the only immunosuppressant in 34 recipients of cadaveric organs: 32 kidneys, 2 pancreases, and 2 livers. *Lancet* 2:1033–1036, 1979.
7. Starzl TE, Weil R III, Iwatsuki S, et al: The use of cyclosporin A and prednisone in cadaver kidney transplantation. *Surg Gynecol Obstet* 151:17–26, 1980.
8. Starzl TE, Todo S, Fung J, Demetris AJ, Venkataramanan R, Jain A: FK 506 for human liver, kidney and pancreas transplantation. *Lancet* 2:1000–1004, 1989.
9. Cosimi AB, Colvin RB, Burton RC, et al: Use of monoclonal antibodies to T-cell subsets for immunologic monitoring and treatment in recipients of renal allografts. *N Engl J Med* 305:308, 1981.
10. Sigal NH, Dumont FJ: Cyclosporin A, FK 506 and rapamycin: pharmacologic probes of lymphocyte signal transduction. *Annu Rev Immunol* 10:519–560, 1992.
11. Thomson AW, Starzl TE (eds): *Immunosuppressive Drugs: Developments in Anti-Rejection Therapy.* London, Edward Arnold, 1996:1–231.
12. Starzl TE: Host-graft adaptation. In: Starzl TE (ed), *Experience in Renal Transplantation.* Philadelphia, Saunders, 1969:164–170.
13. Starzl TE: Effects to mitigate or prevent rejection. In: Starzl TE (ed), *Experience in Hepatic Transplantation.* Philadelphia, Saunders, 1969:203–206, 216–220, 226–233.
14. Monaco AE, Wood ML, Russell PS: Studies of heterologous anti-lymphocyte serum in mice. III. Immunologic tolerance and chimerism produced across the H-2 locus with adult thymectomy and anti-lymphocyte serum. *Ann N Y Acad Sci* 129:190–209, 1966.
15. Monaco AP, Wood ML: Studies on heterologous antilymphocyte serum in mice. VII. Optimal cellular antigen for induction of immunologic tolerance with ALS. *Transplant Proc* 2:489–496, 1970.
16. Monaco AP, Wood ML, Maki T, Gozzo JJ: Post transplantation donor-specific bone marrow transfusion in polyclonal antilymphocyte serum-treated recipients: the optimal cellular antigen for induction of unresponsiveness to organ allografts. *Transplant Proc* 20:1207–1212, 1988.
17. Garnier H, Clot J, Bertrand M, et al: Liver transplantation in the pig: surgical approach *C R Acad Sci* 260:5621-5623, 1965.
18. Peacock JH, Terblanche J: Orthotopic homotransplantation of the liver in the pig. In: Read AE (ed), *The Liver.* London, Butterworth, 1967:333–336.
19. Calne RY, White HJO, Yoffa DE, et al: Observations of orthotopic liver transplantation in the pig. *Br Med J* 2:478–480, 1967.
20. Starzl TE: Rejection in unmodified animals. In: Starzl TE (ed), *Experience in Hepatic Transplantation* Philadelphia, Saunders, 1969:184–190.
21. Porter KA: Pathology of the orthotopic homograft and heterograft. In: Starzl TE (ed), *Experience in Hepatic Transplantation.* Philadelphia, Saunders, 1969:427–437.
22. Corry RJ, Winn HJ, Russell PS: Primary vascularized allografts of hearts in mice: the role of H-2D, H-2K and non-H-2 antigens in rejection. *Transplantation* 16:343–350, 1973.
23. Russell PS, Chase CM, Colvin RB, Plate JMD: Kidney transplants in mice: an analysis of the immune status of mice bearing long-term G-2 incompatible transplants. *J Exp Med* 147:1449–1468, 1978.

24. Weber RA, Cannon JA, Longmire WP: Observations on the regrafting of successful homografts in chickens. *Ann Surg* 139:473–477, 1954.
25. Murray JE, Sheil AGR, Moseley R, Knight R, McGavic Dickinson J, Dammin GJ: Analysis of mechanism of immunosuppressive drugs in renal homotransplantation. *Ann Surg* 160:449–473, 1964.
26. Levey RH: Immunological tolerance and enhancement: a common mechanism. *Transplant Proc* 3:41:48, 1971.
27. Murase N, Kim DG, Todo S, Cramer DV, Fung JJ, Starzl TE: FK 506 suppression of heart and liver allograft rejection. II. The induction of graft acceptance in rat. *Transplantation* 50:739–744, 1990.
28. Streilen JW: Neonatal tolerance of H-2 alloantigens: Procuring graft acceptance the "old-fashioned" way. *Transplantation* 52:1–10, 1991.
29. Eto M, Mayumi H, Nishimura, Maeda T, Yoshikai T, Nomoto K: Similarity and difference in the mechanisms of neonatally induced tolerance and cyclophosphamide-induced tolerance in mice. *J. Immunol* 147:2439–2446, 1991.
30. Starzl TE, Demetris AJ, Murase N, Ildstad S, Ricordi C, Trucco M: Cell migration, chimerism, and graft acceptance. *Lancet* 339:1579–1582, 1992.
31. Starzl TE, Demetris AJ, Trucco M, et al: Systemic chimerism in human female recipients of male livers. *Lancet* 340:876–877, 1992.
32. Starzl TE, Demetris AJ, Trucco M, et al: Chimerism after liver transplantation for type IV glycogen storage disease and Type I Gaucher's disease. *N Engl J Med* 328:745–749, 1993.
33. Starzl TE, Demetris AJ, Trucco M, et al: Chimerism and donor specific nonreactivity 27 to 29 years after kidney allotransplantation. *Transplantation* 55:1272–1277, 1993.
34. Starzl TE, Demetris AJ, Murase N, Thomson AW, Trucco M, Ricordi C: Donor cell chimerism permitted by immunosuppressive drugs is the basis of organ transplant acceptance and tolerance. *Immunol Today* 14:326–332, 1993.
35. Starzl TE, Demetris AJ, Trucco M, et al: Cell migration and chimerism after whole organ transplantation: the basis of graft acceptance. *Hepatology* 17:1127–1152, 1993.
36. Demetris AJ, Murase N, Fujisaki S, Fung JJ, Rao AS, Starzl TE: Hematolymphoid cell trafficking, microchimerism, and GVHD reactions after liver, bone marrow, and heart transplantation. *Transplant Proc* 25:3337–3344, 1993.
37. Woodruff MFA, Woodruff HG: The transplantation of normal tissues: with special reference to auto- and homotransplants of thyroid and spleen in the anterior chamber of the eye, and subcutaneously, in guinea pigs. *Philos Trans R Soc Lond B Biol Sci* 234:559–581, 1950.
38. Woodruff MFA: Evidence of adaptation in homografts of normal tissue. In: Medawar PB (ed), *Biological Problems of Grafting.* Oxford, England, Blackwell Scientific, 1959:83–94.
39. Steinmuller D: Immunization with skin isografts taken from tolerant mice. *Science* 158:127–129, 1967.
40. Randhawa PS, Starzl TE, Ramos H, Nalesnik MA, Demetris AJ: Allografts surviving for 26–29 years following living related kidney transplantation: Analysis by light microscopy, in situ hybridization for the Y chromosome, and anti-HLA antibodies. *Am J Kidney Dis* 24:72–77, 1994.
41. Wilson WEC, Kirkpatrick CH: Immunologic aspects of renal homotransplantation. In: TE Starzl (ed), *Experience In Renal Transplantation.* Philadelphia, Saunders, 1964:239–261.
42. Lawrence HS: The transfer of hypersensitivity of the delayed type in man. In: Lawrence HS (ed), *Cellular and Humoral Aspects of the Hypersensitive States.* New York, Hoeber-Harper, 1959:279.
43. Warburton PE, Greig GM, Haaf T, Willard HG: PCR amplification of chromosome-specific alpha satellite DNA: definition of centromeric STS markers and polymorphic analysis. *Genomics* 11:324, 1991.

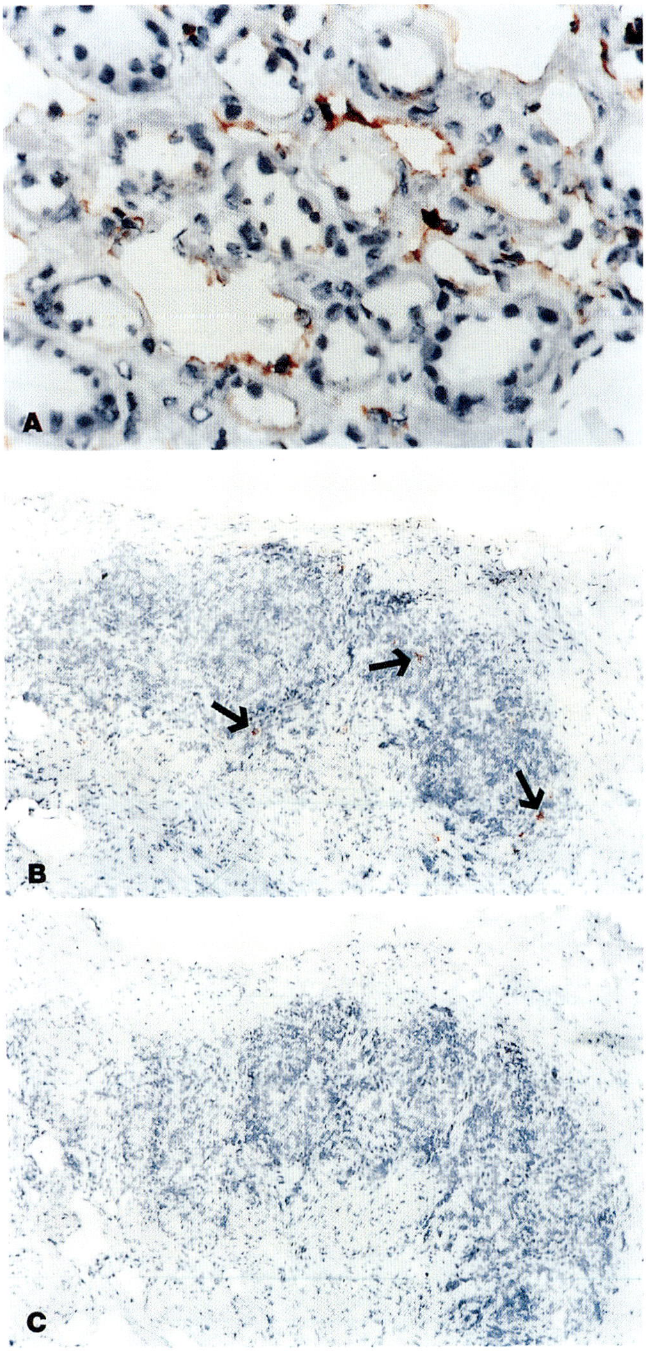

Kidney allograft. (A, ×450) and recipient lymph node (B, ×100) stained with anti-HLA B 7,40 mAb using an avidin-biotin complex method. The rust-colored endothelial cells in the kidney and scattered cells in the lymph node are of donor origin. (C, ×100) The negative control in which anti-A2, 28 (irrelevant class-matched antibody) was used as the primary antibody. (From Starzl TE, et al: Chimerism and donor specific nonreactivity 27 to 29 years after kidney allotransplantation. *Transplantation* 55:1272–1277, 1993.)

44. Nakagome Y, Seki S, Fukutani K, Nagafuchi S, Nakahori Y, Tamura T: PCR detection of distal Yp sequences in an XX true hermaphrodite. *Am J Med Genet* 41:112, 1991.
45. Hsia S, Tong JY, Parris GL, et al: 1992 molecular compatibility and renal graft survival: the HLA DRB1 genotyping. *Transplantation* 55:395–399, 1993.
46. Kashiwagi N, Porter KA, Penn I, Brettschneider L, Starzl TE: Studies of homograft sex and of gamma globulin phenotypes after orthotopic homotransplantation of the human liver. *Surg Forum* 20:374–376, 1969.
47. Murase N, Demetris AJ, Matsuzaki T, et al: Long survival in rats after multivisceral versus isolated small bowel allotransplantation under FK 506. *Surgery* 110:87–98, 1991.
48. Iwaki Y, Starzl TE, Yagihashi A, et al: Replacement of donor lymphoid tissue in human small bowel transplants under FK 506 immunosuppression. *Lancet* 337:818–819, 1991.
49. Qian S, Demetris AJ, Fu F, et al: Murine liver allograft transplantation: tolerance and donor cell chimerism. *Hepatology,* 19:916–924, 1994.
50. Calne RY, Sells RA, Pena JR, et al: Induction of immunological tolerance by porcine liver allografts. *Nature* 233:472–474, 1969.
51. Zimmerman FA, Butcher GW, Davies HS, Brons G, Kamada N, Turel O: Techniques for orthotopic liver transplantation in the rat and some studies of the immunologic responses to fully allogeneic liver grafts. *Transplant Proc* 11:571–577, 1979.
52. Kamada N, Davies HFFS, Roser B: Reversal of transplantation immunity by liver grafting. *Nature* 292:840–842, 1981.
53. Murase N, Demetris AJ, Kim DG, Todo S, Fung JJ, Starzl TE: Rejection of the multivisceral allograft in rats: a sequential and analysis with comparison to isolated orthotopic small bowel and liver grafts. *Surgery* 108:880–889, 1990.
54. Murase N, Kim D, Todo S, Cramer DV, Fung J, Starzl TE: Induction of liver, heart and multivisceral graft acceptance with a short course of FK 506. *Transplant Proc* 22:74–75, 1990.
55. Murase N, Demetris AJ, Woo J, et al: Graft versus host disease (GVHD) after BN to LEW compared to LEW to BN rat intestinal transplantation under FK 506. *Transplantation* 55:1–7, 1993.
56. Nemlander A, Soots A, Willebrand EV, Husberg B, Hayry P: Redistribution of renal allograft responding leukocytes during rejection. II. Kinetics and specificity. *J Exp Med* 156:1087–1100, 1982.
57. Larsen CP, Morris PJ, Austyn JM: Migration of dendritic leukocytes from cardiac allografts into host spleens: a novel route for initiation of rejection. *J Exp Med* 171:307–314, 1990.
58. Demetris AJ, Qian S, Sun H, et al: Early events in liver allograft rejection. *Am J Pathol* 138:609–618, 1991.
59. Forbes RD, Parfrey NA, Gomersail M, Darden AG, Guttmann RD: Dendritic cell-lymphoid aggregation and major histocompatibility antigen expression during rat cardiac allograft rejection. *J Exp Med* 164:1239–1258, 1986.
60. van Schlifgaarde R, Hermans P, Terpstra JL, van Breda Vriesman PJC: Role of mobile passenger lymphocytes in the rejection of renal and cardiac allografts in the rat. *Transplantation* 29:209, 1989.
61. Hayry P, Willebrand B: *Transplantation and Clinical Immunology: Immunosuppression.* Vol 15. Amsterdam, Excerpta Medica, 1983:124–137.
62. von Willebrand E, Taskinen E, Ahonen J, Hayry P: Recent modifications in the fine needle aspiration biopsy of human renal allografts. *Transplant Proc* 15:1195–1197, 1983.
63. Russell PS: Modifications of runt disease in mice by various means. In: Wolstenholme CEW, Cameron MP, London J, Churchill A (eds), *Transplantation: Ciba Foundation Symposium.* Boston, Little Brown, 1962:350–383.
64. Liegeois A, Charreire J, Brennan LB: Allograft enhancement induced by bone marrow cells. *Surg Forum* 25:297–300, 1974.

65. Monaco AP, Gozzo JJ, Wood ML, Liegeois A: Use of low doses of homozygous allogeneic bone marrow cells to induce tolerance with antilymphocyte serum (ALS): tolerance by intra-organ injection. *Transplant Proc* 3:680–683, 1971.
66. Groth C, Collste H, Dreborg S, Hakansson G, Lundgren G, Svennerholm L: Attempts at enzyme replacement in Gaucher disease by renal transplantation. *Acta Paediatr Scand* 68:475–479, 1979.
67. Desnick RJ, Simmons RL, Allen KY, et al: Correction of enzymatic deficiencies by renal transplantation: Fabry's disease. *Surgery* 72:203–11, 1972.
68. Inaba K, Inaba M, Romani N, et al: Generation of large numbers of dendritic cells from mouse bone marrow cultures supplemented with granulocyte/macrophage colony-stimulating factor. *J. Exp Med* 176:1693–1702, 1992.
69. Bandeira A, Coutinho A, Carnaud C, Jacquemart F, Forni L: Transplantation tolerance correlates with high levels of T- and B-lymphocyte activity. *Proc Natl Acad Sci USA* 86:272–276, 1989.
70. Starzl TE, Todo S, Tzakis A, et al: The many faces of multivisceral transplantation. *Surg Gynecol Obstet* 172:335–344, 1991.
71. Slavin S, Strober S, Fuks Z, Kaplan HS: Induction of specific tissue transplantation tolerance using fractionated total lymphoid irradiation in adult mice: long-term survival of allogeneic bone marrow and skin grafts. *J Exp Med* 146:34–48, 1977.
72. Ildstad ST, Sachs DH: Reconstitution with syngeneic plus allogeneic or xenogeneic bone marrow leads to specific acceptance of allografts or xenografts. *Nature* 307:168–170, 1984.
73. Jenkins MD: The role of cell division in the induction of clonal anergy. *Immunol Today* 13:69–73, 1992.
74. Steinman RM, Cohn ZA: Identification of a novel cell type in peripheral lymphoid organs of mice. I. Morphology, quantitation, tissue distribution. *J Exp Med* 137:1142–1162, 1973.
75. Steinman RM, Lustig DS, Cohn ZA: Identification of a novel cell in peripheral lymphoid organs of mice. III. Functional properties in vivo. *J Exp Med* 139:1431–1445, 1974.
76. Steinman RM: The dendritic cell system and its role in immunogenicity. *Annu Rev Immunol* 9:271–296, 1991.
77. Miller JFAP, Morahan G: Peripheral T cell tolerance. *Annu Rev Immunol* 10:51–69, 1992.
78. Coutinho A: Beyond clonal selection and network. *Immunol Rev* 110:63–87, 1989.
79. Cohen IR: The cognitive paradigm and the immunological homunculus. *Immunol Today* 13:490–494, 1992.
80. Jerne NK: Idiotypic networks and other preconceived ideas. *Immunol Rev* 79:5–24, 1984.
81. Zubiaga AM, Munoz A, Huber BT: Superinduction of IL-2 gene transcription in the presence of cycloheximide. *J Immunol* 146:3857–3863, 1991.
82. Isobe M, Yagita H, Okumura K, Ihara A: Specific acceptance of cardiac allograft after treatment with antibodies to ICAM-1 and LFA-1. *Science* 255:1125, 1992.
83. Waldmann H, Cobbold S: The use of monoclonal antibodies to achieve immunological tolerance. *Immunol Today* 14:247–251, 1993.
84. Lechler RI, Batchelor JR: Restoration of immunogenicity to passenger cell-depleted kidney allografts by the addition of donor-strain dendritic cells. *J Exp Med* 155:31–41, 1982.
85. Thomas J, Carver M, Foil B, Haisch C, Thomas F: Renal allograft tolerance induced with ATG and donor bone marrow in outbred rhesus monkeys. *Transplantation* 36:104–106, 1983.
86. Barber WH, Mankin JA, Laskow DA, et al: Long term results of a controlled prospective study with transfusion of donor-specific bone marrow in 57 cadaveric renal allograft recipients. *Transplantation* 51:70–75, 1991.

87. Salvatierra O, Vincenti F, Amend WJC, et al: Deliberate donor-specific blood transfusions prior to living related renal transplantation: a new approach. *Ann Surg* 192:543–552, 1980.
88. Ricordi C, Tzakis AG, Demetris AJ, et al: Reversal of graft versus host disease with infusion of stored autologous bone marrow cells following combined liver-bone marrow allotransplantation in man. *Transplant Sci* 3:73–74, 1993.
89. Harrison DE: Competitive repopulation in unirradiated normal recipients. *Blood* 81:2473–2474, 1993.
90. Stewart FM, Crittenden RB, Lowry PA, Pearson-White S, Quesenberry PJ: Long-term engraftment of normal and post-5-fluorouracil murine marrow into normal nonmyeloablated mice. *Blood* 81:2566, 1993.
91. Carroll PB, Ricordi C, Shapiro R, et al: Frequency of kidney rejection in diabetic patients undergoing simultaneous kidney and islet cell transplantation. *Transplantation* 55:761–765, 1993.
92. Ricordi C, Ildstad ST, Starzl TE: Induction of pancreatic islet graft acceptance: the role of antigen presenting cells. *Transplant Sci* 2:344–38, 1992.
93. Reyes J, Tzakis A, Ramos HC, et al: The frequent achievement of a drug free state after orthotopic liver transplantation. *Transplant Proc* 25:3315–3319, 1993.

10

Clinical Aspects of Renal Transplantation Pathology

Parmjeet S. Randhawa / Anthony J. Demetris

The pathologist plays an indispensable role in any renal transplantation program, both by helping to determine the suitability of a donor kidney before transplantation and by diagnosing varying causes of allograft dysfunction after the operation. This chapter outlines the general principles of pathology on which such determinations are made. Preexisting changes in the donor, manifestations of rejection, drug-induced injuries, ischemia, infections, recurrent glomerulonephritis, and metabolic diseases are considered, with emphasis on pathogenesis, pathologic features, and differential diagnosis. It concludes with a section that discusses the processing of biopsy tissue, with the goal of obtaining the most information possible about the renal allograft.

▲ HISTOLOGIC EVALUATION OF THE DONOR KIDNEY

A biopsy documenting the baseline histology of every donor kidney is a desirable goal. However, we perform pretransplantation biopsies only in donors who are elderly, hypertensive, diabetic, or have some other renal disease of concern to the clinician. Before biopsy, such kidneys should be subjected to gross examination on the back table to assess the degree of scarring in the parenchyma and the amount of atherosclerosis in the renal artery. Localized lesions such as small abscesses or neoplasms also may be recognized at this stage. The back table biopsy should attempt to sample any suspicious lesion seen but at the same time should avoid areas of obvious scarring. There are no established guidelines pertaining to the extent of chronic histopathologic changes permissible in a prospective donor organ. At the

University of Pittsburgh, we are unwilling to use any kidney with more than 20% glomerulosclerosis or with a moderate degree of fibrosis, arteriosclerosis, and arteriolosclerosis.

At times, small renal cortical neoplasms are noted during the examination of the donor kidney. There is evidence that complete excision of small tumors of this kind can be safely performed.[1] However, in general, the presence of documented malignancy in the donor is an absolute contraindication to transplantation.[2]

There are reports of successful transplantation of donor kidneys with evidence of disseminated intravascular coagulation, but many surgeons remain skeptical. Observations on small groups of patients suggest that fibrin thrombi present in the donor organ can resolve after transplantation, even if transient microangiopathic hemolytic anemia is initially transmitted to the recipient.[3]

▲ ISCHEMIC PRESERVATION AND HARVESTING INJURY

Ischemic injury to the donor kidney before or during recovery of the organ, transportation to the recipient institution, and subsequent transplantation into the patient is a common cause of graft dysfunction in the immediate posttransplant period. Oliguria and anuria of varying degree and duration can be observed in as many as 40% of patients, but the process is usually self-limiting, and complete recovery occurs within a few weeks. Biopsies of the allograft kidney performed during the ischemic phase show coarse, irregular cytoplasmic vacuoles in the renal tubular epithelium and focal acute tubular necrosis (ATN) (Fig. 10–1). The necrotic tubular epithelium subsequently undergoes dystrophic calcification. During the resolution phase of the injury, the tubules may show only nonspecific dilatation, cast formation, and regeneration.[4] The peritubular capillaries can be markedly congested and sometimes show extramedullary hematopoiesis.[5] In the glomeruli, severe ischemic injury may manifest itself in the form of capillary thrombi or neutrophilic infiltration. These changes can mimic humoral rejection and acute drug-induced vascular injury.

▲ REJECTION

Hyperacute and Accelerated Rejection

Rapid catastrophic rejection of a transplanted kidney within minutes or the first few hours after transplantation is called *hyperacute rejection.* The term *accelerated rejection* has been used to categorize immunologically mediated episodes of renal dysfunction that occur during the first several days after transplantation. Hyperacute and accelerated acute rejection begin with injury to the endothelium of the arterial and capillary compartments of the renal parenchyma. This type of rejection is most often the result of recipient presensitization to donor-incompatible blood groups or HLA antigens. Such sensitization typically occurs because of prior transplantation, blood transfusions, or pregnancies.[6] Endothelial injury from the ensuing antigen-

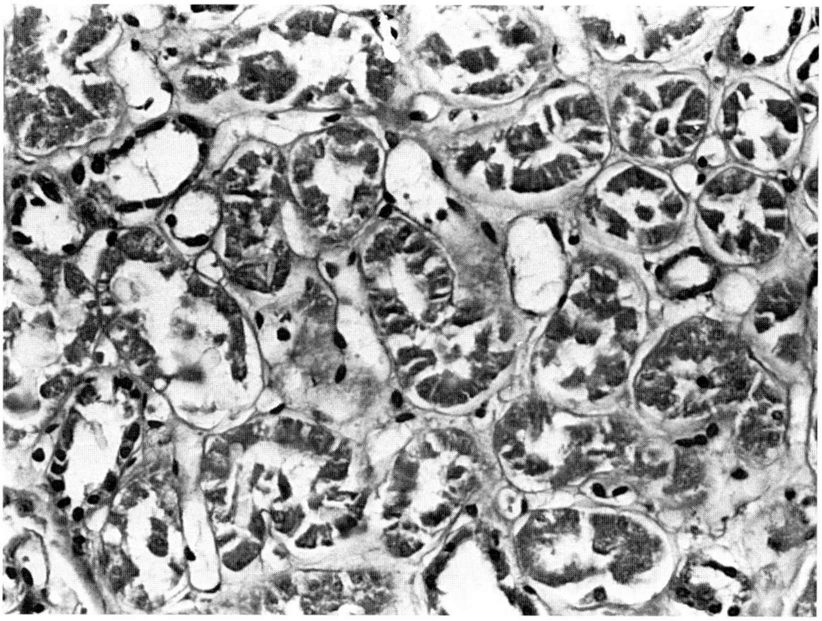

Figure 10–1. Acute tubular necrosis, (ATN). The tubular epithelium in this biopsy specimen is largely necrotic. Cellular outlines are poorly defined and the cytoplasm is filled with irregular masses of eosinophilic material. Nuclei are shrunken, deeply pyknotic, or completely lysed.

antibody reaction leads to activation of complement by the classic pathway, resulting in vascular thrombosis and ischemic necrosis of the allograft. It appears that in some patients with perioperative endotoxinemia, activation of complement can also proceed via the alternate pathway. At present, nothing can be done for hyperacute rejection except to remove the allograft; the goal is to prevent its occurrence by ensuring a negative pretransplant crossmatch. Accelerated rejection can sometimes be treated with intensified immunosuppression, although the effectiveness of such therapy is debatable.

Early stages of hyperacute and accelerated rejection are characterized histopathologically by reactive vascular endothelium and scattered subendothelial lymphocytes present in the arterioles and small arteries. A diffuse margination of neutrophils is seen throughout the peritubular capillaries. Foci of extravasated red blood cells may be noted in the interstitium.[7] The presence of more than five neutrophils in the glomeruli is also a helpful clue to the presence of an underlying antibody-mediated rejection. In severe cases, one sees obvious vasculitis, glomerular thrombosis, and infarction of the renal parenchyma (Fig. 10–2). Immunofluorescence examination helps to confirm the diagnosis of antibody-mediated injury by documenting immunoglobulin and complement deposition at the arteriolar and capillary level (Fig. 10–3). If hyperacute or accelerated rejection is suspected, the transplant surgeon should ensure that a portion of the biopsy specimen

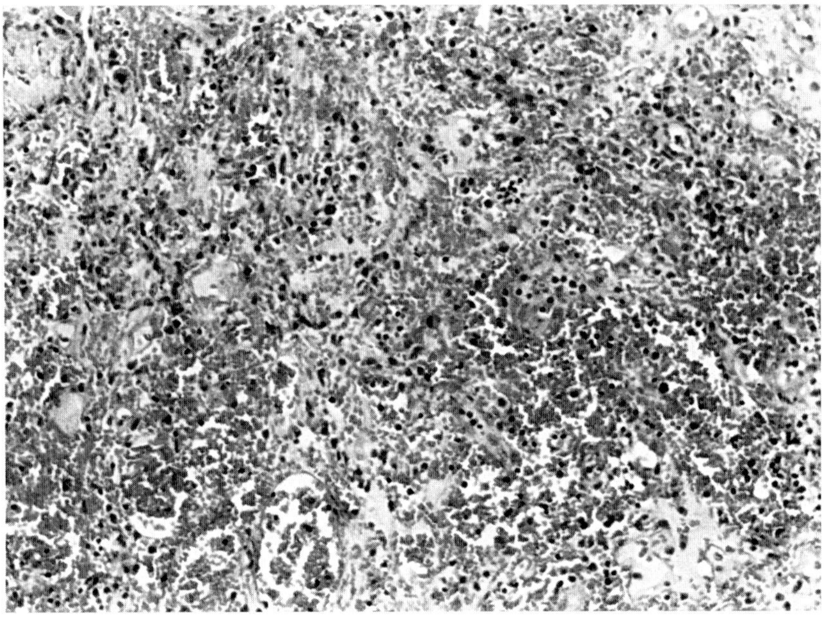

Figure 10–2. Acute infarction in a renal allograft in the early postoperative period. The glomeruli, tubules, and vessels show hemorrhagic necrosis. When tissue destruction is this extensive, differentiation between hyperacute rejection and renal artery thrombosis may not be possible without immunologic studies.

is sent fresh to the pathologist, without formalin fixation, for immunofluorescence studies.

The histopathologic differential diagnosis of hyperacute or accelerated rejection includes infarction of ischemic etiology, drug-induced vascular thrombosis, recurrent hemolytic-uremic syndrome, and vascular fibrinoid necrosis due to severe hypertension. In difficult cases, a review of the patient's panel reactive antibody (PRA) profile and cross-match status can be helpful in establishing the diagnosis of rejection. However, it is important to remember that hyperacute or accelerated rejection can occur in the face of a negative cross match, if it is mediated by antiendothelial antibodies, which are not detected with conventional microcytotoxicity assays. It is also possible to obtain a negative cross match with pretransplant serum, if sensitization to the donor antigens has occurred in the remote past. In such instances, repeating the cross match with posttransplant serum may give a positive result. The cross-match test, however, cannot detect rejection mediated by the alternate pathway through mechanisms independent of preformed antibodies.

Acute Rejection

Immune-mediated dysfunction that develops about 7 or more days after transplantation has been called *acute rejection*. Acute rejection is often characterized by

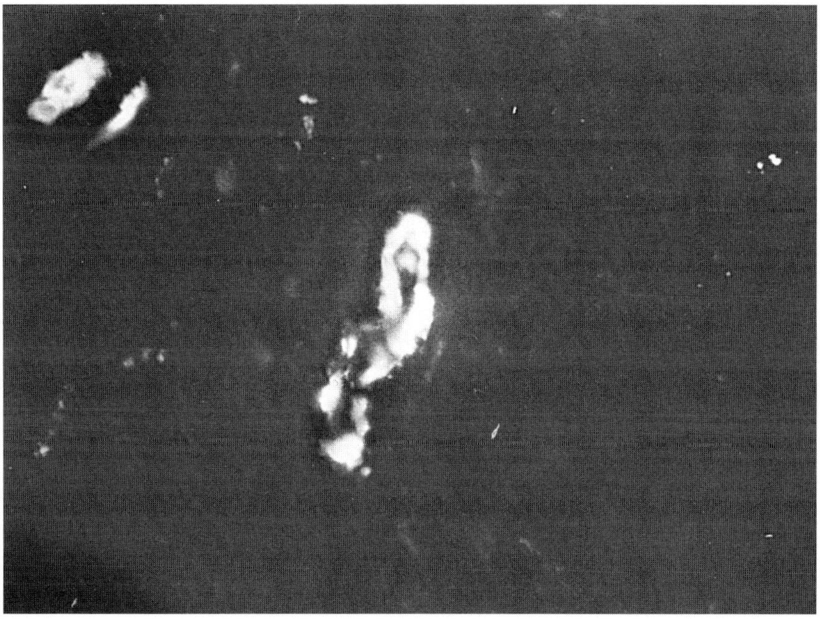

Figure 10–3. Immunofluorescence examination can document immunoglobulin and complement deposition in allograft vessels, as shown in this biopsy specimen 1 week after transplantation. Interpretation of these findings necessitates clinicopathologic correlation. Kidneys from aged, hypertensive donors may show nonspecific IgM and C3 deposits in arterioles. In hyperacute rejection, IgG is the usual immunoglobulin deposited, multiple components of complement are identified, and the interstitial capillaries show diffuse staining.

changes in the tubulointerstitial compartment of the kidney. Acute rejection is a manifestation of cell-mediated immune injury. It is believed that both delayed hypersensitivity and cytotoxicity mechanisms are involved. The immune injury is directed against HLA and possibly other cell-specific antigens expressed by the tubular epithelium and vascular endothelium. The expression of class I and class II human leukocyte (HLA) antigens on these cells can be readily demonstrated by immunoperoxidase studies performed on renal allograft biopsies. Immunophenotypic characterization of lymphocyte populations in situ has generated conflicting data. Various authors report the predominance of CD4-positive cells, CD8-positive cells, or macrophages. It is likely that these differences are due to differences in patient selection or to sampling of tissue at different stages in the evolution of the alloimmune response.[6,7]

Acute rejection is recognized histopathologically by the presence of interstitial infiltrates of activated lymphocytes. These cells breach the tubular basement membrane and extend into the epithelium, producing a lesion referred to as *tubulitis* (Fig. 10–4). The intensity of the infiltrate and tubular injury are used by pathologists to classify the rejection as mild, moderate, or severe. Such a grading system is a useful way of indicating how urgently and intensively a particular episode of rejection needs to be treated.[8] The clinician should recognize that there are cases in which in-

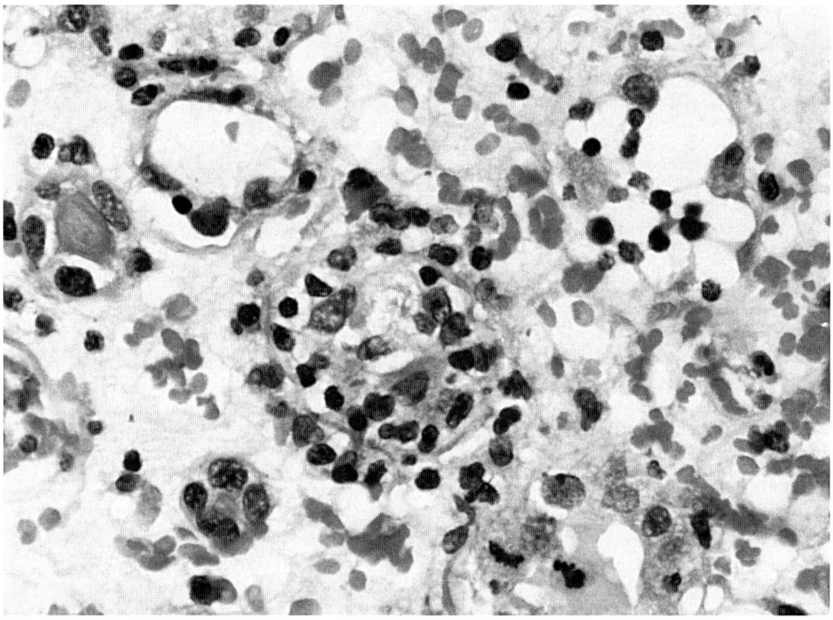

Figure 10–4. A renal tubule with several lymphocytes on the inner aspect of its basement membrane. This lesion is referred to as *tubulitis* and is the sine qua non for the diagnosis of acute rejection.

terstitial lymphocytic infiltrates constitute only a small proportion of the total renal tissue sampled. When only infrequent foci of tubular injury are present but the biopsy is not entirely normal, the pathologist gives a diagnosis of *borderline acute cellular rejection.* Decisions regarding whether patients should be treated are based on a combination of clinical and pathologic findings. In many cases, it may be sufficient to treat the patient with clinical observation. However, clinically significant rejection can be missed or inadequately graded if its distribution within the allograft is focal and patchy. When acute rejection is moderate to severe, there also may be arterial endothelial or smooth muscle wall involvement (Fig. 10–5). Such a manifestation of rejection is most serious and should be treated aggressively.

Chronic Rejection

Chronic rejection is characterized by slowly progressive graft dysfunction that ultimately leads to chronic renal failure. Many patients develop nephrotic-range proteinuria. Histopathologic examination in some cases shows prominent changes within the glomeruli, so-called *transplant glomerulopathy.* In other cases, the essential

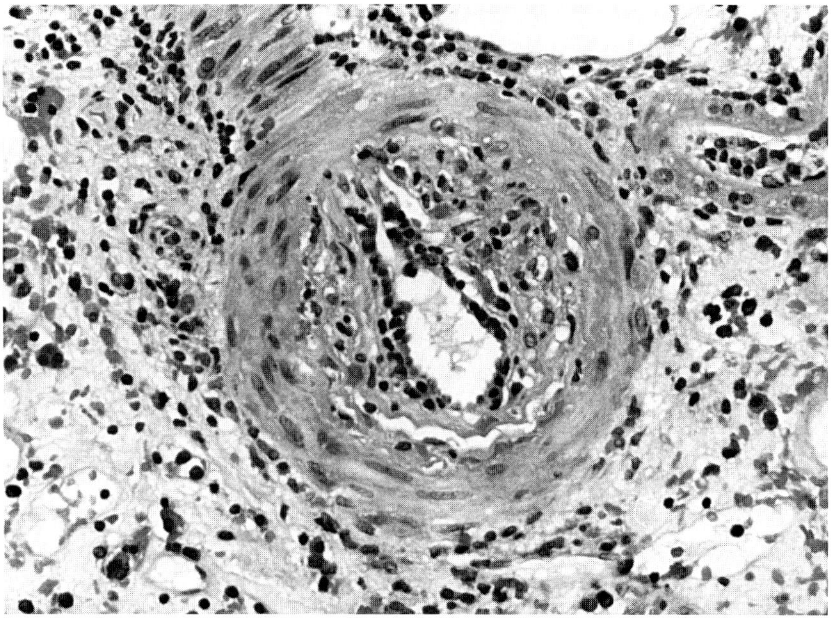

Figure 10–5. Acute rejection complicated by intimal arteritis. Such extension of lymphocytes into the arterial wall puts the allograft at increased risk for thrombotic occlusion and infarction.

change is a marked atherosclerotic narrowing of renal vascular tree, and the term *chronic vascular rejection* seems more appropriate. Glomerular and vascular changes can be seen concomitantly.

The pathogenesis of chronic allograft rejection is believed to be a multifactorial process. When episodes of acute rejection have occurred previously, arteriosclerosis and arteriolosclerosis can be explained on the basis of prior immune injury to the vessels. Vascular narrowing leads to ischemic changes in the glomeruli characterized by progressive mesangial expansion and glomerulosclerosis. The interstitial fibrosis and tubular atrophy seen in long-standing grafts is in part due to prior acute tubulointerstitial rejection. In addition, long-term administration of cyclosporine or tacrolimus probably contributes to the development of interstitial fibrosis and arteriolosclerosis.[6,7]

Chronic transplant glomerulopathy is recognized in allograft biopsies by increased mesangial expansion, accentuation of the normal glomerular lobularity, and a segmental increase in mesangial cellularity (Fig. 10–6). In late stages, thickening of the glomerular basement membrane occurs, a process best demonstrated by the PAS and Jones stains (Fig. 10–7). Lesions of segmental and global glomerulosclerosis may supervene. Hyperplasia of the juxtaglomerular apparatus has been described, though this may only reflect associated hypertension or renal artery stenosis. If immunofluorescence studies are performed, finely granular deposits of immunoglobu-

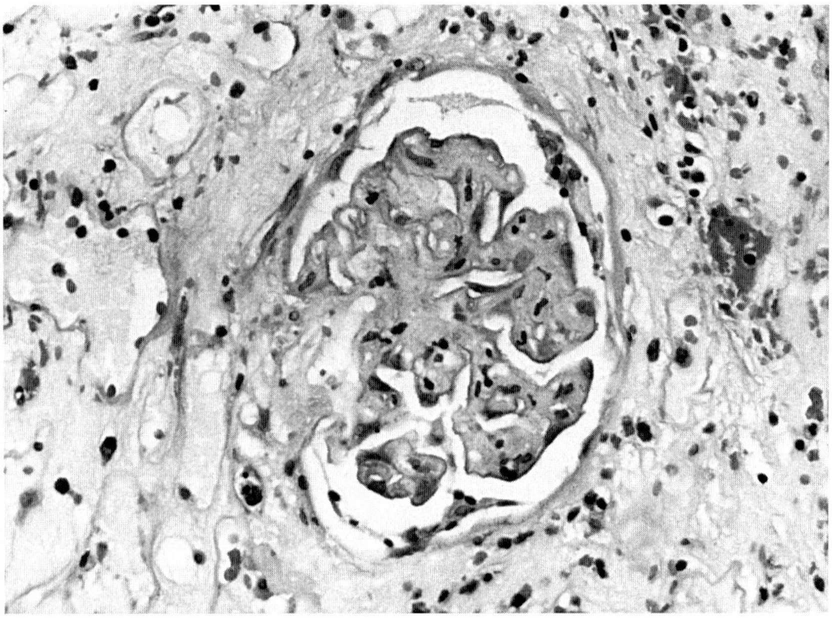

Figure 10–6. This glomerulus from an allograft nephrectomy specimen with chronic rejection shows a marked increase in mesangial matrix. The glomerular capillary loops are mostly collapsed, but a few patent ones with thickened basement membranes are still visualized.

lins and complement can be observed. Electron microscopic studies should be performed when glomerulonephritis is in the differential diagnosis.[9] Transplant glomerulopathy is characterized ultrastructurally by a flocculent electron-lucent material deposited in a subendothelial location. Cytoplasmic processes of the mesangial cells may insinuate between the endothelial and epithelial aspects of the glomerular basement membrane, producing a lesion called mesangial interposition (Fig. 10–8). Large electron dense deposits are not observed.[10]

Chronic vascular rejection is characterized by intimal sclerosis and vessel hyalinosis affecting the arterioles, interlobular and arcuate arteries, and more proximal vessels (Fig. 10–9). Deposition of mucopolysaccharides and hyaluronic acid may cause myxoid degeneration in the vessel wall. Foamy macrophages can be seen infiltrating the intima and the media of the affected arteries. Progressive vascular narrowing leads to patchy interstitial fibrosis and tubular atrophy. The tubular basement membranes can become thickened. Ischemia of the glomerular capillary bed leads to shrinkage and collapse of the capillary tufts (see Fig. 10–6). Mesangial expansion and a segmental or global glomerulosclerosis follow. Associated lymphocytic infiltrates in the interstitium are usually mild and not associated with clinically significant tubulitis. In some cases a prominent population of plasmacytic cells is seen. Lymphoid aggregates with well-defined circumscribed borders also can be seen in these cases.[11]

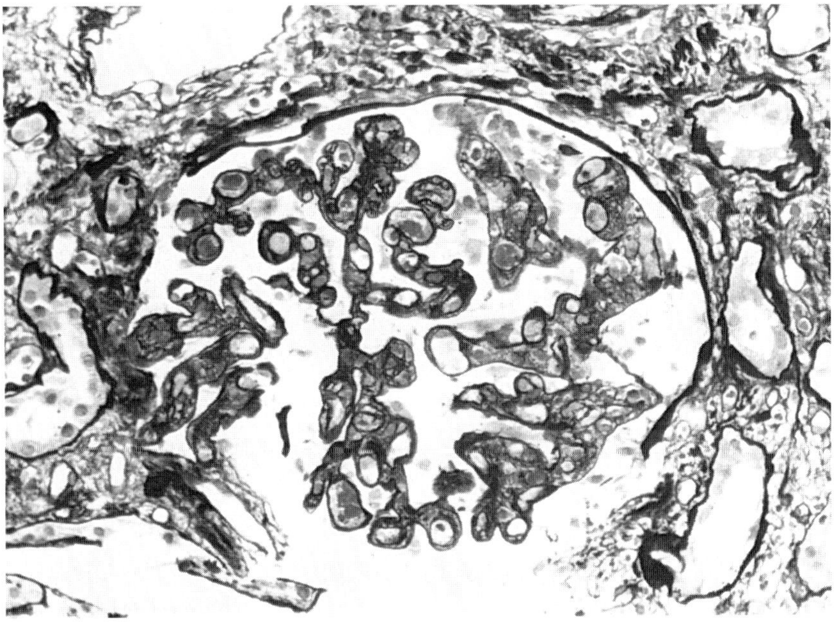

Figure 10–7. Jones stain shows reduplication of the basement membranes in several capillary loops of this glomerulus with chronic transplant glomerulopathy.

▲ DRUG-INDUCED INJURY

Cyclosporine Toxicity

Cyclosporine toxicity is an important cause of renal allograft dysfunction. Clinically, it may be difficult to differentiate between rejection and drug toxicity, and examination of a needle biopsy specimen is frequently performed to resolve the issue. A variety of cyclosporine-associated morphologic changes have been described in the literature.[12]

Cyclosporine toxicity can manifest itself purely as a rise in the serum creatinine. The biopsy may show minimal pathologic changes, and yet reduction in the cyclosporine dosage leads to improvement in allograft function. When this sequence of events is documented, a diagnosis of functional cyclosporine toxicity is made. Most episodes occur within the first few weeks after transplantation and may not be associated with elevated blood levels of cyclosporine.

Cyclosporine has been implicated in the occurrence of acute tubular necrosis in renal allografts.[13] The incidence and duration of posttransplant anuria or oliguria in cyclosporine-treated patients are higher than that observed with azathioprine therapy. This may partly reflect cyclosporine-induced exacerbation of ischemic injury to the tubules, but similar tubular injury is observed after liver, heart, and lung transplantation, in which the kidney has not been subjected to the metabolic insults as-

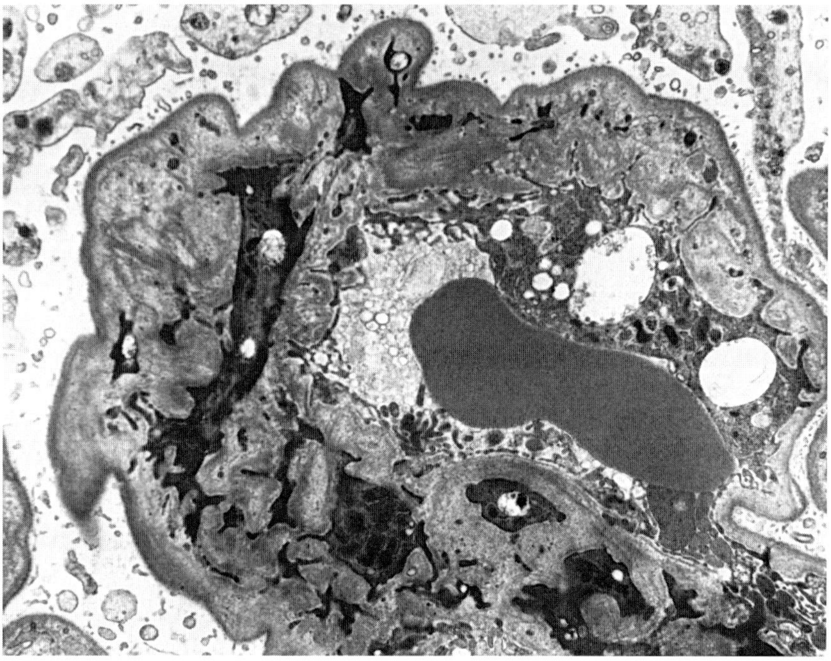

Figure 10–8. Electron microscopic details of a thickened capillary loop from the case illustrated in Figure 10–7. The mesangial cells bear multiple, irregularly branching cytoplasmic processes that insinuate between the endothelial and epithelial aspects of the capillary basement membrane (mesangial interposition).

sociated with harvesting and reimplantation. Tubular necrosis is recognized histopathologically by nuclear pyknosis or karyorrhexis and cytoplasmic eosinophilia in the tubular epithelium. Biopsies performed in the resolving phase may show only tubular dilatation with focal regeneration. The process is generally reversible, but in some cases, the development of a diffuse interstitial fibrosis has been noted.

Cyclosporine toxicity may lead to vacuolization of the tubular epithelium. These vacuoles are typically fine and isometric in nature (Fig. 10–10). The occurrence of such vacuolization in an allograft biopsy specimen in the absence of changes of rejection can be used as an indication to reduce the dosage of cyclosporine. Tubular vacuolization, however, is not always associated with high cyclosporine levels in the blood. Furthermore, isometric tubular vacuolization has been described after administration of mannitol or intravenous radiographic contrast medium.

Cyclosporine can damage the vascular endothelium and lead to thrombosis in the arterioles and the glomerular capillaries. If one looks carefully, occasional thrombi can be seen in as many as one fourth of all allograft biopsy specimens examined within the first month after transplantation. The prevalence of such thrombi is higher in cyclosporine-treated patients than in those receiving azathioprine primarily. Patients with isolated thrombi may have no symptoms, but more widespread endothelial injury may be associated with the hemolytic-uremic syndrome.

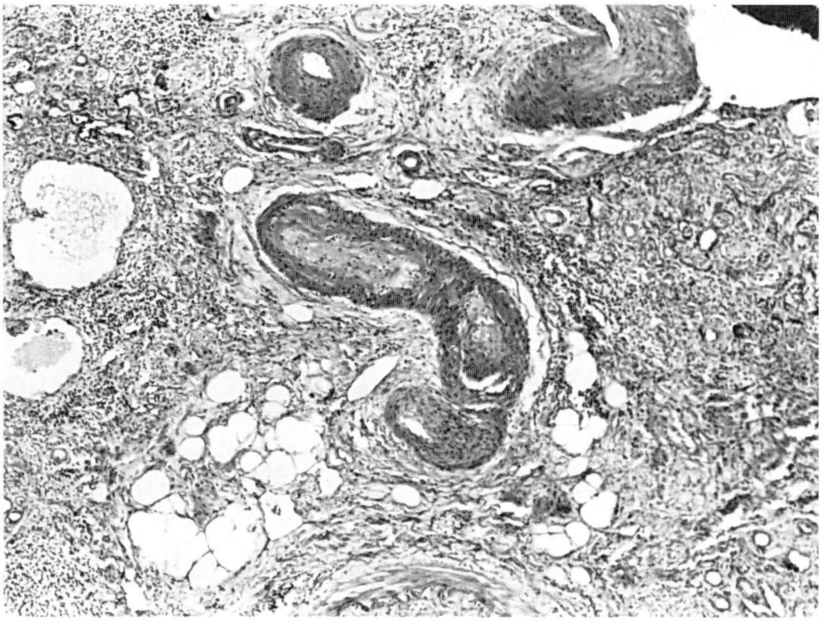

Figure 10–9. Chronic vascular rejection with moderate to severe obliterative arteriopathy affecting arteries in the hilar region. The perivascular soft tissue shows a chronic inflammatory infiltrate and marked fibrosis.

Milder cases recover without any long-term sequelae to the graft. However, other patients develop thickening of the glomerular basement membranes associated with focal segmental or diffuse global glomerulosclerosis.

Cyclosporine can also reportedly cause an acute arteriopathy characterized by endothelial swelling, mucoid degeneration in the intima, and even frank vasculitis.[14] Differentiation from acute vascular rejection may be extremely difficult morphologically. The presence of subendothelial lymphocytic infiltration, proliferative lesions, and associated interstitial hemorrhage or tubulitis should lead one to favor rejection over drug toxicity. In problematic cases, ancillary information such as the cyclosporine level, PRA, and the cross match status of the patient should be taken into account before therapeutic decisions are made. If the lesion is clearly drug-induced, cyclosporine is discontinued, and a different maintenance immunosuppressive agent, such as tacrolimus, mycophenolate mofetil, or azathioprine is used. Acute lesions can reduce or heal with scarring and eventually arteriolosclerosis and hyalinosis (Fig. 10–11). In contrast to vascular rejection, these changes remain confined to small arteries and arterioles with up to three layers of smooth muscle in the media.

The final manifestation of cyclosporine injury to the kidney, which is seen after prolonged administration of the drug, is the occurrence of interstitial fibrosis in a striped pattern.[15] Striped fibrosis is frequently associated with chronic cyclosporine arteriopathy and is therefore believed to be ischemic in origin. Reduction in cyclosporine dosage may result in some improvement in renal function. Before interstitial fibrosis is attributed to a drug-induced insult, it is necessary to exclude other

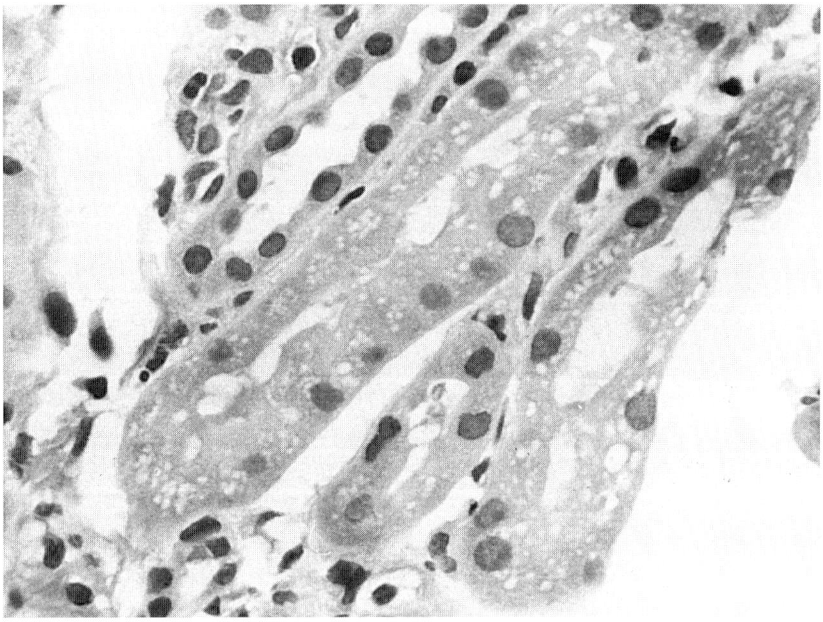

Figure 10–10. Isometric vacuolization of the proximal tubular epithelium in a renal allograft biopsy. This change can be observed with elevated blood levels of cyclosporine or tacrolimus.

causes, such as chronic rejection, glomerulonephritis, persistent urinary obstruction, or renal artery stenosis.

Tacrolimus Toxicity

Tacrolimus (FK 506) is under investigation at several centers around the world as a primary immunosuppressive agent instead of cyclosporine. The principal advantages to tacrolimus therapy are a reduced need for concurrent steroid administration and a lower incidence of hypertension and hypercholesterolemia; graft survival may also be somewhat better. In addition, tacrolimus can "rescue" allografts with refractory acute cellular rejection under cyclosporine therapy. Tacrolimus is qualitatively and quantitatively similar to cyclosporine in its profile of nephrotoxicity. Tubular vacuolation, arterial hyalinosis, functional toxicity, and striped fibrosis all have been documented in patients treated with tacrolimus.[16]

▲ DE NOVO OCCURRENCE OR RECURRENCE OF NATIVE RENAL DISEASE

Several primary glomerular diseases can recur in the allograft; in some cases, this can occur quite rapidly after transplantation. The incidence and severity of recurrent

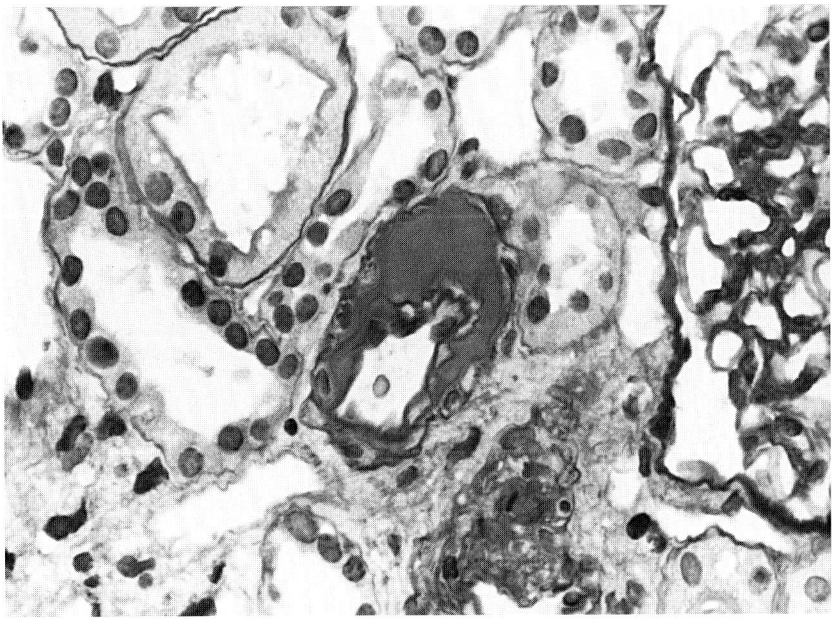

Figure 10–11. An arteriolar vessel with eccentric deposition of an eosinophilic hyaline material. Hyalinosis occurring in the absence of donor disease, hypertension, and diabetes can be ascribed to chronic cyclosporine or tacrolimus toxicity.

renal disease vary according to the disease entity.[17] Primary glomerular diseases also develop after transplantation in allografts implanted into recipients with nonglomerular diseases such as diabetes mellitus, hypertension, or polycystic kidneys. The term *de novo glomerulonephritis* is used to describe these cases. A third and somewhat uncommon mechanism of glomerulonephritis in a transplant kidney is direct transmission of disease present in the donor organ. IgA nephropathy and membranoproliferative glomerulonephritis (MPGN) type I have been shown to be transmitted in this way. Fortunately, the immune complex deposits present in these kidneys resolve spontaneously with time.

Recurrent Focal Segmental Glomerulosclerosis

Focal segmental glomerulosclerosis (FSGS) recurs in 30–50% of patients. In some studies, recurrence has been noted to be more common in children younger than 15 years of age and uncommon in adults older than 30 years.[18,19] Clinical onset is usually within the first few months of transplantation. In some cases, recurrence occurs dramatically on the day of or within a few days of the operation, suggesting involvement of a circulating factor in the pathogenesis of this disease. The typical clinical presentation is proteinuria. Graft loss occurs at a variable rate, and it is possible for patients to become dialysis-dependent within a year of diagnosis. Needle biopsies of the allograft kidney may show no diagnostic abnormality if a sufficient number of glomeruli have not been sampled. In other cases, classic focal segmental lesions may be seen, particularly in the juxtamedullary location. Immunofluorescence examination shows only traces of IgM and C3 in the sclerotic segments. Electron microscopic examination shows nonspecific swelling and degeneration in the visceral epithelial cells of Bowman's capsule.

De Novo Focal Segmental Glomerulosclerosis

De novo FSGS complicates 1–9% of renal transplantations. Some authors report an increased incidence with pediatric en bloc donors. This may be due to the exposure of relatively immature glomeruli to adult glomerular filtration rates. The associated hemodynamic stresses seem to damage the glomerular capillary membranes and result in segmental sclerosing lesions. Unlike recurrent FSGS, de novo disease presents several months after transplantation.[7] Graft loss is slow and progressive. Microscopically, the focal segmental lesions are often associated with chronic vascular rejection and chronic transplant glomerulopathy. It is likely that de novo FSGS is the result of ischemic changes secondary to graft atherosclerosis. Consistent with this explaination is the observation that de novo FSGS begins in a cortical location, in contrast to recurrent FSGS, which begins at a juxtamedullary location.

Recurrent Membranous Glomerulonephritis

Membranous glomerulonephritis (MGN) recurs in 25–50% of patients. The onset is typically 1 year or more after transplantation. Microscopically, one observes glomerular basement membrane (GBM) thickening on sections stained with hematoxylin and eosin.[20] A Jones stain shows the presence of subepithelial silver deposits taking the form of spikes (Fig. 10–12). Immunofluorescence shows diffuse IgG and complement deposits throughout most of the glomeruli (Fig. 10–13). Electron microscopic examination shows subepithelial electron-dense deposits; the spikes seen on the Jones stain are invaginations of the GBM close to the site of immune complex deposition (Fig. 10–14). With the progression of disease, the deposits get completely incorporated into the GBM and may no longer be subepithelial. These changes are associated with gradual graft loss over 2–7 years.

De Novo Membranous Glomerulonephritis

Membranous glomerulonephritis occurs de novo in 1–9% of grafts. The onset is typically 1–2 years after transplantation. The patients may have no symptoms or show persistent proteinuria. The morphologic changes are similar to those of recurrent membranous disease.[21] The clinical course is slow and progressive, and the graft is typically lost to associated chronic rejection rather than the glomerulonephritis. The occurrence of de novo MGN after renal transplantation should prompt investigations

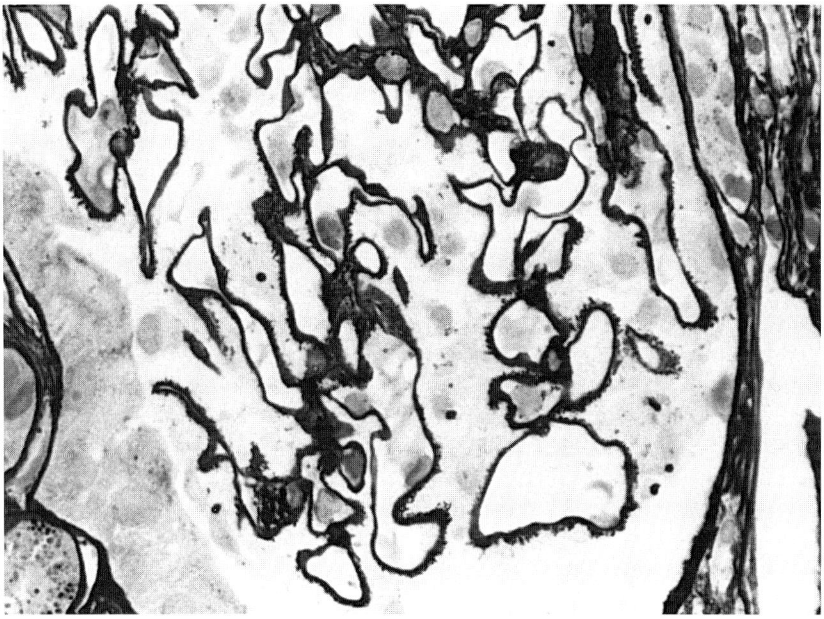

Figure 10–12. Recurrence of membranous glomerulonephritis in an allograft. Immune complex deposits on the epithelial aspect of the glomerular capillary basement membranes appear as spiky projections (Jones stain).

for hepatitis B and C infections. De novo MGN also is described in patients who receive horse antithymocyte globulin therapy for persistent rejection. An etiologic link between the therapy and the glomerular disease can be documented with the demonstration of horse protein within the glomerular immune complex deposits. De novo MGN can coexist with chronic transplant glomerulopathy. In these cases the immune complexes within the glomeruli are believed to contain tubular and endothelial HLA antigens specific to the donor.

Recurrent Membranoproliferative Glomerulonephritis Type I

MPGN type I reportedly recurs in 30–40% of renal allografts.[22] The recurrence may be asymptomatic in as many as 30% of patients. Histopathologic examination shows expansion of the mesangium with varying degrees of mesangial proliferation. The marked increase in mesangial cellularity may accentuate the normal glomerular lobularity. The GBM becomes thickened and shows a double contour on Jones stain. Electron microscopic examination reveals interposition of mesangial cell processes between the epithelial and endothelial sides of the GBM and characteristic subendothelial electron-dense deposits.

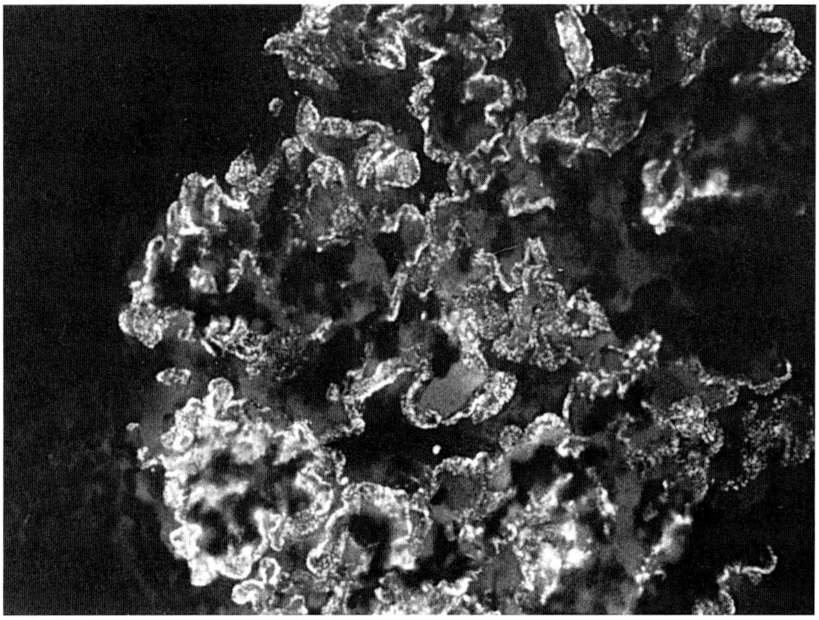

Figure 10–13. Immunoflourescence evaluation of biopsy specimens with recurrent membranous glomerulonephritis shows diffuse granular deposits of immunoglobulins and complement within the glomerular basement membranes.

Recurrent Membranoproliferative Glomerulonephritis Type II

Recurrent MPGN type II (dense deposit disease) has a much higher incidence of recurrence than MPGN type I. Ultrastructural recurrence, evidenced by immune complex deposits in the lamina densa of the GBM, can be demonstrated in more than 90% of patients within 6–9 months of transplantation.[23] Fortunately, 30–40% of such patients remain clinically asymptomatic. However, the remainder have a 40–50% risk of graft loss within 2 years. The light microscopic signs of MPGN type II are difficult to differentiate from those of MPGN type I. The presence of glomerular crescents is more common in type I disease and when present implies a worse prognosis.

Recurrent Anti-GBM Antibody Disease

Renal transplantation performed in patients with anti-GBM disease while circulating antibodies are still demonstrable leads to disease recurrence in as many as 40% of patients. If transplantation is delayed until the disease has regressed, and anti-GBM antibodies have been absent for at least 6 months, recurrent anti-GBM disease becomes rare. Clinical manifestations span the entire spectrum from an asympto-

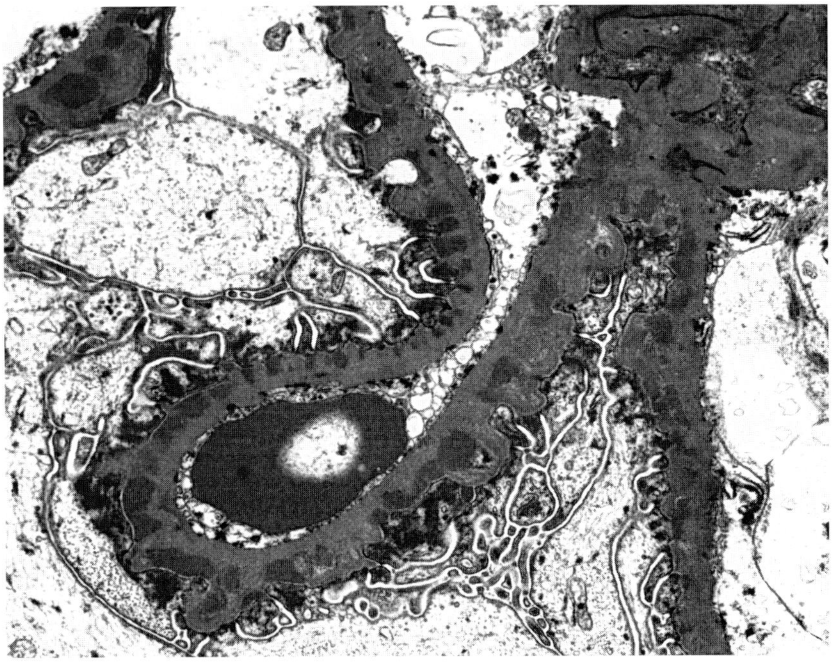

Figure 10–14. Electron microscopic examination is a conclusive way to establish the subepithelial location of immune complexes in membranous glomerulonephritis. Several foci of electron-dense material are shown close to the foot processes of Bowman's capsular epithelium.

matic state to severe proteinuria. Light microscopic examination of kidneys may show segmental proliferative, necrotizing, or crescentic glomerulonephritis.[6,7] Immunofluorescence examination shows IgG deposition within the GBM in a characteristic linear (as opposed to granular) pattern. When there is doubt about whether the immunofluorescence pattern is linear, circulating anti-GBM antibodies may be demonstrated with enzyme-linked immunosorbent assay (ELISA). If sufficient amounts of allograft tissue are available, as at allograft nephrectomy, anti-GBM antibodies may be eluted from the graft tissue itself. The rate of progression of graft dysfunction in recurrent anti-GBM disease is variable and depends on the histopathologic findings. In crescentic glomerulonephritis the graft may be lost rapidly over 6–12 weeks.

De Novo Anti-GBM Disease

De novo anti-GBM disease is a rare occurrence. It has been described in renal transplant recipients with Alport's syndrome. Alport's syndrome is associated with an absence of Goodpasture's antigen within the native kidney GBM. When these individuals are exposed to this antigen for the first time in life through the allograft, induction of anti-GBM antibodies is initiated.[24] Fortunately, this happens only in about 15% of cases, and de novo disease is generally subclinical with excellent prognosis. Some patients, however, rapidly lose their graft within a few months.

Recurrent IgA Nephropathy

Renal transplantation for IgA nephropathy is followed by recurrence of disease within the allograft in as many as 50% of patients. This observation is consistent with the current understanding that the disease is essentially a manifestation of excessive production of IgA immune complexes at various mucosal surfaces in the alimentary and respiratory systems of the patient.[25] Because this basic immune dysfunction is not altered by the transplant procedure, IgA immune complexes are readily redeposited within the allograft. Clinical manifestations are noted 3 months to 4 years after transplantation and generally consist of only mild proteinuria. Histopathologic examination of the kidney shows mild mesangial proliferation. Immunofluorescence confirms the presence of IgA immune complex deposits in a mesangial location.

Recurrent Lupus Nephritis

Renal transplantation for systemic lupus erythematosus (SLE) is not usually followed by the recurrence of the disease within the graft. If, however, there is serologic or clinical evidence of active SLE at the time of transplantation, recurrence rarely may occur.[26] Extrarenal symptoms of SLE in the form of dermatitis or polyarthritis are inconstantly present at the time of recurrent disease. The histopathologic findings in the graft biopsy recapitulate those present in the native kidney. The rate of progression of the disease in the allograft varies widely from patient to patient.

▲ INFECTIOUS DISEASE AFTER RENAL TRANSPLANTATION: RENAL PATHOLOGIC MANIFESTATIONS

Infection after renal transplantation is discussed in Chapter 11. This section is confined to a discussion of how histopathologic examination of the allograft kidney aids in establishing a diagnosis in some of these cases.

Pyelonephritis

Pyelonephritis is recognized because of dilated tubules that contain clusters of neutrophils in the lumen. The interstitium may show polymorphonuclear infiltrates and microabscess formation.[6] A Gram stain may be used to demonstrate cocciform or bacillary organisms in the infected kidney, but specific identification of the organisms involved requires urinary cultures. Lower urinary tract infections also can cause renal dysfunction, but allograft biopsies show no pathologic change.

Cytomegalovirus Infection

Cytomegalovirus (CMV) is commonly cultured from the urine of renal transplant recipients, but clinically significant graft dysfunction occurs rather infrequently.[27] The most common presentation is tubulointerstitial nephritis. CMV inclusions can be seen in the tubular epithelium and vascular endothelium. Classic CMV inclusions are recognized as eosinophilic globules surrounded by a clear halo within a grossly enlarged nucleus. In doubtful cases immunoperoxidase staining for immediate-early and early antigens is helpful in demonstrating the presence of infected cells (Fig. 10–15).

Epstein-Barr Virus Infection

Epstein-Barr virus infection in immunosuppressed recipients of solid organ transplants can result in polyclonal or monoclonal posttransplant lymphoproliferative

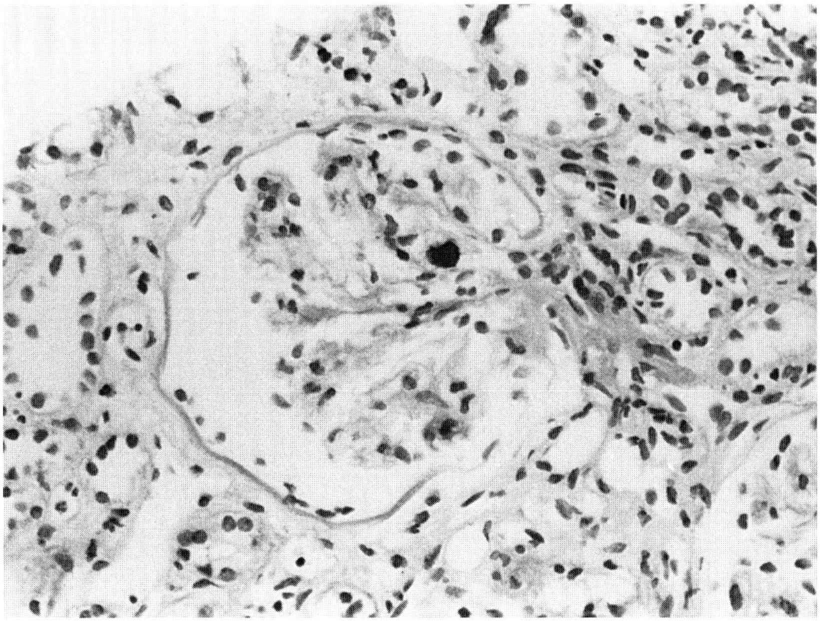

Figure 10–15. Immunoperoxidase staining highlights the presence of an intraglomerular cytomegalovirus-infected cell with marked nuclear enlargement.

disorder (PTLD).[28] These PTLD can involve the allograft kidney and cause severe interstitial nephritis. The presence of large numbers of immunoblasts with nuclear and cytologic atypia alerts the pathologist to the development of this unfortunate complication. Tubular injury and vascular involvement can occur, and differentiation from severe acute cellular rejection is sometimes difficult. Immunoperoxidase and in situ hybridization studies to document Epstein-Barr virus infection are helpful in differential diagnosis. Once a diagnosis of PTLD is established, immunosuppression must be reduced or discontinued, and a course of acyclovir or gancyclovir given.

Fungal Infections

Fungal infections may occasionally involve the renal allograft. The most common example is *Candida* infection, which is recognized by the presence of delicate pseudohyphae accompanied by budding yeast forms (Fig. 10–16). The next most common organism is *Aspergillus,* which is recognized by septate hyphae that branch in a dichotomous pattern. Rarely *Cryptococcus, Histoplasma,* and other fungi may be seen in allografts.

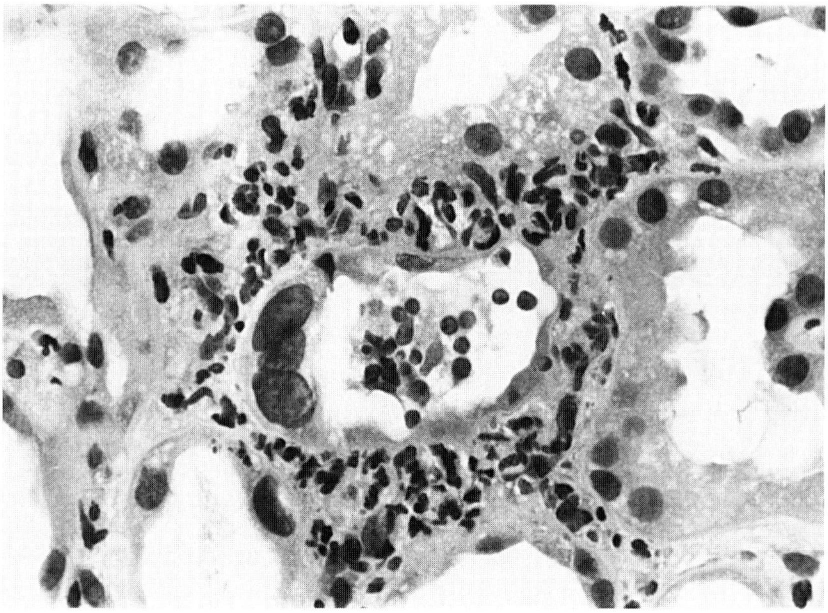

Figure 10–16. Renal allograft biopsy specimen with a neutrophil-rich infiltrate with tubular damage that qualifies for the diagnosis of acute interstitial nephritis. A tubular lumen in the center of the photograph contains numerous *Candida* yeast forms. The marked nuclear enlargement in several tubules is a regenerative response.

▲ METABOLIC DISEASES IN RENAL TRANSPLANTATION

Diabetes Mellitus

Diabetes mellitus is the most common indication for renal transplantation in many medical centers today. Because the underlying defect in glucose metabolism is not corrected by kidney transplantation, progressive structural changes can be demonstrated if serial allograft biopsy specimens are carefully examined with ultrastructural and morphometric techniques.[29] However, clinically significant recurrent diabetic nephropathy is uncommon and occurs only in long-term survivors of renal transplantation. The earliest reported case of nodular glomerulosclerosis in an allograft kidney occurred 8.5 years after transplantation. In general, overall graft survival rates in recipients with and without diabetes are comparable.

Oxalosis

Primary hyperoxaluria frequently recurs in the allograft kidney unless prior or concomitant liver transplantation is performed to correct the underlying enzyme deficiency (see Chapter 3).

Amyloidosis

In amyloidosis, the presence of systemic disease makes the postoperative management of these patients clinically difficult.[30] Patients who do survive 1 year or more after transplantation show recurrent amyloid in the graft about 20% of the time.

Cystinosis

Renal transplantation has been more successful for patients with cystinosis. Although cystine crystals are readily demonstrable in the interstitium and glomeruli of the allograft kidney, this is not associated with clinically significant graft dysfunction. The systemic manifestations of cystinosis are not influenced by transplantation.[31]

▲ RENAL ALLOGRAFT BIOPSY TECHNIQUE

The techniques of renal allograft biopsy have evolved over the past several years. A percutaneous biopsy with an 18-gauge biopsy gun is probably the safest core-biopsy technique to monitor renal allograft function after transplantation. The procedure can be performed under local anesthesia. It is essential to use ultrasound localization of the graft to minimize the risk of injury to the large vessels or pelvicalcyceal system.[6] The surgeon should, as far as possible, obtain sufficient tissue to enable a complete light microscopic, immunofluorescence, and electron microscopic evaluation. The adequacy of a specimen can be readily evaluated by immediate examination of the tissue with a microscope (either low-power or dissecting) kept in the biopsy suite. When only a limited amount of kidney tissue can be obtained, triage of the available material is dictated by the clinical setting. If vascular rejection is an important clinical concern, priority should be given to freezing a portion for immunofluorescence studies. When recurrent or de novo glomerulonephritis is in the differential diagnosis, at least one glomerulus from the biopsy should be fixed in glutaraldehyde for electron microscopic studies. The remaining tissue is fixed in formalin and transported to the pathology laboratory. Rapid biopsy processing protocols are available, and it is possible to prepare paraffin-embedded hematoxylin and eosin–stained sections in about 6 hours. Immediate frozen-section evaluation of the tissue can be requested if the clinical situation is critical.[32] Periodic acid–Schiff and Jones silver stains help in more detailed examination of the GBM.

▲ FINE-NEEDLE ASPIRATION OF RENAL ALLOGRAFTS

The core needle biopsy has become established as a reasonably safe and reliable procedure for serial assessment of renal allografts after transplantation. Nonetheless, it is a traumatic procedure associated with gross hematuria approximately 1–3% of patients. In recent years, fine-needle aspiration has been advocated as a less traumatic alternative to core biopsy. The aspiration procedure can be performed in the outpatient department with or without local anesthesia. If clinically indicated, it can even be repeated daily to allow close monitoring of intragraft events. The three most common causes of renal graft dysfunction—ATN, acute cellular rejection, and acute drug toxicity—can be quite reliably diagnosed with fine-needle aspiration.[33,34] At some transplant centers, fine-needle aspiration has actually replaced core biopsy for the evaluation of renal allograft function during the immediate postoperative period. However, because the procedure is based on reading of cytocentrifuge preparations of cell suspensions, it is not possible to evaluate the anatomic architecture of the kidney. A serious implication of this limitation is that it becomes difficult to diagnose vascular rejection, documentation of which necessitates demonstration of vascular thrombosis or lymphocytic infiltration into the arterial intima. Likewise, glomerular abnormalities associated with transplant glomerulopathy, glomerulonephritis, or hemolytic uremic syndrome cannot be appreciated in fine-needle aspirates. Long-standing grafts with marked interstitial fibrosis are difficult to aspirate and may provide inadequate preparations. For these reasons, use of fine-needle aspiration is restricted to the first several weeks after transplantation, even at experienced centers.

▲ REFERENCES

1. Penn I: Transmission of cancer with donor organs. *Transplant Proc* 20:739–740, 1988.
2. Marsh JW, Jr, Esquivel CO, Makowka L, et al: Accidental transplantation of malignant tumor from a donor to multiple recipients. *Transplantation* 44:449–450, 1987.
3. Curschellas E, Landmann J, Durig M, et al: Morphologic findings in zero-hour biopsies of renal transplants. *Clin Nephrol* 36:215–222, 1991.
4. Olsen S, Burdick JF, Keown PA, Wallace AC, Racusen LC, Solez K: Primary acute renal failure ("acute tubular necrosis") in the transplanted kidney: morphology and pathogenesis. *Medicine* 68:173–187, 1989.
5. Solez K, Kramer KC, Fox JA, Heptinstall RH: Medullary plasma flow and intravascular leukocyte accumulation in acute renal failure. *Kidney Int* 6:24–37, 1974.
6. Croker BP, Salomon DR: Pathology of the renal allograft. In: Tisher CC, Brenner BM (ed), *Renal Pathology with Clinical & Functional Correlations.* Philadelphia, Lippincott, 1989: 1518–1552.
7. Porter KA: Renal transplantation. In: Heptinstall RH (ed), *Pathology of the Kidney.* Boston, Little Brown, 1992:1799-1934.
8. Solez K, Axelsen R, Benediktsson H, et al: International standardization of nomenclature and criteria for the histologic diagnosis of rejection: the Banff working classification of kidney transplant pathology. *Kidney Int* 44:411–422, 1993.
9. Maryniak RK, First MR, Weiss MA: Transplant glomerulopathy: evolution of morphologically distinct changes. *Kidney Int* 27:799–806, 1985.
10. Monga G, Mazzucco G, Novara R, Reale L: Intertubular capillary changes in kidney allografts: an ultrastructural study in patients with transplant glomerulopathy. *Ultrastruct Pathol* 14:201–209, 1990.
11. Busch GJ, Galvanek EG, Reynolds ES: Human renal allografts: analysis of lesions in long-term survivors. *Hum Pathol* 2:253–298, 1971.
12. Mihatsch MJ, Ryffel B, Gudat F, Thiel G: Cyclosporine nephropathy. In: Tisher CC, Brenner BM (eds), *Renal Pathology with Clinical & Functional Correlations.* Philadelphia, Lippincott, 1989:1555–1586.
13. Thiru S, Maher ER, Hamilton DV, Evans DB, Calne RY: Tubular changes in renal transplant recipients on cyclosporine. *Transplant Proc* 15(Suppl 1):2846–2851, 1983.
14. Landmann J, Mihatsch MJ, Ratschek M, Thiel G: Cyclosporine A and intravascular coagulation. *Transplant Proc* 19:1817-1819, 1987.
15. Myers BD, Ross J, Newton L, Luetscher J, Perlroth M: Cyclosporine-associated chronic nephropathy. *N Engl J Med* 311:699–705, 1984.
16. Randhawa PS, Shapiro R, Jordan ML, Starzl TE, Demetris AJ: The histopathological changes associated with allograft rejection and drug toxicity in renal transplant recipients maintained on FK 506: clinical significance and comparison with cyclosporine. *Am J Surg Pathol* 17:60–68, 1993.
17. Mathew TH: Recurrence of disease following renal transplantation. *Am J Kidney Dis* 12:85–96, 1988.
18. Leunissen KML, Kootstra G, Bosman FT, van Hooff JP: Focal glomerulosclerosis in neonatal kidney grafts. *Lancet* 2:1019–1020, 1987.
19. Hayes JM, Steinmuller DR, Streem SB, Novick AG: The development of proteinuria and focal-segmental glomerulosclerosis in recipients of pediatric donor kidneys. *Transplantation* 52:813–817, 1991.

20. Verani R, Dan M: Membranous glomerulonephritis in renal transplant: a case report and review of the literature. *Am J Nephrol* 2:316–320, 1982.
21. Truong L, Gelfand J, D'Agati V, et al: Denovo membranous glomerulonephropathy in renal allografts: a report of ten cases and review of the literature. *Am J Kidney Dis* 14:131–144, 1989.
22. Moritz MJ, Burke JF, Jarell BE, Carabasi RA: The incidence of membranoproliferative glomerulonephritis in renal allografts. *Transplant Proc* 14:2206–2207, 1987.
23. Bennett WM, Fassett RG, Walker RG, Fairley KF, d'Apice AJ, Kincaid-Smith P: Mesangiocapillary glomerulonephritis type II (dense-deposit disease): clinical features of progressive disease. *Am J Kidney Dis* 13:469–476, 1989.
24. Shah B, First MR, Mendoza NC, Clyne DH, Alexander JW, Weiss MA: Alport's syndrome: risk of glomerulonephritis induced by anti-glomerular-basement-membrane antibody after renal transplantation. *Nephron* 50:34–38, 1988.
25. Suganuma T, Morozumi K, Satoh K, et al: Studies of IgA nephropathy in renal transplantation. *Transplant Proc* 21:2123–2127, 1989.
26. Bumgardner GL, Mauer SM, Payne W, et al: Single-center 1–15-year results of renal transplantation in patients with systemic lupus erythematosus. *Transplantation* 46:702–709, 1988.
27. Naraqi S, Jackson GG, Jonasson O, Rubenis M: Search for latent cytomegalovirus in renal allografts. *Infect Immunol* 19:699–703, 1978.
28. Randhawa PS, Magnone M, Jordan M, Shapiro R, Demetris AJ, Nalesnik M: Renal allograft involvement by Epstein-Barr virus associated post-transplant lymphoproliferative disease. *Am J Surg Pathol* 20:563–571, 1996.
29. Osterby R, Nyberg G, Persson H, Hedman L: Early glomerulopathy in kidneys transplanted into diabetic patients. *Transplant Proc* 23:1270, 1991.
30. Isoniemi H, Eklund B, Hockerstedt K, Salmela K, Ahonen J: Renal transplantation in amyloidosis. *Transplant Proc* 21:2039–2040, 1989.
31. Almond PS, Morel P, Troppmann C, Matas A, Najarian JS, Chavers B: Progression of infantile cystinosis after renal transplantation. *Transplant Proc* 23:1386, 1991.
32. Cohen AH, Gonzalez S, Nast CC, Wilkinson A, Danovitch GM: Frozen-section analysis of allograft renal biopsy specimens. *Arch Pathol Lab Med* 115:386–389, 1991.
33. Hayry P, Von Willebrand E: Transplant aspiration cytology. *Transplantation* 38:7–12, 1984.
34. Gray WR, Richardson A, Hughes D, et al: A prospective randomised blind comparison of three biopsy techniques in the management of patients after renal transplantation. *Transplantation* 53:1226–1232, 1992.

11

Complications of Renal Transplantation

Complications after renal transplantation can be broadly classified as medical or surgical. Medical complications include those related to immunosuppressive therapy, namely rejection (see Chapters 1 and 8), infection, malignancy, metabolic derangements, systemic disorders, and neurologic problems, and those related to the original cause of end-stage renal disease. Surgical complications include urologic complications, general surgical complications, and vascular complications.

This chapter will focus on the etiology, diagnosis, and management of the major complications of renal transplantation that the transplant clinician is likely to encounter. Surgical complications will be discussed first, followed by general medical complications, infectious complications, neurologic complications, and posttransplant malignancy.

Surgical Complications

Robert M. Naraghi / Mark L. Jordan

▲ UROLOGIC COMPLICATIONS

Introduction

Urologic complications following renal transplantation can pose a significant challenge to the transplant surgeon in both diagnosis and management. The overall incidence of urologic complications after renal transplantation has been reported to be 0.9–30%, but most centers currently report an incidence of 3% or less.[1–8] The last decade has witnessed a significant decrease in the incidence of urologic complications, probably related both to improved surgical techniques of ureteral implantation and to improved techniques of organ recovery, with careful preservation of the ureteric blood supply. Renal transplant ultrasound and radionuclide scanning, and percutaneous and endourologic surgical techniques also have resulted in earlier detection and improved management of these complications.

Of paramount importance in the prevention of urologic complications is the precise recovery of the kidney. A basic understanding of renal and ureteral vascular anatomy is essential for proper dissection and preservation of ureteric blood supply during organ recovery. It is important to remember that the allograft ureter, unlike the native ureter, receives its blood supply solely from the renal artery, and thus, preservation of branches at the renal hilum is essential to preserve the subsequent viability of the ureter.[9–11] Angiographic studies of cadaveric ureters have revealed two major ureteral vascular patterns: longitudinal and plexiform.[9,10] Both types of vessels arise at the confluence of the segmental arteries at the renal hilum and traverse the entire length of the ureter within the adventitial layer. In anatomic reviews, the longitudinal channel system was found in 76% of ureters,[9] with a single channel at the pseudomesentery as its most common subtype. The plexiform pattern was present in 24% of ureters.[10]

To preserve the ureteral vasculature during donor nephrectomy, the periureteral tissue and a sufficient conical mass of hilar fibrofatty tissue should be removed en bloc with the kidney and the ureter. The shortest possible length of ureter that allows a tension-free anastomosis to the bladder should be used during subsequent implantation. Excessive dissection within the renal hilum should be avoided, as segmental and accessory renal arteries, especially lower pole vessels, may be injured, with resultant ureteral ischemia. Any injured accessory renal arteries (especially to the lower pole) should be repaired, if possible.[3]

A number of techniques for implantation of the transplant ureter have been described (see Chapter 6)[12–19] and are shown in Table 11–1. The most common technique now employed is the extravesical ureteroneocystostomy. In the past, a standard Politano–Leadbetter tunneled ureteral reimplantation was the most commonly performed method. However, the incidence of ureteral complications with the Politano–Leadbetter technique has been reported to be as high as 9.4%.[12,19] Over the last several years, the complication rate with the extravesical technique has been reported to be 3% or less.[12,19] In most reports comparing the traditional Politano–Leadbetter to the extravesical techniques, the complications of leak, ureteral necrosis, and stricture have been similiar. However, a significantly higher incidence of ureterovesical junction obstruction has been observed with the Politano–Leadbetter technique (3.7%) compared with the extravesical technique (0.6%).[12,19] This difference may be related to the tunneling technique used in the intravesical ureteroneocystostomy, which may predispose to obstruction. Ureterovesical junction obstruction may also occur as a result of possible kinking of the ureter at the new muscular hiatus in the bladder.[12] Another potential disadvantage of the

TABLE 11–1 ▲ TECHNIQUES OF URETERAL RECONSTRUCTION

- Ureteroneocystostomy
  - Antireflux (tunneling) technique
    - Intravesical (Politano–Leadbetter)
    - Extravesical (Lich, Gregoir)
  - No tunnel technique
    - Intravesical
    - Extravesical
- Use of the recipient ureter
  - Ureteroureterostomy
  - Ureteropyelostomy
  - Pyelopyelostomy
- Use of the recipient bladder (usually for management of complications)
  - Psoas hitch
  - Boari flap
  - Vesicopyelostomy

Politano–Leadbetter technique is the requirement to open the bladder formally, resulting in a higher risk of vesical leak. Still another additional factor may be the extra length and the additional manipulation of the ureter necessary for its intravesical placement with this technique. By permitting the use of a shorter segment of ureter, the extravesical technique may reduce the risk of these complications by minimizing excessive ureteral manipulation and eliminating the need for a separate open cystotomy. The extravesical technique is usually done as a tunneled antireflux procedure rather than a simple nontunneled ureteroneocystostomy, with the goal of avoiding vesicoureteral reflux (see Chapter 6).

Other options for reestablishing urinary continuity include techniques utilizing the recipient native ureter, including ureteropyelostomy and ureteroureterostomy (Table 11–1).[14–18] The use of the native recipient ureter for primary ureteral reconstruction may necessitate native nephrectomy, although end-to-side anastomosis of the transplant renal pelvis to the native ureter may be performed without native nephrectomy. The use of the native ureter may be necessary when dealing with a short or obstructed transplant ureter or for repair of a subsequent ureteral complication. Ureteroureterostomy and pyeloureterostomy as primary means of urinary reconstruction have been associated with complication rates high as 21%.[1,4,11,15] We therefore recommend preserving the native ureter at the time of transplantation and not using it for primary ureteral reconstruction unless no other choices are available.

Direct anastomosis of the transplant renal pelvis to the recipient bladder (pyelovesicostomy) may be required in the presence of extensive injury to the transplant ureter or when the native ureter is unavailable or unusable. Pyelovesicostomy is usually necessary only when treating urologic complications and not for primary transplantation.[18]

▲ UROLOGIC COMPLICATIONS OF RENAL TRANSPLANTATION

The incidence of urologic complications in renal transplantation has been historically reported to be as high as 30%, with associated patient mortality rates of up to 68%.[1–8] Increasing recognition of the factors predisposing to urologic complications has resulted in a significant decrease in their incidence over the past decade, so that the reported incidence in most centers does not exceed 10%.[1–8,12,13] Urologic complications may be broadly classified as either obstruction or extravasation. Taken together, they account for up to 95% of all urologic complications,[17,20] as classified in Table 11–2. The reported incidence of obstruction ranges from 1 to 10%, and of extravasation from 1.8 to 3%.[20–22] Urologic complications usually (>75%) occur early (<3 months) after transplantation.[1–8] In general, most cases of urinary extravasation occur early after transplantation, whereas obstruction tends to occur later in the posttransplant course, but either type of complication may be seen at any time point.

TABLE 11–2 ▲ CLASSIFICATION OF UROLOGIC COMPLICATIONS OF RENAL TRANSPLANTATION

I. Obstruction
- A. Intrinsic
  - (i) Stricture
  - (ii) Edema
  - (iii) Blood clot
  - (iv) Stone
  - (v) Excess ureteral redundancy
  - (vi) Tumor
  - (vii) Infection—fungus ball, viral
  - (viii) Indwelling ureteral stent
- B. Extrinsic
  - (i) Fluid collection
    - (a) Lymphocele
    - (b) Hematoma
    - (c) Urinoma
    - (d) Tumor
    - (e) Abscess
  - (ii) Kidney itself
  - (iii) Bladder itself

II. Extravasation
- A. Calyceal
- B. Renal pelvic
- C. Ureteral
- D. Ureteroneocystostomy
- E. Vesical

▲ OBSTRUCTION

Etiology

Obstruction of the transplant kidney may be classified as being of either intrinsic or extrinsic origin (Table 11–2). Obstruction may occur at the level of the bladder, the ureterovesical junction, along the course of the transplant ureter, or at the ureteropelvic junction.

Intrinsic ureteral obstruction is most commonly caused by ischemic ureteral stricture.[11,23] This ischemic insult usually results from vascular compromise of the ureter during organ recovery or subsequent back-table dissection, primarily because of excessive dissection of the ureter itself or the renal hilum, leading in either case to compromise of the ureteral blood supply. Other potential causes of intrinsic ureteral obstruction include posttransplant periureteral fibrosis or entrapment, which can be panureteral or segmental.[24–26] Intrinsic ureteral obstruction may also be caused by infection (fungus balls), stones, tumor, blood clot (eg., following renal biopsy), and excessive ureteral length with associated ptosis of the kidney (Table 11–2). On occasion, ureteral stents that have been placed intraoperatively may cause obstruction, especially if they have been inadvertently left for prolonged periods. The most common site of ureteral obstruction is at the ureterovesical junction (63%), followed by the distal ureter (13%), mid ureter (13%), and proximal ureter (10%).[27]

Extrinsic ureteral obstruction may be caused by fluid collections, most commonly lymphocele, hematoma, or urinoma accompanying a urine leak (Table 11–2). Extrinsic obstruction from tumor and peritransplant abscess is less common. Finally, in patients with a hypertrophied bladder wall (as in some cases of neurogenic bladder), or with a high intravesical pressure, the bladder itself may obstruct the transplant ureter.

Diagnosis of Ureteral Obstruction

Obstruction of the renal allograft should be suspected in any patient with an otherwise unexplained fall in urine output, enlargement or tenderness of the allograft, and/or fever. Because the signs and symptoms of obstruction may be easily mistaken for acute allograft rejection, ultrasound examination of the renal allograft is essential to distinguish between these clinical entities. Typically, ultrasound findings associated with obstruction may include hydronephrosis and ureterectasis (Figure 11–1).

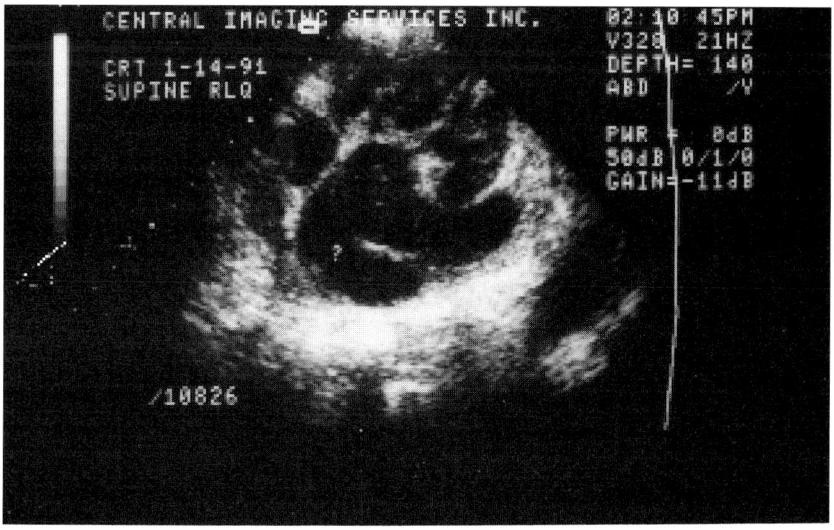

Figure 11–1. Ultrasound examination of transplant kidney demonstrating hydronephrosis and ureterectasis.

However, early obstruction of the allograft may appear normal on ultrasound. A nuclear medicine technetium-99m DPTA or iodine-131 hippurate (OIH) scan may help to define obstruction by demonstrating normal perfusion and parenchymal uptake, but with prolonged pelvic retention (Figure 11–2). Administration of furosemide during nuclear scanning (Lasix® renography) may elicit a prolonged $T_{1/2}$ for clearing of nuclide from the kidney (Figure 11–3). However, radionuclide renal scan can only suggest the diagnosis of obstruction (see Chapter 13). Intravenous pyelography (Figure 11–4), used more often in the past, is now rarely indicated or even necessary for making the diagnosis and is usually contraindicated because of the deterioration in renal function associated with the obstructed allograft. A CT scan without contrast (Figure 11–5) may be helpful in visualizing the collecting system and demonstrating the exact anatomy of any fluid collections, but does not give dynamic functional assessment of the kidney unless contrast is used, and the latter may not be desirable. Cystoscopy may be helpful in assessing the viability of the ureteral orifice and to rule out an obstruction by either a clot, fungus ball, or (rarely) a stone at the ureteral orifice. In addition, retrograde ureterography may be performed to identify the level and possible cause of obstruction. Retrograde ureterography may prove to be technically difficult, especially if the transplant ureteral orifice is located near the bladder dome, as is usually the case after an extravesical ureteroneocystostomy. In the case of a Politano–Leadbetter reconstruction, retrograde ureteral catheterization is usually more feasible (and may be therapeutic). If a retrograde study is not possible, an antegrade study by percutaneous

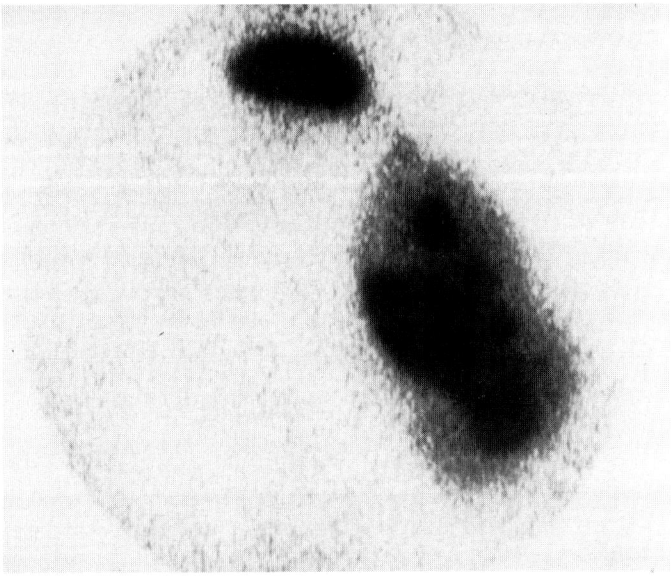

Figure 11–2. Nuclear medicine renal scan (iodohippurate) demonstrating normal perfusion but prolonged renal pelvic retention and excretion of tracer.

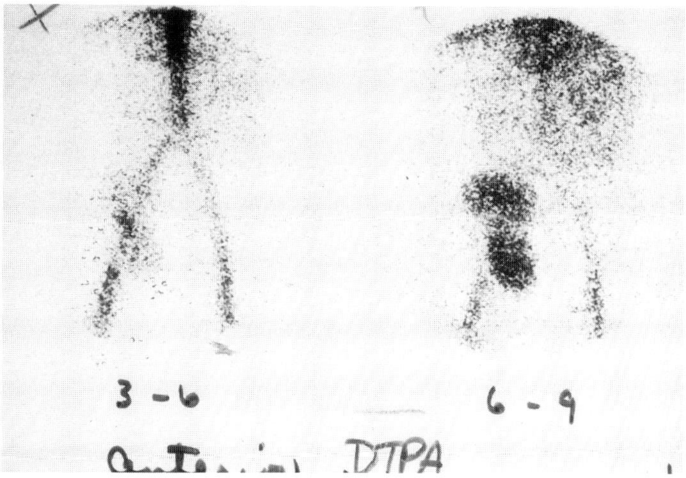

Figure 11–3. Nuclear medicine renal scan (DTPA) with prolonged $T_{1/2}$ of clearing of nuclide after furosemide.

nephrostomy under ultrasound or CT guidance is indicated (Figure 11–6). After placement of a percutaneous nephrostomy tube (we prefer an 8 or 10 French pigtail catheter), further diagnostic workup including a formal nephrostogram and pressure/flow studies (Whitaker test) may then be undertaken to delineate more precisely the site, extent, and functional significance of the obstruction. Percutaneous nephrostomy also allows decompression of the obstruction and stabilization of renal function.[27–28]

Treatment of Ureteral Obstruction

Definitive treatment of ureteral obstruction will, of course, depend on the cause. Intrinsic causes of obstruction, such as blood clots or edema at the ureterovesical junction, may resolve spontaneously with either proximal diversion or stenting. Further radiologic studies performed 1–2 weeks after diversion may show resolution of the obstruction, at which point the nephrostomy tube may be clamped and subsequently removed. Other causes of intrinsic anatomic obstruction, such as ureteral stricture, may require more aggressive intervention. Ureteral obstruction due to a short-segment ureteral stricture may be amenable to percutaneous endourologic techniques, including balloon dilatation or endoureterotomy.[29–35] The long-term effectiveness of percutaneous balloon dilatation and endoureterotomy is reported to be 40–70%. Failures usually manifest within the first year of follow-up.[32–35] Strictures at the ureteroneocystostomy appear to respond most favorably to endoluminal balloon dilatation (Figure 11–7). The length of the stricture, time after transplant and, most importantly, the ureteral vascular supply appear to be the key factors determining the long-term effective-

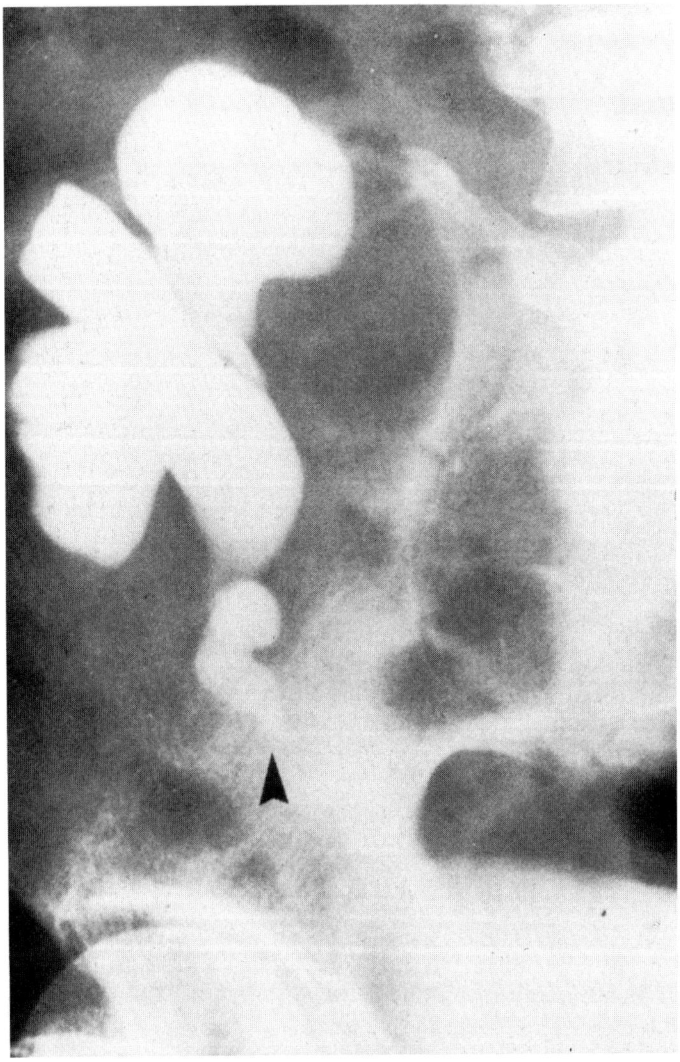

Figure 11–4. Intravenous pyelogram of transplant kidney demonstrating hydronephrosis and ureterectasis to point of obstruction (arrowhead).

ness of endoscopic procedures.[35] In general, strictures greater than 2 cm in length do not respond well to endoluminal dilatation. Long strictures and segments with evidence of vascular compromise are probably best managed with open surgical repair.[34–38]

The use of ureteral stents after endoscopic or surgical repair is advocated by most surgeons. The duration of stenting necessary for complete ureteral healing,

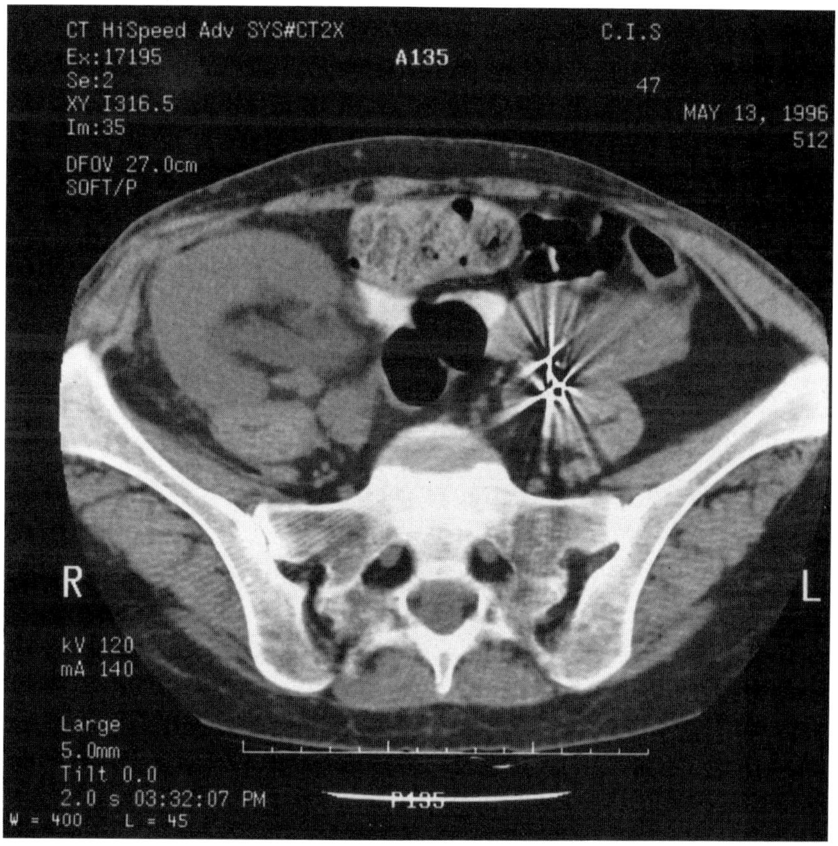

Figure 11–5. Computerized tomography showing obstruction of transplant kidney.

however, remains controversial. Stents are usually left in place for 6 weeks,[39–41] which is the interval required for complete ureteral muscular healing and the return of peristalsis. Stenting is thought to provide a scaffolding around which the ureter heals; on the other hand, all stents can cause irritation and inflammatory changes, which may impede healing or induce scar formation. Currently, internal stents are used for relief of obstruction or urinary leak, and as a prophylactic measure for the implantation of short/injured ureters. Their routine prophylactic use during the transplant procedure has been controversial. Reported outcomes have been good, but it is not clear that the incidence of urologic complications is decreased. The potential complications of internal stenting include infection, obstruction, encrustation, ureteral perforation, and migration.[41] At our institution, we routinely stent the ureter only after repair of ureteral complications.

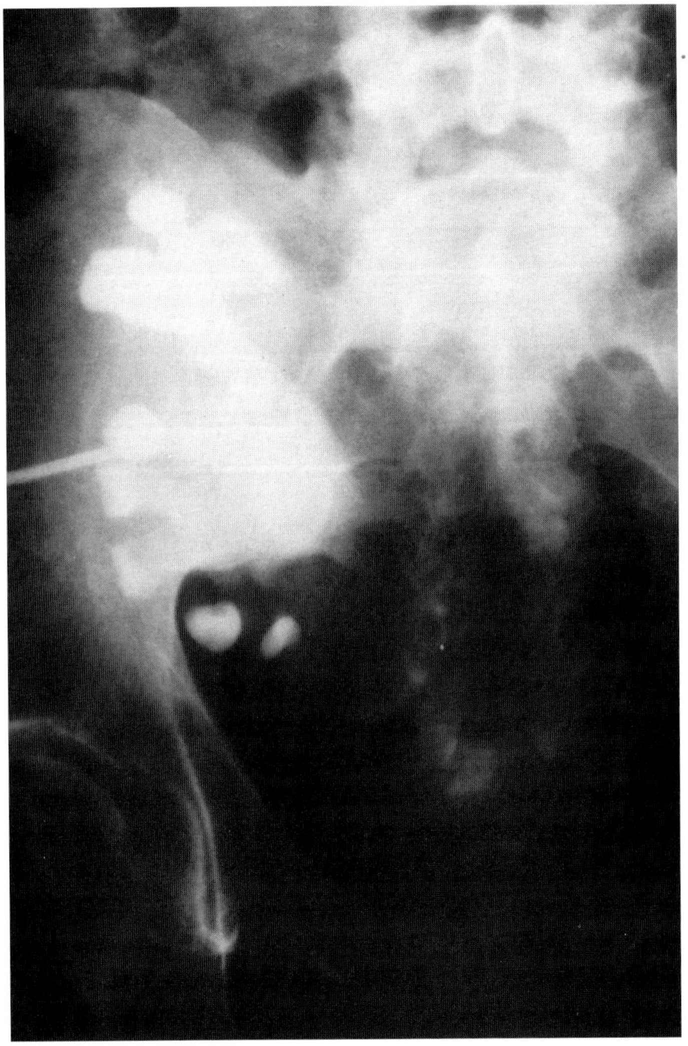

Figure 11–6. Antegrade study performed after percutaneous nephrostomy tube insertion into renal allograft showing high-grade obstruction at the ureteropelvic junction.

Open Surgical Techniques

If endoscopic techniques are unsuccessful in treating obstruction, then open surgical repair is indicated.[36–38,42] Any open repair should include inspection of the ureteroneocystostomy site for evidence of a hematoma or kinking of the intramural segment of ureter. If an ischemic distal ureter is noted and adequate viable length remains, then direct ureteral reimplantation may be possible. If extensive necrosis of the ureter is present, then pyeloureterostomy [transplant renal

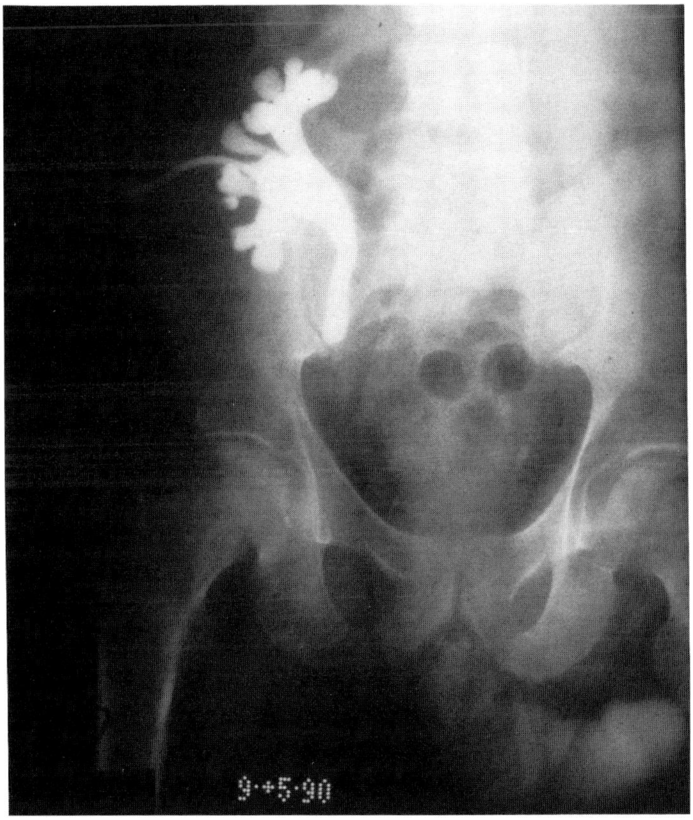

Figure 11–7. A. Antegrade study of midureteral obstruction of renal allograft prior to percutaneous balloon dilatation.

pelvis to native ureter (Figure 11–8),[14–16] ureteroureterostomy to the native ipsilateral (or, rarely, contralateral) ureter, pyelovesicostomy,[17–18] and/or a Boari flap[42] are potential treatment options. Pyeloureterostomy or ureteroureterostomy to the native ureter does not require native nephrectomy if the anastomosis of the transplant renal pelvis or ureter is performed end-to-side to the native ureter. A retrograde study should always precede the open repair to assure patency of the native ureter. If there is insufficient, diseased, or an absent native ureter, a pyelovesicostomy and/or Boari flap may be necessary. On occasion, however, even the contralateral native ureter can be used to perform a pyeloureterostomy.

Late Ureteral Obstruction

Ureteral obstruction secondary to stricture is usually more insidious in onset, producing a gradual deterioration in renal function. The denervated allograft may

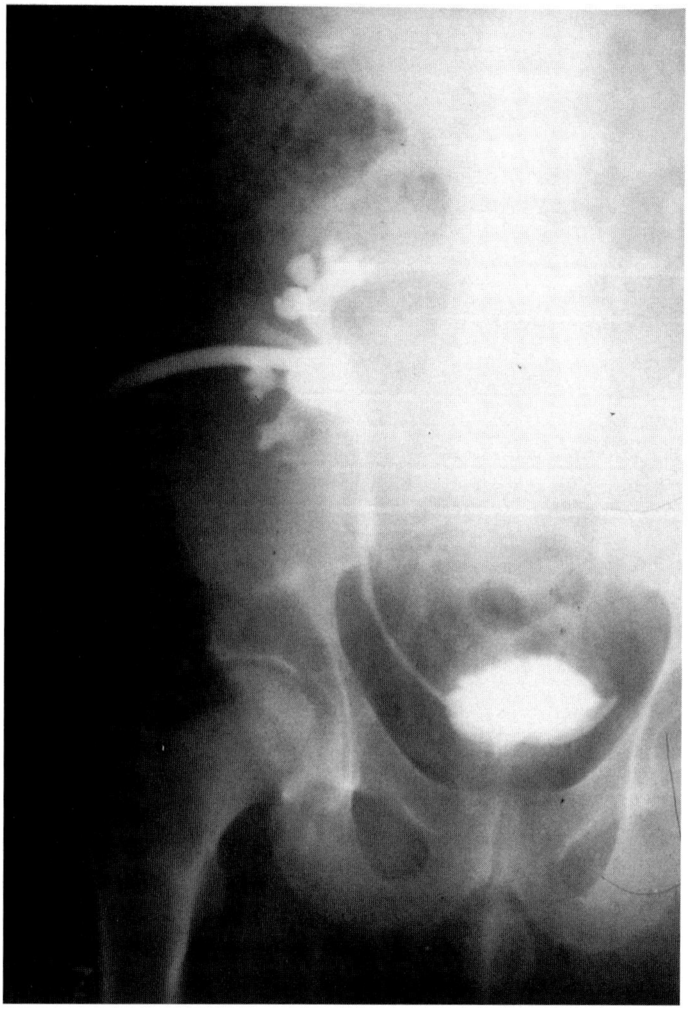

Figure 11–7. B. Antegrade study of same ureter immediately following balloon dilatation.

not manifest the typical pain associated with obstruction, and the patient may remain relatively asymptomatic. Evidence of ureteral obstruction may present only as a deterioration in renal function manifested by an elevated serum creatinine. In this respect, late ureteral obstruction may mimic chronic rejection, and thus, proper evaluation may require a biopsy, in addition to radiologic evaluation. If obstruction is suspected, the most definitive diagnostic modality is antegrade pyelography. Once the site, length, and the degree of obstruction are confirmed with antegrade pyelography, appropriate treatment options can be considered.

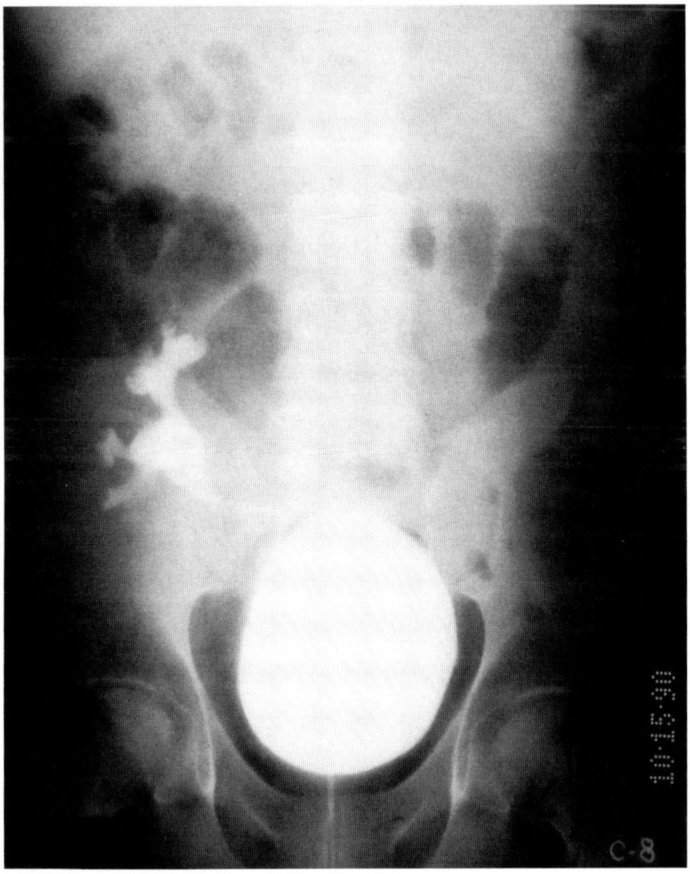

Figure 11–8. IVP 4 weeks following pyeloureterostomy (transplant renal pelvis to native ureter) of renal allograft with obstructed transplant ureter.

▲ URINARY EXTRAVASATION

Urinary extravasation usually presents within the first 7 weeks following transplantation and may arise from the calyceal system, renal pelvis, ureter, or bladder.[20] The reported incidence of urinary extravasation is 2–3%. Most cases of ureteral leaks (>75%) are associated with ureteral ischemia.[20–22,43–45] Extravasation from the bladder is more common following the Politano–Leadbetter technique of ureteral reimplantation than with the extravesical technique.[10–13,19] The incidence of urinary extravasation is not related to extremes of donor age, revascularization, or preservation times.[43] However, this complication is more common in diabetics (6%).[44] The clinical features of urinary extravasation may mimic rejection or obstruction, including graft tenderness or fullness, fever, and decreasing urine output. Early allograft dysfunction in this setting, unassociated with rejection, should prompt a full investigation to rule out a potential urinary leak. Any wound drainage fluid should be promptly analyzed for BUN and creatinine. If these values are not comparable to the corresponding serum levels, a leak should be suspected. It may also be helpful to administer 5 cc of indigo carmine intravenously (preferable to methylene blue, which may stain the sclera permanently) to determine the site of extravasation. Following these initial noninvasive tests, a leak can often be identified but not necessarily ruled out. Cystography should be performed next, with films obtained in both anterior/posterior and oblique projections, both before and after bladder drainage (Figure 11–9). However, the cystogram may be negative even in the presence of a significant bladder or ureterovesical leak. An ultrasound may reveal hydronephrosis and/or a perinephric fluid collection if a urinoma has formed. A nuclear scan may reveal tracer accumulation suggesting a urinoma or

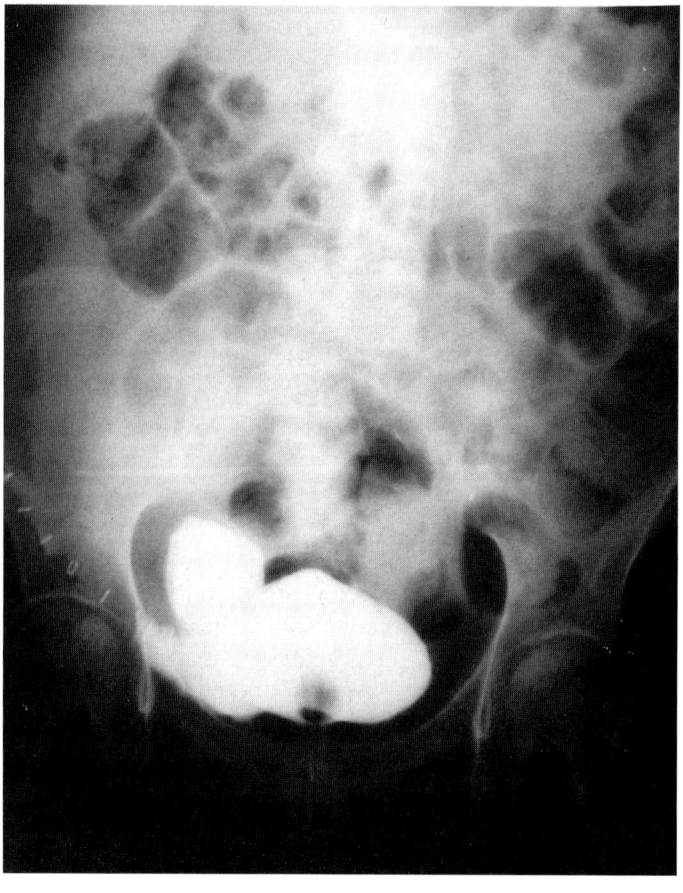

Figure 11–9. A. Cystogram demonstrating retroperitoneal extravasation from bladder at level of ureteroneocystostomy (right side of bladder).

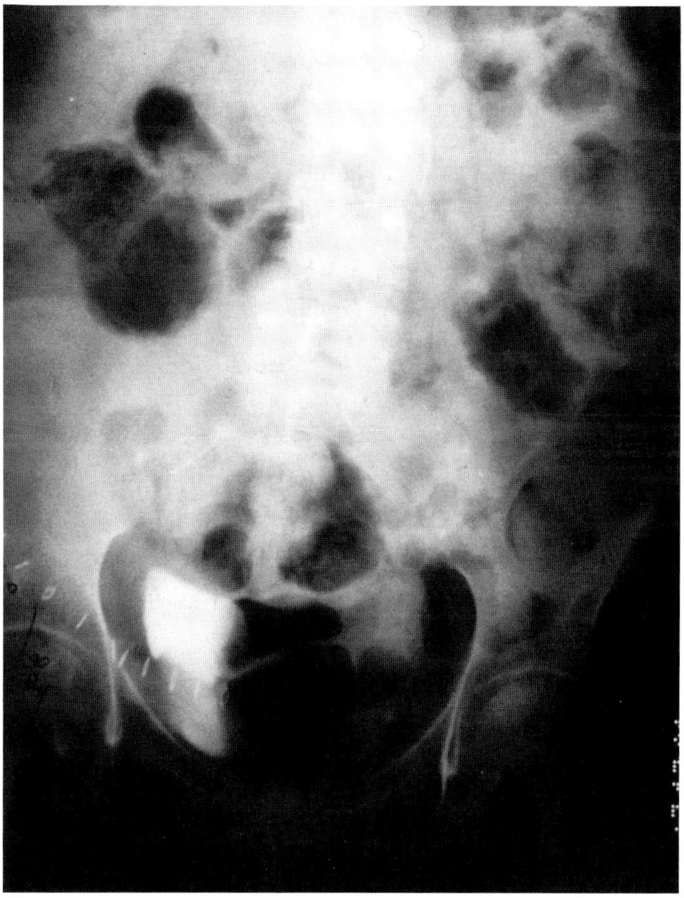

Figure 11–9. *B.* Postdrainage film demonstrating persistence of contrast in retroperitoneum following bladder emptying.

may show decreased uptake and excretion of nuclide if allograft function is impaired. If a perinephric fluid collection is found, ultrasound-guided aspiration and biochemical analysis of the fluid may be helpful in the diagnosis of a urinoma. If extravasation is suspected but cannot be confirmed by the above mentioned tests, antegrade pyelography should be performed. The antegrade pyelographic findings may include extravasation of contrast, segmental ureteral nonvisualization, and/or hydronephrosis.

Treatment of Urinary Extravasation

Small vesicular leaks can be managed with simple Foley catheter placement for decompression. Larger leaks may require operative repair. All open procedures should include placement of a drain. For leaks at or above the ureterovesical junction, placement of a percutaneous nephrostomy provides prompt control of urinary leakage, stabilization of allograft function, and prevention of further increase in the size of the urinoma.[28,29] Further management of small fistulae can be conservative if adequate drainage has been established with a percutaneous nephrostomy or internal stent, since most of these will heal spontaneously.[11] If a large urinoma is present, percutaneous drainage may be initially attempted, but open operative repair and drainage are usually required (see techniques for ureteral obstruction). The method of repair is individualized to the operative findings and depends on the site of obstruction, the viability of the ureter, the usable ureteral length, and bladder mobility. A necrotic distal ureter may be resected and a repeat ureteroneocystostomy attempted if an adequate viable segment of ureter remains. If this is not possible, pyeloureterostomy or ureteroureterostomy to the native ureter may be performed. This may be done end (pelvis)-to-side (native ureter) without need for ipsilateral native nephrectomy. End-to-end anastomosis of the renal pelvis or proximal ureter to the native ureter may be performed, but this may require native nephrectomy in cases where the native kidney has retained urine output. Ureteroureterostomy,[14–16] pyeloureterostomy, Boari flap,[42] psoas hitch, and calyceovesicostomy[17] are all potential options, depending on the operative findings.

▲ OTHER SURGICAL COMPLICATIONS OF RENAL TRANSPLANTATION

Perinephric Fluid Collections

Perinephric fluid collections of greater than 50–100 cc volume are detected in 20–50% of renal transplant recipients on routine follow-up ultrasound examinations.[46–51] The clinical significance of these relate to the composition of the collection and the functional compromise they impose on the kidney and/or adjacent structures. Lymphoceles comprise the majority (40%) of these fluid collections, followed in frequency by hematoma, abscess, and urinoma. The treatment of urinoma is discussed under the management of urinary extravasation (see above).

Lymphoceles

The incidence of clinically significant lymphoceles is reported to be 0.6–18%.[46,51–58] Most lymphoceles present within the first 2–6 months after renal transplantation. Lymphocele formation is thought to be related to inadequate ligation of transected lymphatics during iliac vessel mobilization at the time of the transplant, although the allograft itself may also serve as a significant source of lymphatic fluid, especially during episodes of rejection.[51–54] Lymphoceles have also been associated with the use of anticoagulants, diuretics, and excessive steroid use.[52–57] There does not appear to be any correlation between the incidence of lymphoceles and donor factors or the degree of donor–recipient HLA matching. However, the most consistent observation is a higher incidence of lymphoceles after ipsilateral retransplantation.[54] This is probably related to the additional dissection required to prepare the recipient vessels. Most lymphoceles are asymptomatic but may be detected on routine ultrasound examination (Figure 11–10). Therefore, the frequency with which ultrasonography is performed is important in assessing the incidence reported in any one series. Clinically significant lymphoceles usually present with a mass or fullness around the allograft, but also present with signs of ureteral obstruction. Other presenting features may include ipsilateral lower extremity edema or deep vein thrombosis (as a result of lymphatic or venous obstruction, respectively), urinary frequency or retention (due to bladder neck irritation or obstruction), pain, and/or fever (in the presence of infection). The diagnosis of a symptomatic lymphocele should be confirmed by ultrasonography and needle aspiration with chemical and bacteriologic analysis.[47–49] The concentration of the fluid electrolytes, blood urea nitrogen, and creatinine equal to or less than serum values distinguishes lymphocele from urinoma. Often, CT may be helpful in outlining the exact location and extent of the lymphocele, which is important in evaluating treatment options. The decision to intervene depends on the clinical presentation and functional compromise of allograft function. The optimal mode of therapy is a matter of some controversy. Currently available treatment modalities include fine needle aspiration[59] and percu-

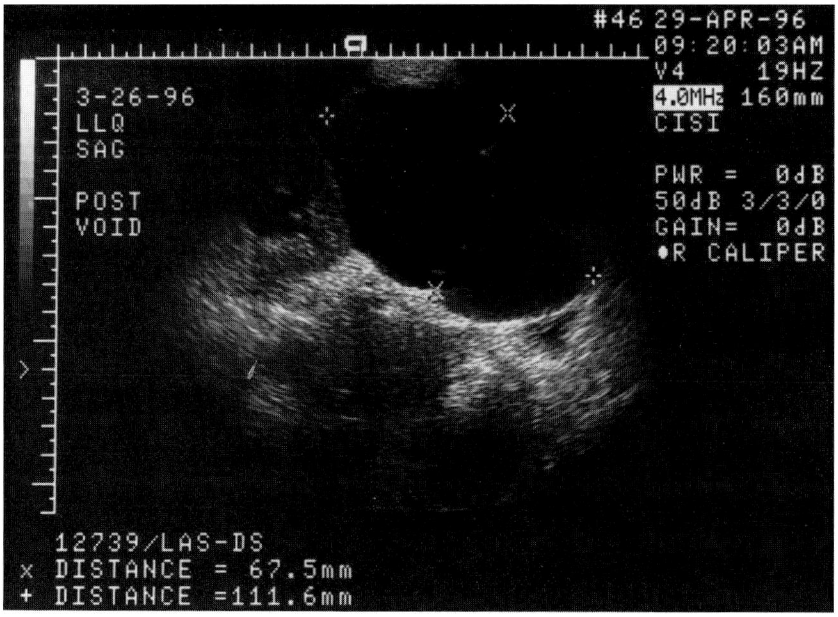

Figure 11–10. Peritransplant lymphocele shown on routine ultrasound examinations.

taneous drainage, drainage with sclerosis, open internal drainage with intraperitoneal marsupialization (peritoneal window)[55–59] and, more recently, laparoscopic internal marsupialization.[56–58] Simple needle aspiration has been previously reported as a safe[53] and effective therapeutic alternative to surgery; however, most studies report a recurrence rate of 80–90%. The necessity for repeat needle aspiration may result in a significant (25–50%) incidence of infection.[53] Currently, we recommend needle aspiration for diagnostic purposes only and not for definitive treatment. Most reports cite internal marsupialization as the definitive form of treatment with a primary success rate of 89%.[51–55,59] The optimal technique of internal marsupialization involves a transperitoneal or retroperitoneal exploration and removal of a wide ellipse of lymphocele wall to avoid intestinal herniation and future closure of the window.[56] Some authors have also recommended simultaneous omentoplasty and placement of internal stents.[60] External percutaneous drainage yields a primary success rate of 60%, with an overall success rate of 73%.[59] The disadvantage of percutaneous drainage includes a high recurrence rate and the need for prolonged extracorporeal drainage, which can be associated with a significant incidence of infection, as well as the risk of lymphatic fistula formation. The use of sclerosing agents (betadine, tetracycline, talc)[53,55] in the management of lymphoceles has met with some success. Some report a primary success rate of 89%,[55] with a rare potential complication of extravasation beyond the lymphocele into the peritoneum, and subsequent chemical peritonitis. Sclerosing agent therapy should probably be reserved for those lymphoceles that are recurrent or have failed to respond to other forms of treatment. Drainage by laparoscopic internal marsupialization is the most recently described treatment option for lymphoceles.[56–58] This minimally invasive procedure is gaining increasing acceptance for a wide range of indications across multiple surgical subspecialties. Laparoscopic drainage is most applicable to lymphoceles that are superior and anterior to the allograft. Omentoplasty can also be performed at the time of laparoscopic drainage. Limitations to laparoscopic drainage may include a thick walled or medially placed lymphocele, which can make identification of nearby vital structures difficult. Preoperative CT scan or MRI should be performed to assess whether the lymphocele is amenable to laparoscopic drainage.

Hematomas

Postoperative perirenal hematomas comprise 5–20% of all aspirated fluid collections.[46–48] Most small perirenal hematomas are asymptomatic; however, larger hematomas can produce significant local wound and flank pain and cause ureteral obstruction. In addition to the obvious changes in vital signs secondary to active bleeding, clinical clues to the presence of a significant hematoma include an appreciable drop in hematocrit along with perigraft fullness and/or rigidity. The findings of a large complex perigraft fluid collection on ultrasound or CT or a displacing perirenal photopenic halo on renal nuclide scan support the diagnosis. Management of small hematomas can be expectant. Larger or expanding hematomas may signal ongoing hemorrhage and require prompt exploration for control of bleeding.

Hematomas producing compromised renal function by obstruction (vascular or ureteric) also should be evacuated.

Abscess

The incidence of peritransplant abscess is difficult to estimate from reported series. Most data collected from prior studies report an incidence of 2–30% of all aspirated fluid collections.[46–50] Classically, these patients present with fever, perigraft pain, and tenderness within the first few days to weeks after transplantation. Most late peritransplant abscesses occur as a consequence of graft pyelonephritis.[50] In addition, other peritransplant fluid collections, such as urinomas, hematomas, or lymphoceles, may become secondarily infected either due to manipulation or to seeding from sepsis. US and CT are the most helpful imaging modalities to detect a peritransplant abscess. In the clinical setting of fever and leukocytosis in a transplant patient, the detection of a perinephric fluid collection is presumptive evidence that the fluid is infected. Under these circumstances, ultrasound- or CT-guided needle aspiration may confirm the diagnosis and permit percutaneous drainage. Although most abscesses are well localized and thick-walled, they may rupture into the peritoneal cavity and result in peritonitis. This serious complication, if not promptly recognized, may carry significant morbidity and mortality. Appropriate treatment of a peritransplant abscess includes drainage, antibiotics, and a judicious reduction in immunosuppression.

Calculi

Urolithiasis is the least well described complication following renal transplantation, with a reported incidence ranging from 0.2 to 1.0%.[61–65] Renal transplant lithiasis is usually a late complication, often occurring at least 6 months after transplantation. Predisposing conditions for the formation of calculi are thought to be present in the majority of cases. Ureteral stricture, hypercalcemia secondary to hyperparathyroidism, glucocorticoid administration, papillary necrosis, hypophosphatemia from overaggressive antacid therapy, chronic infection, use of nonabsorbable suture for the ureteral anastomosis, primary hyperoxaluria, and distal renal tubular acidosis have all been identified as risk factors in the pathogensis of renal transplant lithiasis.[65,66] Long-standing indwelling ureteral stents may become encrusted with subsequent stone formation. Stones may also be present in the donor kidney prior to transplantation. Van Gansbeke[63] estimated the incidence of stones in donor kidneys to be 0.37% (the same as that of asymptomatic stones in the general population). Some authors have advocated that screening radiographs of allograft kidneys be performed to rule out the presence of stones; however, the low incidence of preexisting stones does not justify their attempted identification prior to multiple organ recovery. Renal calculi may be discovered incidentally on routine posttransplant ultrasound, and in many cases, no treatment may be indicated. However, hydronephrosis, infection, and compromised allograft function secondary to obstruction may occur; therefore, patients with untreated stones must be followed closely. If the calculus migrates into the ureter, the patient may experience pain and swelling of the graft (related to peritoneal irritation), simulating acute rejection or pyelonephritis. Diagnosis can best be made by KUB and ultrasound. Treatment options for transplant calculi include ureteral stents to facilitate stone passage, endourologic techniques, and surgical removal.[67–69] Extracorporeal shock wave lithotripsy (ESWL) provides an alternative to these invasive methods and has been successfully employed.[70,71] The long-term effects of ESWL on the transplant kidney are unknown, but it is probably as safe in treating transplant lithiasis as it has been for the treatment of native kidney stones. The position of the allograft kidney renders it ideally suited for treatment with the Siemens Lithostar, which does not require water bath immersion.[70,71] ESWL should probably not be used in poorly or nonfunctioning transplant kidneys because fragment passage may be impaired in such oliguric or anuric grafts.

▲ VASCULAR COMPLICATIONS OF RENAL TRANSPLANTATION

The other major group of posttransplant sugical complications involves the renal and/or recipient vasculature. The overall incidence of such complications ranges from 2 to 10% in most series, and will be discussed in detail in this section.

Arterial Complications

Renal Artery Thrombosis

Thrombosis of the main renal artery is the least common vascular complication seen after transplantation, with a reported incidence ranging from 0.9 to 3.5%.[72–79] It is usually an acute event that may occur intraoperatively or in the early postoperative period. In a large reported series, the majority (>80%) of cases of renal artery thrombosis were recognized within the first month after transplantation, and over 90% presented within the first year after transplantation.[78] Late arterial thrombosis (>3 years posttransplant) has usually been associated with immunologic causes or related to renal artery stenosis.[77–80] Allograft arterial thrombosis may be extensive and involve the main renal artery or may be limited to segmental arterial branches. In the latter situation, prompt diagnosis and therapy may allow partial or even total graft salvage. Thrombosis of the main renal artery usually results in allograft loss.[72–78] Although there have been isolated case reports of successful revascularization of acute renal artery thrombosis within 12 hours of acute occlusion,[79,81] and a few reports of late arterial thrombosis salvaged with streptokinase or heparin,[82] allograft loss is the usual outcome. In general, the greater the interval between transplantation and the occurrence of arterial thrombosis, the better the chance that a successful outcome can be achieved.[78]

Etiology of Renal Artery Thrombosis. Arterial thrombosis is usually the consequence of technical or mechanical factors during recovery, implantation, or both.[72,73] Possible causes of early arterial thrombosis include hyperacute or accelerated rejection, postoperative hypotension, hypercoagulable state, atherosclerosis of the donor or recipient vessels, torsion or kinking of the vessels, trauma to the donor artery during recovery or subsequent perfusion, disparity in vessel size during anastomosis, or dissection of a distal intimal flap.[72] Arterial thrombosis can also result from thrombosis of the renal vein.[72] The use of cyclosporine has also been associated with renal artery thrombosis.[83,84] The exact mechanisms by which cyclosporine may promote renal arterial thrombosis remain to be defined. That native renal vascular thrombosis has not been described in patients on cyclosporine for indications other than renal transplantation suggests that factors other than cyclosporine alone are likely to be involved.[85] Several proposed mechanisms by which cyclosporine is thought to contribute to vascular thrombosis include decreased prostacyclin production by the vascular endothelium, promotion of ADP-induced platelet aggregation, induction of thromboxane A_2 synthesis, and tissue thromboplastin and factor VIII release.[86]

Segmental renal arterial thrombosis may result in limited infarcts and focal scarring and may escape clinical suspicion unless or until renal function deteriorates and/or the patient develops worsening hypertension. A high index of suspicion for any vascular complication, including segmental thrombosis, must be present after transplantation of a kidney with multiple vessels requiring vascular repair at the time of transplantation. Calyceal-cutaneous fistulae or ureteral ischemia may also occur as a consequence of segmental and/or accessory renal arterial thrombosis[76] and may be a clue to the presence of an underlying thrombosed vessel.

Diagnosis of Renal Artery Thrombosis. The clinical findings suggestive of main renal arterial thrombosis can be highly variable. The patient may be asymptomatic or may complain of an acute onset of allograft tenderness and/or gross hematuria. As always, acute diminution and/or cessation of urine output requires urgent histologic and radiographic assessment of the allograft to rule out a graft-threatening vascular complication. The diagnosis of segmental or main renal arterial thrombosis requires proof of absent arterial flow. Duplex Doppler sonography, color Doppler sonography, and renal scintigraphy can all suggest the diagnosis (Figure 11–11); however, the diagnosis should be confirmed angiographically. In the immediate postoperative period, Doppler ultrasound can be invaluable in the confirmation of vascular integrity. In acute arterial thrombosis, the absence of a Doppler signal is usually diagnostic. Nuclear scintigraphic findings of main renal artery thrombosis may include lack of perfusion, absent visualization of the normal scintigraphic nephrogram, poor background clearance of activity, and/or a photopenic defect in the transplant bed. The sensitivity of scintigraphy is limited in that renal vein thrombosis, severe acute tubular necrosis, and hyperacute rejection may all display similar scintigraphic findings.[87] Segmental arterial thrombosis may produce persistent intrarenal photopenic defects that are classically wedge-shaped. Although this appearance is fairly specific, other causes of focal photopenic areas such as intrarenal hematomas, ab-

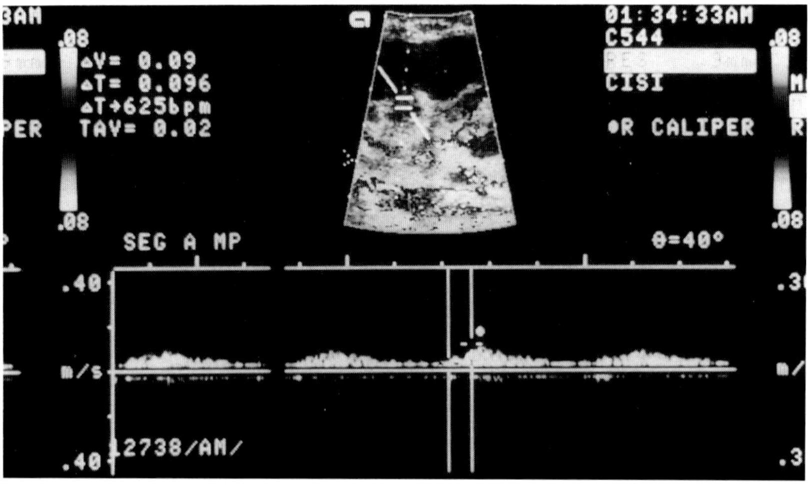

Figure 11–11. Duplex Doppler ultrasound study of renal allograft showing absence of detectable flow velocity in renal allograft.

scesses, and cysts should be included in the differential diagnosis and may be confirmed by ultrasound examination. If arterial thrombosis is clinically suspected by any of these modalities, renal angiography should be performed. The angiographic findings associated with thrombosis of the transplant renal artery vary depending on its location and extent.[88] If the thrombus extends to or near the origin of the vessel, then the vessel may not be visible except for irregularity at its origin or filling of a small stump. Occasionally, contrast will surround a portion of a partially occlusive thrombus, which appears as a filling defect within the lumen of the artery. In cases of an occlusive thrombus, the parenchyma in the distribution of the occluded vessel is not usually visualized, as there are no collateral vessels present in the transplanted kidney. If renal artery thrombosis is confirmed by radiologic studies, the allograft should be explored. Successful thrombectomy with salvage of the allograft has been reported on rare occasions, but in most cases the allograft will be infarcted and will have to be removed. In cases of segmental renal artery thrombosis, attempts at thrombolytic therapy with systemic heparin or streptokinase infusion may lead to recanalization of the involved branches. More commonly, however, segmental infarction of the kidney in the area subtended by the involved branch(es) occurs.

Renal Artery Stenosis

Transplant renal artery stenosis (TRAS) is the most common renal transplant vascular complication, with a reported incidence of 1.6–12%.[72–74,89–92] The true prevalence of TRAS, however, is unknown because reports vary from series to series, depending on the indications for performing renal angiography. In one study where routine postoperative angiography was performed, a 25% incidence of radiographic TRAS was reported.[91] In other series where angiography was performed only when a clinically significant TRAS was suspected, the incidence was in the range of 1.5–5%.[93,94] Several studies have reported a higher incidence of TRAS after cadaveric (17%) compared with living related renal transplantation (5.8%);[91,95] other studies, however, report an equivalent incidence of 5.8%–6.8%, respectively.[96] The interval at which TRAS is detected posttransplant is highly variable, but most cases are identified within 34 months after transplantation.[97] Clinical findings suggestive of TRAS include poorly controlled hypertension, a decrease in allograft function with or without the use of angiotensin-converting enzyme inhibitors, and the appearance, or change in the intensity, of a bruit over the allograft.[98,99] While these clinical findings may be suggestive of TRAS, they nevertheless are of limited diagnostic value. One study reported a positive predictive value of only 20% when clinical parameters suggestive of TRAS were verified by renal angiography.[100]

Although TRAS is a recognized cause of posttransplant hypertension, isolated hypertension in the absence of TRAS is also common in the renal transplant population.[93,101,102] Posttransplant hypertension may be observed in 50–80% of recipients and may result from chronic allograft rejection, recurrence of the primary disease, renin production from native kidneys, de novo renal disease, steroids, and/or the immunosuppressive drugs themselves. (See the section on General Medical Complications in this chapter.) Other causes may include obesity, volume overload, and essential hypertension.[103] It is therefore imperative to distinguish these causes of posttransplant hypertension from that caused by TRAS.

The etiology of TRAS is multifactorial and may include progressive atheroma in the recipient artery, faulty anastomotic suture technique, arterial injury during donor nephrectomy, excessive length of vessel with angulation and stenosis after anastomosis, and disparity in donor–recipient vessel size.[89,96,104] Rejection has also been associated with TRAS, and histologic changes associated with narrowing of wide-caliber renal arteries have been described, as well as complement and immunoglobulin deposition in the vessel wall of stenosed transplant renal arteries.[105] Stenosis may occur in the donor vessel, in the recipient vessel, at the anastomotic site (Figure 11–12), or as multiple stenotic lesions in the involved vessels. Currently, most transplant surgeons use an end-to-side anastomosis of the donor renal artery, with a Carrel patch, to the recipient external iliac artery. However, when a Carrel patch is not available, as in living donor transplants and in some cadaver donor kidneys with excessive aortic atheroma, end-to-end anastomosis of the renal artery to the hypogastric artery may be used instead, although end-to-side is also perfectly feasible. A large series of cases found no correlation between the type of anastomosis used and the site of subsequent stenosis; however, stenosis at any location was encountered less frequently when an end-to-side (3.9% incidence) rather than an end-to-end (9.7% incidence) anastomosis was used.[72]

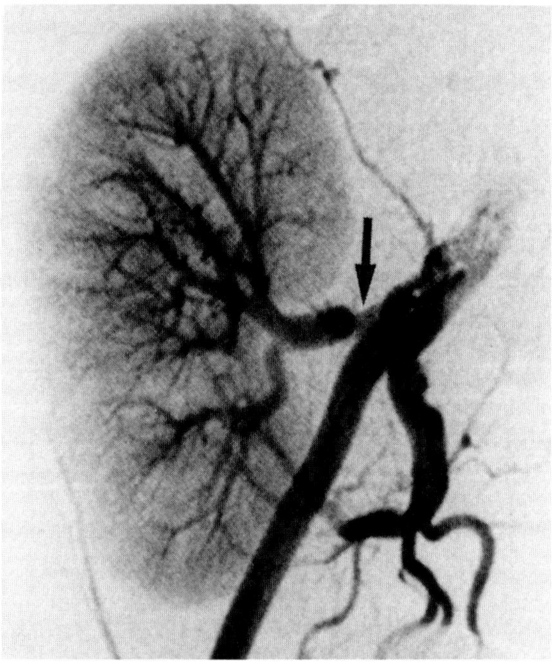

Figure 11–12. Arteriography of renal allograft demonstrating anastomotic stenosis of renal artery (arrow).

Renal Artery Stenosis—Diagnosis and Management

The diagnosis of TRAS may be difficult. This is probably because the transplanted kidney behaves as a "one clip" Goldblatt kidney in which the hypertension is likely volume-mediated and not renin-mediated. Noninvasive screening methods for the diagnosis of TRAS include: (1) determination of peripheral plasma renin and the response to angiotensin-converting enzyme (ACE) inhibition;[106] (2) evaluation of the decline in GFR and ERPF by nuclear medicine scintigraphy after ACE inhibition; and (3) evaluation of the transplant renal artery with duplex color sonography.[86–88,99,100,107–109] These noninvasive screening techniques are useful in ruling out TRAS or in assessing the functional significance of an angiographically demonstrable TRAS. Color Doppler ultrasound has been gaining increased utility in the evaluation of TRAS. Some centers report a diagnostic sensitivity and specificity of 100% and 75%, respectively.[108] With color Doppler ultrasound, an area of luminal narrowing produces a segmental region of abnormal flow typified by increased maximum systolic velocity accompanied by marked turbulence. The diagnostic accuracy of color Doppler is nevertheless limited in that the technique is operator-dependent. Currently, there are no uniformly accepted standard criteria by which the diagnosis of TRAS can be made using color Doppler alone. The peripheral renin response to ACE inhibition by captopril has a reported sensitivity and specificity of 75% and 67%, respectively. Evaluating the allograft with a captopril renal scan may predict TRAS with a sensitivity and specificity of 75% and 84%, respectively.[100] However, the use of ACE inhibitors in the evaluation of TRAS may be dangerous, because of low flow through an already narrowed renal artery, which may result in compromised renal function, and even frank renal failure.[110,111] Factors that may predispose to ACE inhibitor–induced renal failure include a critical stenosis, chronic renal insufficiency, and volume depletion (in most cases secondary to the concurrent use of diuretics). Preserved renal function immediately following ACE inhibition does not necessarily rule out a functionally significant stenosis.[102] Renal functional impairment following ACE inhibition in the presence of TRAS is unpredictable and may occur at any time from hours to months after ACE inhibitor administration. Fortunately, the deleterious effects of ACE inhibition on renal function are usually reversible.[110]

Although the presence of TRAS may be suggested by noninvasive screening methods, confirmation should be obtained by angiography (Figure 11–12). The criteria for performing angiography should include a new onset or progressive hypertension, hypertension resistant to medical treatment, or hypertension accompanied by deterioration of renal function that cannot be explained by rejection. An angiographically significant stenosis generally corresponds to a decrease in luminal diameter of >75% and/or a transstenotic pressure gradient of >40 Torr.[112,113] The functional significance of the stenotic segment can usually be ascertained only after treatment. Once the diagnosis of TRAS is made, a decision should be made promptly whether further medical therapy or interventional therapy (angioplasty or surgical reconstruction) is indicated. Pharmacotherapy may be continued if hypertension can be controlled and if the stenosis does not actually endanger allograft perfusion.[114] In general, angiographically demonstrable lesions are functionally significant and should be treated. In addition, poorly controlled hypertension with multiple drug therapy may be responsible for considerable morbidity, including accleation of cardiovascular and cerebrovascular complications. Furthermore, pharmacologic therapy does not halt the progression of arterial stenosis.

Percutaneous transluminal angioplasty (PTA) should usually be the initial step in the treatment of TRAS (Figure 11–13) and carries an initial success rate of 50–80%. PTA has been used to treat TRAS since 1979.[115–118] The initial use of PTA does not preclude subsequent vascular surgical repair if the initial attempt is unsuccessful. PTA carries an overall technical success rate of up to 84%.[32,34] Failure rates are reported to range from 19 to 50%. Graft loss as an immediate result of PTA has also been reported, with an incidence of 0 to 20%. Serious complications of PTA, such as dissection and thrombosis, may occur in 7–28% of all cases. Other complications reported include reversible renal failure, femoral artery pseudoaneurysm, and arterial perforation.[115–120] We recommend that PTA be carried out with surgical standby immediately available for correction of these potential complications.

Angioplasty is generally quite successful for anastomotic stenoses. Surgical revascularization should be considered for failed angioplasty, or for lesions not amenable to angioplasty. Surgical techniques include resection of the stenotic segment with reanastomosis, various bypass grafting methods, lysis of periarterial adhesions, venous patch angioplasty, and open dilation.[121–123] These procedures are

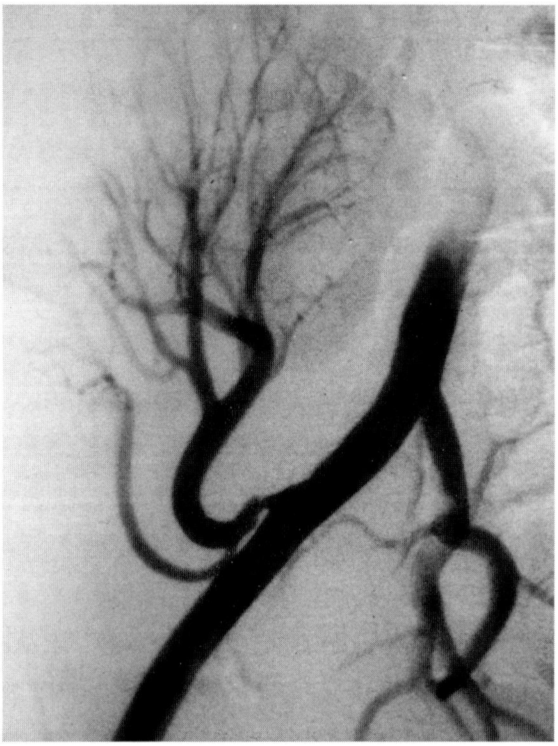

Figure 11–13. Percutaneous transluminal angioplasty (PTA) of renal allograft. A. Before treatment showing high-grade stenosis (post-anastomotic).

technically difficult and have varying degrees of success. Graft loss and significant morbidity following surgical repair of TRAS have been reported in up to 20% of the cases, with mortality rates of up to 20%.[121] Nonetheless, surgical repair in selected cases may be of benefit and yield a higher immediate success rate and a lower recurrence rate when compared to angioplasty.[123]

Other Arterial Complications

Complex vascular reconstructions of the renal artery may be necessitated by the presence of multiple vessels, or in the use of pediatric "en bloc" kidneys from very young (ie, <2 years) donors. In the latter situation, the use of extension grafts to the donor aorta may be necessary to allow sufficient arterial length to permit a satisfactory anastomis. Such extension grafts may be obtained from another ABO-compatible adult donor, in which the common and/or external iliac artery, and on occasion the carotid vessels, may be used. Pseudoaneurysm formation, stenosis, and occasionally, thrombosis of the extension graft may occur. Successful repair of a pseudoaneurysm of the extension graft has been reported.[123a] Infectious (mycotic) pseudoaneurysms (see Infectious Complications, Chapter 12) can be associated with arterial rupture and usually require

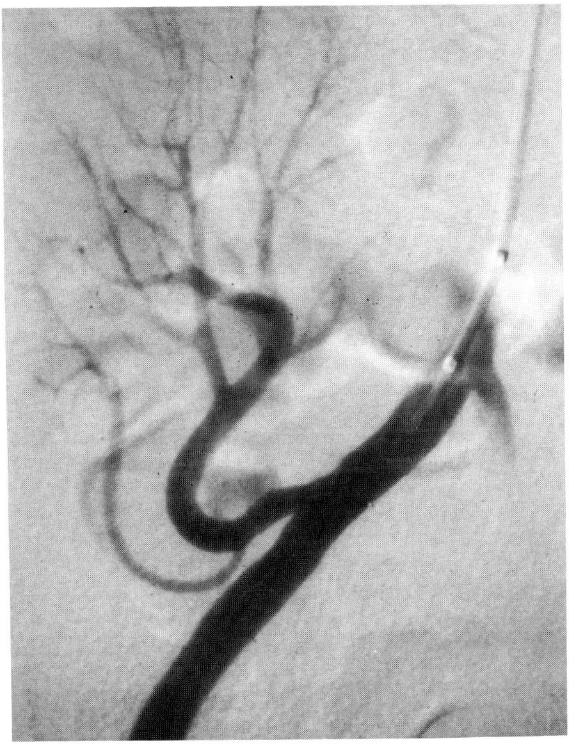

Figure 11–13. B. Following successful angioplasty with marked angiographic improvement in luminal diameter.

allograft nephrectomy, excision and ligation of the external iliac artery, and, if necessary, extra-anatomic bypass.[243,331]

Venous Complications

Renal Vein Thrombosis

The incidence of renal vein thrombosis is reported to be 0.9–7.6%.[72–75] This complication usually occurs early in the postoperative period and almost invariably results in the loss of the transplanted kidney.[72] A number of possible causes for renal vein thrombosis have been proposed and include kinking or angulation of the renal vein, stenosis of the venous anastomosis, postoperative hypovolemia and hypotension, hypercoagulable state, acute rejection, deep venous thrombophlebitis with extension into the allograft, and renal vein compression by a perinephric fluid collection.[124–128] A number of studies have reported an association between cyclosporine and an increased incidence of both arterial and venous thrombosis.[129]

Clinical Presentation, Diagnosis, and Management of Renal Vein Thrombosis. Clinically, renal vein thrombosis may present with acute allograft swelling, pain and tenderness accompanied by oliguria, impaired renal function, and proteinuria. Since the clinical distinction between renal vein thrombosis and acute rejection can be difficult, prompt histologic and radiographic evaluation is indicated. Ultrasonography and renal scintigraphy are currently the mainstays in postoperative allograft evaluation; however, the diagnosis of renal vein thrombosis may be difficult. Venous Doppler examination of the renal vein has a high degree of accuracy in establishing the diagnosis.[88,107,126,130]

Venous occlusion occurring in the early postoperative period almost invariably results in allograft loss. When the diagnosis of renal vein thrombosis is suspected, the most expedient approach is prompt reexploration and attempted venous thrombectomy. Successful venous thrombectomy has been reported sporadically, but in most cases venous thrombosis has led to graft nonviability by the time exploration is undertaken.[72–75,124,125] Late renal vein thrombosis (occurring more than 4 weeks after transplantation) is usually a result of propagation of deep iliac or femoral venous thrombosis into the renal vein. Anticoagulation or use of intravenous streptokinase may be considered.[131,132] Placement of a vena caval filter to prevent pulmonary embolus may also be indicated if the thrombus extends superiorly beyond the allograft. In most cases, late renal vein thrombosis leads to allograft loss despite these measures. The optimal treatment of renal vein thrombosis lies in its prevention by ensuring adequate hydration, precise surgical technique, and avoidance of postoperative complications, especially deep venous thrombosis and perinephric fluid collections.

Arteriovenous Fistula

Percutaneous allograft biopsy is routine in the postoperative assessment of allograft dysfunction. Although relatively safe when assisted with color Doppler ultrasound for localization, biopsies are associated with potential complications. These include formation of arteriovenous fistulas (AVF), arteriocalyceal fistulas (ACF), iliac or mesenteric vascular lacerations, perirenal collections (hematoma), pseudoaneurysms, gross hematuria, and/or intraabdominal organ injuries.[133]

Arteriovenous fistula (AVF) is a well recognized complication of biopsy in both the native kidney and in renal allografts. The incidence of AVF in the allograft kidneys is not well known and is most likely underestimated, because most small fistulas remain clinically silent. Most series report an incidence of 5–10%.[133,134] When clinical symptoms are the indication for performing angiography that discloses a fistula, the incidence is 1–2%.[135,136] When Doppler ultrasound is done routinely shortly after a biopsy, the incidence is 10%.[137] This is not very different from the incidence of 15–18% found with routine angiography performed after biopsy of the native kidney.[138,139]

Most AVF are small and clinically silent and usually resolve in 1–2 years.[139,140] AVF occur as a result of simultaneous injury to the walls of an adjacent artery and vein. When prebiopsy parameters are assessed, it is found that a significantly higher percentage of patients with a prolonged bleeding time and a low platelet count form fistulas than those with nomal parameters.[137] Patients with preexisting hypertension (HTN) and nephro-angiosclerosis also appear to be at greater risk.[133] Other causes of AVF include accidental trauma, infection, local mycosis, rupture of an aneurysm, and technical failure during procurement.[141,142] Consequences of most AVF are limited. Obviously only a small number of these reach clinical relevance. It has been calculated that only 4% of AVF persist, whereas most resolve spontaneously.[142] An AVF may persist without renal dysfunction or signs of a hyperdynamic circulation, but alternatively may lead to deterioration of renal function, uncontrolled hypertension, and/or hemorrhage.[143] These are complications that require treatment. Angiography with selective embolization is the treatment of choice in most AVF.[144] If selective embolization is not possible, it may be necessary to resect the fistula-bearing part of the kidney.[145] According to Lawen et al,[135] most symptomatic AVFs are found in patients who have undergone biopsy more than 1 year after transplantation. They attributed this higher incidence to the histologic features of arterial wall thickening and intimal fibrosis occurring in the graft at this point in time.[135] In cases of an asymptomatic AVF with no coexistent allograft dysfunction, watchful waiting is advisable. Periodic color Doppler exam every 3–6 months is recommended.[146] Ultrasound findings in AVF may include a pulsatile (arterialized) venous flow with increased arterial velocity and a reduced arterial resistive index. An AVF that shows no diminution in size on several interval ultrasound examinations may require correction, since severe bleeding more than 1 year after diagnosis of an AVF has been reported.[146] In general, the more centrally located fistulas are more commonly symptomatic and require intervention.[147]

In our experience, the complication rate associated with percutanteous biopsies is clearly related to the experience of the individual performing the biopsy. It is our policy to perform biopsies as peripherally as possible, directing the needle toward the upper or lower pole, or the most lateral aspect of the kidney, rather than toward the hilum, to minimize the risk of traumatizing a major artery or a calyx.

Medical Complications

Jerry McCauley

Despite improvements in immunosuppression and in other aspects of posttransplant care, many medical problems continue to be encountered after renal transplantation. Some represent a continuation or progression of diseases that were present before transplantation. Others are side effects of the agents needed to control the rejection process. Proper management of these problems may prevent much of the potential morbidity that could limit the full rehabilitation of these patients.

▲ CARDIOVASCULAR

Cardiovascular disease is one of the leading causes of morbidity and mortality in the posttransplant period and may account for 25–50% of deaths.[148,149] Risk factors include pretransplant cardiovascular disease, diabetes, male sex, elevated serum lipids, hypertension, cigarette smoking, and allograft dysfunction.[150] The risk of cardiovascular disease often begins prior to transplantation. Dialysis patients are particularly at risk because of the high prevalence of hypertension, which may cause left ventricular hypertrophy, cardiac chamber dilatation, increased left ventricular wall stress, redistribution of coronary artery flow, myocardial fibrosis, heart failure, and arrhythmias.[151] Abnormalities in lipid metabolism in dialysis patients and in patients with long-standing nephrotic syndrome can increase the risk of accelerated atherosclerotic disease. Other important risk factors for cardiovascular disease include diabetes, obesity, advanced age, hyperuricemia, and hypercholesterolemia, all of which are particularly prevalent after transplantation.[151] The rate of cardiovascular disease is largely dependent upon the selection criteria for transplant candidates. Centers accepting high-risk cardiac patients will have higher rates of death from cardiovascular disease. For patients 45–64 years of age at the time of transplantation, cardiovascular-related mortality was 29.1/1000 overall (11.4 for myocardial infarction, 14.5 for other cardiac diseases, and 3.1 for cerebrovascular disease).

Patients with known pretransplant cardiac disease should be followed closely for progression after transplantation. Many of these patients will have undergone coronary artery angioplasty or bypass surgery prior to transplantation and are at risk for restenosis or progression of lesions in these vessels. Measures to reduce the risk of cardiovascular death are similar to those used in the nontransplant setting and include the obvious interventions, such as routine follow-up stress or pharmacologic thallium studies in patients with known coronary artery disease, but, in addition, should also include those directed at delaying the progression of disease, eg, control of serum cholesterol and of hypertension (discussed below).

▲ HYPERTENSION

Hypertension is a common complication after renal transplantation and has many potential etiologies (Table 11–3). The rate of hypertension has increased from 40–50% in the pre-cyclosporine era to 60–70% in cyclosporine-treated renal allograft recipients.[152] The most common causes of hypertension are cyclosporine and chronic rejection.[153] Cyclosporine causes vasoconstriction of the afferent arteriole, which reduces both GFR and renal blood flow.[154] Cyclosporine-induced hypertension is also, in part, volume dependent and worsens with volume expansion; it is poorly responsive to angiotensin-converting enzyme inhibitors.[152] The vasoconstriction may be related to vasoconstricting prostaglandins and the renin-

TABLE 11–3 ▲ CAUSES OF HYPERTENSION IN RENAL TRANSPLANT RECIPIENT

Immunosuppressive therapy	Steroids
	Cyclosporine
	Tacrolimus (FK 506)
Allograft dysfunction	Acute rejection
	Chronic allograft nephropathy
	Cyclosporine nephrotoxicity
	Tacrolimus nephrotoxicity
	Transplant renal artery stenosis
	Recurrent or de novo glomerulonephritis
Causes prior to transplantation	Renal artery stenosis in native kidneys
	Polycystic kidney disease
	Persistent essential hypertension
Other causes	Dietary sodium loading
	Florinef treatment
	Primary aldosteronism
	Pheochromocytoma
	Hypercalcemia

angiotensin system. Systemic vascular resistance also increases with cyclosporine, but apparently not with tacrolimus. This may explain the somewhat lower rate of hypertension in tacrolimus-treated patients.[155] Prednisone contributes to hypertension with either agent when the adult steroid doses are greater than 10 mg/day.

Hypertension developing from disease in the allograft is generally due to decreased renal function, in addition to the effects of immunosuppressive agents. Renal artery stenosis in the allograft vessels is the exception (see previous section). A sudden onset of severe hypertension or worsening of stable hypertension should suggest this diagnosis. A noninvasive diagnosis using captopril may not be valid in the presence of cyclosporine and may increase the risk of worsening renal function in a patient with renal artery stenosis in a solitary kidney.[156] Renal artery stenosis in the native kidneys as a cause of posttransplant hypertension probably occurs infrequently, so that native nephrectomy as a cure for hypertension should be reserved for patients with well-documented disease.

The treatment of posttransplant hypertension must take into consideration both the pathophysiology of hypertension and potential drug interactions with cyclosporine and tacrolimus. Although cyclosporine-induced hypertension is in part volume mediated, these patients are also more likely to experience a rise in Scr and BUN from diuretic-induced prerenal azotemia. The preferred first-line agents are probably calcium channel blockers. These agents have been shown to vasodilate preferentially the afferent arterioles, increase renal blood flow, and induce a moderate natriuresis.[157] The dihydropyridines (nifedipine and isradipine) do not affect cyclosporine or tacrolimus blood levels and are very effective in lowering blood pressure. Diltiazem, and to a lesser extent verapamil, increase cyclosporine and, possibly, tacrolimus blood levels. This feature has been used to lower the dosage of cyclosporine by approximately 50%, a maneuver that can reduce significantly the cost of this agent.[158] Centrally acting agents (clonidine) are effective in lowering blood pressure and do not interfere with cyclosporine or tacrolimus blood levels. An added advantage, if the patient can tolerate the somnolence and other side effects, is blunting of the tremors and insomnia associated with cyclosporine toxicity. Alpha- and beta-blocking agents can also be used and do not affect cyclosporine or tacrolimus blood levels. Moderate to severe hypertension can often be controlled with oral agents initially (nifedipine 5–10 mg sublingually, clonidine 0.1 mg, or labetalol). Labetalol may cause hyperkalemia in patients with poor renal function, which may be exacerbated by cyclosporine or tacrolimus.

▲ HYPERLIPIDEMIA

Hyperlipidemia is very common after renal transplantation irrespective of the immunosuppressive protocol, and may develop in 50–80% of patients.[159] Factors associated with the risk of hyperlipidemia include (1) elevated lipid levels prior to transplantation, (2) older age, (3) renal dysfunction, (4) diet, (5) hyperglycemia,

(6) hyperinsulinemia, (7) weight gain, (8) diuretic use, (9) proteinuria, (10) steroid therapy, and (11) cyclosporine.[160] Many of these factors may be related to the use of steroids, such as increased appetite, weight gain, and hyperglycemia. In one study, patient age, pretransplant cholesterol levels, steroid therapy, and cyclosporine therapy were independent predictors of hyperlipidemia in a multivariate analysis.[161] Steroids may cause hypertriglyceridemia by increasing peripheral resistance to insulin action, reducing lipolytic activity, and impairing triglyceride clearance.[162] Hypercholesterolemia has not been consistently associated with steroid use when low doses are administered, but elevated levels are associated with adult prednisone dosages of 12.5 mg/day or greater.[163] Cyclosporine may cause hyperglycemia and hyperinsulinemia (see posttransplant diabetes) and may require diuretic use to control hypertension, which may lead to hyperlipidemia. A direct effect of cyclosporine was suggested by Kasiske et al, who noted a 15–20% increase in serum lipid levels with cyclosporine, compared to azathioprine-treated patients.[164] Evidence for the role of cyclosporine is also supported by a fall in lipid levels after conversion to azathioprine.[165,166] Tacrolimus also has been associated with lower cholesterol levels than cyclosporine.[166a]

There is a growing interest in treating hyperlipidemia with lipid-lowering agents when dietary measures have failed. The use of 3-hydroxy-3 methylglutaryl (HMG) coenzyme A (CoA) reductase inhibitors was initially discouraged because of the potential risk of rhabdomyolysis and myopathy. The use of these agents was also potentially complicated by the cyclosporine-induced inhibition of drug metabolism by cytochrome P450, resulting in elevated lovastatin drug levels.[167] Studies using pravastatin,[168,169] simvastatin,[170] and fluvastatin[171,172] suggest that all drugs in this class may have a prolonged half-life because of cyclosporine. Appropriate dosage reduction of these agents has allowed significant improvement in total and LDL cholesterol without muscle damage.[173] One half of the usual starting dose of each agent is a prudent adjustment. These agents are very effective in treating hyperlipidemia but may potentially also improve allograft survival. In a study of cardiac transplant patients, Kobashigawa et al noted that patients treated with HMG CoA reductase inhibitors experienced improved 1-year allograft survival (94% vs 78%), fewer acute rejection episodes, and less vasculopathy (chronic rejection).[174] Natural killer (NK) cell cytotoxicity was also significantly reduced, which may mediate the change in immunoregulation. A subsequent study was performed in 48 primary cadaveric renal transplant patients.[175] Acute rejection episodes were reduced in the treated group (25% vs 58%), and NK cell cytotoxicity was also reduced.

Other lipid-lowering agents may be used but have different potential complications.[160] Bile acid sequestrants (cholestyramine or colestipol) interfere with cyclosporine absorption. Close monitoring of cyclosporine blood levels should be performed if these agents are used. Nicotinic acid may exacerbate the cyclosporine-induced hyperuricemia. Gemfibrozil and clofibrate (fibric acid derivatives) also cause myositis and have been associated with an unexpectedly increased incidence of malignancy.[160]

▲ DRUG TOXICITIES

Many of the medical complications after transplantation are related to the side effects of immunosuppressive agents. The relative severity of these side effects for cyclosporine and tacrolimus are listed in Table 11–4. The toxicities of these drugs are similar, but with some important exceptions. Many of the side effects can be improved or eliminated by reductions in drug dosage.

Nephrotoxicity is one of the limiting side effects of both cyclosporine and tacrolimus. The histologic and functional changes of acute and chronic cyclosporine and tacrolimus nephrotoxicity appear to be similar (see also Chapter 10).[177–179] Acute nephrotoxicity is manifested by a sudden rise in Scr, which is usually associated with elevated drug levels and improves quickly after dosage reduction. Chronic toxicity is typically associated with high drug levels resulting in persistently elevated Scr. Renal function usually stabilizes once drug levels are reduced; however, if the levels remain high, progressive renal failure may develop. The risk of chronic nephrotoxicity has stimulated some clinicians to reduce drug dosage progressively to very low levels.[180] Ultimately, this has led to doses that have been subtherapeutic for cyclosporine-treated patients ($<$4–6 mg/kg/day or 150–400 ng/mL trough HPLC levels), and this may increase the risk of graft loss from chronic allograft rejection.[181] The lower therapeutic limit for dosing of tacrolimus has not been determined to date, although chronic levels of 5–10 ng/mL have been recommended (whole blood IMX).

TABLE 11-4 ▲ TOXICITY OF TACROLIMUS COMPARED TO CYCLOSPORINE

Complication	Tacrolimus	Cyclosporine	Dosage Reduction
Nephrotoxicity	Very common	Very common	Improves
Neurotoxicity			
Tremors	Very common	Very common	Improves
Paresthesia	Common	Unusual	Improves
Insomnia	Common	Common	Improves
Seizures	Rare	Rare	Improves
Hypertension	Uncommon	Very common	? Improves
Hyperlipidemia	Unusual	Very common	? Improves
Hyperglycemia	Initial—fairly common Chronic—uncommon	Uncommon	Improves
Hyperkalemia	Very common	Common	Improves
Hyperuricemia	Common	Common	No change
Gingival hyperplasia	Rare	Very common	Improves
Hypertrichosis	Rare	Very common	Improves
Hepatotoxicity	Unusual	Uncommon	Improves
Anorexia	Unusual	Unusual	Improves
Hemolytic uremic syndrome	Rare	Rare	? Improves

The neurotoxicity of cyclosporine and tacrolimus is a common side effect and will be discussed in a separate section. The symptoms listed in Table 11–4 are manifestations of toxic drug levels and usually resolve with dosage reduction.

Some side effects are seen more often in cyclosporine-treated patients than in tacrolimus-treated patients. These include gingival hyperplasia and hypertrichosis. Both are physically disfiguring complications that distinguish cyclosporine from other known agents. In addition to cyclosporine, other commonly used drugs such as phenytoin, diltiazem, and nifedipine have been reported to cause gingival hyperplasia. Adams and Famili suggested that gingival hyperplasia improved after conversion from cyclosporine to tacrolimus.[182] Hypertrichosis has not been described in tacrolimus-treated patients and gingival hyperplasia occurs rarely, if at all. Hypertension is probably also less common with tacrolimus-based than with cyclosporine-based therapy; this may in part be related to the lower steroid dosages used with tacrolimus.[256]

Hemolytic uremic syndrome (HUS) has been associated with both cyclosporine and tacrolimus therapy.[183,184] The typical presentation includes microangiopathic hemolytic anemia, thrombocytopenia, and renal failure. The onset may be explosive, with oliguric renal failure, severe thrombocytopenia, and rapidly progressive anemia. A subacute presentation is common, which may lead to a delay in clinical recognition, since the rise in creatinine may be slow and hematologic abnormalities subtle. Renal biopsies reveal microthrombi in glomerular capillaries, which can also be seen during acute rejection episodes. The diagnosis of HUS should be made in the presence of an appropriate constellation of clinical findings in association with appropriate pathologic changes on renal biopsy. Several approaches to treatment have been attempted, with variable success. Cessation of the offending agent often is sufficient to correct subacute cases, and occasionally, the drug might be able to be reintroduced.[183] Patients with cyclosporine have been successfully treated by substitution of tacrolimus without recurrence of HUS.[185–187] The difference in molecular structure between these two agents may explain this effect. Plasmapheresis has also been effective in some cases of severe cyclosporine- or tacrolimus-induced HUS, in contrast to its lack of efficacy in other forms of HUS. Recurrent primary HUS after renal transplantation has not been responsive to plasmapheresis.

The complications of steroids are well known and are listed in Table 11–5. Poor wound healing has led most surgeons and physicians to require a long period of healing for the allograft wound in the immediate perioperative period, but may continue to complicate recovery from any procedure when steroids are given at significant doses. The general practice of aggressive reduction in steroid dosage has reduced the frequency of most serious side effects seen historically with azathioprine-based immunosuppression. Osteopenia and avascular necrosis are major causes of morbidity after transplantation.[188] Pathologic fractures due to osteopenia have been noted in 22% of renal transplant patients.[189] Avascular necrosis is characterized by necrosis of marrow cells, trabeculae, and osteocytes in weight-bearing long bones. Approximately 15% of cyclosporine-treated patients develop this problem, which may be multifocal in 50–70% of cases.[190,191] Cataracts, obesity, and cushing-

TABLE 11-5 ▲ COMPLICATIONS OF STEROIDS

Poor wound healing
Obesity
Diabetes
Growth retardation
Osteopenia and osteonecrosis (avascular necrosis)
Psychiatric disorders
Cataracts
Hypertension
Acne
Pancreatitis
Cushingoid features

oid features are associated with high-dose steroids during the early postoperative period. The low maintenance doses (0–7.5 mg/day) used with cyclosporine and tacrolimus contribute less to these problems. Changes in mood from depression to euphoria and psychosis have also been observed with high-dose steroids. These symptoms are seldom seen with maintenance doses.

The spectrum of complications related to azathioprine and mycophenolate mofetil (MMF) are very similar to one another. Three recent randomized trials compared the ability of these two agents to prevent acute rejection and directly compared the toxicities after renal transplantation.[192] Gastrointestinal symptoms were the most common with 3 g/day MMF, with diarrhea (31% MMF, azathioprine 17%) and abdominal pain (31% MMF, 23% azathioprine) being the most common. When MMF was given at 2 g/day, gastrointestinal symptoms were less frequent. Leukopenia was also very common and was dosage dependent. Myelosuppression causing leukopenia developed in 30% of the azathioprine-treated patients, 19% of the 2 g/day MMF-treated patients, and 35% of the 3 g/day MMF-treated patients. Thrombocytopenia developed in 12% of azathioprine-treated patients, 9% of the 2 g/day MMF-treated patients, and 5% of the 3 g/day MMF-treated patients. Other side effects were not significantly different between the two agents.

▲ METABOLIC COMPLICATIONS

Many metabolic derangements develop or persist after renal transplantation. The side effects of immunosuppressive agents can cause many of these problems, but others may be related to other commonly used drugs or the effects of long-standing end-stage renal disease.

Hyperparathyroidism

Hyperparathyroidism may persist after transplantation in approximately 33% of patients.[193] This is usually manifested by hypercalcemia, which can develop during the first week after transplantation but may be delayed by 6 months or more.[194] Hypercalcemia in this setting correlates with the size of parathyroid glands. Severe hypercalcemia has become less common with improved control of hyperphosphatemia during dialysis; however, patients with poor phosphate control remain at risk for severe hypercalcemia after transplantation. Most glands involute after near-normal renal function has been attained, but this may require several months to years if the glands are very large. Approximately 10% of these patients will have hypercalcemia 1 year after transplantation. Patients with severe hyperparathyroidism prior to transplantation will often develop significant hypophosphatemia and hypercalcemia in the early postoperative period if good renal function has been attained. Normalization of serum phosphate is usually sufficient to prevent symptomatic hypercalcemia in mild cases until the glands involute. Evidence for involution includes normalization of serum calcium and alkaline phosphatase levels. Patients with persistent severe hypercalcemia (>12.5 mg/dL) approximately 1 year after transplantation should be considered for parathyroidectomy. Another indication for surgery is in patients with severe symptomatic hypercalcemia in the early postoperative period that does not respond to conservative measures.

Hypocalcemia may have many causes after transplantation. Hypomagnesemia (<0.8 meq/L) causes PTH-induced impairment of calcium release from bone, and greater depressions in serum magnesium may decrease PTH secretion. Severe hypermagnesemia (usually iatrogenic) may also inhibit PTH secretion and cause hypocalcemia. Hypocalcemia developing soon after renal function is normalized in the postoperative period is an occasional problem in patients who have previously undergone subtotal parathyroidectomy on dialysis. In such patients, persistent hypocalcemia may be attentuated by giving high dose vitamin D and calcium supplementation.

Hyperkalemia

Hyperkalemia is very common after renal transplantation. Renal insufficiency, with the resulting slow excretion of dietary potassium, is probably the most common cause in the early postoperative period. In such patients, metabolic acidosis and the resulting transcellular shift of potassium is a contributing factor that should be managed by replacement of bicarbonate orally or intravenously. Hyperkalemia may be present in patients with adequate renal function without significant metabolic acidosis. In this setting, cyclosporine or tacrolimus may be the cause. The reduction in potassium excretion may be due to decreased aldosterone, NA-K ATPase, or other undefined tubular defects. Management centers around reduction in dietary potassium intake. Florinef (fludrocortisone) has been useful in controlling the hyperkalemia of tacrolimus and is initially started at a dose of 0.1 mg/day. A typical dose is 0.1 mg BID.

Hypomagnesemia

Hypomagnesemia is a common complication in hospitalized patients and is particularly prevalent in renal transplant patients. Renal transplant patients are at risk for all of the major causes of hypomagnesemia (Table 11–6).[195] Renal losses of magnesium are the most important causes and may be related to defects in tubular reabsorption of magnesium or inhibition of sodium reabsorption, leading to a reduction in passive transport of magnesium. Both tacrolimus and cyclosporine cause hypomagnesemia, probably related to urinary magnesium wasting.[196,197] Seizures after transplantation have been traced to high cyclosporine levels and low magnesium levels (see the section on Neurologic Complications). Other biochemical abnormalities associated with hypomagnesemia include hypokalemia, hypocalcemia, and metabolic acidosis. The symptoms of hypomagnesemia are predominantly those related to these metabolic changes. In addition, hypomagnesemia may predispose to ventricular arrhythmias. In many cases, hypomagnesemia and associated hypokalemia improve after a reduction in dosage of cyclosporine or tacrolimus. Intravenous or oral repletion of magnesium may be required in severe cases. Other nephrotoxic drugs commonly used in transplant patients increase magnesium wasting, such as amphotericin B, aminoglycoside antibiotics, and pentamidine. High dose pentami-

TABLE 11–6 ▲ POTENTIAL CAUSES OF HYPOMAGNESEMIA AFTER RENAL TRANSPLANTATION

- Renal Magnesium Wasting
  - Nephrotoxic drugs
    - Cyclosporine
    - Tacrolimus
    - Pentamidine
    - Amphotericin B
  - Loop diuretics
    - Lasix
    - Bumex
  - Renal tubular dysfunction
    - Diuretic phase of acute tubular necrosis
    - Postobstructive diuresis
  - Volume expansion
  - Hypercalcemia (ie, hyperparathyroidism)
- Gastrointestinal Losses
  - Diarrhea
  - Malabsorption
  - Acute pancreatitis
- Other
  - Foscarnet
  - Diabetes

dine at doses used in nebulizers has been associated with acute tubular necrosis and may cause tubular wasting of magnesium.[198,199] Loop diuretics decrease the tubular reabsorption of magnesium. Tubular dysfunction can also develop in patients with postobstructive diuresis or with acute tubular necrosis (ATN); magnesium wasting may be significant in patients recovering from ATN. Volume expansion (typically practiced after transplantation) increases magnesium wasting by decreasing sodium reabsorption, and in hypercalcemia, calcium competes with magnesium transport at the thick ascending limb of the loop of Henle. The increased filtered load of calcium reduces magnesium reabsorption and may cause hypomagnesemia in patients with hyperparathyroidism after transplantation. Persistent diarrhea and malabsorption (often seen in diabetics) can be a significant cause of hypomagnesemia, particularly in patients with poor dietary intake. Pancreatitis causes saponification of magnesium and calcium in necrotic fat.[200] Foscarnet therapy for CMV disease causes hypomagnesemia by chelation.[201] Diabetics also develop hypomagnesemia commonly; this may be due to increased renal losses and may reduce glucose disposal, which hypothetically could increase the risk of many diabetic complications.[202]

Hyperuricemia and Gout

Hyperuricemia and gout are common complications after transplantation. Prior to the introduction of cyclosporine these were infrequent problems. Lin et al found that 84% of cyclosporine-treated and 30% of azathioprine-treated patients developed hyperuricemia.[203] Symptomatic gout has been observed in up to 24% of cyclosporine-treated patients and only rarely in azathioprine-treated patients.[204] The reduction in GFR observed in many renal transplant patients is a factor in the reduction in uric acid excretion found in patients with hyperuricemia after transplantation. Diuretic-induced hyperuricemia also plays a major role by directly decreasing uric acid excretion and by causing volume depletion. The rate of hyperuricemia seen in tacrolimus-treated patients is similar to that observed in cyclosporine-treated patients.[205] Management of hyperuricemia should begin with discontinuing diuretics, if possible. Colchicine can be used to treat symptomatic gout. Allopurinol inhibits the metabolism of azathioprine by xanthine oxidase and, ordinarily, the two agents should not be used together. If it is necessary to do so, both drugs should be given at low dosages, with careful monitoring of the white blood cell count.

Posttransplant Diabetes Mellitus

Posttransplant diabetes mellitus (PTDM) develops in 4–20% of renal transplant patients.[206] Many of the most commonly used immunosuppressive agents, steroids, cyclosporine, and tacrolimus, are diabetogenic. Steroids may (1) induce insulin resistance, (2) impair glucose uptake, and (3) decrease insulin receptor number and affinity, in addition to other proposed effects.[206] The rate of PTDM is directly related to the doses of steroids used to maintain allograft function. This problem, in addition to other complications of steroids, has prompted some to attempt complete withdrawal of steroids.[207] De novo PTDM is more common with cyclosporine- (18.6%) than with azathioprine- (9.1%) based immunosuppression.[208] The reported rate of posttransplant hyperglycemia with tacrolimus was similar to that for cyclosporine.[209] In a recent randomized trial of tacrolimus–prednisone versus tacrolimus–prednisone–Imuran, new onset PTDM was noted initially in 18% of non-diabetic recipients, without significant differences between treatment protocols; the final incidence, after reduction of tacrolimus and prednisone doses, was 9%.[210] The phase III multicenter American trial also showed an initial incidence of PTDM of 19.9% with tacrolimus, with a higher incidence in black recipients.[211] This initial incidence was higher than that seen with cyclosporine, 4%. Potential mechanisms of cyclosporine and tacrolimus-induced PTDM include decreased insulin secretion, increased insulin resistance, and a toxic effect on pancreatic beta cells. There is evidence that both FKBP-12 and calcineurin are present in pancreatic islets,[212] and that tacrolimus reversibly inhibits insulin mRNA synthesis. Dosage reduction of prednisone, cyclosporine, and tacrolimus may improve glucose metabolism and allow many patients to discontinue insulin therapy. Approximately 25% of patients with PTDM develop persistent hyperglycemia, and 50% of this group continue to require insulin therapy.[213] Potential risk factors for PTDM include (1) steroid dose, (2) age, (3) weight, and (4) family history of diabetes. No consistent association with HLA type has been confirmed, although studies have suggested an increased frequency of HLA-A28,[214] and the combination of HLA-B8, B18, Bw15, and Dw16.[215] Newer immunosuppressive agents, such as MMF, deoxyspergualin, and sirolimus, have not been reported to cause PTDM.[206,216]

▲ LIVER DISEASE

Liver disease after renal transplantation is an important cause of morbidity and mortality. The prevalence of liver disease has been reported to be 7–24% during the early posttransplant period, and it has been a major factor in patient death in 8–24% of cases.[217–219] Many commonly used drugs may lead to abnormal liver function (Table 11–7).[220] Although these agents have been clearly implicated in liver dysfunction, all drugs should be considered suspect when hepatic dysfunction develops in a transplant patient. Cyclosporine may cause an isolated increase in bilirubin or in serum transaminases. These changes are dose dependent and respond to a reduction in dosage. Azathioprine can cause cholestatic hepatic abnormalities, and there are reported cases of veno-occlusive hepatic disease, and peliosis hepatis. The spectrum of hepatic changes with the other drugs range from mild increases in transaminases to fulminant hepatic failure from hepatic necrosis. The management of most drug-induced hepatic dysfunction is discontinuation of the offending drug.

Viral hepatitis is an important cause of liver dysfunction after renal transplantation. Hepatitis B (HBV) has long been recognized as a potential cause of liver disease and inferior patient and graft survival.[221] Since the introduction of assays for he-

TABLE 11-7 ▲ COMMONLY USED AGENTS IN TRANSPLANTATION CAUSING LIVER DYSFUNCTION

Agent	Hepatic Problem
Immunosuppressive agents	
Cyclosporine	Hyperbilirubinemia, elevated transaminase levels
Azathioprine	Cholestasis, veno-occlusive disease, fibrosis
MMF	Hyperbilirubinemia rarely
Allopurinol	Elevated transaminase levels → hepatic necrosis, may develop vasculitis and renal failure
Anticonvulsants	Elevated transaminase levels → hepatic necrosis
Antimicrobials	
Penicillins	Elevated transaminase levels, cholestasis, acute hepatic and chronic hepatitis
Sulfonamides	Hepatocellular necrosis, chronic liver disease
Antifungals	Elevated transaminase levels → hepatic necrosis
INH	Hepatocellular necrosis, elevated transaminase levels, hyperbilirubinemia
Antihypertensives	
Methyldopa	Elevated transaminase levels, acute and chronic hepatitis
Hydralazine	Granulomatous hepatitis
Captopril	Cholestasis, hepatitic necrosis
Verapamil	Cholestasis

patitis C (HCV), the importance of this virus has become apparent, and it is now considered to be the leading cause of posttransplant liver disease.[222] The presence of prior exposure to HCV has not been shown consistently to impact adversely on allograft or patient survival, but has been demonstrated to increase the risk of developing liver disease and sepsis.[222] Since approximately 10–40% of hemodialysis patients have antibodies to HCV, detection of subclinical hepatic dysfunction in renal transplant recipients is crucial.[223] Routine measurement of liver enzymes should be performed, although only 31% of patients with detectable HCV RNA had elevated transaminases.[224] In addition, any patient with an unexplained rise in cyclosporine or tacrolimus blood levels should be investigated for hepatic insufficiency, which may present as a decreased ability to metabolize these agents. Liver biopsy and HCV PCR may be required to confirm the diagnosis. There is currently no effective treatment. Interferon has been used but has been associated with allograft-destroying rejection.[225]

▲ GASTROINTESTINAL COMPLICATIONS

Gastrointestinal complications may be related either to the persistence of preexisting problems (eg, diabetic gastropathy), or may be caused or exacerbated by immunosuppressive agents (eg, diverticulitis, peptic ulcer disease, or pancreatitis). Steroids can have a particularly deleterious impact on these problems. With the trend toward lower long-term steroid dosages with cyclosporine- and tacrolimus-treated patients, these complications have perhaps become less common. Epigastric discomfort may suggest CMV gastritis, candida esophagitis and gastritis, or peptic ulcer disease. Detection of associated clinical findings such as leukopenia and atypical lymphocytes points toward CMV gastritis, and oral thrush would suggest candida esophagitis. Detection of peptic ulcer disease is particularly important, since massive life-threatening hemorrhage may develop in patients with minimal symptoms. Endoscopy should be performed to confirm the diagnosis in patients with gastritis. The mortality associated with pancreatitis after renal transplantation has been reported to be as high as 70%. Prevention of these complications by maintaining low steroid dosages and prophylaxis with antacids and H2 blockers is important.

Diarrhea is also a common complication after transplantation; it is commonly seen in diabetic patients with gastropathy, and in other patients with antibiotic-induced *Clostridium difficile* (*C. difficile*) colitis. Once these have been ruled out, other, less common diseases should be sought. Potential causes include: osmotic diarrhea (lactase deficiency, laxatives), malabsorption (eg, celiac sprue, giardiasis, amyloidosis, lymphoma or PTLD, AIDS), maldigestion (eg, chronic pancreatitis), exudative diarrhea (eg, ulcerative colitis, Crohn's disease, tuberculosis), secretory diarrhea (eg, VIP-secreting pancreatic tumor, carcinoid, villous adenoma), and motility-related diarrhea (eg, hyperthyroidism, scleroderma, irritable bowel disease). Diarrhea is also a common side effect of MMF and develops in at least 16% patients treated with 2 g/day.[192] The introduction of MMF may exacerbate chronic diarrhea from other causes and may require either a reduction in dosage or discontinuation. Diabetic patients with gastropathy may be particularly sensitive to the diarrhea-inducing effects of MMF.

▲ HEMATOLOGIC COMPLICATIONS

Anemia and leukopenia are common complications seen in the outpatient setting. Patients with anemia usually have poor renal function and are erythropoietin (EPO) deficient. Frequent blood sampling exacerbates this problem. Erythropoietin should be continued in such patients until renal function improves. Deficiencies in iron, folate, and vitamin B_{12} should be investigated in anemic patients with normal renal function or in those refractory to EPO. Parvovirus infection should be suspected in patients with isolated anemia without renal insufficiency or dietary deficiencies. Parvovirus B19 has been documented to cause aplastic anemia in renal transplant recipients.[226] Likewise, hemolytic anemia should prompt a search for medications and other causes, but hemolytic uremic syndrome should always be considered (see Drug Toxicities section). Medications such as azathioprine may cause myelosuppression and result in a megaloblastic anemia and pancytopenia. Leukopenia may be related to azathioprine, mycophenolate, or CMV infection. Discontinuing the offending agent usually corrects leukopenia in drug-related cases, and treatment with ganciclovir (which, paradoxically, can cause leukopenia) effectively treats CMV disease and its related leukopenia.

Polycythemia develops in approximately 15% of renal transplant patients.[227] In general, the risk of thrombotic events and other complications of erythrocytosis increases when the hematocrit exceeds 50%. Polycythemia may be caused by excessive production of erythropoietin (EPO) not only from the allograft but also from the native kidneys.[228] In many cases EPO levels are normal or low.[229] The latter may suggest that other factors that enhance the EPO affect or directly stimulate red cell production may be responsible for the excessive erythropoiesis.

The treatment of polycythemia has recently benefited from the observation that some medications may normalize the hematocrit. Phlebotomy has been the standard therapy but has been only temporarily effective. Angiotensin converting enzyme (ACE) inhibitors can lower the hematocrit to normal in most patients.[227] All agents in this class appear to have this effect. Treatment should be initiated at low doses (captopril 12.5 mg twice per day or enalapril 2.5 mg per day). The reduction in hematocrit usually begins by 6 weeks and stabilizes in 3 to 6 months.[230] This effect of ACE inhibitors appears to be independent of the EPO effect, since reductions in hematocrit develop in patients with low, normal, or high EPO blood levels.[221,232] Withdrawal of ACE inhibitors results in recurrence of polycythemia without corresponding increases in EPO.[233] Although ACE inhibitors do not cause anemia in healthy subjects, they may lead to anemia in otherwise healthy renal transplant patients or patients with chronic renal failure.[234] They may also cause resistance to EPO treatment in these patients.[235]

Theophylline may also be used to treat polycythemia. In one study, the hematocrit fell by 10–15% (59% to 47%).[229] The mechanism of theophylline appears to be as an adenosine antagonist, suggesting that adenosine may play a role in the excessive erythropoiesis of posttransplant erythrocytosis.[233] Theophylline should probably be considered as a second choice, since its effect is less predictable than that of ACE inhibitors, and it may not be as potent.

▲ SKIN

Skin abnormalities not related to cancers are some of the most common complications after transplantation. Acne is a well-known side effect of steroids, as is increased bruising and fragility. Cyclosporine can cause hirsutism, gingival hyperplasia, and facial brutalization in children. Gingival hyperplasia may be more severe in patients with poor dental hygiene.[236] Other lesions, such as human papilloma virus (HPV), leading to common warts on the hands (HPV 2,4), plantar warts (HPV 1), and flat warts (HPV 3,10) may proliferate with immunosuppression.[237] The prevalence of warts has been reported to range from as low as 24% during the first year after transplantation to as high as 87% 5 years posttransplantation. Most small warts on the hands do not require removal; however, there may be an increased risk of squamous cell carcinoma developing in these lesions. Typical lesions can be removed by several methods (salicylic acid, cryosurgery, etc), but suspicious lesions should be excised and examined for malignancy.

Infectious Complications

Shimon Kusne / Rafael Manez

▲ INTRODUCTION

Infectious complications after renal transplantation are associated with significant morbidity and continue to be the most frequent cause of death in the early post-transplant period. This has held true both with azathioprine- and cyclosporine-based therapies, and with the new immunosuppressive agents that have been recently entered into clinical trials (see Chapter 8). Although with time there have been changes made in terms of immunosuppression and surgical techniques, the overall spectrum of infectious complications has remained very similar.[238] In this section, the most common infectious complications after kidney transplantation will be reviewed, and regimens for both treatment and prophylaxis will be discussed.

▲ DIAGNOSIS OF INFECTION

Signs and symptoms of infection, which are usually obvious in the normal host, can be very subtle in the immunosuppressed transplant recipient. Febrile episodes after renal transplantation commonly occur during the first 4 months after transplantation, and the majority are associated with infection.[239] This is true for any series of patients reported, independent of the immunosuppressive regimen used. However, the absence of fever does not rule out infection; some patients with systemic infections may present with a low-grade temperature or may even be afebrile. Similarly, patients with systemic infections may not mount a rise in their white blood cell count. Therefore, infectious complications must be included in the differential diagnosis even when the patient does not present with classical signs and symptoms.

Empiric antimicrobial therapy may be given for a suspected infection, but the goal should be to make an accurate diagnosis as rapidly as possible, so that the most appropriate antimicrobial agents can be administered. Since most infections occurring after transplantation are nosocomial, it is helpful to be familiar with the common hospital microbial isolates specific to a particular institution and to use these data when empiric treatment is given. For example, in our hospital *Enterobacter cloacae* is usually sensitive to imipenem-cilastatin and amikacin and resistant to all other antibiotics; vancomycin-resistant *Enterococcus faecium* has emerged recently as an important pathogen; and occasionally, we encounter cases of *Legionella pneumophila* pneumonia.

Invasive diagnostic procedures are sometimes required to establish a diagnosis. Such procedures are best carried out expeditiously; obviously, the opportunity to achieve a successful outcome diminishes with delay in making an accurate diagnosis.

Transplant recipients may have infections caused by several etiologic agents appearing simultaneously.[240] For example, infections accompanying cryptococcosis in one study included tuberculous meningitis, *Pneumocystis carinii* pneumonia, and nocardiosis.[241] Therefore, concurrent infections should be considered in patients who are not responding to initial treatment.

▲ RISK FACTORS FOR INFECTION

Three major risk factors are associated with infectious complications after renal transplantation: technical problems, the degree of immunosuppression, and recent or remote exposure to infectious agents. Bacterial infections usually occur in the first month following transplantation, and technical factors may play an important etiologic role (see the section on surgical complications in this chapter).[242] Examples include urosepsis associated with ureteral obstruction or leak, or mycotic pseudoaneurysm of the vascular anastomosis.[243] The presence of foreign bodies may also play a role; for example, urinary tract infections are more common when ureteral stents are used.[244] Contaminated allograft preservation solutions may also be associated with an increased incidence of infection, although some studies showed no definite correlation.[245] Documented infection in the donor lower urinary tract usually does not represent a contraindication to the use of the kidney; on the other hand, donor upper tract infection generally contraindicates transplantation.[246]

The type and amount of immunosuppression play an important role in the pathogenesis of infectious complications. Cadaveric kidney recipients tend to develop more frequent and severe infectious complications than living donor recipients because of the increased immunosuppression required in the former group. Recipients of cadaveric kidneys who receive induction antilymphocyte preparations have higher infection rates than recipients who do not.[242] Patients receiving azathioprine as the primary immunosuppressive agent have been reported to have more infections than patients receiving cyclosporine.[247–250] In particular, patients receiving azathioprine had more severe nonviral infections, such as *Staphylococcus pneumonia* and bacteremia.[251,252]

Beginning in 1989, we began using a new immunosuppressive agent, tacrolimus (FK 506), for primary[253] and rescue therapy[254] of renal transplant patients at our institution. Nonviral infection rates in patients receiving tacrolimus have been somewhat lower than in patients receiving cyclosporine-based immunosuppression, probably as a result of lower steroid and antilymphocyte preparation requirements.[255,256]

Finally, it is extremely important to determine during the recipient evaluation if the patient has lived in or visited endemic areas. A patient may acquire a primary infection or may reactivate an infection that had been acquired remotely. For example, certain fungal infections, including histoplasmosis, coccidioidomycosis, and blastomycosis, which are unique to certain geographical areas, may become reactivated after transplantation. *Strongyloides stercoralis,* a helminth, may be carried for many years after visiting or living in an endemic area and cause symptoms when the patient is immunosuppressed.[257]

▲ TIMING OF INFECTION

The timing of infections after transplantation can provide clues to the more likely etiologic agents. Rubin has described three time periods: the first month, when infections are mostly related to technical and mechanical problems; from1 to 6 months, where 2/3 of the febrile illnesses are caused by cytomegalovirus (CMV); and beyond 6 months, when the pattern of infection in patients on stable maintenance immunosuppression with well-functioning allografts is usually similar to that seen in the general population.[257–259] Renal transplant patients who develop opportunistic infections after 6 months usually have higher serum creatinine levels, are receiving higher doses of maintenance steroids, and have had recurrent rejection episodes and chronic viral infections.[260]

▲ BACTERIAL DISEASES

Urinary tract infections and urosepsis are the most common infectious complications after renal transplantation. Most episodes of bacteremia in kidney transplant recipients originate from the urinary tract and occur within the first 3 months after transplantation; almost all occur within 1 year.[261] In one series, 58% of bacteremic episodes originated in or around the urinary tract.[261] Other sources of bacteremia may include the surgical wound, the lungs, and the perinephric space.[262] With the use of perioperative antibiotic prophylaxis, transplant wound infections are now relatively uncommon. In a recent series from our institution, most bacteremic episodes in renal transplant patients occurred more than a year following transplantation, and

44% were community acquired.[263] Aerobic gram-negative bacteria constituted 48% of bacteremia isolates, with *E. coli, Klebsiella,* and other Enterobacteriaceae being the major pathogens and the urinary tract being the primary source.[263] This suggests that the kidney transplant recipient may still be at risk for the development of graft pyelonephritis more than 1 year following transplantation. Transplant vesicoureteral reflux is a known risk factor for graft pyelonephritis and is described elsewhere in this chapter.

Other Bacteria

Listeria monocytogenes. This is, at present, an uncommon pathogen. Most of the reported cases of listeriosis are in kidney transplant recipients.[264] In one series, 7 of 9 patients with listeriosis developed the disease within the first month following transplantation, usually after treatment for rejection.[265] The mortality was 30%, and recurrent disease was relatively common. While CNS infection is always a possibility in *Listeria* bacteremia, primary bacteremia was more common in this population, and a secondary focus of infection was not found in most cases.[265] *Listeria* bacteremia may be associated with gastroenteritis, because the organism may be ingested and transmigrate through the bowel wall.[266] Since listeriosis has been reported after ingestion of cheese and other dairy products,[266] the transplant recipient should be judicious in the consumption of these products, especially when they are obtained from unknown sources. Although *Listeria* fecal carriage is not higher in kidney transplant patients than in the general population, its presence in the gut is associated with cheese consumption and the use of H2 antagonists.[267] It tends to occur seasonally and is more frequent during the summer months (July and August).[267] The treatment of listeriosis usually requires intravenous penicillin or ampicillin, with gentamicin usually added for synergy. In recent years, we have seen a decrease in the incidence of listeriosis among our transplant recipients. This is most likely due to the routine use of trimethoprim-sulfamethoxazole for *Pneumocystis carinii* prophylaxis (discussed below).

Nocardia asteroides. This is a filamentous gram-negative soil organism that can cause pneumonia and can frequently disseminate to the brain and result in an abscess formation. In a patient with both pneumonia and brain abscess, *Nocardia* should be considered as the likely etiologic agent. Although in most of the reported cases, *Nocardia asteroides* was the causative agent, other *Nocardia* species can infect kidney transplant patients, including *Nocardia brasiliensis* and *Nocardia transversalis.*[268] The treatment is typically with sulfa drugs, but combination therapy with amikacin and cefotaxime may be indicated for synergy. Drug sensitivity testing may be useful, but only a few laboratories are able to provide these tests. It is important to remember that nocardiosis tends to relapse after treatment, and, therefore, long treatment courses (6 weeks to 6 months) are usually required.[269] The overall mortality of nocardiosis in kidney transplant recipients is 25% but may increase to 44% in patients with CNS involvement.[270]

Mycobacteria. The incidence of tuberculosis after kidney transplantation is low in the United States but is higher in less well-developed countries. In one series reported from Brazil, it was 5.6%; interestingly, four patients presented with tuberculous interstitial nephritis.[271] In India, the incidence is even higher (>10%). Mycobacterial disease should be considered in any patient with a fever of unclear etiology.[272] The patient should be questioned regarding possible exposure to tuberculosis or travel in endemic areas. There is also an increased incidence of atypical mycobacteria infections among kidney transplant recipients,[273] and all reported cases with cutaneous tuberculosis have been caused by atypical mycobacteria.[274] Cooper reported 10 patients with *M. chelonae* skin lesions, none of whom were systemically ill.[275]

Most cases of *M. tuberculosis* infections in kidney transplant recipients are due to reactivation of old tuberculous lesions.[274] Treatment of active tuberculosis caused by *M. tuberculosis* should be initiated with four antituberculous agents, because of the recent emergence of isoniazid (INH)-resistant and multidrug resistant tuberculosis. It is recommended to start with INH, rifampin, pyrazinamide, and ethambutol or streptomycin, and later to adjust treatment according to sensitivities. It should be remembered that rifampin can accelerate the hepatic metabolism of cyclosporine and tacrolimus, so that rejection can be a sequela to the treatment of tuberculosis. However, it should be pointed out that immunosuppression should usually be stopped as part of the overall therapy of tuberculosis, and that loss of the allograft is generally of secondary importance. Rejection may in theory imply an improved prognosis because its occurrence indicates a preserved or recovering recipient immune response.

Treatment of atypical tuberculosis of the skin generally does not require systemic therapy, but systemic therapy is required for visceral disease. Drug treatment of atypical tuberculosis is not at all similar to that for *M. tuberculosis*.[276]

Salmonellosis. In tropical countries, nontyphoidal salmonellosis occurs commonly in kidney transplant recipients. The patient usually presents with a febrile illness and bacteremia; only 50% of patients have diarrhea. *Salmonella* has a unique vascular tropism and may localize in an arterial stump of a transplanted allograft, in a vascular graft aneurysm, or in an arteriovenous fistula. The usual treatment of *Salmonella* infection consists of ampicillin or amoxicillin, but ampicillin-resistant bacteria can be treated successfully with ciprofloxacin.[277]

▲ VIRAL DISEASES

Cytomegalovirus. Cytomegalovirus (CMV) is the most frequent single cause of infectious complications after kidney transplantation. The reported incidence (50–90%) of CMV infection has remained relatively constant over time.[278–280] This is because of the fact that CMV infection, like the other herpes viruses, results in a latent infection that may reactivate under immunosuppression.[281] Almost all CMV seropositive recipients reactivate their latent virus after kidney transplantation. This can be demonstrated by a rise in antibody titer or by a positive culture of the virus. However, the clinical manifestations of this infection vary widely, and fewer than 20% of patients actually develop symptoms related to CMV infection. These patients most often develop disease with the donor strain of CMV.

Several factors influence the development of symptomatic CMV infection after kidney transplantation. The most important is the CMV serologic status of donor and recipient. Primary infections in seronegative recipients are more often clinically evident and induce more severe disease than reactivation infections. The most severe form is usually observed when a CMV-seronegative recipient receives a graft from a CMV-seropositive donor.[282–284] Superinfection in a CMV-seropositive recipient with a new strain of virus originating from the donor seropositive organ occurs in about 50% of secondary infections according to some studies. Symptomatic CMV infection secondary to superinfection is more common than symptomatic disease secondary to reactivation.[285,286]

A second factor is related to host cell–mediated immunity, which is the main defense against CMV infection. MHC-linked immunologic phenomena may be involved: for example, some CMV antigens possess homology with HLA-DR.[287] Other studies have shown a correlation of symptomatic CMV infection and donor/recipient matching for DR 7[288] or alternatively, an association between HLA-B and DR incompatibilities.[289] Although CMV infection does not produce alterations in lymphocyte subset counts after kidney transplantation,[290] a CD4 count below 200/mm^3 has been associated with the development of CMV pneumonitis, the most severe clinical form of CMV disease.[291] Activation of CD8 lymphocytes and natural killer (NK) cells in peripheral blood appeared to accompany asymptomatic infection, whereas a low CD8 count was associated with a relapse of CMV after ganciclovir therapy.[292]

The third factor that influences the incidence of CMV infection, and probably the most important, is the type and amount of immunosuppressive therapy.[260] Both the cytotoxic drugs, such as azathioprine and cyclophosphamide and the antilymphocyte antibodies, such as ATG and OKT3, have been associated with CMV infection.[281,293] Of these agents, the polyclonal and monoclonal antilymphocyte antibodies have the highest CMV-promoting effect and represent the most important factor in the development of CMV infection after transplantation.[294,295] The use of cyclosporine has not been associated with significant changes in the morbidity of CMV infection, compared to azathioprine.[252] With the new immunosuppressive agent tacrolimus, the incidence of CMV infections has been similar to that observed under cyclosporine.[255,256]

The most common form of CMV disease is a viral syndrome characterized by fever, leukopenia, lymphocytosis, and the presence of atypical lymphocytes in the peripheral blood. Interstitial pneumonia is the most serious manifestation of CMV infection. CMV disease may also produce ulcerations in the gastrointestinal tract (most often in the cecum or colon), which may be complicated by bleeding or, rarely, perforation.

Demonstration of CMV in clinical samples, by isolation of the virus or demonstration of its nucleic acid or antigens in tissues, is the main approach for the diagnosis of CMV infection. The availability of specific antibodies against CMV antigens has permitted an early detection of CMV infection. The most widely used diagnostic technique is the shell vial, which can detect the presence of CMV by indirect immunofluorescence after 16 hours of incubation. An antigenemia test based on the detection of a CMV protein in peripheral blood leukocytes permits even earlier recognition of CMV infection.[292,296] Furthermore, the level of antigenemia seems to correlate with the clinical severity of disease.[297] Another new rapid diagnostic technique is the detection of CMV DNA by amplification using the polymerase chain reaction (PCR). Although this method has been demonstrated to be a rapid technique for monitoring CMV infections after kidney transplantation,[298] its very high sensitivity may yield a significant incidence of false-positive results.[299] The role of these new techniques for routine surveillance, diagnosis, and monitoring of treatment during CMV infection is currently under clinical evaluation.

The treatment of CMV presents several unique problems in comparison with other herpes viruses. As a member of the herpes family, CMV would be expected to respond to the same antiviral agents as herpes simplex. However, CMV lacks virus-specific thymidine kinase, which can activate nucleoside antiviral agents.[300] The antiviral ganciclovir suppresses the virus, but fails to eliminate it, and infection can reappear after the drug is discontinued. Ganciclovir has been effective in suppressing CMV disease after kidney transplantation,[301] even if allograft rejection is present.[302] Leukopenia is the main side effect of the drug, and can occasionally be severe enough to require its discontinuation. The administration of granulocyte colony stimulating factor (G-CSF) in this circumstance can allow rapid reinstitution of antiviral therapy.[303] Foscarnet is also an effective drug to treat CMV disease.[304] However, its nephrotoxicity makes its use problematic after kidney transplantation. Foscarnet is usually used after failure of ganciclovir therapy, or in cases of severe neutropenia not responding to G-CSF. The routine use of cytomegalovirus immunoglobulin in active CMV disease is controversial. In one report of CMV pneumonia in bone marrow recipients, the use of ganciclovir in combination with cytomegalovirus immunoglobulin was associated with much better survival when compared with previous antiviral regimens.[305]

Other Viral Infections.

Epstein-Barr Virus. Epstein-Barr virus (EBV) infection can be found in up to 40–70% of transplant recipients.[260] As in CMV infection, the highest risk is in seronegative recipients of organs from seropositive donors, who can develop primary infection within 3 months after transplantation.[306] It is likely that EBV is transmitted in latent form from the donor organ. Since the prevalence of adults seronegative for EBV is generally less than 5%, the major impact of primary infection is seen in the pediatric population.

The most important manifestation of EBV infection in transplant recipients is posttransplant lymphoproliferative disorder (PTLD). This is a B cell proliferation that may range from a benign polyclonal B cell hyperplasia to a malignant B cell lymphoma.[307] This proliferation is thought to be the result of suppression of cytotoxic T-lymphocyte (CTL) function secondary to immunosuppressive therapy.[308] Active CTL are probably needed to control latently EBV-infected B cells. The duration and the type of immunosuppression, particularly the use of antilymphocyte antibodies, are important factors that have been associated with the development of PTLD.[309] Although acyclovir and ganciclovir show some activity in inhibiting EBV in vitro, there is only anecdotal evidence that these agents are effective clinically. PTLD is usually treated with reduction or elimination of immunosuppression in combination with antiviral therapy. Chemotherapy or radiotherapy are reserved for those patients who do not respond to this conservative therapeutic approach. Some of these patients develop a true monoclonal EBV-induced malignancy. An encouraging experience with an anti-B cell monoclonal antibody has been reported, with 50% of patients disease-free after a median follow-up of three years.[310] Early identification of circulating EBV DNA and EBV antigens before onset of clinical disease may be helpful tools for instituting preemptive therapy for EBV infection in transplant recipients.[311,312]

Herpes Simplex Virus. Herpes simplex virus (HSV) is a common infection in transplant recipients. Over 60% of patients have circulating antibodies, which indicates previous exposure to the virus.[313] This suggests that most HSV infection occurring after kidney transplantation represents reactivation of latent virus. Although HSV infection is usually limited to mucocutaneous areas, systemic infections, such as hepatitis, or even disseminated HSV infection, may occur after kidney transplantation.[314]

Varicella-Zoster Virus. Children who receive a kidney transplant are at higher risk for severe varicella infection compared to nonimmunosuppressed patients. Administration of hyperimmune globulin (varicella-zoster immune globulin—V-ZIG) within 96 hours of a known exposure to varicella-zoster virus (VZV) and prompt institution of intravenous acyclovir therapy once symptoms and signs of varicella develop are recommended and are usually effective in preventing serious complications.[315] Alternative treatments, such as varicella vaccination in transplant candidates and the use of oral acyclovir after contact with VZV have not yet been systematically studied in the ESRD population.

Reactivation of herpes zoster infection (shingles) may occur in as many as 15–30% of kidney transplant patients, most often in the first 6 months after transplantation.[316] These episodes are usually self-limited, but on occasion systemic dissemination may occur. Intravenous, followed by oral, acyclovir therapy will usually prevent such complications and will accelerate healing of cutaneous lesions. Recently, famciclovir and valacyclovir, which are acyclovir analogues, have been introduced into clinical use. The acyclovir analogues have a similar antiviral activity with improved bioavailability after oral administration.[317] Clinical trials are under way.

Hepatitis B and C Virus. Liver disease is an important cause of morbidity and mortality after kidney transplantation. Liver dysfunction has been reported to occur in 7–24% of kidney recipients,[318,319] and end-stage liver disease has been the cause of death in as many as 8–28% of these patients.[320,321] Despite a low frequency of hepatitis B surface antigen (HBsAg) carriage in kidney-allograft recipients (less than 5%),[320] the incidence of chronic liver disease after kidney transplantation has not decreased.[321] This is due to the important role of hepatitis C (HCV) infection in kidney transplant recipients. The prevalence of HCV-antibody positivity is kidney transplant candidates is as high as 50% in some populations[322] and is thought to be the cause of liver disease in as many as 20% of kidney transplant recipients.[322]

The information about the risk of transplanting a kidney from an HCV seropositive donor is contradictory and incomplete. A recent study showed a 48% incidence of HCV hepatitis after organ transplantation when the donor was HCV-antibody positive.[323] On the other hand it has been demonstrated that HCV-positive kidney allografts can be safely transplanted into HCV-positive recipients without a major risk of severe liver disease, at least in the short term[324] (see also Chapter 4). Progression to chronic active hepatitis and cirrhosis occurs in 10–20% of patients infected with HCV, usually over a period of 10 or more years.[325] However, it appears that under immunosuppressive therapy, the course of this disease tends to be more rapid.[326] Long-term follow-up studies comparing the outcomes of transplantation and dialysis in patients with anti-HCV antibodies are necessary to answer questions about the utility of transplantation in these patients.

▲ FUNGAL DISEASE

Although there has been an overall decrease in the rate of systemic fungal infections in kidney transplant recipients, these infections are still associated with very high mortality. In some third-world countries, the rate of systemic fungal infections after KTX is still relatively high (6%), most commonly presenting with prolonged fever not responding to antibiotic therapy.[327] The most frequent fungal infections reported in early series from this country included candidiasis, cryptococcosis, and aspergillosis.[328,329]

Candidida Infection. The most common fungal infection after transplantation is candidiasis. *Candida albicans* usually colonizes mucosa and may cause superficial mucositis, such as esophagitis or cystitis. Rarely, *Candida* may cause deep infections.[330] It may also involve the arterial vascular anastomoses (mycotic pseudoaneurysm) and jeopardize survival of the allograft and/or the patient by causing arterial rupture.[331] The presence of *Candida* in the urine should be investigated to rule out infection of the upper urinary tract and should be treated adequately, even when the colony count is less than 100,000 colonies per mL. A case of *Candida* allograft pyelonephritis has been diagnosed by fine-needle aspiration cytology. The patient was febrile and grew 16,000 colonies/mL of *Candida albicans* in the urine at day 15 after transplantation.[332] *Candida* urinary tract infection may be associated with prolonged use of ureteral stents, and in one report was complicated with *Candida* endophthalmitis.[333]

Amphotericin B is the drug of choice for *Candida* and most other fungal infections in transplant patients, but it is notoriously nephrotoxic. When given in high doses, it may act synergistically with cyclosporine or tacrolimus to impair renal function. The recent introduction into clinical use of liposome-encapsulated amphotericin B is promising. These preparations are expensive, but they do allow treatment with high doses with relatively low nephrotoxicity.[334] Fluconazole is quite effective for treatment of candidiasis in transplant patients, but this agent (and all triazoles) can interfere with the hepatic metabolism of cyclosporine and tacrolimus, thereby raising their respective blood levels.[335,336] Therefore, transplant patients receiving triazoles should have careful monitoring of cyclosporine or tacrolimus levels,[337] with appropriate dosage reduction as needed. Although fluconazole is effective against *C. albicans,* some other *Candida* species, such as *Torulopsis glabrata* and *Candida krusei,* are often resistant to it.

Aspergillosis. This is the second most frequent fungal infection in transplant patients. It is commonly associated with unsealed building construction and remodeling work, which can lead to dispersion of the fungal spores, which are then inhaled. The most common species causing disease in transplant patients are *Aspergillus fumigatus* and *Aspergillus flavus*. The fungus typically causes pneumonia. Vascular invasion leads to central infarction, cavitary lesions, and abscesses. CNS lesions often occur with or without pulmonary disease.[338,339] Since *Aspergillus* is a common contaminant of upper airways and laboratories, the definitive diagnosis of invasive disease may be difficult. Because of the high fatality rate associated with aspergillosis, it should be assumed that the fungus is invasive. It is wise to start treatment with high-dose amphotericin B, 0.5 mg/kg/day or more, while proceeding with further diagnostic procedures to confirm or rule out the diagnosis of invasive disease.

Cryptococcus neoformans. After *Candida*, this is the second most common yeast infection in renal transplant patients, and, in some third-world countries, it is the most common systemic fungal infection after kidney transplantation.[340] Infection usually occurs months or years after transplantation and is associated with a poor prognosis in kidney transplant patients. The symptoms are subtle, most characteristically low-grade fever and headache. In one series the mean time of diagnosis was 48 months after transplantation.[241] Although most cases are diagnosed with meningitis, some are diagnosed with pneumonia or skin lesions. Whenever *Cryptococcus* is recovered from one site, it is always necessary to search for dissemination in other sites. Attempts should be made to grow the yeast from specimens of lumbar fluid, sputum, blood, and urine.

Other Fungal Infections. If the history includes exposure in an area endemic for histoplasmosis, coccidioidomycosis, or blastomycosis, one should consider these in the differential diagnosis of any febrile illness.[341]

▲ PROTOZOAL INFECTION

Pneumocystis carinii. With the introduction of trimethoprim-sulfamethoxazole prophylaxis, the incidence of *Pneumocystis carinii* pneumonia (PCP) has decreased dramatically in most transplant centers. Prior to this prophylaxis, the reported incidence of PCP ranged from 5 to 10%.[342,343] PCP is usually considered a late infection after transplantation. Twelve of 14 cases of PCP in our institution occurred in the third and fourth month after transplantation.[344] The few cases of PCP at our institution that have occurred since the introduction of routine prophylaxis were in patients that did not take (or did not receive) their medication. Treatment is with high-dose trimethoprim-sulfamethoxazole or pentamidine, and reduction or cessation of immunosuppression.

Toxoplasma gondii. While the normal host usually develops a febrile illness or lymphadenopathy after infection with this organism, the immunocompromised host may develop visceral disease with pneumonitis, meningo-encephalitis, or myocarditis.[345] The risk for development of toxoplasmosis is relatively low after kidney transplantation, and most patients will not manifest clinical disease even when they exhibit a rising titer.[346,347] This may be related to the routine use of trimethoprim-sulfamethoxazole prophylaxis in most transplant centers. The diagnosis is usually made on the basis of a rise in titer with a compatible clinical picture. It is possible to grow the protozoa in a fibroblast cell culture of blood or other body fluids.[348] *Toxoplasma* trophozoites may be seen in the brochoalveolar lavage fluid of patients with pulmonary infiltrates using Giemsa or Wright stain,[349] and in cases of dissemination, bone marrow biopsy may show intracellular and extracellular trophozoites.[350] Although quite rare, there have been several reports of toxoplasmosis transmitted from the kidney allograft to seronegative recipients causing disseminated toxoplasmosis.[246,351] The clinician should be aware of this possibility when a seronegative patient receives a kidney allograft from a seropositive donor.

▲ PARASITES

It is important to identify and treat patients with parasitic infections at the time of the transplant evaluation, since undiagnosed infections may become worse on immunosuppression. A good example is infection with *Strongyloides stercoralis*. Of 37 cases reviewed by DeVault, 33 patients traveled to or lived in an endemic area, and onset of strongyloidiasis symptoms occurred between 3 weeks and 114 months after kidney transplantation.[352] The mortality was 50% in the hyperinfection syndrome and 71% with disseminated strongyloidiasis. In the hyperinfection syndrome, there are usually gastrointestinal symptoms, such as diarrhea, vomiting, and abdominal pain, but the larvae remain in the gut. In the dissemination syndrome, the larvae migrate outside of the GI tract, and the patient may present with gram-negative sepsis, lung infiltrates, or gram-negative meningitis, and may not necessarily have eosinophilia.[352] To confirm the diagnosis, larvae need to be isolated from the stool, duodenal aspirate, or respiratory secretions. The treatment is with thiabendazole, which can also be given for prophylaxis (oral thiabendazole 25 mg, twice a day, for 2 days or longer).[352] Prophylaxis with thiabendazole should be considered in transplant candidates who come from an endemic area (southern United States, South America, Africa, Asia, South Pacific).[352]

▲ COMMON SYNDROMES

Urinary Tract Infection

Urinary tract infections usually occur early after transplantation and may or may not be associated with urologic complications. Usually they are secondary to gram-negative organisms such as *Escherichia coli* or *Klebsiella*. Allograft pyelonephritis should be considered in a febrile patient who presents with deterioration of renal function more than a year after transplantation.[263,353] In 1100 consecutive renal transplant patients summarized by Pearson, the presenting symptoms of pyelonephritis included fever, allograft tenderness, and positive urine cultures.[354] *Escherichia coli* was the causative organism in 16 of 20 (80%) episodes of pyelonephritis, and 9 patients had evidence of asymptomatic bacteriuria before the onset of pyelonephritis.[354] After kidney transplantation, vesicoureteral reflux may occur in 10–44% of patients, and 35–79% of patients may have asymptomatic bacteriuria.[355] Some of these asymptomatic lower urinary tract infections may progress to cause pyelonephritis.[355] Although patients with vesicoureteral reflux have an increased incidence of allograft pyelonephritis, using an antireflux surgical technique was not associated with a reduced incidence of UTI, according to some authors.[356,357]

Pneumonia

The most common etiologic agents are nosocomial gram-negative and gram-positive organisms, such as *Klebsiella, Enterobacter, Pseudomonas,* and *Staphylococcus*. Other pathogens include *Legionella, Aspergillus,* and *Mycobacterium tuberculosis*.[358] *Legionella pneumophila* and *Legionella micdadei* are the most common *Legionella* isolates to cause pneumonia in the immunocompromised host, but other *Legionella* species have been reported.[359] The drug of choice for legionellosis has been considered to be erythromycin, an antibiotic which interferes with cyclosporine and tacrolimus metabolism and causes elevation of their blood levels. Recently, we have successfully treated several cases of *Legionella* in transplant patients with ciprofloxacin.[360] As a general rule, if no adequate sputum is obtainable for diagnosis, bronco-alveolar lavage is required, and if it is not revealing, more invasive procedures should be considered, including transbronchial biopsy or thoracoscopic open lung biopsy.

Abdominal Infection

Some infections may originate in the GI tract and secondarily disseminate to other organs.[361] Sutherland et al described a syndrome of gastrointestinal bleeding in kidney transplant patients who were maintained on azathioprine and prednisone and had been treated with 2 weeks of antilymphocyte globulin. The patients developed primary CMV infection, classically of the cecum, and the resected colon specimen showed multiple ulcers.[362]

An early series from the University of Minnesota showed that diffuse peritonitis carries a very high mortality rate after kidney transplantation.[363] Seven of 12 patients in this series had a technical problem associated with their transplant operation, and four patients had deep infections of the retroperitoneal space, which ruptured into the peritoneal cavity.[363]

Colonic rupture with peritonitis after kidney transplantation can be secondary to pseudo-obstruction (see Chapter 7) or diverticulitis;[364] other etiologies include CMV or ischemic colitis. Since the symptoms and signs may be very subtle, the clinician should always consider abdominal sepsis when the source of infection cannot be established.

Wound Infection

Most wound infections after kidney transplantation are caused by staphylococcus and gram-negative organisms, and some infections may derive from contaminated urine.[365] Twenty years ago Kyriakides et al reported a wound infection rate of 6.1% in azathioprine-treated patients, and 3.5% involved the perinephric space.[366] The rate is currently less than 1%, and perinephric infections are rare. Perioperative antibiotic prophylaxis, the use of topical antimicrobials in the operative field, and elimination of bladder contaminants have been highly effective.[367] Deep wound infections are serious and are associated with a high rate of sepsis, mycotic pseudoaneurysm, allograft loss, and mortality.[366] The use of drains is generally associated with an increased rate of wound infection.[365] An unusual organism that may cause purulent infections, including peritonitis and wound infections, is *Mycoplasma hominis*.[368,369] Typically the gram stain in this infection shows many white cells, without organisms. Since this bacteria may be a colonizer of the urinary tract, this infection may be associated with a urinary leak.[369,370]

Meningitis

In transplant patients with clinical evidence of meningitis, *Listeria monocytogenes* and *Cryptococcus neoformans* should be considered as possible etiologic agents. Signs of meningismus may not necessarily be present and, therefore, every patient with symptoms of headache, "slight" confusion, or change in behavior should be assessed carefully, and lumbar puncture should be performed.[371] In one series, 7 of 11 (64%) cases of meningitis after kidney transplantation were due to *Cryptococcus neo-*

formans.[372] In another series, only 1 of 11 (9%) patients with *Cryptococcus neoformans* meningitis had nuchal rigidity, and the most common modes of presentation were fever, headache, confusion, and seizure.[373] Only 50% of patients with *Listeria* meningitis complained of headaches, and only 55% had signs of meningeal irritation; 25% had experienced seizures.[374]

Skin and Soft Tissue

Skin lesions may be primary infections or signs of disseminated infection. All skin lesions in systemically ill patients should be biopsied. Ulcerated or nodular skin lesions may be caused by atypical mycobacteria, *Nocardia,* or fungi (*Cryptococcus, Aspergillus, Candida,* dermatiaceous fungi).[353,375] In diabetics, skin and soft tissue infections present at the usual sites in the distal extremities, but are more severe and difficult to treat.[376] A hand infection in a diabetic may result in involvement of the deep space, osteomyelitis, or tenosynovitis and may require amputation.[371] Unhealed lower extremity wounds in diabetics are always potentially dangerous.

▲ PREVENTION AND PROPHYLAXIS OF INFECTION

Prevention of infectious complications (Table 11–8) after kidney transplantation starts at the time of the pretransplant evaluation, when it is possible to identify and resolve problems that might be exacerbated once the patient is placed on immunosuppression. Dental problems should be identified and treated before transplantation. Bacteremia originating from the oral cavity or fever secondary to an abscessed tooth may be confusing and problematic in the transplant patient. The evaluation is also a good time to discuss vaccination with the patient. Candidates should receive hepatitis B vaccine if they have not been previously immunized. Influenza and pneumococcal vaccines are also recommended by many authors.

Antimicrobial prophylaxis has played an important role in decreasing infectious complications after renal transplantation. The reduction in the incidence of wound infection illustrates this point. Rates of wound infection as high as 36% were reported in the early history of renal transplantation, when patients received no antibiotic wound prophylaxis. Improvement in surgical techniques, together with the use of systemic and topical antibiotics, have reduced the wound infection rate to 1%.[367] Trimethoprim-sulfamethoxazole prophylaxis (TMP-SMZ) has been shown to reduce the incidence of urinary tract infections in kidney transplant recipients during the first 4 months after transplantation.[378] TMP-SMZ prophylaxis is not only useful in the prevention of urinary tract infections and *Pneumocystis carinii* pneumonia, but may also prevent other infections caused by *Legionella, Listeria, Nocardia,* and *Toxoplasma*.[379]

TABLE 11-8 ▲ INFECTION PROPHYLAXIS

Bacterial	
Perioperative	Cefazolin IV 1 g preoperatively and every 8 hr for 3 doses postoperatively, bladder wash with cefazolin and/or neomycin 0.25%, and topical antibiotic irrigation (1 g cefazolin/1 L saline)
Long term	Oral trimethoprim/sulfamethoxazole 80 mg/400 mg per day, dose reduced to every other day when creatinine ≥ 2.5 mg%.
Viral	
CMV	Oral acyclovir 3200 mg/day in four divided doses for 6–12 months (adjusted for renal dysfunction). In seronegative recipients who receive a CMV positive organ, may use CMV hyperimmune globulin, or ganciclovir.
HSV	Oral acyclovir 200 mg bid or tid or 400 mg bid is adequate for prevention. In patients with recurrent oral or genital lesions, may use oral suppressive treatment for the duration of a year.
Fungal	
Candida	Nystatin suspension, 2–4 million units a day in four divided doses, orally or per nasogastric tube, for 3–4 months. Alternatively oral clotrimazole troches 10 mg qid. Oral fluconazole 50–100 mg a day also effective, but interferes with cyclosporine A and tacrolimus metabolism. May use solutions for irrigation of wound and bladder with amphotericin B (50 mg in 1 L of D5W).
Protozoal Parasites	
PCP	Oral trimethoprim/sulfamethoxazole as for bacterial prophylaxis, or oral Dapsone 50–100 mg per day, or aerosolized pentamidine 300 mg diluted in sterile water and given by inhalation every 4 weeks.
Toxoplasma gondii	Usually unnecessary, but in special situations oral pyrimethamine 25 mg a day for 6 weeks.
Strongyloides stercoralis	Oral thiabendazole 25 mg, twice a day, for two days or longer.

Bacterial Prophylaxis

Perioperative antibacterial prophylaxis employs a number of simple strategies. Before the transplant procedure begins, the patient receives an intravenous dose of antibiotic. Antibiotics commonly used include cefazolin, cefamandole, and ampicillin/sulbactam.[380] Prophylaxis is usually given for no more than 24 hours after transplantation. In addition, after placement of the Foley catheter, the bladder is instilled with an antibiotic solution (eg, 0.25% neomycin) and the catheter is clamped. Finally, during the transplant procedure, the wound is frequently irrigated with a topical antibiotic-containing solution (eg, 1 g cefazolin in 1 L saline).

In addition to the above measures, there is evidence that trimethoprim-sulfamethoxazole prophylaxis, which is mainly given to prevent *Pneumocystis carinii* (see below), is also useful in reducing the rate of bacterial infections after kidney transplantation.[381]

With regard to prophylaxis for dental procedures following transplantation, any standard regimen is likely to be useful. Currently, we use the American Heart Association recommendation of amoxicillin, 3.0 g orally one hour prior to, and 1.5 g 6 hours following any dental procedure. Alternative antibiotics include ampicillin, clindamycin, or vancomycin. Erythromycin is not recommended because of its interaction with cyclosporine and tacrolimus.

To test for exposure to tuberculosis, we routinely perform a PPD test and other anergy skin tests at the time of pretransplant evaluation. The antigens used in our center to assess anergy include *Trichophyton* and mumps. Some centers also use tetanus toxoid. It is advisable to retest PPD-negative patients periodically, especially after possible exposure to TB. Patients known to be PPD positive before transplantation should still get tested at the time of evaluation. To prevent an excessive reaction to PPD, the test should initially be done with lower strength (1 tuberculin unit); if negative, the test is repeated with regular strength (5 tuberculin unit). More than 50% of kidney transplant candidates are anergic (not responding to any skin test, including PPD), and skin tests are therefore often not meaningful for assessment of TB exposure. The renal transplant population, however, is highly susceptible to TB infection, with a high risk of progression to active disease.[382,383]

The need for INH prophylaxis should be evaluated on a case-by-case basis. In general we recommend INH prophylaxis in the following patients: (1) those born in endemic areas outside the United States, (2) patients with extensive travel experience, (3) patients who are HIV seropositive, (4) patients who are PPD positive or who have had a recent skin test conversion (from negative to positive), (5) patients with a history of tuberculosis, even if adequately treated in the past, (6) anergic patients with a negative PPD, but with a history of exposure to tuberculosis, or with radiologic changes suggestive of old tuberculosis.

In patients requiring prophylaxis, INH is usually given at a dose of 300 mg together with vitamin B_6 50 mg (for prevention of peripheral neuropathy caused by INH). The optimal duration of INH prophylaxis is unclear. Some recommend prophylaxis for life in immunosuppressed patients. In our institution, we prefer to use 6 months of prophylaxis following transplantation. The issue of whether to give prophylaxis to patients who have had full treatment for active tuberculosis in the past is controversial. We have chosen to give INH prophylaxis in these cases, since it is not clear if past treatment has eradicated all mycobacteria.[273]

Viral Prophylaxis

Prophylaxis with ganciclovir has been reported to be effective in prevention of CMV disease in bone marrow, heart, and liver transplantation.[384–386] In one report in high-risk kidney transplant recipients, prophylaxis with ganciclovir delayed CMV infection but did not prevent its occurrence.[387] In another report, both ganciclovir and immunoglobulin were effective in prevention of CMV in the same population when compared to historical controls.[388] High-dose oral acyclovir and CMV hyperimmune globulin[389,390] have been used separately and together for prevention of CMV disease after KTX. A course of 12 weeks of oral acyclovir, 3200 mg per day, significantly decreased the incidence of symptomatic CMV infection after kidney transplantation.[389] While these results have been confirmed by other authors in seropositive recipients,[391] the beneficial effect of acyclovir prophylaxis in seronegative recipients of seropositive grafts is not universally accepted.[392] Similar contradictory results have been reported with the use of nonspecific hyperimmune globulin[393–396] and CMV hyperimmune globulin.[390,397] These discrepant results may reflect differences in various factors that influence CMV infection (as described above).

Low-dose acyclovir prophylaxis has been demonstrated to prevent reactivation of latent HSV infection after kidney transplantation.[398] However, this policy has been questioned by some authors, who argue that the frequency and severity of HSV disease after kidney transplantation is relatively low and does not justify routine prophylaxis.[399]

Fungal Prophylaxis

Prophylaxis of *Candida* mucositis is generally recommended after renal transplantation. Oral nystatin suspension, 2–4 million units per day, is given for the first 3–4 months after transplantation. In diabetics, nystatin prophylaxis may need to be continued longer or even indefinitely. Clotrimazole troches are a useful alternative to nystatin.

The new triazole, fluconazole, has also been used for fungal prophylaxis. In one center, it is being given for 2 weeks in cases of asymptomatic candiduria.[382] Intravenous amphotericin B may also be used for prophylaxis at low dose of 0.2–0.3 mg/kg/day, up to 20 mg/day, in high-risk patients in intensive care units. It is not clear if this is effective in the prevention of invasive fungal infections.

Protozoal Prophylaxis

To prevent *Pneumocystis carinii* pneumonia, oral trimethoprim-sulfamethoxazole (80 mg trimethoprim + 400 mg sulfamethoxazole) is administered daily. In patients with a serum creatinine $\geq$ 2.5 mg/dL, the same dose may be given every other day. The dose is usually given orally or through an NG tube. In our institution, prophylaxis is given indefinitely because of the continued risk and high morbidity of *Pneumocystis* infections (the dose can be reduced to 3 times a week after 6–12 months). TMP-SMZ is stopped only in cases of true allergy to sulfa or if sensitization to the drug occurs after transplantation.

Other drugs used for prophylaxis are aerosolized pentamidine 300 mg diluted in 6 mL of sterile water given once per month, or oral dapsone at a dose of 100 mg given daily. Since dapsone is a sulfone, patients who manifest an allergy to TMP-SMZ may also develop an allergy to dapsone. Trimethoprim as a single agent without the sulfa component cannot be used for prevention of PCP.

Routine *Toxoplasma gondii* prophylaxis is not indicated. Although there have been some reports of transmission of *Toxoplasma gondii* by a kidney allograft, this is quite rare. In some solid organs, transmission of *Toxoplasma* is known to occur when an organ from a positive donor is transplanted into a seronegative recipient. The classic example is the heart transplant recipient. Prophylaxis with pyrimethamine is used to prevent toxoplasmosis in the seronegative recipient who receives an organ from a seropositive donor. The dose is oral pyrimethamine, 25 mg daily for 6 weeks.[400]

▲ THE FUTURE

Further improvements in morbidity and mortality associated with infection after transplantation hopefully will be accomplished by the development of new immunosuppressive agents potent enough to prevent rejection without the need for steroids and antilymphocyte preparations, development of new viral and fungal prophylactic agents, better handling of nosocomial infections through infection control measures, and earlier recognition of patients with irreversible allograft rejection, leading to prompt withdrawal of immunosuppression before overwhelming sepsis supervenes.

Neurologic Complications

Benjamin Eidelman

▲ INTRODUCTION

Neurologic complications are an important cause of morbidity and mortality in transplant patients. The risk to the nervous system arises even before organ transplantation. Organ failure creates an environment that puts the nervous system at risk, not only from the effects of the loss of function of the organ in question, but also from an accompanying state of disability that predisposes the nervous system to a variety of insults. This precarious state may carry through to, and persist following transplantation. The transplant procedure itself imperils the nervous system, although the risk may vary depending on the organ. Kidney transplantation, which is one of the least stressful, still involves general anesthesia, several hours of surgery, and the use of a variety of pharmacologic agents. These may singly, or in combination, further create stresses to the nervous system. Surgical complications carry over into the immediate posttransplantation phase, and as the patient recovers from the stress of surgery, there is a further period of vulnerability related to the use of immunosuppressive drugs and extending throughout the period of time that the individual keeps the transplanted organ.

Nervous system complications may be overt and readily recognizable, but in some patients the presentation may be quite subtle, and involvement of the nervous system becomes apparent only with the most careful clinical scrutiny. Even then, latent conditions may exist that may show themselves only over time or become apparent with exhaustive testing.

The ramifications of neurologic complications of transplantation are complex, but in most instances are of considerable importance. Neurologic events should not be considered in isolation, but in the overall context of the patient's general clinical picture. Thus, it is critical that the neurologist and the other members of the transplant team work in a collaborative manner. It is also important that the consulting neurologist have some understanding of transplantation, because without this knowledge the neurologic consultation becomes much less meaningful. Of equal importance is a need for other members of the transplant team to be aware of potential neurologic problems. In many instances the evolution of nervous system complications is slow, and signs and symptoms may often be misleading. In these circumstances, careful clinical observations, together with the judicious use of tests, may provide the answers, although the "waiting" phase may be frustrating to the other members of the transplant team.

Neurologists are sometimes regarded as the harbinger of some catastrophic event, and there may be some reluctance to obtain neurologic input or to do so very late. There are many situations where serious neurologic events do indeed occur. However, many neurologic events are of a relatively minor nature, and it is thus important to have a balanced perspective on the spectrum of nervous system complications that may apply to the transplant patient.

▲ GENERAL APPROACH TO NEUROLOGIC COMPLICATIONS OF THE TRANSPLANT PATIENT

Different neurologic complications occur at different times in the course of transplantation. This section will, therefore, be subdivided into the following categories:

1. Neurologic Complications of Renal Failure
2. The Operative and Perioperative Phase
3. Early Posttransplant Phase (First Month)
4. Late Posttransplant Phase (From One Month Onward)
5. Other Neurologic Disorders That May Occur in the Renal Transplant Recipient

▲ NEUROLOGIC COMPLICATIONS OF RENAL FAILURE

A patient whose general medical condition has deteriorated because of kidney failure is subject to an increased risk of neurologic complications. There are conditions related to the kidney failure itself, as well as complications of a more general nature related to the state of disability that develops in the presence of disturbed renal function. Sometimes multiorgan failure occurs, and this further increases the risk to the nervous system. Neurologic complications during this stage may thus be considered as follows.

Infection

There is an increased risk of infection in certain renal transplant candidates, particularly if they have been on dialysis.[401] There are many nervous system complications of infection. While these will be discussed in subsequent sections of this chapter, it is important to appreciate that sepsis may play a role in nervous system complications even prior to the introduction of immunosuppressive agents.

Cerebrovascular Disease

Renal transplant candidates are at risk for cerebrovascular complications of various types. There are many reasons for this. In the renal transplant candidate, hypertension is common,[402] and this predisposes to premature vascular disease, which in turn may lead to ischemic strokes. Diabetes is also prevalent in patients being considered for kidney transplantation,[403] and this also causes an increased risk of cerebrovascular disease and resultant ischemic strokes.

Seizures

Seizures may occur in the pretransplant phase as a complication of renal failure, infection, vascular events, or metabolic disturbances.[404] Toxic exposure can result from the effects of certain pharmacologic agents. There may often be multiple interacting factors giving rise to seizures.

Encephalopathy

Uremic encephalopathy is an important complication of renal failure. Encephalopathy does not relate to specific laboratory abnormalities, but rather appears to be a function of the rate of development of renal impairment. Thus, in acute renal failure, impairment of consciousness may occur in the presence of azotemia, yet in chronic renal failure there may be little or no disturbance of awareness in the presence of far greater metabolic abnormalities. The earliest signs of uremic encephalopathy are those of alterations in concentration and awareness.[405] As the condition progresses, the patient may become more withdrawn and eventually lapses into coma, which may vary in depth, from response to verbal stimulation to a state of complete unresponsiveness to all stimuli, including pain. In the early phases of uremic encephalopathy, a fluctuating level of awareness and consciousness may be evident, with marked variation in reactivity to environmental stimuli occurring over brief periods of time. Agitation, delirium, and hallucinatory behavior may also be apparent.

Movement Disorders

A variety of abnormal movements may be apparent in the presence of renal failure.

Tremulousness

Tremor is a common component of chronic renal failure.[406] Tremor tends to be most apparent during the course of motor activities and not present at rest. This is best demonstrated by having hands held in an outstretched position, where a somewhat irregular, coarse tremor may become apparent. This tremor may intrude into voluntary movements, creating a sense of clumsiness, and there is a resulting impairment of ability to carry out fine-skilled movements.

Asterixis

This will often develop in the wake of an initial tremulousness.[407] This movement is most obvious when the hands are held in an outstretched position with the wrists maintained in a position of hyperextension. There may be an initial period of latency, followed by a brief flexion movement of the fingers and wrist, and then an immediate extension maneuver that restores the hand to its previous posture. Asterixis is regarded as an inability to maintain a sustained extension posture, and it is apparent that the flexion component relates to an abolition of muscle contraction, as evidenced by complete electrical silence during the downward flexion phase. It is believed that asterixis relates to a central disturbance of motor control.

Myoclonus

Multifocal myoclonus commonly occurs in renal failure.[408] This is characterized by coarse twitching of various muscle groups, resulting in asymmetrical, multifocal muscle contractions. Any muscle may be affected, but the disturbance tends to be more prominent about the face and in proximal muscles.

Disturbances of Resting Posture

Increased muscle tone becomes apparent with prolonged renal failure.[409] Initially, the manifestations of this may relate to hyperactive tendon reflexes and accompanying clonus. As muscle tone increases, disturbed posturing of the limbs may become apparent. This may affect all limbs, resulting in a decortical type of posturing, and in some cases, an opisthotonos may also be apparent.

Peripheral Nervous System Complications

Peripheral neuropathy is a common neurologic complication of chronic renal failure.[409] The neuropathy is of the mixed sensory motor type, usually affecting the lower limbs, although the arms may also be involved. The neuropathy usually develops insidiously but in some situations may evolve rapidly. Distal sensory loss together with weakness and muscle atrophy are the hallmarks of the condition. In some patients sensory symptoms may be quite prominent, and these take the form of the "restless legs syndrome." This condition is characterized by uncomfortable dysesthetic symptoms, usually affecting the lower limbs, and the symptoms tend to be most obvious when the extremities are at rest. Patients may thus develop the habit of constantly moving their limbs in an attempt to decrease the intensity of these unpleasant sensory symptoms.

Damage to isolated peripheral nerves may occur during the course of placement of an arteriovenous shunt. This may result from direct trauma to the nerve, but "ischemic neuropathy" on the basis of a "steal syndrome" may also occur.[410] Neuropathy may also develop as a result of the general state of disability that occurs in renal failure. For example, patients who have lost a considerable amount of weight may also be prone to pressure palsy.[411] The peroneal nerve is frequently affected, producing a "foot drop."

Complications of Dialysis

Dialysis is an important cause of neurologic disability in the transplant candidate.

Dysequilibrium Syndrome

This is typically seen when hemodialysis is first initiated, particularly if fluid and electrolyte shifts occur too rapidly.[412] The characteristics of this syndrome are dehydration, weakness, nausea, vomiting, hypertension, muscle cramping, irritability, agitation, delirium, convulsions, and obtundation.

Headache

Headache is a common symptom in patients supported by dialysis.[413] Headache may be related to an exacerbation of preexisting migraine. There are many causes, but headaches may also occur as a specific complication of hemodialysis; they usually develop during the course of treatment but may sometimes become apparent after dialysis has been completed. The pain tends to be fairly diffuse and sometimes may have a throbbing characteristic. The development of a new headache or change in headache characteristic during the course of dialysis may be indicative of a structural disorder, such as a subdural hematoma.[414] This should prompt urgent evaluation, including imaging studies of the head.

Dialysis Dementia

A progressive decline in intellect may be encountered in patients who require chronic dialysis.[415] This syndrome usually becomes evident after a year or more of treatment, and there are many components to the syndrome.[416,417] One of the earlier symptoms relates to hesitancy of speech. This may in the early phases only be apparent during dialysis, but as time progresses abnormalities continue, even after dialysis is discontinued. The condition progresses to dysarthria, where speech may be unintelligible. There is usually an accompanying cognitive decline, and in some cases, delusional thinking, hallucinatory behavior, and convulsions may complicate the clinical picture. Movement disorders, specifically tremulousness and myoclonus, may also be present. Aluminum in the dialysate may be operative in causing the dementia.[418] The disorder may improve when the aluminum is removed from the dialysate. However, this may not be the only factor in the causation of dialysis dementia; although aluminum levels are generally higher in patients on dialysis,[419] specific experimental evidence linking aluminum to dementia is lacking.[420]

▲ THE OPERATIVE AND PERIOPERATIVE PHASE

The renal transplant procedure itself carries relatively little risk to the nervous system. The operation does not usually produce profound blood loss and hypotension, which could potentially lead to the development of central nervous system complications. Renal transplant patients, however, may be vulnerable to certain neurologic conditions that may be precipitated or unmasked by the stress of anesthesia and surgery. Thus, a cerebrovascular event, such as an ischemic stroke, may first manifest immediately after transplantation. End-stage renal failure may produce encephalopathy,[405] which may be mild and barely evident clinically, yet may manifest more dramatically in the postsurgical phase due to the effects of sedatives and other drugs used in the customary management of anesthetic and surgical procedures.[421] Similarly, seizures due to an underlying latent epileptogenic focus may manifest in the face of electrolyte disturbances, which may alter the seizure threshold.[422] There are additional conditions that may occur in the perioperative phase and impact on the nervous system.

Metabolic and Electrolyte Disturbances

Metabolic and electrolyte disturbances are common in the transplant patient. They may result from single or multiple organ failure, but pharmacologic agents, including the use of immunosuppressive drugs, may also play a role. Electrolyte imbalance, frequently encountered in the ICU or transplant unit, can have a profound effect on cerebral function. The following are the important metabolic and electrolyte complications with neurologic sequelae that have been described in transplant patients:

1. Hypercalcemia
2. Hypomagnesemia
3. Hypocalcemia
4. Hypokalemia
5. Hypernatremia
6. Hypophosphatemia

Hypercalcemia

Hypercalcemia may be encountered following kidney transplantation and may relate to a variety of mechanisms, including persistent hyperparathyroidism,[423] steroid therapy, vitamin D therapy, and magnesium deficiency. Changes in mental status are common accompaniments of hypercalcemia, particularly when levels rise above 14 mg/dL. Frequently seen features include lethargy and confusion, which may eventually merge into a state of coma.[424,425] Convulsions are rarely seen. These symptoms resolve promptly when the hypercalcemia is treated.

Hypomagnesemia

Hypomagnesemia is a common complication of renal transplantation and can be related to protein calorie malnutrition before and after transplantation,[426] hypercalcemia,[427] steroid therapy, and cyclosporine or tacrolimus.[428] The clinical manifestations include irritability, confusion, convulsions, hyperreflexia, tremulousness, myoclonic jerking, and upon examination, hyperreflexia, tetany, and a positive Chvostek's sign.[429] These neurologic manifestations are similar to those seen in hypocalcemia. Treatment requires the slow parenteral administration of magnesium (to avoid hypermagnesemia).

Hypocalcemia

Hypocalcemia is not common but may complicate renal transplantation when massive blood transfusion is required, resulting in a decrease in both total and ionized serum calcium.[430] The manifestations of hypocalcemia include disturbances of consciousness, which may begin as irritability followed by confusion, delirium, delusional state, and then frank psychosis. In some instances, there may be a marked depression with severe psychomotor retardation.[431,432] Examination will often reveal evidence of tetany with a positive Chvostek's sign. Tonic muscle spasms may occur with involvement of the laryngeal muscles, producing stridor,[433] and in the most acute cases, an opisthotonos may occur. Severe cardiovascular depression may occur. Parenteral calcium replacement is usually necessary to correct the deficiency.

Hypokalemia

Hypokalemia may be encountered in renal transplant patients due to excessive use of diuretics, inadequate diet, or potassium-losing nephropathy.[434] While chronic mild hypokalemia is generally well tolerated, the condition may be exacerbated by hyperventilation and rapid correction of metabolic acidosis, infusion of potassium-free fluid, or the administration of insulin, glucose, or catecholamines. Cerebral symptoms are uncommon in hypokalemia, but lethargy, drowsiness, confusion, and coma have been described.[435,436]

Hypernatremia

Hypernatremia, for the most part, is not a common complication of renal transplantation but may occasionally develop immediately after surgery[437] as a result of overzealous sodium replacement in a patient who had been previously hyponatremic. The main feature of hypernatremia is disturbed consciousness, ranging from mild drowsiness to deep coma,[438,439] sometimes accompanied by seizures,[440] or tremulousness, chorea, and an increase in muscle tone.[440]

Hypophosphatemia
Phosphate depletion early after transplantation is common in renal transplant patients with a successful graft. Many mechanisms may be operative in inducing this metabolic abnormality. Secondary hyperparathyroidism may continue after transplantation in the presence of a functioning kidney, resulting in tubular loss of phosphorus.[441] Antacids, which reduce phosphorus absorption in the gut, are commonly used in these patients.[442–444] Both mechanisms can result in a marked loss of phosphorous. The clinical features of hypophosphatemia include irritability, marked anxiety, weakness, numbness, slurred speech, and disturbed consciousness; deep coma may eventually ensue.[445,446]

▲ EARLY POSTTRANSPLANT PHASE (FIRST MONTH)

Additional sources of neurologic complications arise as the patient progresses from the perioperative to the early posttransplant period. These may stem from the immunosuppressive agents, the overall state of immunosuppression, and complications arising from rejection. There are also a host of other neurologic disorders that may impact on the renal transplant recipient.

Neurologic Complications of Immunosuppressive Agents

Immunosuppressive therapy is essential for the survival of the transplanted organ. Currently, cyclosporine (CyA) is the most common immunosuppressive drug in most transplant centers. Tacrolimus, formerly known as FK 506, is a newer agent that is being used with increasing frequency in renal transplantation. Other drugs that may be used include corticosteroids, OKT3, azathioprine, and mycophenolate mofetil. Except for azathioprine and mycophenolate mofetil, all of these immunosuppressive drugs have the potential for inducing nervous system complications.

Cyclosporine
Cyclosporine was first introduced in 1978.[447] While it has proved to be a very effective immunosuppressive agent, a number of neurologic side effects have been described with its use. These range from the relatively mild complication of tremor[448] to life-threatening encephalopathic states.[449] The important neurologic side effects are listed in Table 11–9.

Tremor. Tremor is a common side effect of cyclosporine and is generally seen soon after the agent is introduced; it tends to improve after prolonged administration.[448] The tremor is not obvious at rest, tends to develop during the course of activity, and is best demonstrated by observing the patient with the hands outstretched.

Sensory Symptoms. Patients frequently complain of burning and tingling in the extremities after initiation of cyclosporine therapy. Objective sensory changes may not be pre-

TABLE 11–9 ▲ NEUROLOGIC COMPLICATIONS OF CYCLOSPORINE

1. Tremor
2. Sensory symptoms
3. Seizures
4. Encephalopathy
5. Movement disorders
6. Disturbances of speech
7. Disturbances of affect
8. Peripheral nervous system complications

sent, but it is possible cyclosporine may indeed induce a neuropathy that could explain the clinical presentation, at least in some subjects.[449]

Seizures. Seizures have been described in association with the use of cyclosporine. These may occur in the context of encephalopathy (see below) but may also develop in the absence of other neurologic abnormalities.[450] There may be many interacting factors responsible for the development of seizures in renal transplant patients, including rejection[451] and electrolyte disturbances.[452] Seizures may also be related to an underlying pathologic process associated with renal disease. Thus, cyclosporine should not be implicated in the pathogenesis of seizures without excluding other etiologies.

Encephalopathy. Cyclosporine-induced encephalopathy may develop as a nonspecific syndrome of apathy, agitation, disorientation, and delusional thinking. However, there may also be striking features in the form of cortical blindness, motor dysfunction, seizures,[453–455] and visual hallucinations.[456] Imaging studies reveal abnormalities best seen on MRI. Diffuse white matter changes may be seen on T2-weighted magnetic resonance (MR) images.[454] The syndrome will usually improve following withdrawal or a decrease in the dosage of cyclosporine, after which the MRI disturbances also tend to resolve. Encephalopathy is usually seen soon after the medication is introduced and may recur if the drug is subsequently restarted. Another variation of cyclosporine–induced central nervous system toxicity takes the form of an encephalopathic picture complicated by the development of severe ataxia, dysarthria, and diffuse weakness.[457] These complications are not necessarily related to high blood cyclosporine levels, but low serum cholesterol levels may play a role in their pathogenesis.[454]

Movement Disorders. Tremor is the most common of the movement disorders associated with the use of cyclosporine. Other movement disorders have also been encountered, including a cerebellar-like tremor.[448] The latter, however, may be part of a more severe complication termed cerebro-cerebellar syndrome.[457]

Disturbances of Speech. Transient aphasia has been reported with the use of cyclosporine, although this may be related to hypomagnesemia.[452] A striking syndrome characterized by an apraxia of speech has also been reported in a number of patients.[458] The predominant feature related to the development of an almost mute state is a marked apraxia of buccal and lingual function. These patients have no demonstrable abnormality on imaging studies, and there is no immediate explanation for this strikingly focal disorder, which tends to improve with withdrawal of cyclosporine.

Disturbances of Affect. Patients may become withdrawn and overtly depressed following the introduction of cyclosporine.[448] Such patients demonstrate the affective disorder and psychomotor retardation seen in patients with depression, and in many instances, may not progress beyond this state. In some instances, however, these manifestations may reflect the onset of an encephalopathy, and in time, these patients may progress and develop the frank encephalopathic features outlined above.

Peripheral Nervous System Complications. Neuropathy may occur as a complication of transplantation. This is usually in the form of single nerve involvement and arises directly from the surgical procedure, probably as a result of direct trauma.[459] There is some suggestion that cyclosporine may be implicated in the development of neuropathy, although this usually occurs in combination with other agents. While sensory symptoms such as burning, tingling, and uncomfortable dysthestetic phenomena are common with the use of cyclosporine, there is little evidence to indicate that the agent alone causes neuropathy.[460] Myopathy, which usually presents as an acute proximal weakness, has been attributed to cyclosporine, although this complication probably occurs only in combination with other agents, particularly colchicine.[461]

Tacrolimus (FK 506)

Tacrolimus is a relatively new immunosuppressive agent, and a number of neurologic complications have been described with its use.[462,463] They are similar to those seen with cyclosporine. Like the latter, tacrolimus binds to intracellular proteins, namely the immunophilins.[464] This common mechanism of action could possibly explain the similarity in neurologic side effects. Common neurologic complications are listed in Table 11–10.

Tremor. Tremor may be seen in as many as 20% of patients receiving tacrolimus[462] and is similar to that seen with cyclosporine. The abnormal movements are not usually evident at rest but are seen during the course of activity, especially when the hands are held in an outstretched position. Tremor tends to become less severe with time.

TABLE 11–10 ▲ NEUROLOGIC COMPLICATIONS OF TACROLIMUS

1. Tremor
2. Headache
3. Insomnia
4. Peripheral neuropathy
5. Encephalopathy
6. Akinetic mutism

Headache. Many patients experience headaches after introduction of tacrolimus.[462] The pain tends to be nonspecific and somewhat generalized in nature and improves over the course of time. In some instances, migraine-like headaches may occur with the development of a typical throbbing headache and accompanying photophobia. This latter may reflect an unmasking of an underlying migraine disorder rather than a specific complication of tacrolimus.

Insomnia. Sleep disorders may also occur; these tend to be relatively minor and are usually not a major source of disability.[462]

Peripheral Neuropathy. As with cyclosporine, sensory symptoms are frequently encountered with this agent. There are also indications that tacrolimus may induce a rapid demyelinating neuropathy.[465] The onset of this disorder is typically often asymmetric, and motor findings predominate. Plasma exchange has been demonstrated to be an effective treatment.

Encephalopathy. Tacrolimus-associated encephalopathy is characterized by a disturbance of consciousness, in some cases heralded by initial agitation.[462] There may be accompanying seizure activity. The level of disturbed consciousness may range from mild lethargy to deep coma. This condition appears to be related to high levels of tacrolimus, and recovery occurs fairly rapidly after it is withdrawn or the dose decreased. There are no characteristic imaging changes. A less common syndrome, characterized by cortical blindness without other encephalopathic features and accompanying white matter lesions on the MRI, has also been described.[466]

Akinetic Mutism. This usually occurs within several days of transplantation.[462] The patient appears awake, but makes no attempt to communicate or respond to verbal stimuli. Eye contact is not maintained. Motor responses to painful stimuli are generally reduced and may be absent, although posturing may occur in reaction to noxious stimuli. Reflexes of release are prominent. Recovery is the rule following withdrawal or a decrease in the dose of tacrolimus. The course may be protracted, extending over many weeks. There are no specific MRI abnormalities; in particular, the white-matter changes accompanying cyclosporine encephalopathy[454] have not been associated with this complication.

OKT3

OKT3 is a murine monoclonal antibody directed against the CD3 portion of the T cell receptor. This antibody is used for induction and as an adjunctive agent for the treatment of acute rejection.[467] The therapeutic rationale for the use of this antibody is to block T cell action, but OKT3 also induces the release of cytokines, which can lead to significant systemic as well as neurologic side effects.[468,469] OKT3 has been implicated in the development of a meningeal syndrome[470] and an encephalopathic state.[471] The former presents as an aseptic meningitis, with consciousness usually preserved; the encephalopathy is characterized by fever, obtundation, hypertonia, nuchal rigidity, involuntary movements, and reflex abnormalities. Cerebrospinal fluid (CSF) examination reveals a predominantly lymphocytic pleocytosis. This syndrome is usually seen over the first 2–3 days of administration of OKT3, and brain edema may be evident on computed tomographic (CT) scanning.

The prognosis is good, and patients usually recover fully, even when OKT3 therapy is not withdrawn.

Corticosteroids

Corticosteroids are used in combination with other immunosuppressive agents to augment immunosuppression. Intravenous methylprednisolone is also employed in the treatment of acute rejection. Thus, transplant patients are at risk for developing corticosteroid-related complications. An encephalopathic-like state may occur as a direct neurologic complication of corticosteroid use, particularly with high doses of the drug such as may be required for the treatment of acute rejection.[472,473] The clinical picture varies, but in its most florid presentation, severe agitation or marked mood lability and frank psychotic behavior become apparent. The marked irritability, impaired concentration, and changes in memory may mimic the onset of a toxic encephalopathy. These patients do not usually lapse into coma.

Chronic steroid use may induce a myopathy, which presents with proximal muscle weakness.

Infection

Some aspects of central nervous system infections have already been discussed in the section on infectious complications. Infections in this early phase (ie, the first month) relate to a variety of causes. These include the immediate effects of the transplant procedure, prolonged hospitalization, and multiple vascular access sites. Conventional infections arise from these sources, and these rarely involve the central nervous system, although a general state of sepsis may give rise to septic encephalopathy[474,475] and can further lead to the development of bacterial meningitis. The state of immunosuppression induced to prevent transplant rejection can further enhance the development of such infections. Other infections that may involve the nervous system arise from a latent infection present prior to transplantation that continues in the posttransplant phase, often exacerbated by posttransplant immunosuppression. The viral infections are most commonly represented in this category. Cytomegalovirus,[476] Epstein-Barr virus,[477] and herpes simplex virus infections may all be activated following transplantation.[478] While they for the most part produce constitutional symptoms, they may occasionally cause encephalitis. The clinical presentation of an encephalitis may be modified in the transplant patient because of the state of immunosuppression, but common presenting features include headache, fever, signs of nuchal rigidity, and disturbances of consciousness. Seizures may also be a manifesting feature. Nervous system involvement, however, may be quite subtle, and the onset of headache or disturbed awareness, even in the absence of the traditional signs of meningeal irritation, should prompt evaluation for an underlying infection.

Viral infection may induce other syndromes. CMV has been implicated in the development of a myelitis, which may present as an acute motor loss with sensory signs.[479] CMV infection may also involve the lumbosacral plexus, producing focal, motor, and sensory signs referable to the lower limbs and has been implicated in the causation of the Guillain-Barré syndrome,[480] which may develop after renal transplantation.[481] Recognition and treatment of these disorders results in clinical improvement.

Rejection Encephalopathy

This syndrome has for the most part been described in renal transplant recipients.[457] It occurs during the course of acute rejection of the transplanted kidney, and the essential features include headache, irritability, altered mental status, and seizures; papilledema was also present in one subject who manifested features of the syndrome. Signs of rejection were also present in the form of fever, weight gain, hypertension, and swelling of the graft. The series of patients in whom this was described were for the most part on azathioprine and steroids. It is less common with cyclosporine immunosuppression and has not been described with tacrolimus. A similar clinical picture may occur with the use of OKT3,[471] thus raising the possibility that cytokines, at least during the course of acute rejection, may play a role in the pathogenesis of the encephalopathy. The paucity of reports of this condition subsequent to the introduction of the more effective immunosuppressive agents, cyclosporine and tacrolimus, suggest that better immunosuppression is indeed the key to preventing the syndrome.

Cerebrovascular Disease

Renal transplant recipients are at risk for cerebrovascular complications of various types. There are many reasons for this. In the renal transplant candidate, hypertension is common,[462] and this predisposes to premature vascular disease, which in turn may lead to ischemic strokes. Diabetic patients who have received kidney transplants also carry an increased risk of cerebrovascular disease, and this predisposes to the development of ischemic strokes. Thus, strokes may be apparent early after transplantation,[482] but the risk continues to be high even in patients many years after transplantation.[483] There are many risk factors that predispose renal transplant patients to stroke,[484] and these include hypertension, diabetes, and systemic lupus erythematosus. Various types of cerebrovascular events may occur:[484] cerebral hemorrhage, spontaneous subdural hemorrhage, and subarachnoid hemorrhage related to rupture of an aneurysm have all been reported by Adams and his coworkers.[484] Of interest, in this series, a number of patients with polycystic kidney disease had cerebrovascular events, but none had subarachnoid hemorrhage. There are a number of risk factors predisposing to cerebrovascular disease in the renal transplant patient, and these include accelerated atherosclerosis,[485] hypertension,[486] and disturbances in serum cholesterol and triglycerides.[487]

Strokes typically present as a sudden catastrophic event, usually leading to permanent neurologic deficits. In some instances, the presentation may be in the form of a transient ischemic attack, where the deficit is of short duration and usually resolves completely. In some instances, ischemic strokes may be preceded by transient ischemic attacks. The development of strokes in a renal transplant recipient requires traditional management strategies, including the identification and treatment of risk factors,[488] as well as the employment of appropriate medical or surgical interventional measures.

Seizures

Seizures may occur at any stage following transplantation. They may develop as the result of preexisting disease, but there are many conditions in the posttransplant phase that could lead to the development of seizures. Renal failure itself may lead to the development of seizures.[409] Cerebrovascular disease is common in renal transplant recipients, and strokes of various types may be complicated by the development of seizures.[489] Following transplantation, the many metabolic disturbances may be complicated by seizures (see section on metabolic and electrolyte disturbances in this section). Immunosuppressive agents, particularly cyclosporine, tacrolimus, and OKT3, may induce seizures. In renal transplant recipients in particular, rejection may be associated with the neurologic syndrome of rejection encephalopathy, and seizures may be the first manifestation of this.[451] Seizures may be the only sign or could be part of the complex clinical presentation of an underlying central nervous system infection, either bacterial such as *Listeria monocytogenes*[490] or fungal such as aspergillus.[491] In the late posttransplant phase, seizures may be the manifestation of posttransplant lymphoproliferative disorder.[492] The approach to a seizure will be dictated by the specific clinical circumstances. The time of onset of seizures in relation to the transplant is of importance. In the early posttransplant phase, metabolic and electrolyte disturbances dominate as the cause of seizures, but immunosuppressive agents and preexisting structural central nervous system disorders may also play a role in the development of seizures in this early phase. In the late transplant phase, particularly after the first month, infections tend to dominate as the cause of seizures. The new onset of seizures or a change in seizure pattern should be regarded very seriously, as these developments may be harbingers of a serious underlying neurologic disorder. Thus, appropriate testing, including imaging studies and lumbar puncture, may be required.

Movement Disorders

The majority of movement disorders encountered in the transplant population are related to the use of immunosuppressive agents. Cyclosporine and tacrolimus are the principal immunosuppressive agents that may induce a variety of movement disorders.[449,493] The most common abnormality encountered in this category is tremor. This usually affects the upper limbs and is seen when the arms are held in a position of sustension, but an action tremor may also be present. This disturbance of movement is most prominent early on after the introduction of immunosuppressive therapy and tends to subside over time, but may never entirely disappear. These agents have also been implicated in the development of orofacial dyskinesias, which may become quite severe and even cause distortion of speech. A Parkinson-like syndrome has also been reported.[494] This may often herald the onset of akinetic mutism. As the latter evolves, patients become withdrawn and, where there is a general decrease in voluntary activity, the face will become expressionless, and reflexes of release will also appear. As the state of akinetic mutism evolves, blepharospasm and other involuntary movements about the face may become apparent. Cerebellar tremor has also been described with prominent speech and limb ataxia.[448,495]

Headache

There are many potential causes of headache in the transplant patient. The causes may vary from transplant type to transplant type. Headache may herald a catastrophic central nervous system complication such as intracerebral hemorrhage, infection, or a space-occupying lesion. In some patients, signs of the causative pathologic event will be evident and the diagnosis readily established. In many instances, headache may be the only feature of any underlying serious cerebral condition. Thus, the onset of a headache should always be viewed with great suspicion, and particular attention should be directed toward the exclusion of an underlying intracranial structural disorder. There are many other causes of headache in the transplant patient. Cyclosporine and tacrolimus have been implicated as a cause of headache,[448,462] and a reduction in the dosage of these agents may result in improvement. Hypertension, which may sometimes complicate renal transplantation,[496] may also induce headache.

Peripheral Nervous System Complications

Injuries to the peripheral nerves supplying the lower limbs will occasionally be encountered as a complication of the renal transplant procedure. This relates to the proximity of these nerves to the surgical site. The femoral and lateral femoral cutaneous nerves are the most frequently involved structures.[497] These are usually injured as a result of pressure caused by retraction. The femoral nerve is usually injured in its intrapelvic course.[498,499] These patients present with unilateral postoperative weakness of knee extension relating to decreased or absent function of the quadriceps muscle. Sensory loss is usually confined to the anterior thigh with extension into the region of the medial calf. The prognosis is usually favorable, with return of function occurring in weeks to months after the procedure.

Spinal cord symptoms may develop following transplantation as a result of disruption of the blood supply.[500] This occurs when the internal iliac artery is used for revascularization of the graft. Paraplegia with marked loss of lower limb function may be evident, although less severe deficits may also occur.

Lumbosacral plexopathy may also occur, and this is more common in the diabetic patient.[501] The presentation is usually one of buttock and thigh pain. The accompanying weakness may vary in distribution, depending on which segments are involved. Common presentations include weakness of foot dorsiflexion and plantar flexion with accompanying loss of strength in the knee flexors. Sensory findings may also be present, and the involvement tends to be most obvious below the knee on the lateral aspect of the calf, although sensory findings may also be present in the posterior proximal thigh region. Recovery is generally the rule, but occasionally deficits may persist.

Peroneal nerve palsy is a further complication sometimes encountered in the renal transplantation recipient. This may occur as a result of weight loss,[411] but may also develop as a consequence of maintaining the patient in a fixed position. Peroneal palsy results from compression of the peroneal nerve at the fibular head. The signs and symptoms include foot drop with accompanying sensory loss, which usually involves the lateral calf and the dorsum of the foot.[502] Early diagnosis is important, as splinting is required to prevent contractures at the ankle. Prognosis for recovery is usually good.

▲ LATE POSTTRANSPLANT PHASE (FROM ONE MONTH ONWARD)

This period may be considered to extend from the first month after transplantation.

Infection

The most important complication occurring during this stage relates to the development of infection. The risk of infection is greatest in the first 6 months, and it is during this stage that opportunistic pathogens may manifest themselves. The risk to the central nervous system may parallel the state of the allograft.[503] There tend to be few neurologic complications in those patients who have good kidney function and whose immunosuppression requirements are relatively modest. Chronic allograft rejection can be associated with higher doses of immunosuppressive agents, and this can increase the risk of opportunistic infection. The most important neurologic infections that face the renal transplant patient in this later posttransplant phase include the following: *Listeria monocytogenes, Cryptococcus neoformans, Toxoplasma gondii,* aspergillus, *Nocardia asteroides,* and *Mycobacterium tuberculosis.* Viral infections may also involve the nervous system at this stage.[504]

Opportunistic infections have variable clinical manifestations. They may present as an acute meningitis, or an encephalitic-like picture may dominate. In some instances, a subacute or chronic meningitic picture may occur, and organisms presenting in this manner include *Cryptococcus neoformans* and *Mycobacterium tuberculosis.* A focal presentation mimicking a tumor may occur with aspergillus, *Nocardia asteroides,* and *Toxoplasma gondii.* Localizing signs referable to the area of involvement are usually evident. It is important to recognize that infections in the renal transplant recipient may have protean manifestations. There may be florid, overt signs of infections, which are easily recognized, but very often the state of immunosuppression may modify the clinical picture to the point where traditional signs of infection may not be apparent.[503] The picture may further be complicated by coexisting conditions such as organ failure, a generalized state of disability, and the effects of pharmacologic agents. These may mask signs of infection or make it difficult to dissect out the specific effects of an underlying infectious disorder. Several syndromes of infection may be recognized.

Acute Meningitis

An important cause of acute meningitis is *Listeria monocytogenes*,[505] but other organisms can be involved. Headache and fever are the initial presenting features, followed by signs of meningeal irritation, although the latter may not always be present. The patient may rapidly become obtunded and focal signs, typically referable to the brain stem in the case of *Listeria monocytogenes*, may be present. Fever, headache, meningeal irritation, and impaired level of consciousness, with or without focal neurologic signs, are of ominous significance and require immediate attention. The usual approach will be a CT scan followed by a spinal tap, the former being necessary to exclude a mass lesion, which may contraindicate the lumbar puncture. Florid presentations may not always be the rule, and in some instances, immunosuppression may mask the typical features of a meningeal infection, and only fragments of the syndrome may be evident. Thus, any unexplained fever, subtle change in level of consciousness, or the development of focal signs should be regarded with great suspicion, and appropriate investigations should be carried out.

Subacute and Chronic Meningitis

The clinical presentation of subacute or chronic meningitis is much less dramatic, and the features are often those of a mild headache that gradually increases in severity, fever, and disturbances of cognitive function. The latter may be nonspecific, taking the form of lack of interest, impaired concentration, memory disturbances, and a general sense of lethargy and disinterest. Nuchal rigidity may be absent. As the condition progresses, disturbances of consciousness may become apparent, and focal neurologic deficits may develop. Thus, the presence of any one of these symptoms or signs should be viewed with great suspicion and should prompt an immediate, thorough evaluation for any underlying opportunistic infection.

The organisms that may be involved include fungi—Aspergillus species, *Cryptococcus neoformans, Blastomyces dermatitis,* and *Histoplasma capsulatum.*[503] *Mycobacterium tuberculous* and *Nocardia asteroides* are less commonly encountered, but may nonetheless present in this manner.

Focal Presentation

In some instances, infection presents as a mass lesion and the accompanying clinical findings are of a focal nature, such as unilateral weakness, aphasia, visual field disturbance, or focal onset of a seizure disorder. There may be accompanying headache and altered mental status. Toxoplasmosis may present in this manner.[506]

Other fungal diseases, namely aspergillosis, may manifest as a rapidly evolving focal lesion, often mimicking a stroke syndrome.[507] Nocardia may present in a similar manner.[503] Most focal presentations relate to fungal disease, although *Listeria monocytogenes* may also present as a focal syndrome, often referable to the brain stem.[508]

In some patients, focal cranial nerve palsies may be an indication of a basilar meningitis, and this is quite common in patients who develop tuberculous infections. Thus it is important to recognize that infections may present in a focal manner, and the syndromes that may result from these are quite varied.

Nonspecific Clinical Presentation

The state of immunosuppression that is induced in transplant patients may mask the common features of a central nervous system infection. Thus, fever may be absent or minimal, and there may be no evidence of meningeal irritation. It may be extremely difficult to diagnose infection under these circumstances, as illustrated by Estol et al,[509] who demonstrated a higher neuropathologic incidence of infection than was suspected on the basis of the clinical findings alone. Infection should thus always be considered in patients who present with an unexplained alteration in level of consciousness, particularly if there are systemic signs of an infectious process. Headache alone may also provide a clue to the diagnosis of infection, even if fever is absent. The presence of fever and headache suggests the possibility of infection. Other presentations that may point toward an infection include seizures, either generalized or focal, the presence of unexplained focal neurologic findings, cranial nerve palsy, and behavioral aberrations. The latter may be subtle and may be mistaken for depression, anxiety, or even psychiatric illness. Thus, the presence of any one of these syndromes should prompt a vigorous search for an underlying central nervous system infection.

The Approach to a Suspected CNS Infection

In general, when infection is suspected, an initial imaging study should be carried out. It is usually more convenient to obtain a CT scan, but in some instances, an MRI may yield more information. In the absence of an abnormality on CT scan, particularly where infection is strongly suspected, an MRI should be obtained. It is essential to follow the imaging study with a spinal tap, which is usually obtained by conventional lumbar puncture. The spinal fluid is examined microscopically by Gram stain in addition to obtaining the cell count and chemical analysis for glucose and protein concentration. Serologic testing for fungal infection as well as specialized staining techniques are also required in most instances. Cultures should be obtained for bacterial infections, tuberculosis, and fungi. Where specific viral infections are suspected, specific organisms may be identified using polymerase chain reaction techniques. In the instance of a suspected infection with initially negative studies, several of the investigations may need to be repeated, and this particularly applies to the examination of the spinal fluid. In the latter situation, there may be some merit in obtaining the spinal fluid from a level closer to basal meninges, and thus a high cervical spinal tap should be considered. This should typically be done under fluoroscopy by a radiologist familiar with the procedure of inserting needles into the cervical spinal canal. Meningeal biopsy may occasionally be required to diagnose an infectious process and may yield valuable information regarding the nature of the offending organism.

▲ OTHER NEUROLOGIC DISORDERS THAT MAY OCCUR IN THE RENAL TRANSPLANT RECIPIENT

Progressive Multifocal Leukoencephalopathy (PML)

Progressive multifocal leukoencephalopathy (PML) is an infectious complication caused by the human papovaviruses, BK virus, and JC virus. These are commonly encountered in the population at large, and for the most part, do not cause clinical illness.[510,511] These agents, however, induce the syndrome of PML in an immunocompromised individual where the state of immunosuppression has been present for a prolonged period of time. The condition is encountered relatively infrequently in renal transplant recipients.[512,513] The clinical feature is one of a slowly evolving clinical syndrome. Hemiparesis may be the dominant feature, and there may be an accompanying decline in cognitive function. Aphasia may also be evident in some patients, and some patients may present with cortical blindness. In some instances, confusion may be the dominant feature. Seizures may also occur. The course is one of relentless progression, with death occurring within several months of diagnosis.[514,515]

The diagnosis rests on a brain biopsy. There are no specific spinal fluid findings, but the MRI may be quite helpful in delineating the extensive white-matter changes that are characteristic of the disease. There is no effective treatment other than to withdraw immunosuppression, which may result in recovery but at the expense of loss of the graft.

Posttransplant Lymphoproliferative Disorder

Posttransplant lymphoproliferative disorder may also complicate renal transplantation.[516] This condition results from the abnormal proliferation of B lymphocytes, usually induced by Epstein-Barr virus.[517,518] As time progresses, the proliferation will take on a monoclonal histopathology, and the condition will then take on malignant characteristics.[519] The central nervous system may be involved in the presence of systemic disease[520] but occasionally may be the only site of invasion.[521] The white matter of the brain is usually first involved, and this may be focal or multicentric. There are no specific clinical features, and the presentation may include impaired cognition, disturbance of consciousness, focal deficits, and seizures.[521] Imaging studies may be useful in detecting the site of involvement, but the diagnosis rests on stereotactic biopsy. Treatment involves discontinuation of immunosuppression, antiviral agents, radiation, and chemotherapy.[522] These modalities may or may not be effective.

Central Pontine Myelinolysis

Central pontine myelinolysis (CPM) is a condition that relates to an acute demyelination of brain stem structures,[523] but extensive extra-pontine disease may also be evident.[524] The clinical features include facial palsy, bulbar symptoms, long-tract signs, and altered mental status. Cranial nerve and motor signs may not be obvious, particularly in an intubated patient, but a rapid rise in the serum sodium is believed to be operative in the development of the syndrome.[525] CPM may be difficult to detect clinically in some cases but should also be suspected in a patient presenting with an altered state of consciousness, particularly when there are accompanying signs of bulbar dysfunction.

Malignancy After Renal Transplantation

Mark L. Jordan

Because of the immunosuppressed state of the transplant recipient, the risk of developing a posttransplant malignancy is higher than that in the general population. Malignancy in transplant patients can occur in several circumstances. First, malignancies may be inadvertently transplanted with the donor organ. Second, malignancies in the recipient that were present prior to transplantation may recur after transplantation. Finally, de novo malignancy may develop after transplantation. Each of these categories will be discussed in this section.

▲ MALIGNANCY TRANSMITTED FROM THE DONOR

When a recipient is identified as having a transmitted malignancy, the proper approach for the renal transplant patient should be allograft removal and discontinuation of immunosuppression, with return to dialysis therapy. While unsuspected transmission of malignancy with the donor kidney is uncommon today, it can still occur. In a review by Penn, the Cincinnati Transplant Tumor Registry (CTTR) identified 236 patients who had received organs from donors with cancers, excluding those donors who had been treated for a major malignancy 10 years or more prior to donation.[526] A total of 181 cancers were identified in 174 donors; 38 (21%) were primary renal cell carcinomas. In an earlier series reported by Penn, consisting of 201 patients who had received organs from donors with cancer, over 80% of the donors were cadaver donors, and 40% provided two or more organs to different recipients.[527] Forty-four percent of the transplanted organs were associated with subsequent malignancy in the recipient. These tumors were discovered anywhere from several days up to 38 months posttransplantation. The transmitted tumors were generally identical histologically to those found in the original donors. Fifty-six percent of the recipients developed distant metastases; the most common metastases were from transmitted carcinomas of the lung, choriocarcinomas, malignant melanomas, and renal carcinomas. Of the recipients who did develop distant metastases, 72% died of their cancers, 25% had complete remissions, and the remainder continued ongoing therapy. In 14 donors reported by Penn in whom a primary renal cell carcinoma or an oncocytoma was found at organ recovery, the lesion was widely excised in 8 cases, and the kidney was successfully transplanted.[526] In 5 cases, the initial frozen section examination was not diagnostic, but permanent sections later showed the presence of renal carcinoma. In the last case, an equivocal diagnosis showing "pleomorphic adenoma" was made. The recipient of this kidney underwent partial nephrectomy 3 months after transplantation to excise a carcinoma. In the 14 recipients of these 14 donor kidneys, there was no recurrent malignancy reported, with an average follow-up of 79 months. In these cases, the presenting renal tumor at the time of organ recovery was felt to be small enough to allow wide excision and subsequent transplantation of the organ. In most cases, however, an organ with a macroscopic lesion greater than 1 cm in diameter that is pathologically consistent with the diagnosis of renal cell carcinoma should probably not be used for transplantation.

In 17 cases where no apparent tumor was present at the time of organ recovery, but was later found in the transplanted kidney, 9 recipients underwent transplant nephrectomy at an average of 3 months post transplantation.[526] The transplant nephrectomies were necessitated by rejection, hemorrhage, thrombosis, and, in the case of 2 of these 9 recipients, the discovery at donor autopsy of a brain metastasis from an unsuspected renal cell carcinoma. In a tenth recipient in this group, an enlarging allograft mass was noted, and the specimen removed at the time of allograft nephrectomy 2 years after transplantation was found to contain renal cell carcinoma. In this group of 10 recipients undergoing transplant nephrectomy, 8 kidneys contained renal cell carcinoma, 1 contained transitional cell carcinoma, and 1 contained a carcinoma of the renal pelvis; no recurrences were reported with a mean follow-up of 59 months. In the remaining 7 recipients, malignancy was diagnosed only after metastatic disease had occurred. All of these recipients died of disseminated cancer at a mean of 15 months following transplantation.

These results underscore the importance of careful screening of the donor for malignancy prior to transplantation. It is necessary to ascertain correctly the exact cause of brain death, which has been reported to be misdiagnosed in at least 18% of cadaveric donors.[527] In particular, cerebral metastases, which may result from choriocarcinoma, bronchogenic carcinoma, renal carcinoma, or malignant melanoma, may be mistaken for primary brain tumors or may present with the same clinical signs and symptoms as an intracranial hemorrhage. Unfortunately, in the scenario of most organ recovery situations, a detailed past medical history is often not available, and detailed previous hospital records may not be available for review prior to the decision to recover the organ. As a result, an effort should be made to rule out metastatic disease as a cause of intracranial hemorrhage in a donor who has no previous history of hypertension, no known intracranial aneurysm, or no known arteriovenous malformation. In general, any patient with a history of malignancy should not be considered for organ donation, with a few exceptions as recommended by Penn: low-grade skin cancers, including basal cell carcinoma and squamous cell carcinoma; carcinoma in situ of the cervix; and primary brain tumors that have not been treated with radiation, chemotherapy, or ventriculoperitoneal or ventriculoatrial shunts.[527] Of over 8000 patients reported to the CTTR, 5 donors with primary brain tumors transmitted cancer to 9 recipients, 4 of whom died. However, two of these five donors had previous craniotomies, 1 had a ventriculoatrial shunt, and an additional patient had unspecified previous treatment.[527]

In certain situations, a potential donor may have had a history of treatment of a malignancy in the remote past. Although a 5-year disease-free interval would be accepted in most cases as evidence of "cure," it has been recommended that patients with a history of carcinoma of the breast or colon, or malignant melanoma, should not be considered because of the high incidence of late metastases from these particular tumors. Obviously, during organ recovery the donor surgeon should perform a careful laparotomy, and, on the back table dissection of the kidneys, a careful examination should be performed to rule out any unusual lesions. If any are found, these must be biopsed and submitted for frozen section examination. In some cases, of course, micrometastases will not be detected, and intrarenal tumors that may not be palpable will be missed. Although some of these lesions may be documented by intraoperative or back table ultrasound, this is often not practical in the donor or the recipient hospital. In addition, since the incidence of transplanted malignancy without microscopic evidence of tumor is quite low, it is doubtful whether this would be a cost-effective approach. Autopsy examination is not performed in every cadaver donor, except in coroner's cases. However, because the time elapsed until the completion of the autopsy is usually longer than the interval in which the organs are transplanted, any information learned from the autopsy that would preclude transplantation is usually not available in time to halt the transplant procedure. If information arises that indicates that the donor had evidence of cancer, subsequent allograft removal should be performed. Alternatively, one could consider leaving the organ in place, intensively monitor the recipient with ultrasound and/or CT examinations at frequent intervals posttransplantation, and attempt to minimize the dosage of immunosuppression once stable allograft function has been achieved.

▲ PREEXISTING MALIGNANCY IN THE RECIPIENT (SEE ALSO CHAPTER 3)

The question of when (or if) end-stage renal disease patients with preexisting cancer should be transplanted is still a matter of some controversy. Most clinicians would agree that a 5-year waiting period after curative therapy should be sufficient to rule out most recurrent cancers. However, previous studies have shown that 10% of patients treated for cancer 5 years or more before transplantation still may develop recurrences.[528] In general, a 2-year waiting period following lack of detectable cancer recurrence has been recommended as a minimum interval after which transplantation can safely be performed. However, Penn has determined that a 2-year waiting period will eliminate only 13% of recurrences of colorectal cancer, 19% of recurrences of breast cancer, 40% of recurrences of prostate cancer, and 50% of the recurrences of malignant melanoma.[527] He has proposed that, with these types of primary cancers, a longer waiting period may be justified. Certain other primary cancers, on the other hand, may not require even a 2-year waiting period. For example, a recent study has shown that incidentally detected renal cell carcinomas may not require any waiting time following the removal of the tumor.[526] Seventy-one such patients were reported by Penn and no recurrences were seen, irrespective of the time between nephrectomy and transplantation.[526] In contrast, of 279 patients with symptomatic renal tumors, 25% had recurrences, 63% of which occurred in patients with less than a 2-year interval between excision of the tumor and transplantation. It therefore appears that in case of renal cell carcinoma, incidentally discovered tumors do not require a waiting period before transplantation, but symptomatic tumors should have a waiting period of at least 2 years. Other cancers that may not require the mandatory 2-year waiting period probably include focal neoplasms of the uterus, prostate, nonmuscle invasive bladder tumors, and some skin cancers, including basal cell carcinomas.

Because in some cases preexisting carcinomas are discovered only after transplantation, intensive screening for certain tumors is indicated at the time of evaluation, especially in older patients. This is especially true with prostate cancer, and we have instituted a policy of screening all male patients over the age of 40 with PSA determinations. If the PSA is elevated, prostate ultrasound and biopsy are performed prior to activating the patient on the transplant waiting list. If prostate cancer is discovered, we offer the patient curative therapy if this is indicated. Furthermore, patients who remain on the waiting list for a prolonged period, such as those who are highly sensitized or awaiting retransplantation, should be reevaluated annually to screen for de novo malignancies that may otherwise preclude transplantation.

▲ MALIGNANCY DEVELOPING AFTER TRANSPLANTATION

The overall incidence of posttransplant malignancy is much higher than in the general population and has been reported to range from 4% to 18%, with a mean of 6%.[527] The higher end of the spectrum probably is due to reports from Australia that contain a relatively high incidence of skin cancer.[529] The largest data base accumulated of posttransplant malignancies is that of the Cincinnati Transplant Tumor Registry maintained by Penn.[527] Many of the cancers in the posttransplant population parallel the incidence of those seen in the general population, with certain exceptions. Posttransplant lymphomas account for 23% of all posttransplant malignancies, versus 5% in the general population, and lip cancers account for 7% of posttransplant malignancies, versus 0.3% in the general population.[527,530,531] By far the most common tumors after transplantation involve the skin and lips (37% of the total). The incidence of these cancers is directly related to the degree of sun exposure. Unlike the general population, in which basal cell carcinomas are more common than squamous cell carcinomas, the reverse is true in transplant patients. Malignant melanomas are also more common in transplant patients than in the general population, by a ratio of approximately 2 to 1.

Approximately 94% of posttransplant lymphomas are non-Hodgkin's lymphomas. They are also called posttransplant lymphoproliferative disorder (PTLD). Most of these are of B lymphocyte origin and are related to Epstein-Barr virus infection; they are discussed in another section of this chapter. The treatment of most cases of PTLD involves reduction or cessation of immunosuppressive therapy with or without antiviral therapy directed against EBV. This most commonly involves the use of acyclovir or ganciclovir. In patients with monoclonal PTLD, surgical extirpation and/or chemotherapy may also be required to eradicate the lesion.

The 6% incidence of Kaposi's sarcoma in the transplant population is much higher than that seen in the general population, 0.02–0.07%. In fact, the incidence of Kaposi's sarcoma reported by Penn is greater than that of colorectal or breast carcinoma in the posttransplant population. Although Kaposi's sarcoma is also quite common in AIDS patients, it is very rare for posttransplant patients who have Kaposi's sarcoma to test positive for HIV. Most cases of Kaposi's sarcoma in transplant patients occur in Arabic, Jewish, Black, or Mediterranean patients. Over half of the affected patients have nonvisceral Kaposi's sarcoma confined to the skin or the oropharyngeal mucosa. Of those patients with nonvisceral disease, approximately half have complete remissions following treatment, which consists of reduction or cessation of immunosuppressive therapy. However, those patients with visceral disease experience only a 19% remission rate. Sixty-two percent of patients with visceral Kaposi's sarcoma die.[527]

Carcinoma of the vulva and perineum is increased in incidence in transplant patients by approximately 100-fold compared to the general population.[527] One third of the patients have in situ lesions. One third have a history of condyloma acuminatum, which can be regarded as a premalignant lesion. Most patients with superficial lesions respond well to local excision; however, metastatic disease may still occur. Cervical carcinoma occurs in 11% of women with posttransplant malignancy, and 72% of these are in situ carcinomas. It is therefore recommended that all postadolescent female patients have regular pelvic examinations and pap smears both pre- and posttransplantation on a yearly basis.

▲ SUMMARY OF MALIGNANCIES IN TRANSPLANTATION

The key to the problem of malignancy in transplant patients lies in early detection and prevention. The first line of defense is screening the dialysis patient for malignancy at the time of evaluation, prior to activation on the transplant waiting list. This involves careful evaluation of the lower GI tract and lungs, and, in females, the breasts and pelvic organs, and, in males, the prostate. Care must be taken to evaluate the donor thoroughly for malignancy, especially for metastatic tumors to the brain that may masquerade as intracranial events and are otherwise intrepreted as cerebrovascular accidents. Meticulous attention must be paid to the intra-abdominal findings during organ recovery, and a careful evaluation of the recovered organs for unsuspected malignancies must be performed. When suspicious lesions are encountered, these should be biopsied and subjected to frozen section examination before any consideration is given to using the organ. In the posttransplant period, several cancers, specifically skin and lip cancers and lymphomas, are much more common than in the general population, and transplant recipients must be monitored carefully, with a high index of suspicion for their occurrence. Most transplant malignancies should be treated with a reduction or cessation of immunosuppressive therapy, in addition to specific treatment as indicated for the type of malignancy.

▲ REFERENCES

Complications of Renal Transplantation

1. Thomalla JV, Lingeman JE, Leapman SB, Filo RS: The manifestation and management of late urological complications in renal transplant recipients. Use of the urological armamentarium. *J Urol* 134:944, 1985.
2. Dreikorn K, Rohl L, Horsch R, Rossler W: Urologic complications in renal transplantation. *Transplant Proc* 14:77, 1982.
3. Salvatierra O Jr, Olcott CIV, Amend WJ Jr, Cochrum KC, Feduska NJ: Urological complications of renal transplantation can be prevented or controlled. *J Urol* 117:421, 1977.
4. Holden S, O'Brien DP III, Lewis EL, Green BG, Walton KN: Urological complications in renal transplantation. *Urology* 5:182, 1975.
5. Colfry AJ Jr, Schlegel JU, Lindsey ES, McDonald J: Urological complications in renal transplantation. *J Urol* 112:564, 1974.
6. Malek GH, Uehling DT, Daouk AA, Kisken WA: Urological complications of renal transplantation. *J Urol* 109:173, 1973.
7. Anderson EE, Glenn JF, Seigler HF, Stickel DL: Urologic complications in renal transplantation. *J Urol* 107:187, 1972.
8. Starzl TE, Groth CG, Putnam CW, et al: Urological complications in 216 human recipients of renal transplants. *Ann Surg* 172:1, 1970.
9. Shafik A: A study of the arterial pattern of the normal ureter. *J Urol* 107:720, 1972.
10. De Sousa LA: Microangiographic aspects of the ureter. *J Urol* 95:179, 1965.
11. Dreikorn K: Problems of the distal ureter in renal transplantation. *Urol Int* 49:76, 1992.
12. Thrasher JB, Temple DR, Spees EK: Extravesical versus Leadbetter-Politano ureteroneocystostomy: A comparison of urological complications in 320 renal transplants. *J Urol* 144:1105, 1990.
13. Shah S, Nath V, Gopalkrishnan G, Pandey AP, Shastri JCM: Evaluation of extravesical and Leadbetter-Politano ureteroneocystostomy in renal transplantation. *Br J Urol* 62:412, 1988.
14. Donohue JP, Hostetter M, Glover J, Madura J: Ureteroneocystostomy vs. ureteropyelostomy: a comparison in the same renal allograft series. *J Urol* 114:202, 1975.
15. Greenberg SH, Wein AJ, Perloff LJ, Barker CF: Ureteropyelostomy and ureteroneocystostomy in renal transplantation: postoperative urological complications. *J Urol* 118:117, 1977.
16. Jaffers GJ, Cosimi AB, Delmonico FL, et al: Experience with pyeloureterostomy in renal transplantation. *Ann Surg* 196:188, 1982.

17. Van Son JW, Hooykass AP, Slooff MJH, et al: Vesicocalicostomy as ultimate solution for recurrent urological complications after cadaveric renal transplantation in a patient with poor bladder function. *J Urol* 136:889, 1986.
18. Kennelly MJ, Konnak JW, Herwig KR: Vesicopyeloplasty in renal transplant patients: A twenty year followup. *J Urol* 150:1118, 1993.
19. Hooghe L, Kinnaert P, Schulman CC, et al: Ureteroneocystostomy in renal transplantation: Comparison of endo- and extravesical anastomoses. *World J Surg* 1:231, 1977.
20. Cullman HJ, Prosinger M: Necrosis of the allograft ureter—Evaluation of different examination methods in early diagnosis. *Urol Int* 45:164, 1990.
21. Gianello P, Squifflet JP, Pirson Y, et al: Ischemic necrosis of the allograft ureter. *Transplant Proc* 16:1304, 1984.
22. Goldstein I, Cho SI, Olsson CA: Nephrostomy drainage for renal transplant complications. *J Urol* 126:159, 1981.
23. Robertshaw GE, Madge GE, Kauffman HM Jr: Ureteral pathology in treated and untreated renal homografts. *Surg Forum* 17:236, 1966.
24. Haber MH, Putong PB: Ureteral vascular rejection in human renal transplantation. *JAMA* 192:417, 1965.
25. Schweizer RT, Bartus SA, Kahn CS: Fibrosis of a renal transplant ureter. *J Urol* 117:125, 1977.
26. Freed SZ: The ureter in renal transplantation. In: Bergmann H, (ed), *The Ureter.* New York, Springer, 1981: 669.
27. Jones JW, Hunter DR, Matas AJ: Successful percutaneous treatment of ureteral stenosis after renal transplantation. *Transplant Proc* 25(I):1038, 1993.
28. Ehrlichman RJ, Bettman M, Kirkman L, Tilney NL: The use of percutaneous nephrostomy in patients with ureteric obstruction undergoing renal transplantation. *Surg Gynecol Obstet* 162:121, 1986.
29. Streem SB, Novick AC, Steinmuller DR, Musselman PW: Percutaneous techniques for the management of urological renal transplant complications. *J Urol* 135:456, 1986.
30. Finnerty DP, Trulock TS, Berkman W, Walton KN: Transluminal balloon dilation of ureteral strictures. *J Urol* 131:1056, 1984.
31. Farah NB, Roddie M, Lord RHH, Williams G: Ureteric obstruction in renal transplants: The role of percutaneous balloon dilatation. *Nephrol Dial Transplant* 6:977, 1991.
32. Kim J, Banner MP, Ramchandani P, Grossman RA, Pollack HM: Balloon dilation of ureteral strictures after renal transplantation. *Radiology* 186:717, 1993.
33. Meretyk S, Albala DM, Clayman RV, Denstedt JD, Kavoussi LR: Endoureterotomy for treatment of ureteral strictures. *J Urol* 147:1502, 1992.
34. Streem SB, Novick AC, Steinmuller DR, et al: Long-term efficacy of ureteral dilation for transplant ureteral stenosis. *J Urol* 140:32, 1988.
35. Lang EK, Glorioso LW III: Antegrade transluminal dilatation of benign ureteral strictures: long term results. *AJR* 150:131, 1988.
36. Kinnaert P, Hall M, Janssen F, et al: Ureteral stenosis after kidney transplantation: true incidence and long-term follow up after surgical correction. *J Urol* 133:17, 1985.
37. Helling TS, Thomas CY, Moore JD, Koontz PG Jr: The surgical approach to obstructive problems of the transplant ureter. *Transplant Proc* 14(4)751, 1982.
38. Smolev JK, McLoughlin MG, Rolley R, Sterioff S, Williams GM: The surgical approach to urological complications in renal allotransplant recipients. *J Urol* 117:10, 1977.
39. Thomalla JV, Leapman SB, Filo RS: The use of internalized ureteric stents in renal transplant recipients. *Br J Urol* 66:363, 1990.
40. Pocock RD, Stower MJ, Ferro MA, Smith PJB, Gingell JC: Double J stents: A review of 100 patients. *Br J Urol* 58:629, 1986.

41. Nicholson ML, Veitch PS, Donnelly PK, Bell PR: Urological complications of renal transplantation: the impact of Double J ureteric stents. *Ann R Coll Surg England* 73:316, 1991.
42. Motiwala HG, Shah SA, Patel SM: Ureteric substitution with Boari bladder flap. *Br J Urol* 66:369, 1990.
43. Bretan PN Jr, Hodge E, Streem SB, Steimuller DR, Novick AC: Diagnosis of renal transplant urinary fistulas. *Transplant Proc* 21(1):1962, 1989.
44. Eklund B, Edegren J, Laasonen L, Ahonen J: Percutaneous nephrostomy: A therapeutic procedure for the management of urinary leakage and obstructon in renal transplantation. *Transplant Proc* 16(5):1304, 1984.
45. Decurtins M, Vogt N, Largiader F: Secondary pyeloureterostomy after ureter necrosis in renal transplant recipients. *Urol Int* 49:90, 1992.
46. Pollak R, Veremis SA, Maddux MS, Mozes MF: The natural history of and therapy for perirenal fluid collections following renal transplantation. *J Urol* 140:716, 1988.
47. Yap R, Madrazo B, Oh HK, Dienst SG: Perirenal fluid collection after renal transplant. *Am Surg* 47:287, 1981.
48. Silver TM, Campbell D, Wicks JD, et al: Peritransplant fluid collections. Ultrasound evaluation and clinical significance. *Radiology* 138:145, 1981.
49. Morley P, Barnett E, Bell PRF, et al: Ultrasound in the diagnosis of fluid collections following renal transplantation. *Clin Radiol* 26:199, 1975.
50. Kyriakides GK, Simmons RL, Najarian JS: Wound infections in renal transplant wounds: Pathogenetic and prognostic factors. *Ann Surg* 182:770, 1975.
51. Malovrh M, Kandus A, Buturovic-Ponikvar J, et al: Frequency and clinical influence of lymphoceles after kidney transplantation. *Transplant Proc* 22(4):1423, 1990.
52. Khauli RB, Stoff JS, Lovewell T, Ghavamian R, Baker S: Post-transplant lymphoceles: A critical look into the risk factors, pathophysiology, and management. *J Urol* 150:22, 1993.
53. Shaver TR, Swanson SJ III, Fernandez-Bueno C, Kocandrle V: The optimal treatment of lymphoceles following renal transplantation. *Transplant Int* 6:108, 1993.
54. Stephanian E, Matas AJ, Gores P, Sutherland DE, Najarian JS: Retransplantation as a risk factor for lymphocele formation. *Transplantation* 53(3):676, 1991.
55. Gilliland DJ, Spies JB, Brown SB, Yrizarry JM, Greenwood LH: Lymphoceles: Percutaneous treatment with Povidone-iodine sclerosis. *Intervent Radiol* 171:227, 1989.
56. Khauli RB, Mosenthal AC, Caushaj PF: Treatment of lymphocele and lymphatic fistula following renal transplantation by laparoscopic peritoneal window. *J Urol* 147:1353, 1992.
57. Fahlenkamp D, Raatz B, Schonberger B, Loening SA: Laparoscopic lymphocele drainage after renal transplantation. *J Urol* 150:316, 1993.
58. Ancona E, Rigotti P, Zaninotto G, et al: Treatment of lymphocele following renal transplantation by laparoscopic surgery. *Int Surg* 76:261, 1991.
59. Langle F, Schurawitzki H, Muhlbacher F, et al: Treatment of lymphoceles following renal transplantation. *Transplant Proc* 22(4):1420, 1990.
60. Nicholson ML, Veitch PS: Treatment of lymphoceles associated with renal transplant. *Br J Urol* 65:240, 1990.
61. Lucas BSC, Castro JE: Calculi in renal transplant. *Br J Urol* 50:302, 1978.
62. Normann E, Fryjordet A, Halvorsen S: Stones in renal transplants. *Scand J Urol Nephrol* 14:73 1980.
63. Van Gansbeke D, et al: Lithiasic complications of renal transplantation: The donor graft lithiasis concept. *Urol Radiol* 7:157, 1985.
64. Rosenberg JC, Arnstein AR, Ing TS, et al: Calculi complicating a renal transplant. *Am J Surg* 129:326, 1975.

65. Motayne GG, Jindal SL, Irvin AH, Abele RP: Calculus formation in renal transplant patients. *J Urol* 132:448, 1984.
66. Christensen MS, Nielsen HE, Torring S: Hypercalcemia and parathyroid function after renal transplantation. *Acta Med Scand* 201:35, 1977.
67. Fisher MF, Haaga JR, Persky L, Eckel RE, LiPuma J: Renal stone extraction through a percutaneous nephrostomy in a renal transplant patient. *Radiology* 144:95, 1982.
68. Hulbert JC, Reddy P, Young AT, et al: The percutaneous removal of calculi from transplanted kidneys. *J Urol* 134:324, 1985.
69. Caldwell TC, Burns JR: Current operative management of urinary calculi after renal transplantation. *J Urol* 140:1360, 1988.
70. Wheatley M, Ohl DA, Sonda LP III, Wang SC, Konnak JW: Treatment of renal transplant stones by extracorporeal shock-wave lithotripsy in the prone position. *Endouro* XXXVII(1):57, 1991.
71. Atala A, Steinbock GS, Harty JI, Klein JB: Extracorporeal shock-wave lithotripsy in transplanted kidney. *Urology* 41(1):60, 1993.
72. Jordan ML, Cook GT, Cardella CJ: Ten years of experience with vascular complications in renal transplantation. *J Urol* 128:689, 1982.
73. Rijksen JFVB, Koolen MI, Walaszewski JE, et al: Vascular complications in 400 consecutive renal allotransplants. *J Cardiovasc Surg* 23:91, 1986.
74. Palleschi J, Novick AC, Braun WE, Magnusson MD: Vascular complications of renal transplantation. *Urology* 16:61, 1980.
75. Vidne BA, Leapman SB, Butt KM, Kountz SL: Vascular complications in human renal transplantation. *Surgery* 79:78, 1976.
76. Goldman MH, Tilney NL, Vineyard GC, et al: A twenty year survey of arterial complications of renal transplantation. *Surg Gynecol Obstet* 141:758, 1975.
77. Nerstrom B, Ladefoged J, Lund F: Vascular complications in 155 consecutive kidney transplantations. *Scand J Urol Nephrol* 15(Suppl.)(6):65, 1972.
78. Groggel GC: Acute thrombosis of the renal transplant artery: a case report and review of the literature. *Clin Nephrol* 36(1):42, 1991.
79. Lee HM, Mendez-Picon G, Pierce JC, Hume DM: Renal artery occlusion in transplant recipients. *Am Surg* 43:186, 1977.
80. Swanson DA, Sullivan MJ: Thromboendarterectomy for anuria 4½ years post-renal transplant: A case report. *J Urol* 116:799, 1976.
81. Gerard DF, Devin JB, Halasz NA, Collins GM: Transplant renal artery thrombosis. Revascularization after 5½ hours of ischemia. *Arch Surg* 117:361, 1982.
82. Zajko AB, McLean GK, Grossman RA, et al: Percutaneous transluminal angioplasty and fibrinolytic therapy for renal allograft arterial stenosis and thrombosis. *Transplantation* 33:447, 1982.
83. Remuzzi G, Bertani T: In-depth review: Renal vascular and thrombotic effects of CSA. *Am J Kidney Dis* 13:261, 1982.
84. Dodhia NB, Rodby RA, Jensik SC, Korbet SM: Renal transplant arterial thrombosis: Association with cyclosporine. *Am J Kidney Dis* XVII(5):532, 1991.
85. Gruber SA, Chavers B, Payne WD, et al: Allograft renal vascular thrombosis—lack of increased thrombosis with cyclosporine immunosuppression. *Transplantation* 47:475, 1989.
86. Voss BL, Hamilton KK, Samara EN, et al: Cyclosporine suppression of endothelial prostacyclin generation: A possible mechanism for nephrotoxicity. *Transplantation* 45:793, 1988.
87. Manier SM, Van Nostrand D, Kyle RW: Primer and atlas for renal transplant scintigraphy: flow, Tc-99m DTPA, I-131, Hippuran. *Clin Nucl Med* 10:118, 1985.

88. Dodd GD III, Tublin ME, Shah A, Zajko AB: Imaging of vascular complications associated with renal transplants. *AJR* 157:449, 1991.
89. Ricotta JJ, Schaff HV, Williams GM, et al: Renal artery stenosis following transplantation: Etiology, diagnosis, and prevention. *Surgery* 84:595, 1978.
90. Doyle TJ, McGregor WR, Fox PS, et al: Homotransplant renal artery stenosis. *Surgery* 77:53, 1975.
91. Lacombe M: Arterial stenosis complicating renal allotransplantation in man. A study of 38 cases. *Ann Surg* 13:283, 1975.
92. Morris PJ, Yadav RVS, Kincaid-Smith P, et al: Renal artery stenosis in renal transplantation. *Med J Aust* 1:1255, 1971.
93. Glassock RJ, Feinstein EI, Campese VM, et al: Hypertension in a renal transplant recipient. *Am J Nephrol* 4:262, 1984.
94. Huysmans FT, Hoitsma AJ, Koene RAP: Factors determining the prevalence of hypertension after renal transplantation. *Nephrol Dial Transplant* 2:34, 1987.
95. Texon M, Imparato AM, Lord JJ: Experimental production of arterial lesions. *Arch Intern Med* 110:50, 1962.
96. Sutherland RS, Spees EK, Jones JW, Fink DW: Renal artery stenosis after renal transplantation: The impact of the hypogastric artery anastomosis. *J Urol* 149:980, 1993.
97. Oakes DD, Spees EK Jr, Light JA, Flye WM: Renal perfusion preservation without cannulation. Prevention of post-transplantation renal artery stenosis. *Arch Surg* 113:654, 1978.
98. Smellie WA, Vinik M, Hume DM: Angiograhic investigation of hypertension complicating human renal transplantation. *Surg Gynecol Obstet* 128:963, 1969.
99. Dubovsky EV, Curtis JJ, Luke RG, et al: Captopril as a predictor of curable hypertension in renal transplant recipients. *Contrib Nephrol* 56:117, 1987.
100. Erley M, Duda H, et al: Noninvasive procedures for diagnosis of renovascular hypertension in renal transplant recipients—A prospective analysis. *Transplantation* 54(5):863, 1992.
101. Smith RB, Cosimi AB, Lordon R, Thompson AL, Ehrlich RM: Diagnosis and management of arterial stenosis causing hypertension after successful renal transplantation. *J Urol* 115:639, 1976.
102. Luke RG: Hypertension in renal transplant recipients. *Kidney Int* 31:1024, 1987.
103. Waltzer WC, Turner S, Frohnert P, Rapaport FT: Etiology and pathogenesis of hypertension following renal transplantation. *Nephron* 42:102, 1986.
104. Oakes DD, Spees EK, McAllister HA, Saddler W: Arterial injury during perfusion preservation: a possible cause of post-transplantation renal artery stenosis. *Surgery* 89:210, 1981.
105. Kincaid-Smith P, Hare WSC, Morris PJ, Marshall V: Renal artery stenosis due to the vascular lesions of rejection in cadaveric allografts. *Proc Eur Dial Transplant Assoc* 6:235, 1969.
106. Curtis JJ, Luke RG, Whelchel JD, Diethelm AG, Jones P, Dustan HP: Inhibition of angiotensin-converting enzyme in renal-transplant recipients with hypertension. *N Engl J Med* 308:377, 1983.
107. Ferretti G, Salomone A, Malfi B, Segoloni GP: Duplex scanning and the transplanted kidney. *Lancet* 2:219, 1986.
108. Snider JF, Hunter DW, Moradian GP, Castaneda-Zuniga WR, Letourneau JG: Transplant renal artery stenosis: Evaluation with duplex sonography. *Radiology* 172:1027, 1989.
109. Linas SL, Miller PD, McDonald KM, et al: Role of renin-angiotensin system on post-transplant hypertension in patients with multiple kidneys. *N Engl J Med* 298:1440, 1978.

110. Farrow PR, Wilkinson R: Reversible renal failure during treatment with captopril. *Br Med J* 2:1680, 1979.
111. Van der Woude FJ, Van Son WJ, Tegzess AM, et al: Effect of captopril on blood pressure and renal function in patients with transplant renal artery stenosis. *Nephron* 39:184, 1985.
112. Mann FC, Herrick JF, Essex HE, et al: The effect of the blood flow of decreasing lumen of a blood vessel. *Surgery* 4:249, 1938.
113. Selkurt EE: The effect of pulse pressure and mean arterial pressure modification of renal hemodynamics and electrolyte and water excretion. *Circulation* 4: 541, 1951.
114. Merkus JWS, Dun GC, Reinaerts et al: Renal allograft artery stenosis: Results of medical treatment and intervention. A retrospective analysis. *Transplant Int* 6:111, 1993.
115. Raynaud A, Bedrossian J, Remy P, et al: Percutaneous transluminal angioplasty of renal transplant arterial stenosis. *Am J Roentgenol* 146:853, 1986.
116. Grossman RA, Dafoe DC, Schoenfeld RB, et al: Percutaneous transluminal angioplasty treatment of renal transplant artery stenosis. *Transplantation* 34:339, 1983.
117. Lohr JW, MacDougall ML, Chonko AM, et al: Percutaneous transluminal angioplasty in transplant renal artery stenosis: Experience and review of the literature. *Am J Kidney Dis* VII(5):363, 1986.
118. Sniderman KW, Sos TA, Sprayregen S, et al: Percutaneous transluminal angioplasty in renal transplant arterial stenosis for relief of hypertension. *Radiology* 135:23, 1980.
119. Thomas CP, Riad H, Johnson BF, Cumberland DC: Percutaneous transluminal angioplasty in transplant renal arterial stenoses: A long-term follow-up. *Transplant Int* 5:129, 1992.
120. Benoit G, Hiesse C, Icard P, et al: Treatment of renal artery stenosis after renal transplantation. *Transplant Proc* 19:3600, 1987.
121. Osborn DE, Castro JE, Shackman R: Surgical correction of arterial stenosis in renal allografts. *Br J Urol* 48:221, 1976.
122. Margules RM, Blezer FO, Kountz SL: Surgical correction of renovascular hypertension following renal allotransplantation. *Arch Surg* 106:13, 1973.
123. De Meyer M, Pirson Y, Dautrebande J, et al: Treatment of renal graft artery stenosis. Comparison between surgical by-pass and percutaneous transluminal angioplasty. *Transplantation* 47:784, 1989.
123a. Henry ML, Elkhammas EA, Tesi RJ, Ferguson RM: Mycotic aneurysm following kidney transplantation (discussion). *Transplantation Sci* 2(1):16–17, April 1992.
124. Merion RM, Calne RY: Allograft renal vein thrombosis. *Transplant Proc* 17:1746, 1985.
125. Delbeke D, Sacks GA, Sandler MP: Diagnosis of allograft renal vein thrombosis. *Clin Nucl Med* 14:415, 1989.
126. Duckett T, Bretan PN Jr, Cochran ST, Rajfer J, Rosenthal JT: Noninvasive radiological diagnosis of renal vein thrombosis in renal transplantation. *J Urol* 146:403, 1991.
127. Hilfiker ML, Feddersen RM, Gibel LJ, et al: Allograft renal vein thrombosis in a kidney with two veins. *Transplantation* 54(4):738, 1992.
128. Hammoudi Y, Benoit G, Bensadoun H, et al: Benefits of vena cava removal with the renal vein in cadaver kidney procurement: incidence of arterial complications. *Transplant Proc* 20:762, 1988.
129. Kahan BD: Cyclosporine. *N Engl J Med* 321:1725, 1989.
130. Myerly KF, Kirchner PT: Renal scintigraphic findings in a case of transplant renal vein thrombosis. *Clin Nucl Med* 13:426, 1988.
131. Chiu AS, Landsberg DN: Successful treatment of acute transplant renal vein thrombosis with selective streptokinase infusion. *Transplant Proc* 23(4):2297, 1991.
132. Robinson JM, Cockrell CH, Tisnado J, et al: Selective low-dose streptokinase infusion

in the treatment of acute transplant renal vein thrombosis. *Cardiol Intern Radiol* 9:86, 1986.
133. Baquero A, Morris MC, Cope C, Raja R, Bannett A: Selective embolization of vascular complications following renal biopsy of the transplant kidney. *Transplant Proc* 17/2, 1985.
134. Boschiero LB, Saggin P, Galante O, et al: Renal needle biopsy of the transplant kidney: Vascular and urologic complications. *Urol Int* 48:130–133, 1992.
135. Lawen JD, vanBuren CT, Lewis RM, Kahan BD: Arteriovenous fistulas after renal allograft biopsy: A serious complication in patients beyond one year. *Clin Transplant* 4:357, 1990.
136. Thistlethwaite JR Jr, Woodle ES, Yayes JT, et al: Aggressive needle biopsy protocol prevents loss of renal allografts to undetected rejection during early posttransplant dysfunction. *Transplant Proc* 21, 1980.
137. Merkus JWS, Zeebregts CJAM, Hoitsma AJ, et al: High incidence of arteriovenous fistula after biopsy of kidney allograft. *Br J Surg* 80:310, 1993.
138. Bennett AR, Wiener SN: Intrarenal arteriovenous fistula and aneurysm: a complication of percutaneous renal biopsy. *AJR* 95:372, 1965.
139. Ekelund L, Limdholm T: Arteriovenous fistulae following percutaneous renal biopsy. *Acta Radiol* 11:38, 1971.
140. Herschman A, Klein MJ, Blumberg AG: Spontaneous disapperance of iatrogenic renal arteriovenous fistula: report of a case. *J Urol* 105:4, 1971.
141. Pigott JP, Schab WV: Arteriovenous fistula involving a transplant kidney. *Transplantation* 44:156, 1987.
142. Wallace S, Schwarten DE, Smith DC, Gerson LP, Davis LJ: Intrarenal arteriovenous fistulas—transcatheter steel coil occlusion. *J Urol* 120:282, 1978.
143. Sarramon JP, Cerene A, Gorodetski N, Bernadet P, Durand D: Spontaneous renal arteriovenous fistula and arterial hypertension—conservative treatment and healing. *Eur Urol* 4:214, 1978.
144. Morse SS, Sniderman KW, Strauss EB, Bia MJ: Postbiopsy renal allograft arteriovenous fistula: Therapeutic embolization. *Urol Radiol* 7:161, 1985.
145. Schmid T, Sandbichler P, Ausserwinkler M, Pernthaler H, Margreiter R: Vascular lesions after percutaneous biopsies of renal allografts. *Transplant Int* 2:56–58, 1989.
146. Hubsch P, Schurawitzki H, Traindl O, Karnel R: Renal allograft arteriovenous fistula due to needle biopsy with late onset of symptoms—Diagnosis and treatment. *Nephron* 59:482–485, 1991.
147. Renowden SA, Blethyn J, Cochlin DL: Duplex and colour flow sonography in the diagnosis of post-biopsy arteriovenous fistulae in the transplant kidney. *Clin Radiol* 45:233–237, 1992.

Medical Complications

148. US Renal Data System: USRDS 1994 Annual Data Report. National Institute of Health, National Institute of Diabetes and Digestive and Kidney Diseases. Bethesda, MD, July 1994, Table D.47.
149. Matas AJ, Gillingham KJ, Sutherland DER: Half-life and risk factors for kidney transplant outcome: Importance of death with function. *Transplantation* 55(4):757–761, 1993.
150. Kasiske BL: Risk factors for cardiovascular disease after renal transplantation [Review]. *Miner Electrolyte Metab* 19(3):186–195, 1993.
151. Rostand SG, Brunzell JD, Cannon RO, Victor RG: Cardiovascular complications in renal failure. *J Am Soc Nephrol* 2:1053–1062, 1991.

152. First RM, Neylan JF, Rocher LL, Tejani A: hypertension after renal transplantation. *J Am Soc Nephrol* 4:S30–S36, 1994.
153. Luke RG: Pathophysiology and treatment of posttransplant hypertension. *J Am Soc Nephrol* (Suppl 1):S37–S44, 1991.
154. Curtis JJ, Luke RG, Dubovsky E, et al: Cyclosporine in therapeutic doses increases renal allograft vascular resistance. *Lancet* 2:447–479, 1986.
155. McCauley J, Fung J, Jain A, Todo S, Starzl, TE: The effects of FK 506 on renal function after liver transplantation. *Transplant Proc* 22(1):17–20, 1990.
156. Laskow DA, Curtis JJ: Post-transplant hypertension. *Am J Hypertens* 3:721–725, 1990.
157. Curtis JJ: Hypertension following kidney transplantation. *Am J Kidney Dis* 23(3):471–475, 1994.
158. McCauley J, Ptachcinski RJ, Shapiro R: The cyclosporine-sparing effects of diltiazem in renal transplantation. *Transplant Proc* Dec; 21(6):3955–3957, 1989.
159. Kasiske BL, Umen AJ: Persistent hyperlipidemia in renal transplant recipients. *Medicine* 66:309–316, 1987.
160. Hricik DE. Posttransplant hyperlipidemia: the treatment dilemma [Review]. *Am J Kidney Dis* 23(5):766–771, 1994.
161. Hricik DE, Mayes JT, Schulak JA: Independent effects of cyclosporine and prednisone on posttransplant hypercholesterolemia. *Am J Kidney Dis* 18:353–358, 1991.
162. Ibels LS, Alfrey AC, Weill R: Hyperlipidemia in adult, pediatric and diabetic renal transplant recipients. *Am J Med* 64:634, 1978.
163. Lowry RP, Soltys G, Mangel R, Kwiterovitch P, et al: Type II hyperlipidemia hyperapobetaliproteinemia and hyperalphalipoproteinemia following renal transplantation: prevalence and precipitating factors. *Transplant Proc* 17:2229, 1987.
164. Kasiske BL, Tortorice KL, Heim-Duthoy KL, et al: The adverse impact of cyclosporine on serum lipids in renal transplant recipients. *Am J Kidney Dis* 17:700, 1991.
165. Harris KPG, Russell GI, Pavin SD, et al: Alterations in lipid and carbohydrate metabolism attributable to cyclosporine A in renal transplant recipients. *Br Med J* 292:16, 1986.
166. Gonwa T, Atkins C, Velez R, et al: Metabolic consequences of cyclosporine to azathioprine conversion in renal transplantation. *Clin Transplant* 2:91–96, 1988.
167. Smith PF, Eydelloth RS, Grossman SJ, et al: HMG-CoA reductase inhibitor induced myopathy in rat: Cyclosporine A interaction and mechanism studies. *J Pharmacol Exp Ther* 257:1225–1235, 1991.
168. Kainuma O, Asano T, Ochiai T, Isono K: Lipid disorders in renal transplant recipients. *Transplant Proc* 24:1585–1587, 1992.
169. Al' Halawani MH, Larsen JL, Miller S, et al: Pravastatin reduces serum cholesterol and low density lipoprotein concentrations following pancreas transplantation. *Transplantation* 58:1204–1209, 1994.
170. Castelao Am, Grino JM, Andres E, et al: HMGCoA reductase inhibitors lovastatin and simvastatin in the treatment of hypercholesterolemia after renal transplantation. *Transplant Proc* 25:1043–1046, 1993.
171. Goldberg RB, Roth D: A preliminary report of the safety and efficacy of fluvastatin for hypercholesterolemia in renal transplant patients receiving cyclosporine. *Am J Cardiol* 76:107A–109A, 1995.
172. Li PKT, Mak TWL, Chan TH, et al: Effect of fluvastatin on lipoprotein profiles in treating renal transplant recipients with dyslipoproteinemia. *Transplantation* 60:652–656, 1995.
173. Cheung AK, DeVault GA, Gregory MC: A prospective study on treatment of hypercholesterolemia with lovastatin in renal transplants receiving cyclosprine. *J Am Soc Nephrol* 3:1884–1891, 1993.

174. Kobashigawa JA, Katznelson S, Laks H, et al: The effect of pravastatin on outcomes after cardiac transplantation. *N Engl J Med* 333:621–627, 1995.
175. Katznelson, A, Wilkinson AH, Wang XM, et al: The effect of pravastatin on acute rejection and natural killer cell cytotoxicity after kidney transplantation. *Transplantation* 1996 (In Press).
176. Fung JJ, Alessiani M, Abu-Elmagd K, et al: Adverse effects associated with the use of FK 506 [Review]. *Transplant Proc* 23(6):3105–3108, 1991.
177. McCauley J: The nephrotoxicity of FK 506 as compared with cyclosporine. *Curr Opin Nephrol Hyperten* 2:662–666, 1993.
178. Puschett JB, Greenberg A, Holley J, McCauley J: The spectrum of cyclosporin nephrotoxicity. *Am J Nephrol* 10:296–309, 1990.
179. Randhawa P, Shapiro R, Jordan M, Starzl T: The histologic changes associated with allograft rejection and drug toxicity in renal transplant recipients maintained on FK 506: Clinical significance and comparison with cyclosporine. *Am J Surg Pathol* 17, 1993.
180. Solomon DR: An alternative view minimizing the significance of cyclosporine nephrotoxicity in favor of enhanced immunosuppression for long-term kidney transplant recipients. *Transplant Proc* 23:2115–2118, 1991.
181. Bennett WM, Burdmann EA, Andoh TF, et al: Nephrotoxicity of immunosuppressive drugs [Review]. *Nephrol Dial Transplant* (Suppl) 4:141–145, 1994.
182. Adams CK, Famili P: A study of the effects of the drug FK 506 on gingival tissues. *Transplant Proc* 23(6):3193–3194, 1991.
183. Bolin P. Jr, Jennette JC, Mandel SR: Cyclosporin-associated thrombotic microangiopathy: successful retreatment with cyclosporin [Review]. *Ren Fail* 13(4):275–278, 1991.
184. Schmidt RJ, Venkat KK, Dumler F: Hemolytic-uremic syndrome in a renal transplant recipient on FK 506 immunosuppression. *Transplant Proc* 23(6):3156–3157, 1991.
185. McCauley J, Bronsther O, Fung J, Todo S, Starzl TE: Treatment of cyclosporin-induced hemolytic uraemic syndrome with FK506 [Letter] [see comments]. *Lancet* 2(8678–8679):1516, 1989.
186. McCauley J, Shapiro R, Bronster O, et al: Renal transplantation under FK 506 in patients with previous loss of renal function due to hemolytic uremic syndrome. *Transplant Proc* 23(6):3068–3070, 1991.
187. Abdalla AH, al-Sulaiman MH, al-Khader AA: FK 506 as an alternative in cyclosporin-induced hemolytic uremic syndrome in a kidney transplant recipient. *Transplant Int* 7(5):382–384, 1994.
188. Julian BA, Benfield M, Quarles LB: Bone loss after organ transplantation. *Transplant Rev* 7:82, 1993.
189. Nielsen HE, Melsen F, Christensen MS: Bone lesions following renal transplantation. Bone mineral density and amount of trabecular bone. *Scandinavian Journal of Urology & Nephrology. Supplementum.* (42):127–9, 1977.
190. Zizic TM: Osteonecrosis. *Curr Opin Rheumatol* 3:481, 1991.
191. Gauthier VJ, Barbosa LM: Bone pain in transplant recipients responsive to calcium channel blockers. *Ann Intern Med* 121:863, 1994.
192. Tricontinental Mycophenolate Mofetil Renal Transplant Study Group: A blinded, randomized clinical trial of mycophenolate mofetil for the prevention of acute rejection in cadaveric renal transplantation. *Transplantation* 61:1029–1037, 1996.
193. Julian BA, Quarles LD, Niemann KM: Musculoskeletal complications after renal transplantation: Pathogenesis and treatment. *Am J Kidney Dis* 19:99, 1992.
194. D'Alessandro AM, Melzer JS, Pirch D, et al: Tertiary hyperparathyroidism after renal transplantation: Operative indications. *Surgery* 106:1049, 1989.

195. Shah GM, Kirschenbaum MA: Renal magnesium wasting associated with therapeutic agents. *Miner Electrolyte Metab* 17(1):58–64, 1991.
196. Allen RD, Hunnisett AG, Morris PJ: Cyclosporin and magnesium. *Lancet* 1:1283, 1985.
197. McCauley J, Fung JJ, Todo S, et al: Changes in renal function after liver transplantation under FK 506. *Transplant Proc* 23(6):3143–3145, 1991.
198. Lachaal M, Venuto RC: Nephrotoxicity and hyperkalemia in patients with acquired immune deficiency syndrome treated with pentamidine. *Am J Med* 87:260, 1989.
199. Miller RF, Delany S, Semple SJ: Acute renal failure after nebulized pentamidine (Letter). *Lancet* 1:1271, 1989.
200. Ryzen E, Rude RK: Low intracellular magnesium in patients with acute pancreatitis and hypocalcemia. *West J Med* 152:145, 1990.
201. Palestine AG, Polis MA, De Smet MD, et al: A randomized, controlled trial of foscarnet in the treatment of cytomegalovirus retinitis in patients with AIDS. *Ann Intern Med* 115:665, 1991.
202. White JR, Campbell RK: Magnesium and diabetes: a review. *Ann Pharmacother* 27:775, 1993.
203. Lin HY, Rocher LL, McQuillan MA, et al: Cyclosporine induced hyperuricemia and gout *N Engl J Med* 321:287, 1989.
204. Noordzij TC, Leunissen KM, Van Hooff JP: Renal handling of urate and the incidence of gouty arthritis during cyclosporine and diuretic use. *Transplanation* 52:64, 1991.
205. Shapiro R, Jordan M, Scantlebury V, Fung J, et al: FK 506 in clinical transplantation. *Transplant Proc* 23:3065–3067, 1991.
206. Jindal RM: Posttransplant diabetes mellitus: A review. *Transplantation* 58:1289–1298, 1994.
207. Hricik DE, Almawi WY, Strom TB: Trends in the use of glucocorticoids in renal transplantation. *Transplantation* 57:979–989, 1994.
208. Roth D, Milgrom M, Esquenazi V, et al: Post-transplant hyperglycemia. *Transplantation* 47:278, 1989.
209. Shapiro R, Jordan Scantlebury V, Fung J, et al: FK 506 in clinical transplantation. *Transplant Proc* 23:3065–3067, 1991.
210. Shapiro R, Jordan M, Scantlebury V, Vivas C, et al: A prospective randomized trial of FK 506 based immunosuppression after renal transplantation. *Transplantation* 59:485–490, 1995.
211. Pirsch J, and The FK 506 U.S. Kidney Transplant Multicenter Study Group, Madison, WI: FK 506 in kidney transplantation: Results of the U.S. Randomized, comparative, phase III study. Presented at the ASTP/ASTS Joint Symposium, May, 1996.
212. Tamura K, Fujimura T, Tsutsumi T, et al: Transcriptional inhibition of insulin by FK506 and possible involvement of FK506 binding protein-12 in pancreatic b-cell. *Transplantation* 59(11):1606–1613, 1995.
213. Arner P, Gunnarsson R, Blomdahl S, et al: Some characteristics of steroid diabetes: a study in renal transplant recipients receiving high dose corticosteroid therapy. *Diabetes Care* 6:23, 1983.
214. David SS, Cheigh JS, Brown DW, et al: HLA-A28 and steroid induced diabetes in renal transplant patients. *JAMA* 243:532, 1980.
215. D'Apice AJF, Mathews JD, Tait BD, et al: Association of HLA antigens with glucose tolerance following renal transplantation. *Tissue Antigens* 11:423, 1978.
216. Sollinger HW, Deierhoi MH, Belzer FO, et al: RS-61443 phase 1 clinical trial and pilot rescue study. *Transplantation* 53:428, 1992.
217. Weir MR, Kirkman RL, Strom TB, et al: Liver disease in recipients of long surviving renal allografts. *Kidney Int* 28:839–844, 1985.

218. Pereira BJ: Hepatitis C in organ transplantation: its significance and influence on transplantation policies. *Curr Opin Nephrol Hyperten* 2:912–922, 1993.
219. Braun WE: Nephrology Forum: Long term complications of renal transplantation. *Kidney Int* 37:1363–1378, 1990.
220. Bass NM, Ockner RK: In Zakim D, Boyer TD (eds), *Drug Induced Liver Disease. Hepatology: A Textbook of Liver Disease.* Philadelphia, Saunders, 1990.
221. Parfrey PS, Forbes RDC, Hutchinson TA, et al: The impact of renal transplantation on the course of hepatitis B liver disease. *Transplantation* 39:610–615, 1985.
222. Periera BJG, Wright TL, Schmid CH, et al: The impact of pretransplantation hepatitis C infection on the outcome of renal transplantation. *Transplantation* 60:799–805, 1995.
223. Chan TM, Lok ASF, Cheng IKP, Chan RT: Prevalence of hepatitis C virus infection in hemodialysis patients: A longitudinal study comparing the results of RNA and antibody assays. *Hepatology* 17:5–8, 1993.
224. Pol S, Romeo R, Zins B, et al: Hepatitis C virus RNA in anti-HCV positive hemodialysis patients: Significance and therapeutic implications. *Kidney Int* 44:1097–1100, 1993.
225. Magnone M, Holley JL, Shapiro R, et al: Interferon-alpha-induced acute renal allograft rejection. *Transplantation* 59(7):1068–1070, 1995.
226. Bertoni E, Rosati A, Zanazzi M, et al: Severe aplastic anaemia due to B19 parvovirus infection in renal transplant recipients. *Nephrol Dial Transplant* 10(8):1462–1463, 1995.
227. Gaston RS, Julian BA, Curtis JJ: Posttransplant erythrocytosis: An enigma revisited. *Am J Kidney Dis* 24:1, 1994.
228. Aeberhard JM, Schneider PA, Vollotton MB, et al: Multiple site estimates of erythropoietin and renin in polycythemic kidney transplant patients. *Transplantation* 50:613, 1990.
229. Ilan Y, Dranitzki-Elhallel M, Rubinger D, et al: Erythrocytosis after renal transplantation. The response to theophylline treatment. *Transplantation* 57:661, 1994.
230. Torregrosa JV, Campistol JM, Montesinos M, et al: Efficacy of captopril on posttransplant erythrocytosis. *Transplantation* 58:311, 1994.
231. Danovitch GM, Jamgotchian NJ, Eggena PH, et al: Angiotensin-converting enzyme inhibition in the treatment of renal transplant erythrocytosis. *Transplantation* 60:132, 1995.
232. Parazella M, Mcphedran P, Kliger A, et al: Enalapril treatment of post transplant erythrocytosis: Efficacy independent of circulating erythropoietin levels. *Am J Kidney Dis* 26:495, 1995.
233. OK E, Akcicek F, Toz H, et al: Comparison of the effects of enalapril and theophylline on polycythemia after renal transplantation. *Transplantation* 59:1623, 1995.
234. Vlahakos DV, Canzanello VJ, Madaio MP, Madias NE: Enalapril associated anemia in renal transplant recipients treated for hypertension. *Am J Kidney Dis* 17:199, 1991.
235. Dhondt AW, Vanholder RC, Ringoir SM: Angiotensin converting enzyme inhibitors and higher erythropoietin requirement in chronic hemodialysis patients. *Nephrol Dial Transplant* 10:2107, 1995.
236. Tyldesley WR, Rotter E: Gingival hyperplasia induced by cyclosporin A. *Br Dent J* 157:305, 1984.
237. Gassenmaeier A, Fuchs P, Schell H, Pfister H: Papillomavirus DNA in warts of immunosuppressed renal allograft recipients. *Arch Dermatol Res* 278:219, 1986.

Infectious Complications

238. Rifkind D: Infectious diseases associated with renal transplantation. In: *Experience in Renal Transplantation* Starzl TE (ed), Philadelphia, Saunders, 1964:213.
239. Peterson PK, Balfour HH, Fryd DS, Ferguson RM, Simmons RL: Fever in renal transplant

recipients: causes, prognostic significance and changing patterns at the University of Minnesota Hospital. *Am J Med* 71:345, 1981.
240. Carter JM, Green WR, Callender CO, Peters B: Pulmonary cavitation with *Nocardia* and *Aspergillus,* in a renal transplant patient. *J Natl Med Assoc* 82:527, 1990.
241. Shaariah W, Morad Z, Suleiman AB: Cryptococcosis in renal transplant recipients. *Transplant Proc* 24:1898, 1992.
242. Brayman KL, Stephanian E, Matas AJ, et al: Analysis of infectious complications occurring after solid-organ transplantation. *Arch Surg* 127:38, 1992.
243. Yoshimura N, Oka T: Medical and surgical complications of renal transplantation: Diagnosis and management. *Med Clin North Am* 74:1025, 1990.
244. Nicholson ML, Veitch PS, Donnelly PK, Bell PRF: Urological complications of renal transplantation: the impact of double J ureteric stents. *Ann R Coll Surg Engl* 73:316, 1991.
245. Mora M, Wilms H, Kirste G: Significance of bacterial contamination of cadaver donor renal allografts before transplantation. *Transplant Proc* 23:2648, 1991.
246. Gottesdiener KM: Transplanted infections: donor-to-host transmission with the allograft. *Ann Intern Med* 110:1001, 1989.
247. Shaffer D, Hammer SM, Monaco AP: Infectious complications with the use of cyclosporine versus azathioprine after cadaveric kidney transplantation. *Am J Surg* 153:381, 1987.
248. Najarian JS, Fryd DS, Strand M, et al: A single institution, randomized, prospective trial of cyclosporine versus azathioprine—antilymphocyte globulin for immunosuppression in renal allograft recipients. *Ann Surg* 201:142, 1985.
249. Henry ML, Sommer BG, Ferguson RM: Beneficial effects of cyclosporine compared with azathioprine in cadaveric renal transplantation. *Am J Surg* 150:533, 1985.
250. The Canadian Multicenter Transplant Study Group: A randomized clinical trial of cyclosporine in cadaveric renal transplantation. *New Engl J Med* 309:809, 1983.
251. Ho M, Wajszczuk CP, Hardy A, et al: Infections in kidney, heart and liver transplant recipients on cyclosporine. *Transplant Proc* 15:2768, 1983.
252. Dummer JS, Hardy A, Poorsattar A, Ho M: Early infections in kidney, heart, and liver transplant recipients on cyclosporine. *Transplantation* 36:259, 1983.
253. Shapiro R, Jordan ML, Scantlebury VP, et al: A prospective, randomized trial of FK506-based immunosuppression after renal transplantation. *Transplantation* 59:485, 1995.
254. Jordan M, Shapiro R, Vivas C, et al: FK506 rescue for resistant rejection of renal allograft under primary cyclosporine immunosuppression. *Transplantation* 57:860, 1994.
255. Kusne S, Martin M, Shapiro R, et al: Early infection in kidney transplant recipients under FK506. *Transplant Proc* 23:956, 1991.
256. Shapiro R, Jordan M, Scantlebury V, et al: FK 506 in clinical kidney transplantation. *Transplant Proc* 23:3065, 1991.
257. Rubin RH: Infectious disease complications of renal transplantation. *Kidney Int* 44:221, 1993.
258. Tolkoff-Rubin NE, Rubin RH: Clinical approach to viral and fungal infections in the renal transplant patient. *Semin Nephrol* 12:364, 1992.
259. Rubin RH, Tolkoff-Rubin NE: Opportunistic infections in renal allograft recipients. *Transplant Proc* 20:12, 1988.
260. Rubin RH: Infection in the renal and liver transplant patient. In: Rubin RH, Young LS (eds), *Clinical Approach to Infection in the Compromised Host,* 2nd ed. New York, Plenum Press, 1988:557–621.
261. Myerowitz RL, Medeiros AA, O'Brien TF: Bacterial infection in renal homotransplant recipients. *Am J Med* 53:308, 1972.

262. Masur H, Cheigh JS, Stubenbord WT: Infection following renal transplantation: a changing pattern. *Rev Infect Dis* 4:1208, 1982.
263. Wagener MM, Yu VL: Bacteremia in transplant recipients: a prospective study of demographics, etiologic agents, risk factors, and outcomes. *Am J Infect Control* 20:239, 1992.
264. Ascher NL, Simmons RL, Marker S, Najarian JS: *Listeria* infection in transplant patients. *Arch Surg* 113:90, 1978.
265. Skogberg K, Syrjanen J, Jahkola M, et al: Clinical presentation and outcome of listeriosis in patients with and without immunosuppressive therapy. *Clin Infect Dis* 14:815, 1992.
266. Lunde NM, Messana JM, Swartz RD: Unusual causes of peritonitis in patients undergoing continuous peritoneal dialysis with emphasis on *Listeria monocytogenes*. *J Am Soc Nephrol* 3:1092, 1992.
267. Macgowan AP, Marshall RJ, Mackay IM, Reeves DS: *Listeria* faecal carriage by renal transplant recipients, hemodialysis patients and patients in general practice: its relation to season, drug therapy, foreign travel, animal exposure and diet. *Epidemiol Infect* 106:157, 1991.
268. McNeil MM, Brown JM, Magruder CH, et al: Disseminated *Nocardia transvalensis* infection: an unusual opportunistic pathogen in severely immunocompromised patients. *J Infect Dis* 165:175, 1992.
269. King CT, Chapman SW, Butkus DE: Recurrent nocardiosis in a renal transplant recipient. *South Med J* 86:225, 1993.
270. Wilson JP, Turner HR, Kirchner KA, Chapman SW: Nocardial infections in renal transplant recipients. Medicine 68:38, 1989.
271. Goncalves ARP, Caetano MA, Paula FJ, et al: Tuberculous interstitial granulomatous nephritis in renal transplants: report of three cases. *Transplant Proc* 24:1911, 1992.
272. Mansour AM: Renal allograft tuberculosis. *Tubercle,* 71:147, 1990.
273. Higgins RM, Cahn AP, Porter D, et al: Mycobacterial infections after renal transplantation. *Q J Med* 78:145, 1991.
274. Qunibi WY, Al-Sibai MB, Taher S, et al: Mycobacterial infection after renal transplantation—report of 14 cases and review of the literature. *Q J Med* 77:1039, 1990.
275. Cooper JF, Lichtenstein MJ, Graham BS, Schaffner W: *Mycobacterium chelonae:* a cause of nodular skin lesions with a proclivity for renal transplant recipients. *Am J Med* 86:173, 1989.
276. Wallas RJ, O'Brien R, Glasroth J, et al: Diagnosis and treatment of disease caused by nontuberculous mycobacteria. *Am Rev Respir Dis* 142:940–953, 1990.
277. Dhar JM, Al-Khader AA, Al-Sulaiman M, Al-Hasani MK: Nontyphoid *Salmonella* in renal transplant recipients: a report of twenty cases and review of the literature. *Q J Med, New Series* 78:235, 1991.
278. Human cytomegalovirus infection in immunosuppressed patients. In: Ho M: *Cytomegalovirus Biology and Infection,* ed 2. New York, Plenum Press, New York, 1991:249–270.
279. Pouteil-Noble C, Ecochard R, Landrivon G, et al: Cytomegalovirus infection, an etiological factor for rejection? A prospective study in 242 renal transplant recipients. *Transplantation* 55:851, 1993.
280. Bosch FH, Hoitsma AJ, Janssen HP, van Loon AM, Koene RA: Cytomegalovirus infection and disease in renal transplant patients treated with cyclosporin. A prospective study. *Transplant Int* 2:92, 1989.
281. Simmons RL, Lopez CL, Balfour H Jr, et al: Cytomegalovirus: clinical virological correlations in renal transplant recipients. *Ann Surg* 180:623, 1974.

282. Ho M, Suwansirikul S, Dowling JN, Youngblood LA, Armstrong JA: The transplanted kidney as a source of cytomegalovirus infections. *N Engl J Med* 293:1109, 1975.
283. Suwansirikul S, Rao N, Dowling JN, Ho M: Clinical manifestations of primary and secondary cytomegalovirus infection after renal transplantation. *Arch Intern Med* 137:1026, 1977.
284. Betts RF, Freeman RB, Douglas RG Jr, Talley TE: Clinical manifestations of renal allograft derived primary cytomegalovirus infection. *Am J Dis Child* 131:759, 1977.
285. Chou S: Acquisition of donor strains of cytomegalovirus by renal-transplant recipients. *N Engl J Med* 314:1418, 1986.
286. Grundy JE, Lui SF, Super M, et al: Symptomatic cytomegalovirus infection in seropositive kidney recipients: Reinfection with donor virus rather than reactivation of recipient virus. *Lancet* 2:132, 1988.
287. Fujinami RS, Nelson JA, Walker L, Oldstone MBA: Sequence homology and immunologic cross-reactivity of human cytomegalovirus with HLA-DR beta chain: A means for graft rejection and immunosuppression. *J Virol* 62:100, 1988.
288. Blancho G, Josien R, Douillard D, et al: The influence of HLA A-B-DR matching on cytomegalovirus disease after renal transplantation. Evidence that HLA-DR7-matched recipients are more susceptible to cytomegalovirus disease. *Transplantation* 54:871, 1992.
289. Pouteil-Noble C, Betuel H, Raffaele P, et al: Influence of HLA compatibility on cytomegalovirus infection in kidney transplantation. *Press Med* 20:2022, 1991.
290. Rinaldo CR Jr, DeBiasio RL, Hamoudi WH, et al: Effect of herpesvirus infection on T-lymphocyte subpopulations and blastogenic responses in renal transplant recipients receiving cyclosporine. *Clin Immunol Immunopathol* 38:366, 1986.
291. Bourbigot M, Bensoussan T, Garo B, et al: CD4 T-lymphocyte counts as predictors of pneumonia after kidney transplantation. *Transplant Proc* 25:1491, 1993.
292. van den Berg AP, van Son WJ, Haagsma EB, et al: Prediction of recurrent cytomegalovirus disease after treatment with ganciclovir in solid-organ transplant recipients. *Transplantation* 55:847, 1993.
293. Ho M: Virus infections after transplantation in man. *Arch Virol* 55:1, 1977.
294. Bowmans JS III, Angstadt JD, Waymack JP, Jaffers GJ: A comparison of triple-therapy with double-therapy immunosuppression in cadaveric renal transplantation. *Transplantation* 53:556, 1992.
295. van Dorp WT, van Es LA, Thompson J, van der Woude FJ: The effects of a maintenance immunosuppressive protocol after renal transplantation on infectious complications, comparing cyclosporine/prednisone, cyclosporine/azathioprine/prednisone, and conversion. *Transplantation* 51:193, 1991.
296. Gerna G, Zipeto D, Parea M, et al: Monitoring of human cytomegalovirus infections and ganciclovir treatment in heart transplant recipients by determination of viremia, antigenemia, and DNAemia. *J Infect Dis* 164:488, 1991.
297. van den Berg AP, van Son WJ, van der Bij W, van der Giessen M, The TH: Early identification of patients at high risk of severe cytomegalovirus disease after renal transplantation using the immediate early antigenemia assay. *Transplant Proc* 22:1800, 1990.
298. van Dorp WT, Vlieger A, Jiwa NM, et al: The polymerase chain reaction, a sensitive and rapid technique for detecting cytomegalovirus infection after renal transplantation. *Transplantation* 54:661, 1992.
299. Delgado R, Lumbreras C, Alba C, et al: Low predictive value of polymerase chain reaction for diagnosis of cytomegalovirus disease in liver transplant recipients. *J Clin Microbiol* 30:1876, 1992.

300. Elion GB, Furman PA, Fyfe JA, et al: Selectivity of action of an antiherpes agent, 9-(2-hydroxyethoxymethyl) guanine. *Proc Nat Acad Sci USA* 74:5716, 1977.
301. Jordan M, Hrebinko RL Jr, Dummer JS, et al: Therapeutic use of ganciclovir for invasive cytomegalovirus infection in cadaveric renal allograft recipients. *J Urol* 148:1388, 1992.
302. de Koning J, van Dorp WT, van Es LA, van't Wout JW, van der Woude FJ: Ganciclovir effectively treats cytomegalovirus disease after solid-organ transplantation, even during rejection treatment. *Nephrol Dial Transplant* 7:350, 1992.
303. Kutsogiannis DJ, Crowther MA, Lazarovits AI: Granulocyte macrophage colony-stimulating factor for the therapy of cytomegalovirus and ganciclovir-induced leukopenia in a renal transplant recipient. *Transplantation* 53:930, 1992.
304. Andersson J, Akesson-Johansson A, Brattstrom C: Evaluation by immune scanning electron microscopy of foscarnet treatment of cytomegalovirus infection in patients with renal transplants. *Scand J Infect Dis* 21:605, 1989.
305. Reed EC, Bowden RA, Dandliker PS, Lilleby KE, Meyers JD: Treatment of cytomegalovirus pneumonia with ganciclovir and intravenous cytomegalovirus immunoglobulin in patients with bone marrow transplants. *Ann Intern Med* 109:783, 1988.
306. Ho M, Ronald J, Miller G, et al: The frequency of Epstein-Barr virus infection and associated lymphoproliferative syndrome after transplantation and its manifestations in children. *Transplantation* 45:719, 1988.
307. Hanto DW, Gajl-Peczalska KJ, Frizzera G, et al: Epstein-Barr virus (EBV) induced polyclonal and monoclonal B-cell lymphoproliferative disease occurring after renal transplantation. Clinical, pathologic, and virologic findings and implications for therapy. *Ann Surg* 198:365, 1983.
308. Yao QY, Rickinson AB, Gastron JS, Epstein MA: In vitro analysis of the Epstein-Barr virus: Host balance in long-term renal allograft recipients. *Int J Cancer* 35:43, 1985.
309. Swinnen LJ, Costanzo-Nordin MR, Fisher SG, et al: Increased incidence of lymphoproliferative disorder after immunosuppression with the monoclonal antibody OKT3 in cardiac-transplant recipients. *N Engl J Med* 323:1723, 1990.
310. Fischer A, Blanche S, Le Bidois J, et al: Anti-B-cell monoclonal antibodies in the treatment of severe B-cell lymphoproliferative syndrome following bone marrow and organ transplantation. *N Engl J Med* 324:1451, 1991.
311. Riddler SA, Breining MK, McKnight JLC: Increased levels of circulating Epstein-Barr Virus (EBV)-infected lymphocytes and decreased EBV nuclear antigen antibody responses are associated with the development of posttransplant lymphoproliferative disease in solid organ transplant recipients. *Blood* 84:972, 1994.
312. Hornef MW, Wagner HJ, Fricke L, Bein G, Kirchner H: Immunocytochemical detection of Epstein-Barr Virus Antigen in peripheral B-lymphocytes after renal transplantation. *Transplantation* 59:138, 1995.
313. Straus SE, Rooney JF, Sever JL, et al: Herpes simplex virus infection: biology, treatment, and prevention. *Ann Intern Med* 103:404, 1985.
314. Kusne S, Schwartz M, Breinig MK, et al: Herpes simplex virus hepatitis after solid organ transplantation in adults. *J Infect Dis* 165:1001, 1991.
315. Lynfield R, Herrin JT, Rubin RH. Varicella in pediatric renal transplant recipients. *Pediatrics* 90:216, 1992.
316. Ho M, Dummer JS, Pasculle WA, McMahon DK, Kusne S: Infections in the transplant recipient. In: Makowka L (ed), *The Handbook of Transplantation Management,* Austin, TX, RG Landes Company, 1991:448.

317. Easterbrook P, Wood MJ: Successors to acyclovir. *J Antimicrob Chemother* 34:307, 1994.
318. LaQuaglia MP, Tolkoff-Rubin NE, Dienstag JL, et al: Impact of hepatitis on renal transplantation. *Transplantation* 32:504, 1981.
319. Boyce NW, Holdsworth SR, Hooke D, Thomson NM, Atkins RC: Nonhepatitis B-associated liver disease in a renal transplant population. *Am J Kidney Dis* 11:307, 1988.
320. Strom TB: Hepatitis B, transfusions, and renal transplantation—five years later. *N Engl J Med* 307:1141, 1982.
321. Fernandez JA, Roth D, Burke G, Esquenazi V, Miller J: Detection of antibody to hepatitis C virus (HCV) in renal transplant recipients. *J Am Soc Nephrol* (abs) 1:757, 1990.
322. Ponz E, Campistol JM, Bruguera M, et al: Hepatitis C infection among kidney transplant recipients. *Kidney Int* 40:748, 1991.
323. Pereira BJG, Milford EL, Kirkman RL, Levey AS: Transmission of hepatitis C virus by organ transplantation. *N Engl J Med* 325:454, 1991.
324. Morales JM, Campistol JM: Hepatitis C virus and organ transplantation (Letter to the editor). *N Engl J Med* 328:511, 1993.
325. Koretz RL, Abbey H, Coleman E, Gitnick G: Non-A, non-B post-transfusion hepatitis. Looking back the second decade. *Ann Intern Med* 119:110, 1993.
326. Wright TL, Donegan E, Hsu HH, et al: Recurrent and acquired hepatitis C viral infection in liver transplant recipients. *Gastroenterology* 103:317, 1992.
327. Chugh KS, Sakhuja V, Jain S, et al: Fungal infections in renal allograft recipients. *Transplant Proc* 24:1940, 1992.
328. Gallis HA, Berman RA, Cate TR, et al: Fungal infection following renal transplantation. *Arch Intern Med* 135:1163, 1975.
329. Howard RJ, Simmons RL, Najarian JS: Fungal infections in renal transplant recipients. *Ann Surg* 188:598, 1978.
330. Nemec DK, Lederer ED, Samo T: Candidal splenic abscess in a renal transplant patient. *Am J Kidney Dis* 14:408, 1989.
331. Pluemecke G, Williams J, Elliott D, Paul LC: Renal transplant artery rupture secondary to *Candida* infection. *Nephron* 61:98, 1992.
332. Palmer BF, Hernandez J, Sagalowsky A, Dawidson I, Helderman JH: Documentation of fungal pyelonephritis of the renal allograft by fine needle aspiration cytology. *Transplant Proc* 21:3598, 1989.
333. Nicholson ML, Veitch PS, Donnelly PK: Systemic candidiasis caused by a renal transplant ureteric stent. *Br J Urol* 70:448, 1992.
334. Wiebe VJ, DeGregoris MW: Lipsosome-encapsulated amphotericin B: a promising new treatment for disseminated fungal infections. *Rev Infect Dis* 10:1097, 1988.
335. Tolkoff-Rubin NE, Conti DJ, Doran M, DelVecchio A, Rubin RH: Fluconazole in the treatment of invasive candidal and cryptococcal infections in organ transplant recipients. *Pharmacotherapy* 10:159S, 1990.
336. Manez R, Martin M, Raman V, et al: Fluconazole therapy in transplant recipients receiving FK 506. *Transplantation* 57:1521, 1994.
337. Barbara JAJ, Clarkson AR, LaBrooy J, McNeil JD, Woodroffe AJ: *Candida albicans* arthritis in a renal allograft recipient with an interaction between cyclosporin and fluconazole. *Nephrol Dial Transplant* 8:263, 1993.
338. Beal MF, O'Carroll CP, Kleinman GM, Grossman RI: Aspergillosis of the nervous sytem. *Neurology* 32:473, 1982.
339. Walsh TJ, Hier DB, Caplan LR: Aspergillosis of the central nervous system: clinicopathological analysis of 17 patients. *Ann Neurol* 18:574, 1985.

340. Chugh KS, Sakhuja V, Jain S, et al: High mortality in systemic fungal infections following renal transplantation in third-world countries. *Nephrol Dial Transplant* 8:168, 1993.
341. Sridhar NR, Tchervenkov JI, Weiss MA, Hijazi YM, First MR: Disseminated histoplasmosis in a renal transplant patient: a cause of renal failure several years following transplantation. *Am J Kidney Dis* 17:719, 1991.
342. Elinder CG, Andersson J, Bolinder G, Tyden G: Effectiveness of low-dose cotrimoxazole prophylaxis against *Pneumocystis carinii* pneumonia after renal and/or pancreas transplantation. *Transplant Int* 5:81, 1992.
343. Eickhoff TC: Infectious complications in renal transplant recipients. *Transplant Proc* 5:1233, 1973.
344. Hardy AM, Wajszczuk CP, Hakala TR, et al: Infection in renal transplant recipients on cyclosporine: *Pneumocystis* pneumonia. *Transplant Proc* 15:2773, 1983.
345. Watson AJ, Yang A, Olson JL, Bastacky SI: A 37-year-old man with diabetes mellitus renal transplant, fever, pulmonary infiltrates, and mental status alterations. *Md Med J* 42:51, 1993.
346. Renoult E, Biava MF, Aimone-Gastin I, et al: Evolution and significance of *Toxoplasma gondii* antibody titers in kidney transplant recipients. *Transplant Proc* 24:2754, 1992.
347. Salt A, Sutehall G, Sargaison M, et al: Viral and *Toxoplasma gondii* infections in children after liver transplantation. *J Clin Pathol* 43:63, 1990.
348. Calico I, Caballero E, Martinez O, et al: Isolation of *Toxoplasma gondii* from immunocompromised patients using tissue culture. *Infection* 19:340, 1991.
349. Jacobs F, Depierreux M, Goldman M, et al: Role of bronchoalveolar lavage in diagnosis of disseminated toxoplasmosis. *Rev Infect Dis* 13:637, 1991.
350. Feron D, Goldman M, Jacobs F, et al: Bone marrow aspiration as a diagnostic tool for acute toxoplasmosis in a kidney transplant recipient. *Transplantation* 50:1054, 1990.
351. Renoult E, Chabot F, Aymard B, et al: Generalized toxoplasmosis in two renal transplant recipients who received a kidney from the same donor. *Rev Infect Dis* 13:180, 1991.
352. DeVault GA, King JW, Rohr MS, et al: Opportunistic infections with *Strongyloides stercoralis,* in renal transplantation. *Rev Infect Dis* 12:653, 1990.
353. Peterson PK, Anderson RC: Infection in renal transplant recipients. *Am J Med* 81(Suppl 1A):2, 1986.
354. Pearson JC, Amend WJC Jr, Vincenti FG, Feduska NJ, Salvatierra O Jr: Post-transplantation pyelonephritis: factors producing low patient and transplant morbidity. *J Urol* 123:153, 1980.
355. Gill IS, Hayes JM, Hodge EE, Novick AC: Clean intermittent catheterization and urinary diversion in the management of renal transplant recipients with lower urinary tract dysfunction. *J Urol* 148:1397, 1992.
356. Matthew TH, Kincaid-Smith P, Vikraman P: Risks of vesicoureteric reflux in the transplanted kidney. *N Engl J Med* 297:414, 1977.
357. Franz M, Klaar U, Hofbauer H, et al: Incidence of urinary tract infections and vesicorenal reflux: a comparison between conventional and antirefluxive technique of ureter implantation. *Transplant Proc* 24:2773, 1992.
358. Ramsey PG, Rubin RH, Tolkoff-Rubin NE, et al: The renal transplant patient with fever and pulmonary infiltrates: etiology, clinical manifestations, and management. *Medicine* 59:3, 1980.
359. Humphreys H, Marshall RJ, Mackay I, Caul EO: Pneumonia due to *Legionella bozemanii* and *Chlamydia psittaci*/TWAR following renal transplantation. *J Infect* 25:67, 1992.
360. Williams P, Yu LV: Successful use of ciprofloxacin and rifampin for treatment of *Legionella* pneumonia in a heart transplant recipient. *Transplant Sci* 2:73, 1992.

361. Van Laethem JL, Bourgeois N, Gelin M, et al: Digestive tract infections in kidney and liver transplantation in a single institution. *Transplantation* 55:433, 1993.
362. Sutherland DER, Chan FY, Foucar E, et al: The bleeding cecal ulcer in transplant patients. *Surgery* 86:386, 1979.
363. Hau T, Van Hook EJ, Simmons RL, Najarian JS: Prognostic factors of peritoneal infections in transplant patients. *Surgery* 84:403, 1978.
364. Guice K, Rattazzi LC, Marchioro TL: Colon perforation in renal transplant patients. *Am J Surg* 138:43, 1979.
365. Hoy WE, May AG, Freeman RB: Primary renal transplant wound infections. *NY State J Med* 81:1469, 1981.
366. Kyriakides GK, Simmons RL, Najarian JS: Wound infections in renal transplant wounds: pathogenetic and prognostic factors. *Ann Surg* 182:770, 1975.
367. Simmons RL, Migliori RJ: Infection prophylaxis after successful organ transplantation. *Transplant Proc* 20:7, 1988.
368. Mokhbat JE, Peterson PK, Sabath LD: Peritonitis due to *Mycoplasma hominis* in a renal transplant recipient. *J Infect Dis* 146:713, 1982.
369. McMahon DK, Kusne S: *Mycoplasma hominis* infections in transplant patients. *Transplant Sci* 2:68, 1992.
370. McMahon DK, Dummer JS, Pasculle AW, Cassell G: Extragenital *Mycoplasma hominis* infections in adults. *Am J Med* 89:265, 1990.
371. Tilney NL, Kohler TR, Strom TB: Cerebromeningitis in immunosuppressed recipients of renal allografts. *Ann Surg* 5:104, 1982.
372. Murphy JF, McDonald FD, Dawson M, et al: Factors affecting the frequency of infection in renal transplant recipients. *Arch Intern Med* 136:670, 1976.
373. Kong NCT, Shaariah W, Morad Z, Suleiman AB, Wong YH: Cryptococcosis in a renal unit. *Aust NZ J Med* 20:645, 1990.
374. Stamm AM, Dismukes WE, Simmons BP, et al: Listeriosis in renal transplant recipients: report of an outbreak and review of 102 cases. *Rev Infect Dis* 4:665, 1982.
375. Benedict LM, Kusne S, Torre-Cisneros J, Hunt SJ: Primary cutaneous fungal infections after solid organ transplant, a report of five cases and review of the literature. *Clin Infect Dis* 15:17, 1992.
376. Peterson PK, Ferguson R, Fryd DS, et al: Infectious diseases in hospitalized renal transplant recipients: A prospective study of a complex and evolving problem. *Medicine* 61:360, 1982.
377. Francel TJ, Marshall KA, Savage RC: Hand infections in the diabetic and the diabetic renal transplant. *Ann Plastic Surg* 24:304, 1990.
378. Tolkoff-Rubin NE, Cosimi AB, Russell PS, Rubin RH: A controlled study of trimethoprim-sulfamethoxazole prophylaxis of urinary tract infection in renal transplant recipients. *Rev Infect Dis* 4:614, 1982.
379. Peters C, Peterson P, Marabella P, Simmons RL, Najarian JS: Continuous sulfa prophylaxis for urinary tract infection in renal transplant recipients. *Am J Surg* 146:589, 1983.
380. Rubin RH, Tolkoff-Rubin NE: Antimicrobial strategies in the care of organ transplant recipients. *Antimicrob Agents Chemother* 37:619, 1993.
381. Fox BC, Sollinger HW, Belzer FO, Maki DG: A prospective, randomized, double-blind study of trimethoprim-sulfamethoxazole for prophylaxis of infection in renal transplantation: clinical efficacy, absorption of trimethoprim-sulfamethoxazole, effects on the microflora, and the cost-benefit of prophylaxis. *Am J Med* 89:255, 1990.
382. Sundberg R, Shapiro R, Darras F, et al: A tuberculosis outbreak in a renal transplant program. *Transplant Proc* 23:3091, 1991.

383. Jereb JA, Burwen DR, Dooley SW, et al: Nosocomial outbreak of tuberculosis in a renal transplant unit: application of a new technique for restriction fragment length polymorphism analysis of *Mycobacterium tuberculosis* isolates. *J Infect Dis* 168:1219, 1993.
384. Schmidt GM, Horak DA, Niland JC, et al: A randomized, controlled trial of prophylactic ganciclovir for cytomegalovirus pulmonary infection in recipients of allogeneic bone marrow transplants. *N Engl J Med* 324:1005, 1991.
385. Merigan TC, Renlund DG, Keay S, et al: A controlled trial of ganciclovir to prevent cytomegalovirus disease after heart transplantation. *N Engl J Med* 326:1182, 1992.
386. Martin M, Manez R, Linden P, et al: A prospective randomized trial comparing sequential ganciclovir-high dose acyclovir to high dose acyclovir for prevention of cytomegalovirus disease in adult liver transplant recipients. *Transplantation* 58:779, 1994.
387. Rondeau E, Bourgeon B, Peraldi MN, et al: Effect of prophylactic ganciclovir on cytomegalovirus infection in renal transplant recipients. *Nephrol Dial Transplant* 8:858, 1993.
388. Conti DJ, Freed BM, Gruber SA, Lempert N: Prophylaxis of primary cytomegalovirus disease in renal transplant recipients. *Arch Surg* 129:443, 1994.
389. Balfour HH, Chace BA, Stapleton JT, Simmons RL, Fryd DS: A randomized, placebo-controlled trial of oral acyclovir for the prevention of cytomegalovirus disease in recipients of renal allografts. *N Engl J Med* 320:1381, 1989.
390. Snydman DR, Werner BG, Heinze-Lacey B, et al: Use of cytomegalovirus immune globulin to prevent cytomegalovirus disease in renal-transplant recipients. *N Engl J Med* 317:1049, 1987.
391. Vasquez EM, Sanchez J, Pollak R, et al: High-dose oral acyclovir prophylaxis for primary cytomegalovirus infection in seronegative renal allograft recipients. *Transplantation* 55:448, 1993.
392. Legendre C, Ducloux D, Ferroni A, et al: Acyclovir in preventing cytomegalovirus infection in kidney transplant recipients: a case-controlled study. *Transplant Proc* 25:1431, 1993.
393. Boland GJ, Ververs C, Hene RJ, et al: Early detection of primary cytomegalovirus infection after heart and kidney transplantation and the influence of hyperimmune globulin prophylaxis. *Transplant Int* 6:34, 1993.
394. Conti DJ, Freed BM, Lempert N: Prophylactic immunoglobulin therapy improves the outcome of renal transplantation in recipients at risk for primary cytomegalovirus disease. *Transplant Proc* 25:1421, 1993.
395. Steinmuller DR, Novick AC, Streem SB, Graneto D, Swift C: Intravenous immunoglobulin infusions for the prophylaxis of secondary cytomegalovirus infection. *Transplantation* 49:68, 1990.
396. Kasiske BL, Heim-Duthoy KL, Tortorice KL, et al: Polyvalent immune globulin and cytomegalovirus infection after renal transplantation. *Arch Intern Med* 149:2733, 1989.
397. Pakkala S, Salmela K, Lautenschlager I, Ahonen J, Hayry P: Anti-CMV hyperimmune globulin prophylaxis does not prevent CMV disease in CMV-negative renal transplant patients. *Transplant Proc* 24:283, 1992.
398. Dorsky D, Crumpacker C: Drugs five years later: acyclovir. *Ann Intern Med* 107:859, 1987.
399. Tomlanovich SJ, Sabatte-Caspillo J, Melzer J, et al: The incidence and impact of herpes simplex virus infections in the first month following renal transplantation. *Transplant Proc* 21:2091, 1989.
400. Hakim M, Esmore D, Wallwork J, English TAH: Toxoplasmosis in cardiac transplantation. *Br Med J* 292:1108, 1986.

Neurologic Complications

401. US Renal Data System: USRDS 1992 Annual Data Report. National Institute of Diabetes and Digestive and Kidney Diseases: Bethesda, MD, 1992.
402. Rostand SG, Brunzell JD, Cannon RO, Victor RG: Cardiovascular complications in renal failure. *J Am Soc Nephrol* 2:1053, 1991.
403. DeFronzo RA, Andres R, Edgar P, Walker WG: Carbohydrate metabolism in uremia: A review. *Medicine* (Baltimore) 52:469, 1973.
404. Gilmore RL. Seizures and antiepileptic drug use in transplant patients. *Neurol Clin* 6:279-296, 1988.
405. Tyler HR, Tyler KL: Neurologic complications, In: Eknoyan G, Knochel JP (eds), *The Systemic Consequences of Renal Failure*. New York, Grune & Stratton, 1984:311.
406. Leavitt S, Tyler HR: Studies in asterixis. *Arch Neurol* 10:360, 1964.
407. Adams RD, Foley JM: The neurologic changes in the more common types of severe liver disease. *Trans Am Neurol Assoc* 74:217, 1949.
408. Stark RJ: Reversible myoclonus with uraemia. *Br Med J* 282:1119, 1981.
409. Tyler HR: Neurologic disorders in renal failure. *Am J Med* 44:734, 1968.
410. Bolton CF, Driedger AA, Lindsay RM. Ischemic neuropathy in uremic patients caused by bovine arteriovenous shunt. *J. Neurol Neurosurg, Psychiatr* 42:810–814, 1979.
411. Sherman DG, Easton JD. Dieting and peroneal nerve palsy. *JAMA* 238:230, 1977.
412. Rosen SM, O'Connor K, Shaldon S: Haemodialysis disequilibrium. *Br Med J* 2:672, 1964.
413. Bana DS, Yap AU, Graham JR: Headache during hemodialysis. *Headache* 12:1, 1972.
414. Leonard A, Shaprio FL: Subdural hematoma in regularly hemodialyzed patients. *Ann Intern Med* 82:650–658, 1975.
415. Alfrey AC, Mishell JM, Burks J, et al: Syndrome of dyspraxia and multifocal seizures associated with chronic hemodialysis. *Trans Am Soc Artif Intern Organs* 18:257, 1972.
416. Fraser CL, Arieff AI: Nervous system complications in uremia. *Ann Intern Med* 109:143, 1988.
417. Mahoney CA, Arieff AI: Uremic encephalopathies: Clinical, biochemical, and experimental features. *Am J Kidney Dis* 2:324, 1982.
418. Alfrey AC, LeGendre GR, Kaehney WD: The dialysis encephalopathy syndrome: Possible aluminum intoxication. *N Engl J Med* 294:184, 1976.
419. Rovelli E, Luciani L, Pagani C, et al: Correlation between serum aluminum concentration and signs of encephalopathy in a large population of patients dialyzed with aluminum-free fluids. *Clin Nephrol* 29:294, 1988.
420. Mahoney CA, Arieff AI: Uremic encephalopathies: Clinical, biochemical, and experimental features. *Am J Kidney Dis* 2:324, 1982.
421. Delinger JK: Prolonged emergence and failure to regain consciousness. In: Orkin FK, Cooperman LH, (eds). *Complications in Anesthesiology.* Philadelphia, JB Lippincott, 1983:369.
422. O'Hare SA, Callaghan NM, Murnaghan DJ: Dialysis encephalopathy: Medical, electroencephalographic and interventional aspects. *Medicine* 62:129–141, 1983.
423. Parfitt AM: Hypercalcemic hyperparathyroidism following renal transplantation: differential diagnosis, management, and implications for cell population control in the parathyroid gland. *Mineral Electrolyte Metab* 8:91–112, 1982.
424. Karpati G, Frame B: Neuropsychiatric disorders in primary hyperparathyroidism: clinical analysis with review of the literature. *Arch Neurol* 10:387, 1964.
425. Hensen RA: The neurological aspects of hypercalcemia with special reference to primary hyperparathyroidism. *J R Coll Phys Lond* 1:41, 1966.

426. Wacker WEC, Parisi AF: Magnesium metabolism. *N Engl J Med* 278:658, 712, 772, 1968.
427. MacIntyre I: Magnesium metabolism. *Adv Intern Med* 13:143, 1967.
428. Massry SG, Coburn JW, Chapman LW, Kleeman CR: The effect of long-term desoxycorticosterone acetate administration on the renal excretion of calcium and magnesium. *J Lab Clin Med* 71:212, 1968.
429. Fishman RA: Neurological aspects of magnesium metabolism. *Arch Neurol* 12:562, 1965.
430. Borland LM, Roule M, Cook DR: Anesthesia for pediatric liver transplantation. *Anesth Analg* 64:117–124, 1985.
431. Frame B, Carter S: Pseudohypoparathyroidism: clinical picture and relation to convulsive seizures. *Neurology* 5:297, 1955.
432. Rose GA, Vas CJ: Neurological complications and electroencephalographic changes in hypoparathyroidism. *Acta Neurol Scand* 42:537, 1966.
433. Sharief N, Matthew DJ, Dillon MJ: Hypocalcemic stridor in children. How often is it missed? *Clin Pediatr* 0:51, 1991.
434. Knochel JP, Seldin DW: The pathophysiology of uremia. In: Brenner BM, Rector FE (eds), *The Kidney*. Philadelphia, W. B. Saunders, 1976:1448, 1485.
435. Elman R, Shatz BA, Keating RE, Weichselbaum TE: Intracellular and extracellular potassium deficits in surgical patients. *Ann Surg* 136:111, 1952.
436. Mitchell W, Feldman F: Neuropsychiatric aspects of hypokalemia. *Can Med Assoc J* 98:49, 1968.
437. Estrin JE, Buckley JJ: Complications of anesthesia. In: Toledo-Pereyra CM (ed). *Complications of Organ Transplantation*. New York, Marcel Dekker, 1987:1–35.
438. Epstein FH: Signs and symptoms of electrolyte disorders. In: Maxwell MH, Kleeman CR (eds), *Clinical Disorders of Fluid and Electrolyte Metabolism,* ed. 3 New York, McGraw-Hill, 1979:499.
439. Arieff AI: Central nervous system manifestations of disordered sodium metabolism. *Clin Endocrinol Metab* 13:269, 1984.
440. Sparacio RR, Anziska B, Schutta HS: Hypernatremia and chorea: a report of two cases. *Neurology* 26:46, 1976.
441. Herdman R, Vernier RL, Michael AF, Kelly WP, Good RA: Renal function and phosphorus excretion after human renal homotransplantation. *Lancet* 1:121–123, 1966.
442. Stanbury SW: Bone disease in uremia. *Am J Med* 44:714–724, 1968.
443. Coburn JW, Brickman AS, Hartenbower DL, Norman AW: Intestinal phosphate absorption in normal and uremic man: effects of 1,25-$(OH)_2$ vitamin D_3 and 1∞(OH)-vitamin D_3. *Adv Exp Med Biol* 81:549–557, 1977.
444. Peacock M, Aaron JE, Walker GS: The effect of plasma phosphate on the action of 1-∞-hydroxyvitamin D_3 in hemodialysis patients. *Adv Exp Med Biol* 81:559–570, 1977.
445. Silvis SE, DiBartolomeo AG, Aaker HM: Hypophosphatemia and neurological changes secondary to oral caloric intake. *Am J Gastroenterol* 73:215, 1980.
446. Silvis SE, Paragas PD: Paresthesias, weakness, seizures and hypophosphatemia in patients receiving hyperalimentation. *J Lab Clinic Med* 62:513, 1972.
447. Calne RY, White DJG, Thiru S, et al: Cyclosporine A in patients receiving allografts from cadaver donors. *Lancet* 2:1323–1327, 1978.
448. Kahan DB, Flechner SM, Lorber MI, et al: Complications of cyclosporine-prednisone immunosuppression in 402 renal allograft recipients exclusively followed at a single center for from one to five years. *Transplantation* 43:197, 1987.
449. Walker RW, Brochstein JA: Neurologic complications of immunosuppressive agents. *Neurol Clin* 6:261, 1988.

450. O'Sullivan DP: Convulsions associated with cyclosporine A. *Br Med J* 290:858, 1985.
451. Gross MLP, Sweny P, Pearson RM, et al: Rejection encephalopathy: an acute neurological syndrome complicating renal transplantation. *J Neurol Sci* 56:23–24, 1982.
452. Thompson CB, June CH, Sullivan KM, Thomas ED: Association between cyclosporine neurotoxicity and hypomagnesaemia. *Lancet* 2:1116–1120, 1984.
453. Berden JHM, Hoitsma AJ, Merx JL, et al: Severe central nervous system toxicity associated with cyclosporine. *Lancet* 1:219–220, 1985.
454. DeGroen PC, Aksamit AJ, Rakela J, et al: Central nervous system toxicity after liver transplantation: The role of cyclosporine and cholesterol. *N Engl J Med* 317:861–866, 1987.
455. Rubin AM, Kang H: Cerebral blindness and encephalopathy with cyclosporine A toxicity. *Neurology* 37:1072, 1076, 1987.
456. Noll RB, Kulkarni R: Complex visual hallucinations and cyclosporine. *Arch Neurol* 41:329–330, 1984.
457. Stein DP, Lederman RJ, Vogt DP, Carey WD, Broughan TA: Neurological complications following liver transplantation. *Ann Neurol* 31:644–649, 1992.
458. Bronster DJ, Boccagnii P, O'Rourke M, et al: Loss of speech after orthotopic liver transplantation. *Transplant Int* 8(3):234–237, 1995.
459. Wijdicks E, Litchy WJ, Wiesner RH, Krom R: Neuromuscular complications associated with liver transplantation. *Muscle Nerve* 19:696–700, 1996.
460. Amato AA, Barohn RJ, Sahenk Z, et al: Polyneuropathy complicating bone marrow and solid organ transplantation. *Neurology* 43:1513–1518, 1993.
461. Wijdicks EFM, Weisner RH, Dahlke RN, et al: FK 506-induced neurotoxicity in liver transplantation. *Ann Neurol* 35:498–501, 1994.
462. Eidelman BH, Abu-Elmagd K, Wilson J, et al: Neurologic complications of FK 506. *Transplant Proc* 23:3175–3178, 1991.
463. Wijdicks EFM, Weisner RH, Dahlke RN, et al: FK 506-induced neurotoxicity in liver transplantation. *Ann Neurol* 35:498–501, 1994.
464. Thomson AW, Starzl TE: FK 506 and autoimmune disease: perspective and prospects. *Autoimmunity,* 00:000–000, 1992.
465. Wilson JR, Conwit RA, Eidelman BH, Starzl T, Abu-Elmagd K: Sensorimotor neuropathy resembling CIDP in patients receiving FK 506. *Muscle Nerve* 17:1–5, 1994.
466. Shutter LA, Green JP, Newman NJ, et al: Cortical blindness and white matter lesions in a patient receiving FK 506 after liver transplantation. *Neurology* 43:2417–2418, 1993.
467. Norman DJ: The clinical role of OKT3. *Immunol Allergy Clin North Am* 9:95–107, 1989.
468. Chatenoud L, Ferran C, Legendre C, et al: In vivo cell activation following OKT3 administration. *Transplantation* 49:697–702, 1990.
469. Agarwal RK, Ostaszewsjum Feld LG, et al: Tumor necrosis factor and interleukin-6 in cerebrospinal fluid of a patient with recurrent adverse central nervous system events following OKT3. *Transplant Proc* 25:2143–2144, 1993.
470. Adair JC, Woodley SI, O'Connell JB, et al: Aseptic meningitis following cardiac transplantation: clinical characteristics and relationship to immunosuppressive regimen. *Neurology* 41:249–252, 1991.
471. Shihab FS, Barry JM, Norman DJ: Encephalopathy following the use of OKT3 in renal allograft transplantation. *Transplant Proc* 25:31–34, 1993.
472. Boston Collaborative Drug Surveillance Program: Acute adverse reactions to prednisone in relationship to dosage. *Clin Pharmacol Ther* 13:694–698, 1972.
473. Lewis DA, Smith RE: Steroid-induced psychiatric syndromes: a report of 14 cases and a review of the literature. *J Affective Disord* 5:319–332, 1983.

474. Bolton CF, Young GB, Zochodne DW: The neurological complications of sepsis. *Ann Neurol* 33:94, 1993.
475. Young GB, Bolton CF, Austin TW, et al: The encephalopathy associated with septic illness. *Clin Invest Med* 13:297, 1990.
476. Simmons RL, Lopez CL, Balfour H Jr, et al: Cytomegalovirus: clinical virological correlations in renal transplant recipients. *Ann Surg* 180:623, 1974.
477. Rubin RH: Infection in the renal and liver transplant patient. In: Rubin RH, Young LS (eds). *Clinical Approach to Infection in the Compromised Host,* ed 2. New York, Plenum Press, 1988:557–621.
478. Kusne S, Schwartz M, Breinig MK, et al: Herpes simplex virus hepatitis after solid organ transplantation in adults. *J Infect Dis* 165:1001, 1991.
479. Spitzer PG, Tarsy D, Eliotoulos GM: Acute transverse myelitis during disseminated cytomegalovirus infection in renal transplant recipient. *Transplantation* 44(1):151–153, 1987.
480. Klemola E, Weckman H, Haltia K, et al: The Guillain-Barré syndrome associated with acquired cytomegalovirus infection. *Acta Med Scand* 181:603–607, 1967.
481. Bale JF Jr, Rote NS, Bloomer LC, et al: Guillain-Barré-like polyneuropathy after renal transplant. *Arch Neurol* 37:784, 1980.
482. Ibels LS, Stewart JH, Mahoney JF, Sheil AGR: Deaths from occlusive arterial disease in renal allograft recipients. *Br Med J* 3:552, 1974.
483. Mahoney JF, Sheil AGR, Etheridge SB, Storey BG, Stewart JH: Delayed complications of renal transplantation and their prevention. *Med J Aust* 2:426, 1982.
484. Adams HP, Dawson G, Coffman TJ, Corry RJ: Stroke in renal transplant recipients. *Arch Neurol* 43:113, 1986.
485. Lindstrom BJ: Late complications after primary successful kidney transplantation. *Scand J Urol Nephrol* 12:(Suppl):165, 1977.
486. Ingeltinger JR, Grupe WE, Levey RH: Post-transplant hypertension in the absence of rejection or recurrent disease. *Clin Nephrol* 15:236–239, 1981.
487. Ibels LS, Simons LA, King JO, et al: Studies on the nature and causes of hyperlipidemia in uremia, maintenance hemodialysis and renal transplantation. *Q J Med* 176:601, 1975.
488. Kaplan LR: *Stroke: A Clinical Approach.* Boston, Bullerworth Heinman, 1993:518–523.
489. Olsen TS, Hagenhave H, Thage O: Epilepsy after stroke. *Neurology* 37:1209–1211, 1987.
490. Nicklasson PM, Hambraeus A, Lundgren G, et al: Listeria encephalitis in five renal transplant recipients. *Acta Med Scand* 203:181–185, 1978.
491. Rifkind D, Marchioro TL, Schneck SA, et al: Systemic fungal infectious complicating renal transplantation and immunosuppressive therapy. *Am J Med* 43:28–38, 1967.
492. Briggs JD, Hamilton DNH, MacSween RNM, Pennington TH: Infectious mononucleosis, herpes simplex infection, and diffuse lymphoma in a renal transplant recipient. *Transplantation* 25:227–228, 1978.
493. Reichard A, Eidelman BH: Cyclosporine A-induced dysarthria and tremulousness. *Neurology* 39:208, 1989.
494. Mueller AR, Platz HP, Bechstein WO, et al: Neurotoxicity after orthotopic liver transplantation. *Transplantation* 58:155–169, 1994.
495. European Multicenter Trial Group: Cyclosporine in cadaveric renal transplantation: One year follow-up of a multicentre trial. *Lancet* 2:986–989, 983.
496. McGonigle RJS, Trafford JAP, Bewick M, Parsons V: Hypertensive encephalopathy complicating transplant renal artery stenosis. *Postgrad Med J* 60:356–358, 1984.
497. Junaid I, Kwan JTC, Lord RHH: Femoral neuropathy in renal transplantation. *Transplantation* 56:240–241, 1993.
498. Meech PR: Femoral neuropathy following renal transplantation. *Aust NZ J Surg* 60:117, 1990.

499. Vasiri ND, Barton CH, Ravikumar GR, et al: Femoral neuropathy: a complication of renal transplantation. *Nephron* 28:30, 1981.
500. Jablecki CK, Aguilo JJ, Piepgras DG, et al: Paraparesis after renal transplantation. *Ann Neurol* 2:154–155, 1977.
501. Hefty TR, Nelson KA, Hatch TR, Barry JM: Lumbosacral plexopathy in diabetic women after renal transplantation. *Urology* 143:107, 1990.
502. Dawson DM, Hallett M, Millender LH: *Entrapment Neuropathies,* ed 2. Boston, Little Brown and Company, 1990.
503. Hooper DC, Pruitt AA, Rubin RH: Central nervous system infection in the chronically immunosuppressed. *Medicine* (Baltimore) 61:166–188, 1982.
504. Conti DJ, Rubin RH: Infection of the central nervous system in organ transplant recipients. *Neurol Clin* 6:241–260, 1988.
505. Ashinsky D: Listerial meningitis. *Postgrad Med* 92(8):191–193, 1992.
506. Millar JW, Horne NW: Tuberculosis in immunosuppressed patients. *Lancet* 1:1176, 1979.
507. Bennett JE: Diagnosis and therapy of systemic mycoses in the immunosuppressed host. *Transplant Proc* 5:1255, 1973.
508. Alper G, Knepper L, Kanal E: MR findings in listerial rhombencephalitis. *AJNR* 17:593–596, 1996.
509. Estol CJ, Pessin MS, Martinez AJ: Cerebrovascular complications after orthotopic liver transplantation: a clinicopathologic study. *Neurology* 41:815–819, 1991.
510. Brown P, Tsai T, Gadjusek DC: Seroepidemiology of human papovaviruses. *Am J Epidemiol* 102:331, 1975.
511. Padgett BL, Walker DL: Prevalence of antibodies in human sera against C virus, an isolate from a case of progressive multifocal leukoencephalopathy. *J Infect Dis* 127:467, 1973.
512. Manz HJ, Dinsdale HB, Morrin PAF: Progressive multifocal leukoencephalopathy after renal transplantation. *Ann Intern Med* 75:77, 1971.
513. Zu Rhein GM, Varakis J: Progressive multifocal leukoencephalopathy in a renal-allograft recipient. *N Engl J Med* 291:798, 1974.
514. Faris AA, Martinez AJ: Primary progressive multifocal leukoencephalopathy. A central nervous system disease caused by a slow virus. *Arch Neurol* 27:357, 1972.
515. Richardson EP Jr: Our evolving understanding of progressive multifocal leukoencephalopathy. *Ann NY Acad Sci* 230:358, 1974.
516. Hanto DW, Gajl-Peczalska KJ, Frizzera G, et al: Epstein Barr virus induced polyclonal and monoclonal B-cell lymphoproliferative diseases occurring after renal transplantation. *Ann Surg* 198:356–369, 1983.
517. Thomas JA, Allday MJ, Crawford DH: Epstein-Barr virus-associated lymphoproliferative disorders in immunocompromised individuals. *Adv Cancer Res* 57:329–380, 1991.
518. Hanto DW, Frizzera G, Gail-Peczalska KJ, et al: Epstein-Barr virus, immunodeficiency, and B-cell lymphoproliferation. *Transplantation* 39:461–472, 1985.
519. Hanto DW, Frizzera G, Gail-Peczalska KJ, et al: Epstein-Barr virus, immunodeficiency, and B-cell lymphoproliferation. *Transplantation* 39:461–472, 1985.
520. Cohen JI: Epstein-Barr virus lymphoproliferative disease associated with acquired immunodeficiency. *Medicine* 70:137–160, 1991.
521. Patchell RA: Primary central nervous system lymphoma in the transplant patient. *Neurol Clin* 6:297–303, 1988.
522. Benkerrou M, Durandy A, Fischer A: Therapy for transplant-related lymphoproliferative diseases. *Hematol Oncol Clin North Am* 7:467–475, 1993.
523. Wright DG, Laureno R, Victor M: Pontine and extrapontine myelinolysis. *Brain* 102:361–385, 1979.

524. Wszolek ZK, McComb RD, Pfeiffer RF, et al: Pontine and extrapontine myelinolysis following liver transplantation. *Transplantation* 48:1006–1012, 1989.
525. Noremberg MD: A hypothesis of osmotic endothelial injury: a pathogenic mechanism in central pontine myelinolysis. *Arch Neurol* 40:66–69, 1983.

Malignancy After Renal Transplantation

526. Penn I: Primary kidney tumors before and after renal transplantation. *Transplantation* 59:480–485, 1995.
527. Penn I: The problem of cancer in organ transplant recipients: an overview. *Transplant Sci* 4:23–32, 1994.
528. Penn I: Effects of immunosuppression on preexisting cancers. *Transplantation* 55:742–747, 1993.
529. Sheil AGR, Disney APS, Mathew TH, et al.: Cancer development in cadaveric donor renal allograft recipients treated with azathioprine (AZA) or cyclosporine (CYA) or AZA/CYA. *Transplant Proc* 23:1111–1112, 1991.
530. Mullen DL, Silberger SG, Penn I, et al.: Squamous cell carcinoma of the skin and lip in renal homograft recipients. *Cancer* 37:729–734, 1976.
531. Penn I.: Posttransplant kidney cancers and skin cancers (including Kaposi's sarcoma). In: Schmahl D, Penn I, (eds), *Cancer in Organ Transplant Recipients.* Berlin, Springer-Verlag, 1991:46–53.

12

Allograft Nephrectomy

Carlos A. Vivas

The performance of an allograft nephrectomy to remove a failed renal allograft may not necessarily be straightforward or uncomplicated. Although it is a reasonably safe procedure, with a mortality of 0–1% and a morbidity of 4–10%, it was historically a dangerous undertaking, with a mortality of 20–46% and a reported morbidity of 14–35% in earlier series.[1–5] This chapter discusses the indications and timing, preoperative preparation, technical aspects, and complications of allograft nephrectomy.

▲ INDICATIONS AND TIMING

The need for allograft nephrectomy is related to the time course and cause of graft failure after renal transplantation and the condition of the patient (Table 12–1). Renal allograft failure within the first year after transplantation is often secondary to irreversible acute rejection and is best managed by prompt removal of the graft to avoid complications related to graft rupture or necrosis and resultant sepsis. Graft failure that occurs more than 1 year after transplantation is usually due to chronic rejection. In this setting, the progressive withdrawal of immunosuppression may allow the surgeon to avoid removal of the allograft in 50–90% of instances.[4–7] The development of superimposed acute rejection, with local symptoms of graft tenderness, hematuria, thrombocytopenia related to platelet consumption by the allograft, or fever without obvious other cause necessitates allograft nephrectomy.[8]

The causes of allograft failure include acute or chronic rejection, vascular or urologic technical complications, or recurrence of the primary renal disease in the allograft. Other indications for nephrectomy can include poorly controlled hypertension or the need to make room for a new kidney.

TABLE 12–1 ▲ INDICATIONS FOR ALLOGRAFT NEPHRECTOMY

Rejection
Hyperacute
Acute
Chronic with associated graft tenderness, hematuria, or fever
Technical complications
Renal arterial or venous thrombosis
Uncontrollable bleeding
Persistent urinary extravasation
Graft sepsis
Mycotic pseudoaneurysm
Thrombocytopenia
Hypertension, poorly controlled
Recurrence of native renal disease in the allograft

These indications usually necessitate elective or semiurgent nephrectomy. Emergency allograft nephrectomy is indicated in the setting of a mycotic pseudoaneurysm, a rare but life-threatening complication related to bacterial or fungal infection of the arterial suture line.

An additional factor that affects the timing of nephrectomy is the ability of the recipient to tolerate the procedure. An overimmunosuppressed patient with sepsis secondary to an opportunistic infection may be a poor surgical candidate, and it may be advisable to wait until the patient's medical condition has stabilized.

▲ PREOPERATIVE CONSIDERATIONS

Preoperative preparation is straightforward but requires attention to a few details. Patients should, of course, be adequately dialyzed preoperatively. It is also important to assess the platelet and coagulation status; patients with renal failure may have impaired platelet function secondary to uremia. Correction of coagulation abnormalities with fresh frozen plasma, cryoprecipitate, platelets, and/or desmopressin acetate (DDAVP) simplifies the technical performance of the allograft nephrectomy.

The use of stress doses of steroids, although usually unnecessary, may occasionally be indicated for patients who have been on chronic maintenance steroids for a long period of time. A cosyntropin (Cortrosyn) stimulation test can help to determine the need for stress doses of steroids, but is rarely performed. If the anesthesiologist is adamant about the need for stress steroids, prophylaxis for peptic ulcer disease also is indicated.

Routine antibiotic prophylaxis with a first-generation cephalosporin is usually sufficient, unless graft sepsis is suspected. Topical wound irrigation with the same antibiotic also helps minimize the incidence of wound infection.

Finally, it is important to assess the peripheral pulses in the lower extremities before nephrectomy. Inadvertent damage to or ligation of the native iliac artery can occur and may require prompt surgical intervention to prevent limb loss.

▲ TECHNIQUE OF ALLOGRAFT NEPHRECTOMY

There are two surgical decisions to make during the performance of an allograft nephrectomy. The first concerns whether to dissect out the kidney in an extracapsular or an intracapsular manner. The second focuses on control of the blood supply to the allograft, either by individual ligation of the vessels and ureter or by mass clamping and oversewing of the hilum. The goal is to remove the allograft safely and efficiently without injuring the native iliac vessels. To some extent, the decisions are based on how long the allograft has been in place.

All approaches begin with reopening of the original transplant incision and division of the fascial layers. It is best to divide the fascia at the same point it was originally opened at the time of transplantation.

When the allograft nephrectomy is performed soon after transplantation, up to 6–8 weeks postoperatively, the renal allograft is easily mobilized in an extracapsular manner. The entire ureter can often be removed from its insertion into the bladder, and the bladder is closed in two layers with a long-lasting absorbable suture (eg, 3-0 or 4-0 polyglyconate). The blood vessels can be identified separately and ligated and divided individually.

When the nephrectomy is performed late after transplantation, 2 or more months postoperatively, the renal allograft may have considerable scarring and adhesions to the peritoneum and iliac vessels. Extracapsular dissection may be attempted, but it is usually difficult to perform. In this circumstance, an intracapsular approach minimizes the risk of complications. The incision is taken through the fascial layers down to the capsule of the allograft, which is incised from pole to pole (Fig. 12–1). Using blunt finger dissection, the surgeon dissects free the kidney just below the renal capsule; it is preferable to avoid entering the renal parenchyma. The plane is relatively easy to develop, and it should be possible to mobilize the kidney quickly. Once the dissection has approached the hilum of the kidney, the capsule can be incised again, although this is not always necessary. At this point, each vessel and the ureter may be dissected, ligated, and divided individually, or the whole pedicle can be cross clamped with two vascular clamps (Fig. 12–2). After applying the vascular clamps, the surgeon should check the femoral or distal iliac pulse to ensure that the patient's own iliac vessels have not been clamped. The kidney is then removed deep in the hilum so as to leave about 1 cm of hilum beyond the clamps. The whole vascular pedicle is oversewn in two layers with 2-0 or 3-0 monofilament nonabsorbable continuous suture (Fig. 12–3). After removal of the vascular clamps, individual bleeders are controlled with suture ligature, or the hilum can be oversewn again. Although this technique leaves a relatively long remnant of donor vessels and ureter in the patient, it has not been associated with serious complications other than transient hematuria.[9,10]

After the allograft is removed and the hilum controlled, meticulous hemostasis is required in the retroperitoneum before wound closure. This is particularly impor-

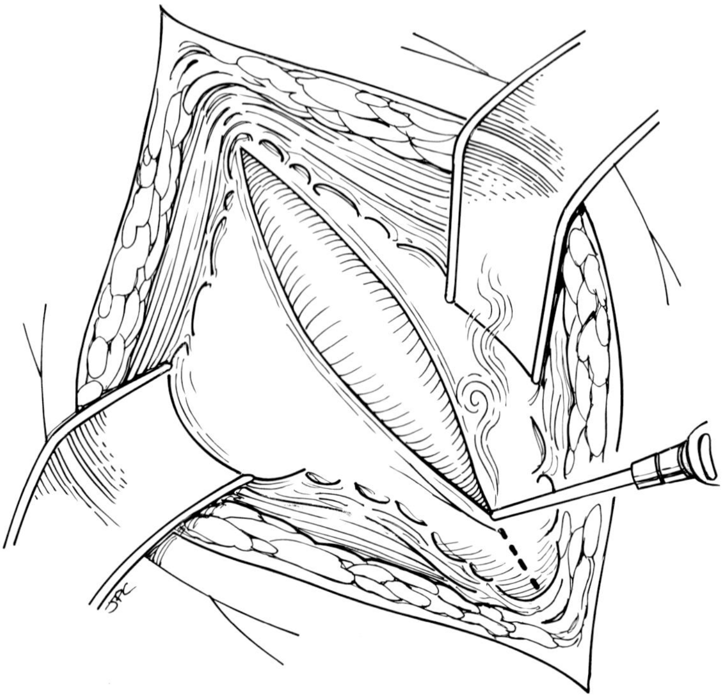

Figure 12–1. The nephrectomy incision is taken through the fascial layers down to the capsule of the allograft, which is incised from pole to pole.

tant when the kidney has been removed in an intracapsular manner, because numerous capsular bleeders must be cauterized. The field should be completely dry before wound closure. Routine placement of a closed suction drain is generally advisable; care should be taken to ensure that the tip does not touch the hilum. The fascia often can only be closed in one full-thickness layer; fortunately, this is usually sufficient.

▲ MYCOTIC PSEUDOANEURYSM

Mycotic aneurysm is a rare complication. It most often occurs when there has been a peritransplant deep wound infection. When present, the techniques described above are inadequate. The iliac artery must be ligated proximal and distal to the allograft arterial anastomosis. The segment of iliac artery containing the pseudoaneurysm is excised with the allograft. Rarely is the iliac vein threatened. Often a separate transperitoneal incision is required to achieve proximal and distal control, particularly if the pseudoaneurysm has ruptured. If arterial reconstruction such as femorofemoral bypass is required, it must be performed through separate incisions.[11]

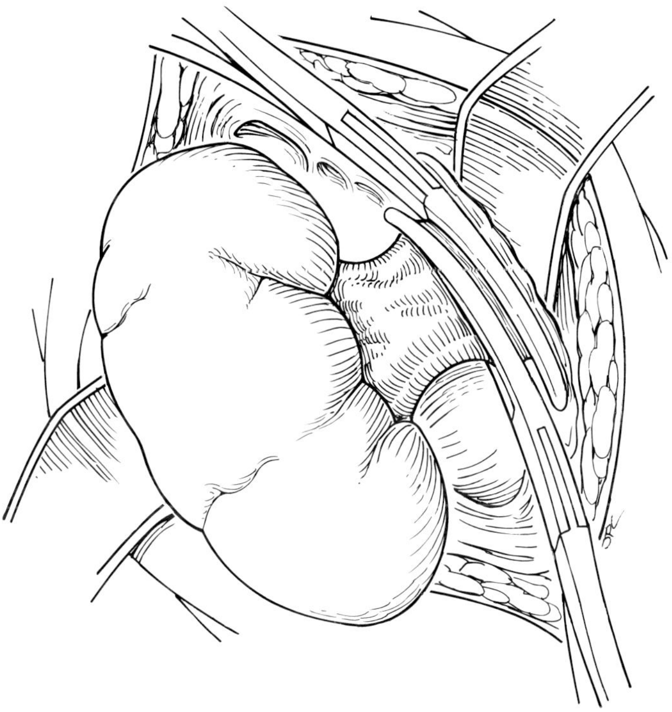

Figure 12–2. Each vessel and the ureter may be dissected, ligated, and divided individually, or the whole pedicle can be cross clamped with two vascular clamps.

It should be noted that there have been two case reports of mycotic pseudoaneurysms that were treated successfully with intravenous antibiotics and surgical repair, but this is a potentially dangerous course of action.[12]

▲ POSTOPERATIVE CARE

General postoperative care is fairly routine. The drain is removed as soon as possible, and a diet is resumed when the patient has return of gastrointestinal function. Patients can usually be discharged within 1 week or less of the operation.

An important issue concerns steroid tapering. Even though most patients have been receiving long-term steroid therapy, the dosages are often low enough that patients have normal adrenal reserve. In that situation, steroids can be stopped immediately after allograft nephrectomy.[13] A cosyntropin (Cortrosyn) stimulation test[14] helps determine which patients can have steroids abruptly discontinued and which patients require a slow taper over several months.

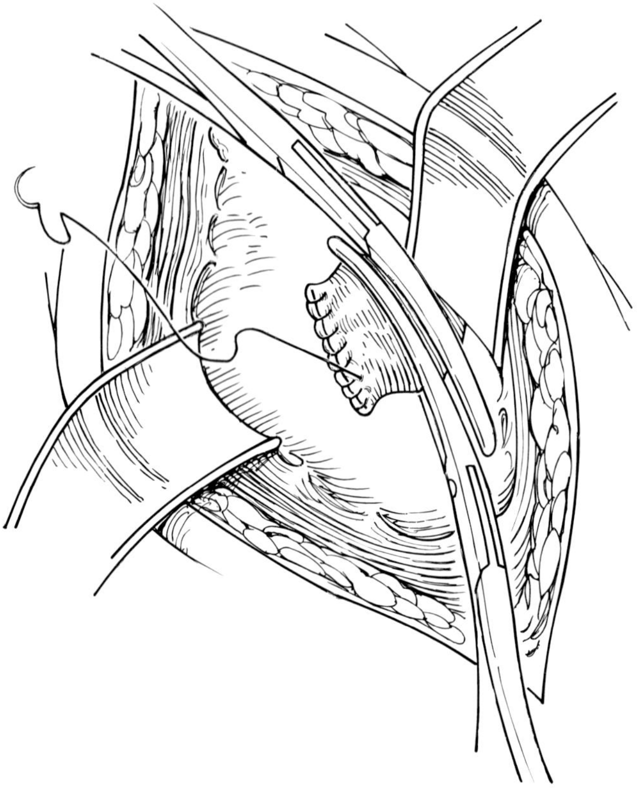

Figure 12–3. The whole vascular pedicle is oversewn into two layers with 2-0 or 3-0 monofilament nonabsorbable continuous sutures.

▲ COMPLICATIONS

The two complications of allograft nephrectomy are bleeding and infection. The incidence of bleeding is 4–6%.[2–7] Bleeding usually arises from the area of dissection and presents as a hematoma; re-exploration generally is necessary. Bleeding occasionally may originate from the oversewn hilar suture line.

The incidence of wound infection is as high as 6%.[4] It may be secondary to allograft infection or a contaminated hematoma. It is best prevented by careful hemostasis during surgery and antibiotic prophylaxis. When gross contamination is present, wound healing by secondary intention may be necessary.[3]

▲ REFERENCES

1. Sharma DK, Pandey AP, Nath V, Gopalakrishnan G: Allograft nephrectomy: a 16 year experience. *Br J Urol* 64:122–124, 1989.

2. Sinha SM, Castro JE: Allograft nephrectomy *Br J Urol* 48:413–417, 1976.
3. Voester HG, Slooff HJ, Kaas JA, Tegzess AM, Kootstra G: Safe removal of failed transplanted kidney. *Br J Surg* 69:480–481, 1982.
4. Chiverton SG, Murie JA, Allen RD, Morris PJ: Renal transplant nephrectomy. *Surg Gynecol Obstet* 164:324–328, 1987.
5. Rosenthal JT, Peaster ML, Laub D: The challenge of kidney transplant nephrectomy. *J Urol* 149:1395–1397, 1993.
6. Thomas PP, Jacob CK, Kirubakaran MG, Pandey AP, Gopalakrishnan G, Shastry JCM: Indications for routine allograft nephrectomy in cases of irreversible rejection (Brief Communication). *Transplantation* 48:155, 1989.
7. Gallo CD, Grino JM, Seron D, Castelao AM, Franco E, Alsino J: Routine allograft nephrectomy in late renal failure (Brief Communication). *Transplantation* 49:1204, 1990.
8. Gustafsson A, Groth CG, Halgrimson CG, Penn I, Starzl TE: The fate of failed renal homografts retained after retransplantation. *Surg Gynecol Obstet* 137:40–42, 1973.
9. Sutherland DE, Simmons RL, Howard RJ, Najarian JS: Intracapsular technique of transplant nephrectomy. *Surg Gynecol Obstet* 146:950–951, 1978.
10. Dumler F: Gross hematuria caused by ureteral remnant hemorrhage in a renal transplant recipient. *South Med J* 74:81, 1981.
11. Starnes HF, McWhinnie DL, Bradley JA, Bramwell SP, Hamilton DM, Briggs JD: Delayed major arterial hemorrhage after transplant nephrectomy. *Transplant Proc,* 16:1320, 1984.
12. Henry ML, Elkhammas EA, Tesi RJ, Ferguson RM: Mycotic aneurysm following kidney transplantation. *Transplantation Sci* 2(1):16–17, 1992.
13. Shapiro R, Carroll PB, Tzakis AG, Cemaj S, Lopatin WB, Wakazato P: Adrenal reserve in renal transplant recipients with cyclosporine, azathioprine and prednisone immunosuppression. *Transplantation* 49:1011, 1990.
14. May ME, Amey RM: Rapid ACTH test in practice. *Am J Med* 79:679, 1985.

13

Radiologic Evaluation of the Renal Transplant Patient

James H. Oliver, III / Philip D. Orons / Ajit N. Shah / Albert B. Zajko

Despite continuing improvement in patient and graft survival rates as a result of advances and refinements in organ preservation, immunosuppressive therapy, and surgical technique, complications after renal transplantation still occur. The clinical signs and symptoms of many causes of graft dysfunction are nonspecific, making radiologic evaluation of the allograft essential. Duplex Doppler ultrasound studies of the allograft and of the renal vasculature are regularly performed on all renal transplant patients. Scintigraphic evaluation of allograft perfusion and function also is utilized, although perhaps less often. Depending on the findings of these studies, other imaging procedures may be indicated. Cystography, percutaneous nephrostomy, and angiography are used to confirm and occasionally manage the complications that can occur after renal transplantation. This chapter discusses the radiologic evaluation of patients after renal transplantation.

▲ ULTRASOUND EVALUATION OF THE RENAL TRANSPLANT

Abnormalities of the Parenchyma and Collecting System

Ultrasound evaluation was originally limited to descriptions of morphologic changes in the allograft kidney. Several investigators believed that certain morphologic changes in the allograft echotexture could be used to differentiate acute rejection from acute tubular necrosis (ATN). Prominent pyramids, increased cortical thickness, increased cortical echogenicity, indistinctness of the corticomedullary junction, and enlargement of the transplant kidney were all considered to be specific findings in patients with acute rejection.[1,2,3–8] Over time, however, there came to be increasing doubt about the accuracy of using morphologic criteria to detect acute rejection.[7–15] Hricak et al,[16] one of the initial proponents of using morphologic criteria to detect rejection, concluded in 1987 that the negative predictive value of a non-Doppler sonographic examination of the kidney was only 30–50%. Although some morphologic changes can be seen in patients with acute rejection, there is too much overlap with other potential diagnoses, such as ATN and cyclosporine toxicity, for morphologic criteria to be of much clinical utility.

With the advent of duplex Doppler ultrasound, many investigators looked at renal vascular waveforms to detect rejection and to differentiate acute rejection from ATN. Rifkin et al,[17] stated that a resistive index (RI) greater than 0.90 was 100% specific for rejection. Conversely, if the RI was less than 0.70, rejection was unlikely. Other investigators concluded that ultrasound Doppler examinations were more reliable than morphologic features in the detection of rejection. Although some research indicated that Doppler ultrasound could be used to differentiate among acute rejection, ATN, and cyclosporine nephrotoxicity,[18,19] later reports were unanimous in finding no consistent Doppler changes associated with acute rejection or cyclosporine nephrotoxicity.[20,21] The consensus now is that Doppler ultrasound is both insensitive and nonspecific in the detection of acute rejection.[15,22,23] Even among patients with markedly elevated RI readings, multiple etiologies other than rejection have been documented.[26]

Ureteral Obstruction

Immediately after renal transplantation it is not uncommon to see mild dilatation of the urinary collecting system. This condition is usually transient and can be related to postoperative edema at the site of the ureteroneocystostomy. In addition to post-surgical edema, extrinsic compression by perinephric or periureteral fluid collections and strictures resulting from ischemia can cause ureteral obstruction. The most common site of obstruction is the ureterovesical anastomosis, followed by the midureter and ureteropelvic junction.

The sonographic observation of dilated calyces does not always imply obstruction. Reflux from the bladder may be a more common cause. In addition, as the transplanted kidney and ureter are denervated, the collecting system might lose its tone and become mildly to moderately dilated over time (although in practice this is rare). In addition, acute rejection can cause atony, which can result in functional dilatation of the collecting system (also rare).

Peritransplant Fluid Collections

Peritransplant fluid collections are common after renal transplantation. Small collections are common in the immediate postoperative period. These are usually small, self-limited hematomas or seromas that require no intervention. It is important to document and measure all perinephric fluid collections during the sonographic evaluation. Any fluid collections that increase in size on subsequent studies should be followed closely and viewed with concern. Most postoperative fluid collections are asymptomatic. However, large collections can compress the ureter, iliac vein, or renal vein. This can lead to urinary obstruction, lower extremity edema, venous stenosis, or, rarely, thrombosis. Large fluid collections can also distort the contour of the allograft kidney. For these reasons, large fluid collections should be drained. Although hematomas are the most common perinephric fluid collections that occur after renal transplantation, lymphoceles, abscesses, and extravasation of urine also can occur (see Chapter 11).

Lymphoceles

During exposure of the iliac vessels for arterial and venous anastomoses, lymphatic channels are disrupted. If they are not ligated carefully, a focal collection of lymph can arise at the surgical site—a lymphocele. Lymphoceles are usually asymptomatic. If lymphoceles become large, they may cause leg or scrotal edema, a palpable mass, ureteral compression, or renal malfunction. At sonography, most lymphoceles are found to be fluid collections with multiple septations and some internal echoes (Fig. 13–1). The sonographic appearance is not specific.

Lymphoceles may enlarge or remain stable, but they generally do not resorb over time. Although percutaneous aspiration and drainage can be performed, and is useful diagnostically, recurrence is common. The most effective therapy for lymphocele is surgical and involves marsupialization of the lymphocele to the peritoneal cavity (see Chapter 11).

Urine Collections

Urine collections (*urinomas,* in the vernacular) are not common. They most often are found in the immediate or early postoperative period in association with leaks at the ureteral anastomosis, either from technical problems or ureteral ischemic necrosis. Urine leaks sometimes close if the bladder is decompressed by Foley catheter drainage, stented with a ureteral catheter, or diverted by percutaneous drainage of the kidney in combination with Foley catheter drainage. Extensive leaks necessitate reoperation for repair. The ultrasound appearance of urinomas is nonspecific; they are usually anechoic and do not have septae. Aspiration of fluid with a high creatinine level is diagnostic.

Abscesses

Abscesses usually occur adjacent to the allograft but can occur elsewhere in the pelvis or abdomen. Although abscesses generally occur early in the postoperative period, they can also be seen many months after transplantation. Unexplained fever or generalized sepsis should lead to percutaneous aspiration of any perinephric fluid collection to exclude the possibility of abscess. The ultrasound appearance of abscesses is variable and nonspecific. Low-level echoes are generally present. If one sees gas within a fluid collection on ultrasound examination or computed tomography (CT), an abscess should be strongly suspected.

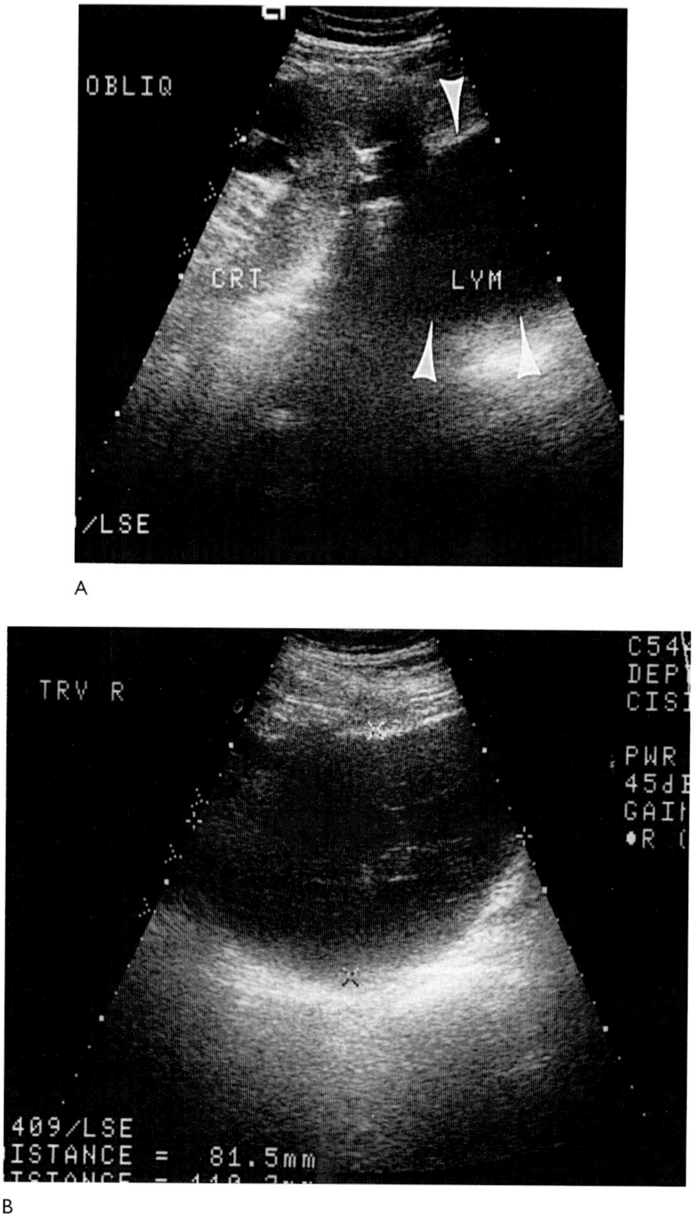

Figure 13–1. Lymphocele. A. Oblique ultrasound image demonstrates a fluid collection inferior to the lower pole of the transplanted kidney (arrowheads). B. Closer inspection of this fluid collection reveals multiple septations within the collection. Although the appearance is not specific for a lymphocele, percutaneous aspiration confirmed the diagnosis.

Hematomas

Hematomas usually occur in the immediate posttransplantation period or after percutaneous needle biopsy. The ultrasound appearance can be quite varied. Hematomas may be anechoic, have low-level echoes, or have areas that have midlevel echoes because of clotted blood. Large, expanding hematomas may lead to a fall in the hematocrit. They may compress the allograft, impairing function and necessitating surgical evacuation. Hematomas that are sterile may become infected. If the patient develops an unexplained fever, ultrasound-guided needle aspiration is recommended to rule out abscess formation.

Vascular Complications

Vascular complications are reported in as many as 10% of renal transplants.[27–30] Although rejection is the most common cause of graft dysfunction, vascular complications in renal transplants remain a serious cause of problems. The most common types of vascular complications are arterial and venous stenoses, intrarenal and extrarenal arteriovenous (AV) fistulas, and pseudoaneurysms. Arterial and venous thromboses occur less frequently and invariably result in graft loss unless discovered and corrected emergently. If detected early, many of the other vascular complications are correctable with interventional radiologic or surgical techniques. The clinical presentation of the various vascular lesions is often ambiguous. However, radiologic imaging often provides a sensitive and specific means of establishing the diagnosis. Angiography has long been accepted as the standard for imaging vascular complications. However, nuclear scintigraphy and, more recently, duplex and color Doppler ultrasound are being used more frequently as screening tests and are often the first to detect and diagnose vascular complications.[30,31]

The most appropriate use of Doppler ultrasound for screening renal grafts for possible vascular complications is to image the graft and associated vascular structures using color Doppler sonography followed by duplex Doppler sonographic evaluation of any flow abnormalities detected by color Doppler. The advantage of color Doppler sonography is its ability to sample larger fields of view, which allows the examiner to sample long segments of one or more vessels at a time. Color Doppler sonography is faster and less likely to miss vascular complications than duplex Doppler sonography. However, color Doppler sonography cannot accurately quantitate flow disturbances. Therefore, all flow abnormalities detected with color Doppler ultrasonography should be evaluated and quantified with duplex Doppler sonography.[32–34]

Accurate Doppler sonographic screening necessitates appropriate adjustments of the Doppler controls. In the evaluation of possible transplant vascular complications, both color and duplex Doppler imaging should be performed using the lowest filter setting, the maximum gain without background noise, and the smallest scale without introducing aliasing from the peak velocities of normal vessels.[34]

It is important to note that a Doppler signal can be displayed in terms of frequency shift (kHz) or velocity (m/sec). One must recognize, however, that frequency shift varies with changes in the insonating Doppler frequency, whereas flow velocity remains constant.

Renal Artery Stenosis

Renal artery stenosis (RAS) is the most common vascular complication of renal transplantation, occurring in 1.5–10% of patients.[27,28,35,36] RAS occurs more commonly in cadaveric kidneys than in living-related donor grafts.[30,37,38] Patients with clinically significant arterial stenoses commonly have hypertension. However, most transplant patients with hypertension do not have arterial stenosis. Arterial stenosis should be considered in any patient with graft dysfunction or hypertension. Suspicion of and sonographic screening for arterial stenosis are indicated in patients with newly developed or progressive hypertension, hypertension with graft dysfunction without biopsy evidence of rejection, or hypertension resistant to medical therapy.[28,30] Bruits over the renal graft are so common that they are not helpful clues to stenosis.

There are three locations for arterial stenoses in renal transplant patients—anastomotic, distal donor, and recipient (native). The anastomotic stenoses are short-segment strictures that are often technical in etiology and are seen more commonly in patients with end-to-end anastomoses. Distal donor stenoses tend to be long-segment strictures that can be caused by intimal injury, turbulence distal to the anastomosis, or destruction of the vasa vasorum. Although both anastomotic and distal donor stenoses can be related to previous rejection, it is believed that most stenoses caused by rejection are of the distal donor type. Distal donor stenoses occur more commonly in patients with end-to-side arterial anastomoses. Recipient stenoses are uncommon and are related to clamp injury during the operation or native atherosclerotic disease or scarring from previous operations.[27,28,30,31,34–36]

Ultrasonography is the most commonly used screening test for RAS. Taylor et al[39] described specific criteria for clinically significant arterial stenoses in the renal transplant population. They found that peak Doppler shifts of greater than 7.5 kHz (2 m/sec) at the stenosis and turbulence in the immediately poststenotic segment were indicative of clinically significant arterial stenosis (Fig. 13–2). Snider et al[40] corroborated these findings in a prospective study, found an overall sensitivity of 94% and a specificity of 87% for stenoses with greater than 50% luminal narrowing.[40]

Examination of the entire length of the main renal artery and the segmental arteries is essential. The success of ultrasound examination depends on direct insonation of the stenosis. Because visualization of these vessels often is difficult, duplex Doppler examinations can sometimes be quite long. Color Doppler sonography, with its larger field of view, allows more rapid examination for arterial stenosis. If the color controls are properly set, stenoses appear as focal regions of aliasing due to the increased velocities at the stenoses. If any areas of aliasing are detected with color Doppler ultrasonography, they can be examined with duplex Doppler ultrasonography to assess the nature and quantify the degree of flow disturbance.[34]

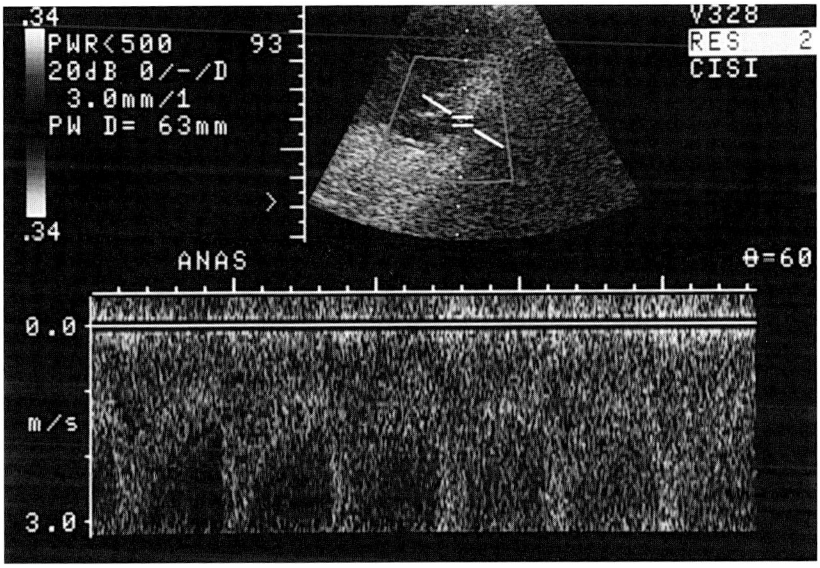

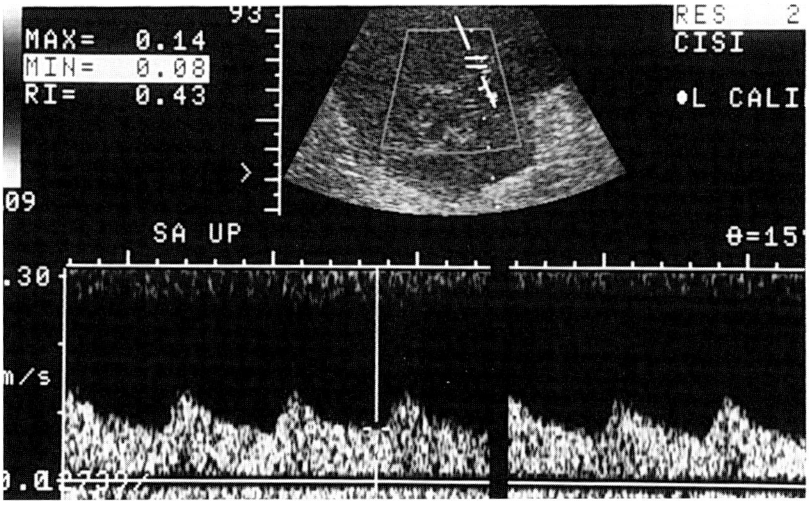

Figure 13–2. Renal artery stenosis. A. A duplex Doppler waveform demonstrates a focal region of increased velocity, greater than 3 m/sec in the main renal artery just downstream from the anastomosis with the iliac artery. This waveform is highly suggestive of clinically significant stenosis. B. In the same patient, duplex Doppler insonation of the intrarenal branches of the renal artery shows an arterial waveform with an abnormally low resistive index (0.43). Maximal velocity is approximately 0.15 m/sec.

The combination of duplex and color Doppler techniques provides a highly sensitive and fairly specific screening study that, unlike angiography, is noninvasive and risk-free for the patient. All flow abnormalities that meet or exceed the criteria of Taylor et al should be further evaluated by angiography to confirm or rule out the diagnosis and allow for precise therapeutic intervention (see Chapter 11).

Renal Artery Thrombosis

Thrombosis of the main renal artery occurs early in the postoperative period and almost always results in graft loss. It is an uncommon complication, occurring among less than 1% of renal transplant recipients.[28,30] The cause is usually assumed to be technical, although hyperacute or acute rejection, disparity in vessel size, vascular kinking, hypercoagulable states, hypotension, cyclosporine toxicity, and intraoperative intimal trauma all have been implicated as causative factors.[40–43] There is a case report of selective intra-arterial thrombolytic drug therapy that resulted in successful reperfusion of a renal graft after arterial thrombosis, although almost all cases require graft nephrectomy.[44]

Segmental renal artery thrombosis also occurs rarely and may present with no clinical symptoms. However, graft tenderness, hematuria, and decreased graft function may be seen. Thrombosis of a segmental renal artery most commonly causes a limited infarct, which does not result in loss of the graft.

The diagnosis of renal artery thrombosis is made when arterial flow cannot be identified. If the Doppler equipment is functioning properly, the absence of arterial Doppler flow is highly sensitive for renal arterial thrombosis. False-positive results can occur with poorly calibrated Doppler equipment. If poor calibration is suspected, Doppler sampling of the adjacent iliac artery can be performed to adjust the Doppler settings. Although both duplex Doppler and color Doppler ultrasonography can be used, color Doppler is more likely to detect segmental arterial thrombosis because of its larger field of insonation.[32] For thrombosis of the main renal artery, both techniques can be used with equally good results.

Intrarenal Arteriovenous Fistulas and Pseudoaneurysms

Almost all AV fistulas and pseudoaneurysms result from injuries sustained during percutaneous needle biopsies. Pseudoaneurysms occur with isolated arterial injury, and AV fistulas occur if there is concomitant laceration of adjacent arteries and veins. Most fistulas and pseudoaneurysms are quite small and resolve spontaneously. Because these lesions generally have a benign and asymptomatic course, they are usually found incidentally. Reported prevalences are 1–18%.[45–47] If AV fistulas become large enough, they can decrease renal perfusion because of marked arteriovenous shunting. AV fistulas that communicate with the calyceal system produce hematuria. Symptoms occur with pseudoaneurysms when they rupture into the calyceal or the perinephric space.[48] Most patients with intrarenal AV fistulas and pseudoaneurysms are not treated unless the fistulas become symptomatic or quite large. These lesions can be treated with transcatheter embolization techniques.[48–50]

The imaging of AV fistulas and pseudoaneurysms is predominantly confined to duplex and color Doppler sonography and angiography. Nuclear scintigraphy can be used to detect large pseudoaneurysms and AV fistulas but the sensitivity is quite low for smaller lesions.

The duplex Doppler findings of AV fistulas and pseudoaneurysms are specific.[39,51] AV fistulas show high-velocity, low-impedance arterial waveforms in association with arterialized venous tracings (Fig 13–3). Pseudoaneurysms have highly turbulent pulsatile flow in the lumen. However, during sampling in the region of the neck of the pseudoaneurysms, classic to-and-fro flow is detected[34,51] (Fig 13–4). This to-and-fro flow is seen when the orifice at the neck is narrow. If the pseudoaneurysm has a broad-based neck, the to-and-fro flow may not be seen. Gray scale sonography misses most AV fistulas, and pseudoaneurysms look like focal cysts. Unfortunately, duplex Doppler evaluation as a screen for AV fistulas is a painstaking process because all segments of the kidney must be examined. The study is fraught with sampling error. Color Doppler sonography, owing to its wide field of view, greatly increases the detection rate of AV fistulas and can be performed in a fraction of the time of duplex Doppler sonography.[32,34,52,53]

Small AV fistulas appear as focal areas of color aliasing on color Doppler. The aliasing reflects the increased arterial velocities. Large AV fistulas can produce a large amount of tissue vibration adjacent to the fistula. This causes an area of disorganized color at normal Doppler settings. With adjustment of the color scales and wall filters, the feeding artery and draining vein of large AV fistulas may be visualized[32,34,52,53] (Fig. 13–3B). AV fistulas detected with color Doppler sonography, regardless of size, should be verified with duplex Doppler sonography to exclude similar color aberrations that may be caused by segmental stenoses or focally prominent normal vessels.[34,53]

The color Doppler appearance of a pseudoaneurysm is virtually diagnostic. It consists of disorganized color flow within an apparent cyst. Surrounding parenchymal vibration color also may be seen. Careful interrogation may reveal the communicating neck, which appears as alternating jets of forward and reverse color.[32,34,51,53]

Extrarenal Arteriovenous Fistulas and Pseudoaneurysms

Extrarenal AV fistulas and pseudoaneurysms are commonly asymptomatic and found as unsuspected lesions on imaging studies obtained for other reasons. They are much less common than their intrarenal counterparts and have a worse prognosis. The most serious complication of these rare extrarenal lesions is exsanguination due to spontaneous rupture of a pseudoaneurysm. The serious nature of this potential complication makes extrarenal pseudoaneurysms a relative clinical emergency necessitating prompt intervention.[34,54–56] Extrarenal AV fistulas and pseudoaneurysms occasionally can cause renal dysfunction due to marked arteriovenous shunting or direct compression of the main renal artery.[34]

The most common cause of extrarenal pseudoaneurysms and AV fistulas is an imperfect surgical vascular anastomosis. Less common causes include perigraft infection and percutaneous biopsies.[57–59] Lesions caused by infection or surgical tech-

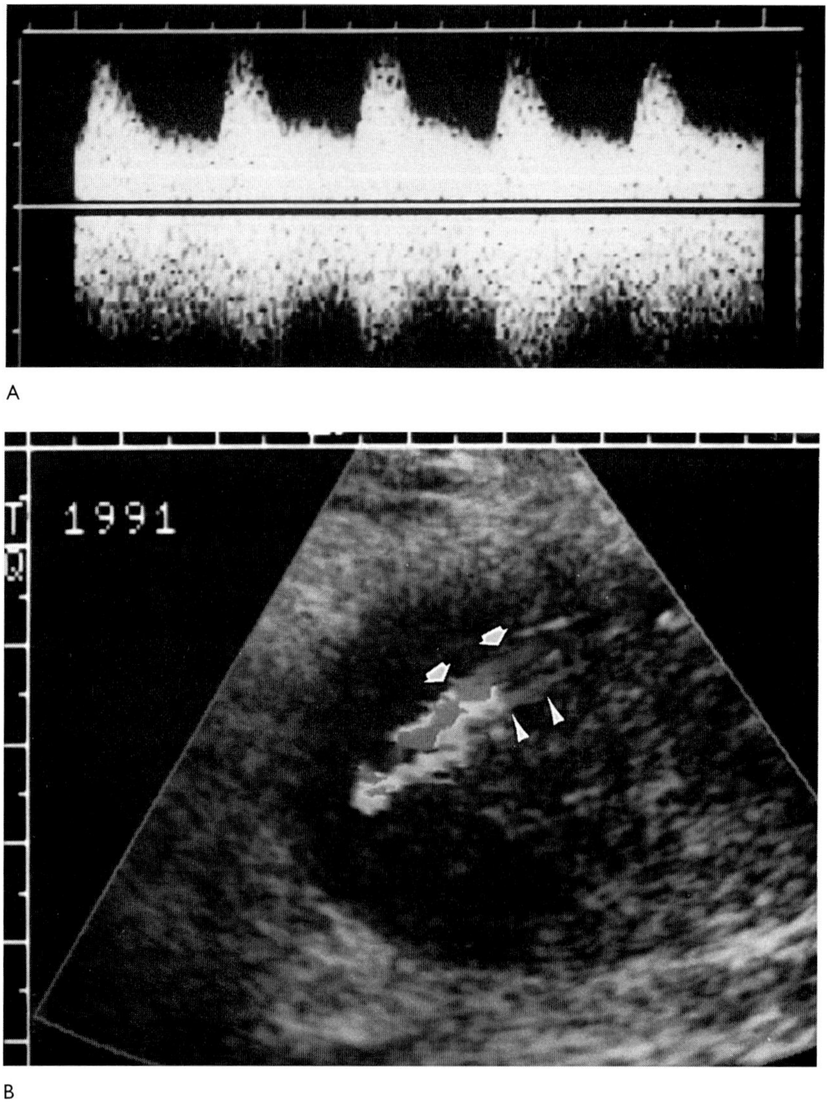

Figure 13–3. Intrarenal arteriovenous fistula. A. A duplex Doppler ultrasound waveform of a segmental artery and vein shows high diastolic arterial flow and pulsating arterialized venous flow. B. Color Doppler scan (shown in black and white) demonstrates the feeding artery (arrows) and draining vein (arrowheads) of the fistula.

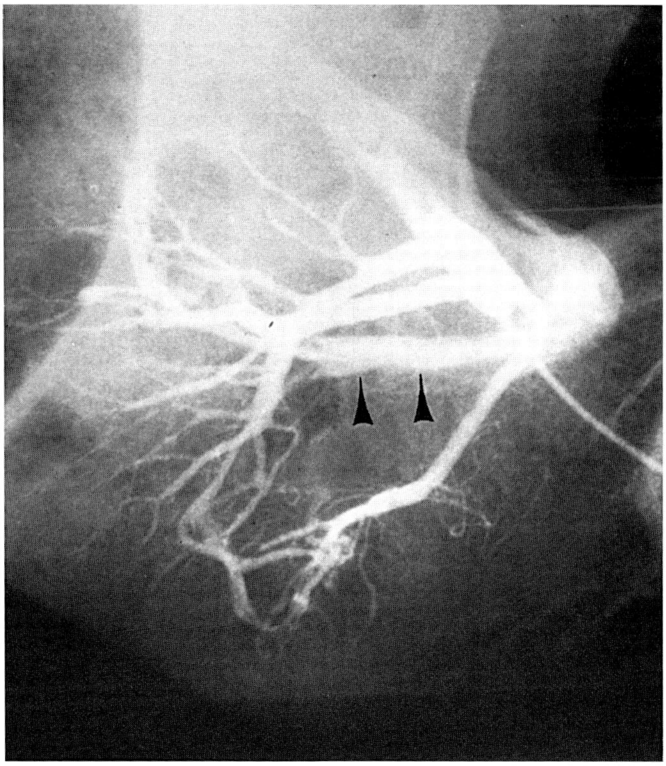

C

Figure 13–3. (*Continued*) C. Image from arterial phase of renal arteriogram shows early venous filling of the draining of the AV fistula (arrowheads).

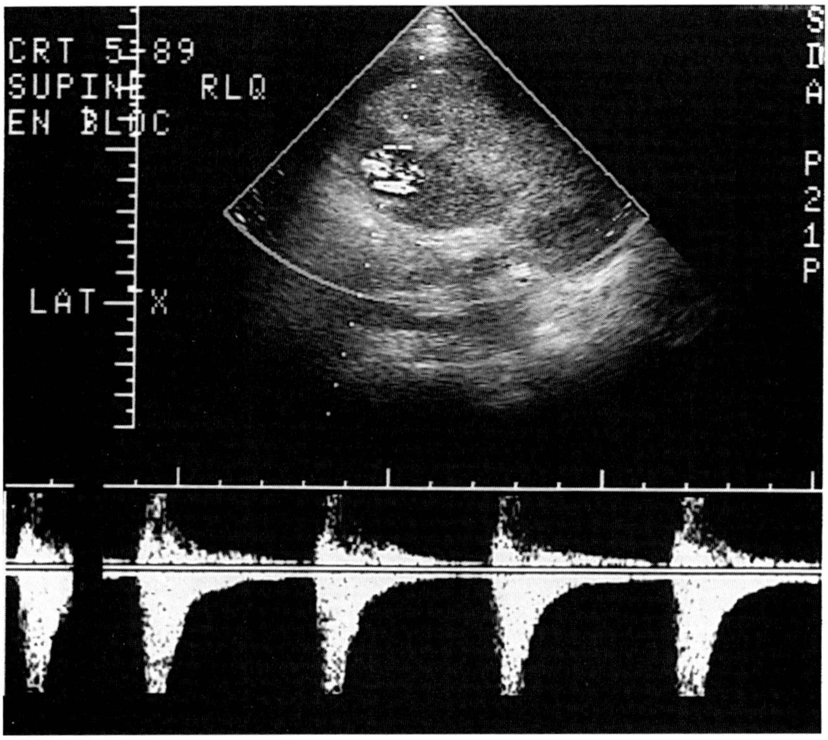

Figure 13–4. Pseudoaneurysm. Color Doppler image with duplex Doppler waveform shows the classic to-and-fro flow pattern.

nique are usually located at the surgical anastomosis. Those due to biopsy error can occur anywhere along the main renal vessels or iliac vessels. In patients with infected extrarenal pseudoaneurysms, not only the pseudoaneurysm but also the renal transplant must be removed, although there have been case reports of successful combined surgical and medical management with salvage of the allograft (see Chapter 12).

The diagnosis of extrarenal pseudoaneurysm can be made definitively with duplex Doppler sonography, color Doppler sonography, and angiography. It may be suggested by contrast-enhanced CT or scintigraphy. The diagnosis of extrarenal AV fistula is much more difficult and is best made with angiography, but it can be suggested by duplex Doppler and color Doppler sonography as well as scintigraphy.

Extrarenal pseudoaneurysms appear as anechoic, spherical, perinephric fluid collections on gray-scale sonography. The Doppler and color Doppler characteristics are identical to those of intrarenal pseudoaneurysms.[34] Therefore, when performing a duplex Doppler examination, unless one examines all perinephric fluid collections, one can mistake a pseudoaneurysm for other more common perinephric collections, such as seromas or lymphoceles.

Extrarenal AV fistulas exhibit Doppler characteristics similar to those of their intrarenal counterparts. However, extrarenal AV fistulas are more difficult to recognize, in part because of involvement of larger vessels. The increased velocity and turbulence seen in the feeding arteries of extrarenal AV fistulas can easily be mistaken for the abnormal waveforms seen in renal artery stenosis. Recognition of the associated increased diastolic flow of an AV fistula suggests the correct diagnosis. Arterialization of the draining vein tends to be diffuse rather than focal. This diffuse venous pulsation can be confusing because it also occurs in normal transplanted kidneys. The diagnosis of an extrarenal AV fistula requires careful inspection of both the arterial and venous Doppler spectra. Final confirmation usually is made by angiography.

Renal Vein Thrombosis and Stenosis

Renal vein thrombosis is one of the rarer vascular complications of renal transplantation; the incidence is 0–4%.[27,28,30] Predisposing factors include hypovolemia, renal venous compression by postoperative fluid collections, extension of ipsilateral common femoral or iliac venous thrombosis, and technical error. Early diagnosis of renal vein thrombosis is critical because thrombectomy, if performed early, can restore graft function. Most cases, however, remain undetected and result in graft loss.

The duplex Doppler findings of renal vein thrombosis consist of no demonstrable venous flow and reversed plateauing diastolic arterial flow[26,60,61] (Fig. 13–5). When these two findings are seen together, they are virtually diagnostic of renal vein thrombosis. Color Doppler sonography can show the absence of venous flow, but this finding alone lacks diagnostic specificity because of its inability to help detect the altered arterial flow.

Renal vein stenosis can be caused by perivascular fibrosis and compression by adjacent perinephric fluid collections. It is a rare complication, and little has been written about it. Venous stenoses are readily detected by color Doppler sonography as regions of focal aliasing that reflect the increased velocities associated with stenosis.[39] Duplex Doppler sonography can help confirm and quantitate the change in velocity at the site of stenosis. A velocity greater than three times that in the prestenotic region is highly suggestive of clinically significant stenosis.

▲ SCINTIGRAPHIC EVALUATION OF RENAL TRANSPLANTS

To a large extent, nuclear medicine flow studies have been supplanted by ultrasonographic techniques. The latter have generally provided more information with greater accuracy. Nevertheless, nuclear scans have some utility in terms of describing qualitative flow and function and are used routinely in some centers. In that setting, a baseline study is obtained during the first few days after transplan-

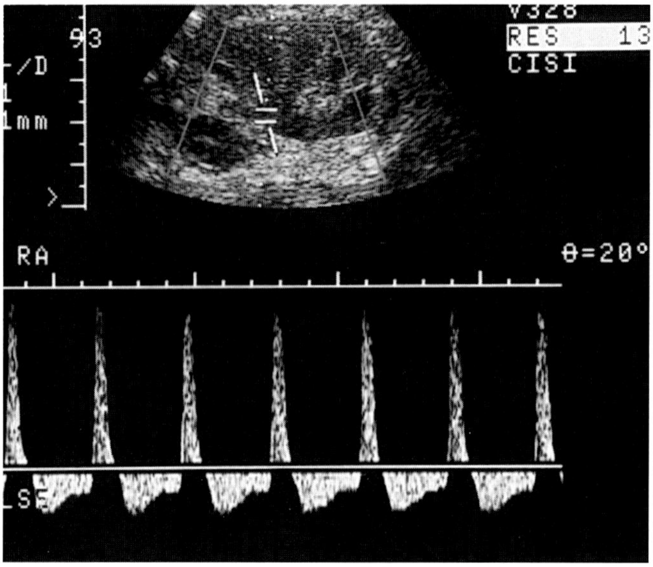

Figure 13–5. Renal vein thrombosis. Duplex Doppler waveform of a segmental renal artery showing reversal and plateauing of the diastolic arterial flow.

tation. A common technique is to give 10 mCi of technetium-99m diethylenetriamine-pentacetic acid (DTPA) intravenously as a bolus injection and acquire data in a computer at one frame per second for 60 frames. This is followed by one frame per minute acquisition for the next 30 minutes. Many quantitative analytic techniques are available, but none of these methods has shown consistently good results.[62–64]

The most widely used agents in nuclear medicine studies after renal transplantation today are technetium Tc 99m DTPA or technetium Tc99m mercaptoacetyltriglycine (MAG3). ^{99m}TcDTPA is produced routinely in the nuclear medicine laboratory by the simple addition of sodium pertechnetate to a sterile kit. The shelf-life of ^{99m}Tc DTPA is generally 6 hours after preparation and depends on the amount of activity, presence of oxygen, and levels of stannous ion. Approximately 3–5% is protein-bound, and nearly 100% filters through the glomerulus.

Radiopharmaceuticals that are predominantly secreted by the tubules are orthoiodohippurate (OIH) and the recently approved technetium-based agent, ^{99m}Tc-MAG3. In each pass through the kidneys, 5–10% of MAG3 passes through the glomerulus and 50–55% is actively secreted by way of the tubules. Approximately 40% leaves the kidney through the renal veins, giving an overall 60% extraction efficiency.[65] The advantage of MAG3 is that it is labeled with the technetium Tc 99m, so that larger doses can be given. In addition, MAG3 is biologically more efficient than DTPA, which has a renal extraction efficiency of approximately 20%. Eshima and Taylor[65] showed that in healthy volunteers, urine extraction of MAG3 is more rapid than that of OIH, but that time to peak concentration activity for MAG3 and OIH is approximately the same. Hepatic extraction of MAG3 might be a problem for patients with poor renal function.[66–70]

A normally functioning graft shows fast uptake of tracer with maximum activity reached at about 5 minutes. Bladder activity should be seen by 5 minutes. The flow portion of the study shows other structures transiently within the abdomen.

Technetium sulfur colloid imaging has been used in an attempt to detect acute rejection. The acute rejection pattern consists of a decreased and delayed arterial peak, followed by more prominent sulfur colloid uptake than that by adjacent bony structures. However, false-negative results were found in patients with nonfunctioning kidneys and patients on anticoagulation. False-positive findings were found among patients with ATN and chronic rejection. Overall the sensitivity of sulfur colloid studies for acute rejection was 70% and the specificity was 85%.[71,72] Indium 111 labeling of leukocytes has been found to have little utility.[73–76]

Renal Artery Thrombosis

The scintigraphic findings of renal artery thrombosis are fairly specific.[77] The absence of renal arterial flow prevents a normal scintigraphic nephrogram. In addition, a large avascular kidney in the pelvis produces a focal ipsilateral decrease in isotope intensity that is less than the background intensity of the contralateral side. This cold spot is highly suggestive of an infarcted kidney, although hyperacute or accelerated rejection may cause a similar appearance. Segmental arterial thromboses produce persistent intrarenal photopenic defects that are classically wedge-shaped.[77] Although their appearance is fairly specific, other causes of focal photopenic areas such as hematomas, abscesses, and cysts should be included in the differential diagnosis.

Renal Artery Stenosis

Routine transplant scintigraphy is not useful in the diagnosis of renal artery stenosis. The findings cannot be differentiated from those of rejection and cyclosporine toxicity. All cause a progressive decrease in renal perfusion and function that can be identified at serial imaging.[77] Some reports indicate that scintigraphy before and after the administration of captopril can be used to detect native renal arterial stenoses with a high degree of confidence.[78] These claims have yet to be substantiated in renal transplants.[79]

Arteriovenous Fistulas and Pseudoaneurysms

Intrarenal

Intrarenal AV fistulas cannot be visualized directly with scintigraphy. Rather, the presence of these fistulas can be suggested with a high degree of confidence if premature isotope activity is detected within the inferior vena cava during the flow phase of the study. After the flow phase, the fistulas become invisible (Fig. 13–6). Large intrarenal pseudoaneurysms are detectable as focal hot spots that appear in the early flow phase and often persist into the functional phase of the study. Their appearance is diagnostic.[77]

Extrarenal

Except for location, the scintigraphic features of extrarenal lesions are identical to those of intrarenal pseudoaneurysms and AV fistulas. In fact, intrarenal and extrarenal AV fistulas are nearly impossible to differentiate from each other. The appearance of extrarenal pseudoaneurysms is fairly diagnostic. However, because of their location they can be confused with focal urine leaks. The two are differentiated by recognition of the early or flow-phase appearance of a pseudoaneurysm as opposed to the delayed or functional-phase appearance of a urine leak. Pseudoaneurysms also tend to wash out sooner than urinomas.[77]

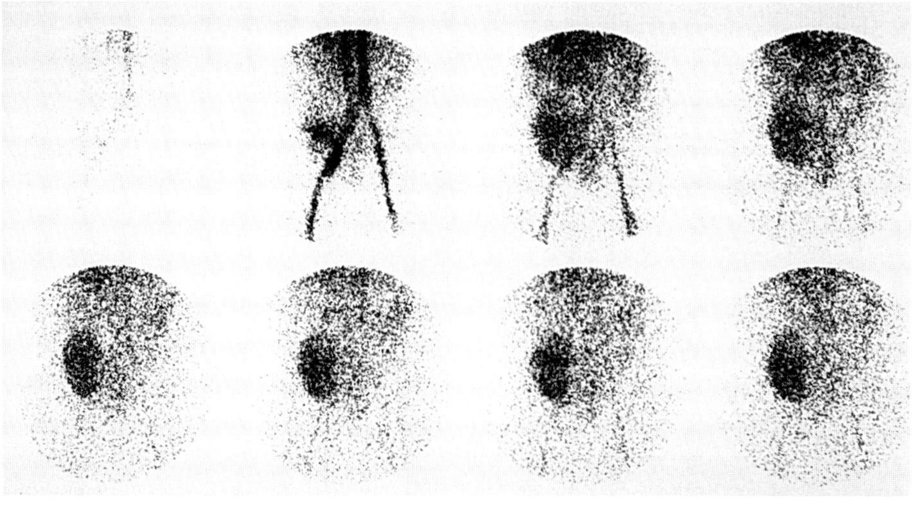

Figure 13–6. Renal flow study of arteriovenous fistula shows premature isotope activity in the inferior vena cava during early flow phase. The inferior vena cava is not visible in the later flow phase.

Renal Vein Thrombosis and Stenosis

The scintigraphic findings of renal vein thrombosis are difficult to differentiate from other causes of decreased perfusion and function. The exact appearance depends on the degree and age of the thrombus. Myerly and Kirchner[80] reported that absence of a nephrogram without a cold spot (ie, isotope intensity of transplant bed equal to background intensity of the contralateral pelvis) is characteristic of renal vein thrombosis. The absence of the cold spot implies that renal perfusion is present but markedly diminished. Other causes, such as rejection, can cause a similar appearance; however, identification of this finding as an acute event in a series of scintigrams warrants immediate clinical attention.

Urinary Obstruction

Diuretic renography is a pharmacologic technique useful for differentiating obstructive from nonobstructive dilatation. With this technique, a diuretic, usually furosemide (0.4 mg/kg), is given intravenously approximately 20 minutes after injection of the radiopharmaceutical (^{99m}Tc-MAG3 at our center).

Diuretic renography can be performed visually by observing the changes in dynamic images or quantitatively by determining the half-life of the radiopharmaceutical after administration of furosemide. A half-life of 10 minutes or less is considered normal, whereas 20 minutes or more is considered abnormal and represents obstruction. Values between 10 and 20 minutes are considered equivocal. Diuretic renography can be used successfully to differentiate an extrarenal pelvis or congenital, postinflammatory, or postobstructive ureterectasis from clinically significant obstruction.

Urinary Leak

The typical scintigraphic finding in a urinoma is a photopenic area adjacent to the allograft that gradually fills in (Fig. 13–7). We prefer to use ^{99m}Tc-MAG3. Occasionally we place markers on the patient's skin and then perform an ultrasound examination to locate the area of extravasation. We also look at the cinematic representation of the study on a computer screen. However, false-positive findings can be seen. Therefore, scintigraphy should never be the only modality used to diagnose a urine leak.

Rejection

In general scintigraphy is not useful in the diagnosis of rejection. Associated findings of hyperacute rejection are the absence of flow or function in the renal allograft. In acute rejection a nuclear medicine flow study shows poor uptake and poor excretion.

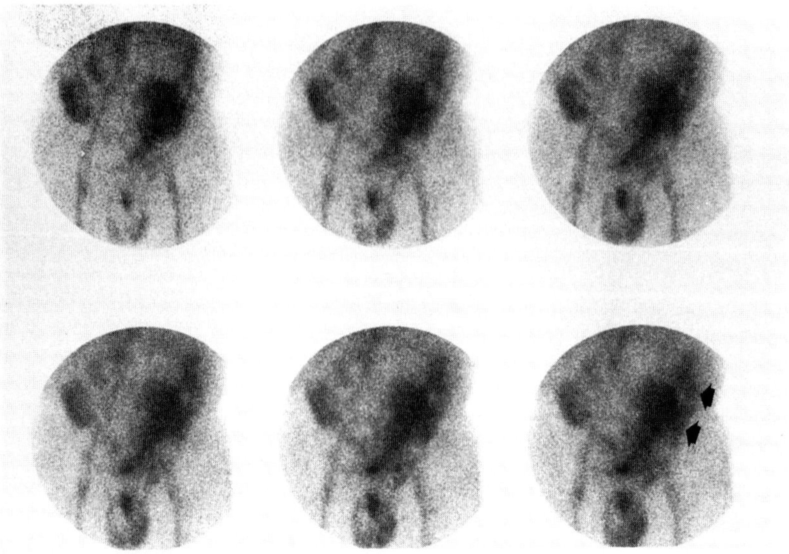

Figure 13–7. Renal functional images showing right lower quadrant transplanted kidney with evidence of gradual accumulation of activity in the left lower quadrant (arrows), highly suggestive of leak.

Serial examination of flow shows a greater perfusion abnormality than is typically seen with ATN. In chronic rejection, the renal flow study shows delayed flow and function.

Cyclosporine and Tacrolimus Toxicity and Acute Tubular Necrosis

Scintigraphy is not a useful modality in the diagnosis of cyclosporine or tacrolimus (FK 506) toxicity or in differentiating either from ATN. Renal flow studies demonstrate findings similar to those seen in ATN; that is, diminished flow and function.

Summary

Scintigraphy is of limited usefulness in renal transplantation. Adverse events are difficult to differentiate from one another with scintigraphic techniques, and the complications in which scintigraphy is diagnostic are usually seen with sonographic studies. In general, we have largely abandoned routine scintigraphy. In spite of these limitations, however, there are occasional situations in which scintigraphy can be of some use.

▲ ANGIOGRAPHY AND INTERVENTIONAL RADIOLOGY

Although ultrasonographic and, to a lesser extent, scintigraphic studies are useful screening tests in the diagnosis of specific complications after renal transplantation, angiography is often necessary to establish a definitive diagnosis. In addition, angiographic and other interventional techniques can be useful therapeutically. Prompt intervention can often either obviate the need for surgical intervention or convert an urgent situation into one amenable to more elective surgical repair.

Vascular Intervention

Arterial stenosis may affect either the donor renal artery or the recipient iliac artery. Compromise of renal blood flow may result from atherosclerosis, arterial kinking due to redundancy or perivascular adhesions, anastomotic stenosis due to fibrosis, faulty suturing technique, or trauma during harvest or reperfusion. Nonanastomotic stenoses also may occur secondary to rejection.[81]

Treatment of renal allograft arterial stenosis traditionally has been surgical.[82] However, as a result of its relative ease and safety compared with the risk of reoperation, percutaneous transluminal angioplasty (PTA) has become the procedure of first choice in the management of both intra- and extrarenal stenoses (Fig. 13–8). Clinical success rates resulting in initial improvement or cure average 73%.[81–85] Improvement in renal function may often be seen within 24 hours of PTA.[83] Although renal allograft PTA is not a completely benign procedure,[82] there is a lower incidence of complications than with surgical correction.[81,85,86] In addition, failure of PTA does not preclude surgical intervention. As many as 20% of successfully dilated stenoses may require repeat dilation for long-term patency.[83,85] There is a relative paucity of long-term follow-up data after renal allograft PTA, but one series showed that 67% of grafts were patent 1 year after PTA.[83] End-to-end anastomoses to the internal iliac artery may be difficult to access because of vascular tortuosity.[83] It is often easier to cannulate an end-to-side (external iliac artery) anastomosis from an ipsilateral femoral arterial approach; end-to-end (internal iliac artery) anastomoses are more accessible from a contralateral approach. Systemic anticoagulation is almost always used during renal allograft PTA. Intraarterial nitroglycerine is helpful in the prevention of arterial spasm.

Another area in which interventional radiologic techniques may be useful is in the management of renal allograft arterial or venous thrombosis. Depending on the

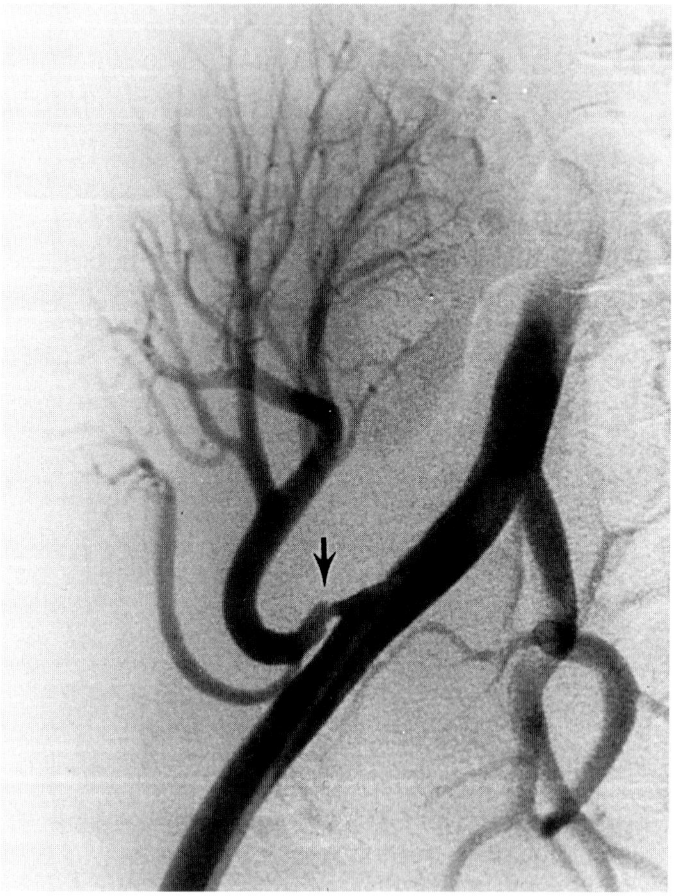

A

Figure 13–8. Percutaneous transluminal angioplasty (PTA) of renal allograft arterial stenosis. A. External iliac arteriogram shows marked stenosis of the allograft renal artery (arrow).

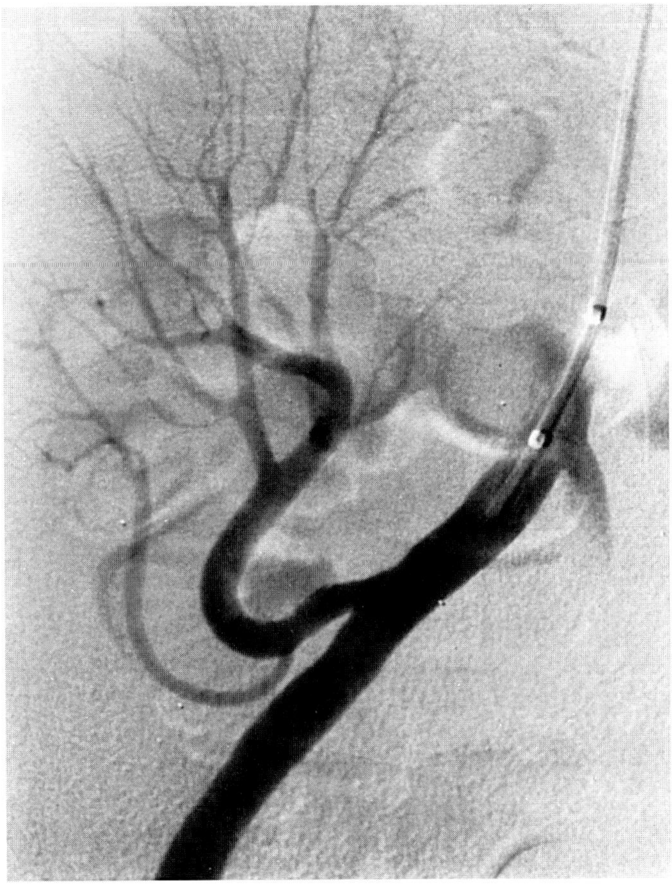

B

Figure 13–8. (*Continued*) B. Post-PTA arteriogram shows widely patent renal artery.

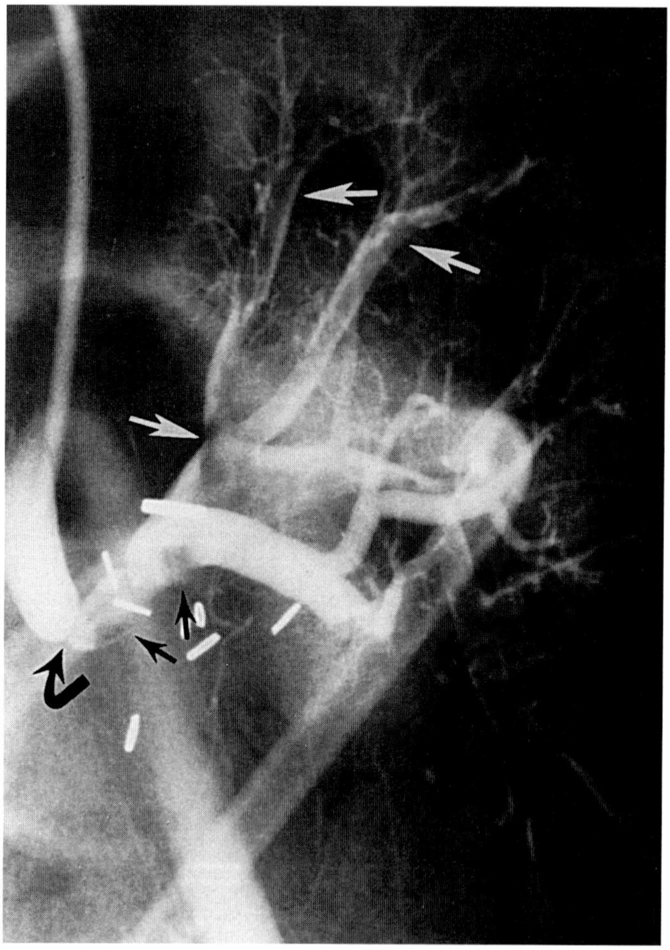

A

Figure 13–9. Intraarterial thrombolytic therapy for treatment of renal allograft arterial thrombosis. A. Selective internal iliac arteriogram shows severe stenosis of the renal allograft arterial anastomosis (curved arrow) and thrombus within the main renal artery and intrarenal branch arteries (straight arrows). Serum creatinine level was 10 mg/dL (880 μmol/L). The patient was treated with balloon angioplasty of the arterial anastomotic stenosis followed by low-dose streptokinase (5000 units/hour) directly into the renal artery for 40 hours resulting in complete thrombolysis. *(From Griffin JF, et al: Diagnosis of disease in renal allografts: correlation between ultrasound and histology.* Clin Radiol *37:59–62, 1986.)*

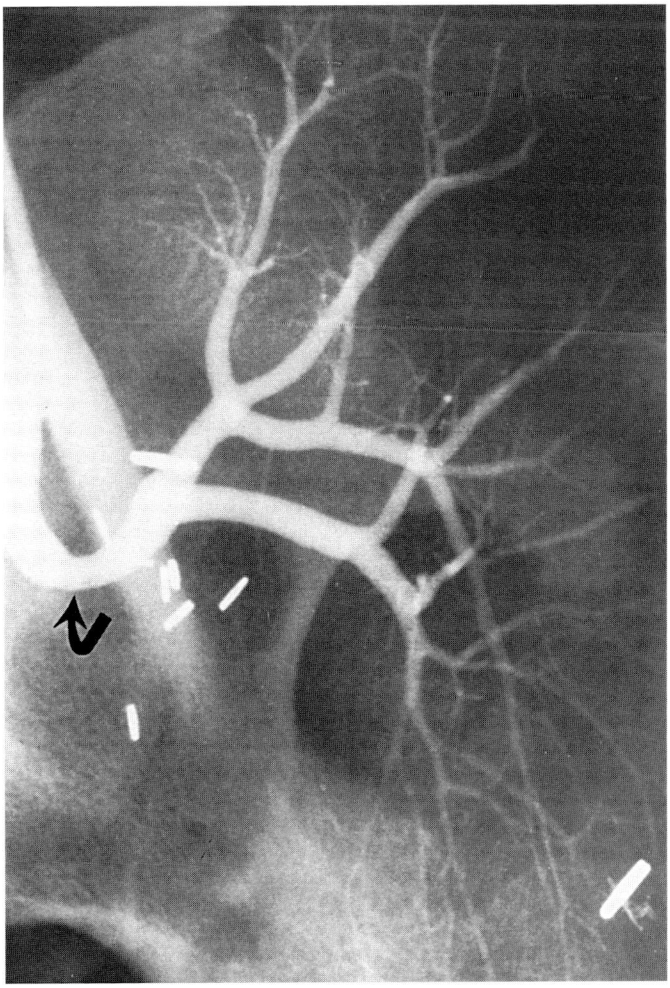

B

Figure 13–9. (*Continued*) B. Follow-up arteriogram 5 weeks after thrombolytic therapy shows complete absence of thrombus. The anastomosis (curved arrow) is widely patent. Serum creatinine level gradually decreased to 3.5 mg/dL (310 umol/L) over the following 5 weeks.

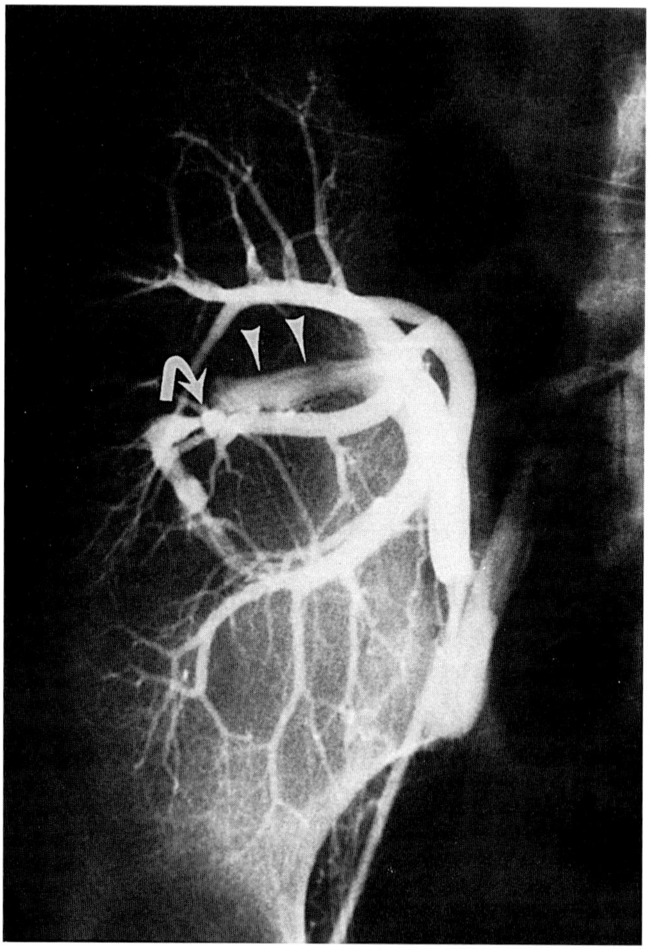

A

Figure 13–10. Transcatheter embolization therapy for control of gross hematuria caused by percutaneous needle biopsy. A. Renal allograft arteriogram shows arteriovenous fistula (curved arrow) and associated rapid venous filling (arrowheads).

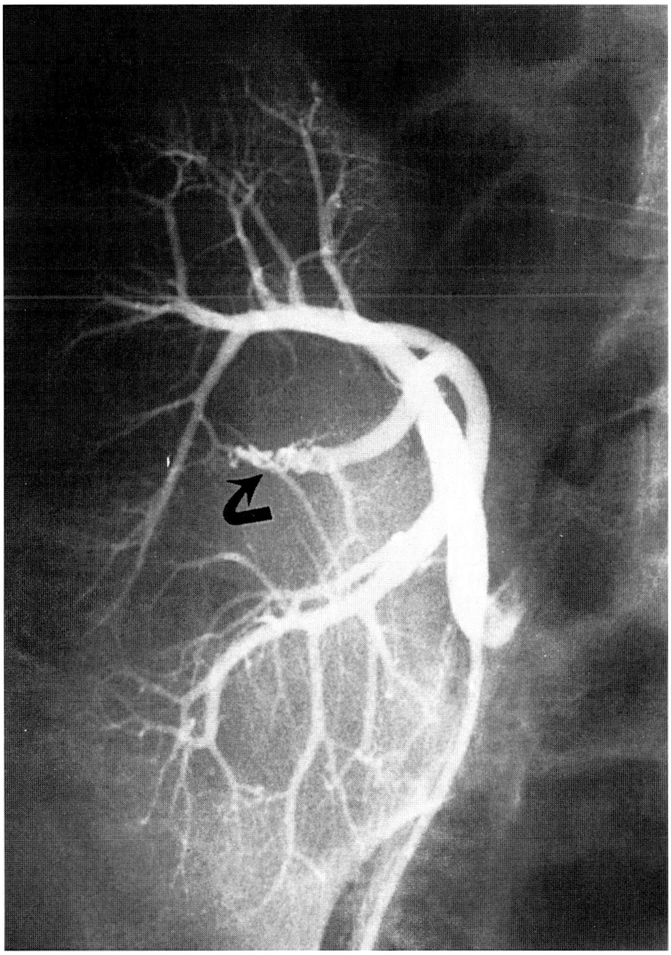

B

Figure 13–10. (*Continued*) B. Arteriogram after selective embolization with stainless steel coils shows occlusion of arteriovenous fistula (curved arrow).

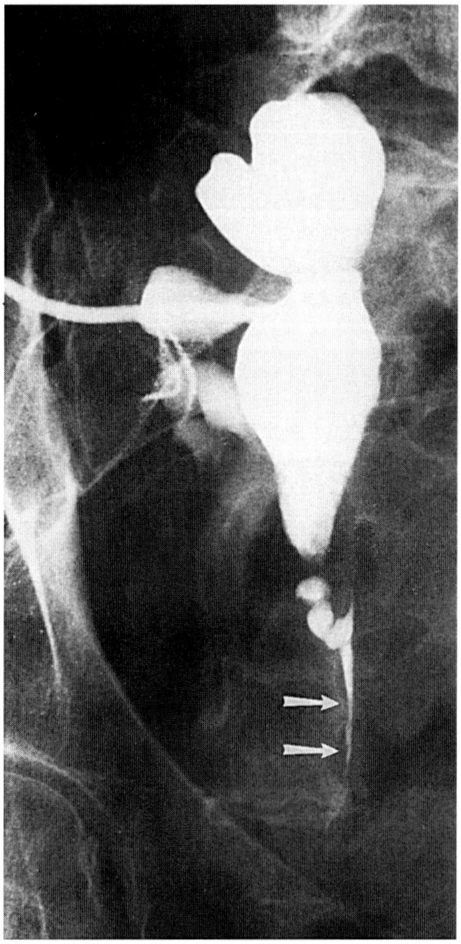

Figure 13–11. Nephrostomy placement for ureteral obstruction. Nephrostogram after catheter placement shows hydronephrosis due to severe stricture of distal ureter (arrowheads).

duration of the occlusion and whether arterial thrombosis is complete, successful thrombolytic therapy and allograft salvage might be feasible, although it must be emphasized that the usual outcome is loss of the allograft[44,87] (Fig. 13–9). Early diagnosis is important in salvage, whether with percutaneous or surgical techniques.[88–90] Thrombolytic therapy also has been used successfully in acute allograft renal vein thrombosis.[87]

Percutaneous allograft biopsies are commonly performed to establish the cause of graft dysfunction. Gross hematuria complicating percutaneous biopsy occurs in approximately 7% of patients and is most often transient and self-limiting, but massive or persistent hematuria occasionally may occur.[91] Although bleeding after a biopsy once was associated with graft loss or even patient death, selective transcatheter embolization techniques have the potential to stop the bleeding with minimal loss of renal tissue (Fig. 13–10).

Other Interventional Modalities

Percutaneous nephrostomy for urinary obstruction (Fig. 13–11) is the interventional procedure most commonly performed in renal transplant patients.[81,92,93] Causes of obstruction include ureteral stricture or kinking, edema or stricture at the ureteroneocystostomy, pelvic fibrosis, ureteral stone or blood clot, and external compression by lymphocele. Nephrostomy placement is usually performed with sonographic guidance.

If obstruction is caused by ureteroneocystostomy edema or ureteral blood clot, a nephrostomy can provide relief of obstruction until the edema subsides or the clot passes.[93] More commonly, a nephrostomy is placed because of a ureteral or anastomotic stricture. In these patients, surgical revision traditionally has been necessary, but a number of small series have shown the successful management of ureteral stricture can be achieved with percutaneous balloon dilation.[93,94–98]

Urinary leak most commonly occurs at the level of the distal ureter or the ureteroneocystostomy.[92,99] Leaks also may occur from more proximal ureter, renal pelvis, or calyces. In addition to relief of urinary obstruction, percutaneous nephrostomy provides external diversion of urinary flow, occasionally allowing urine leaks to heal without surgical intervention[93,100] (Fig. 13–12). Placement of ureteral stents may be of value in the treatment of urine leaks.[100]

Periallograft fluid collections have been reported in as many as 15% of renal transplants.[99] Differential diagnoses of early postoperative collections include urinoma, hematoma, or abscess. Lymphoceles, the most commonly seen periallograft collections, usually occur later in the postoperative period.[99] Percutaneous aspiration under ultrasound guidance is safe and allows biochemical and bacteriologic evaluation of the fluid. Abscesses can be treated effectively with ultrasound-guided placement of drainage catheters in most patients.

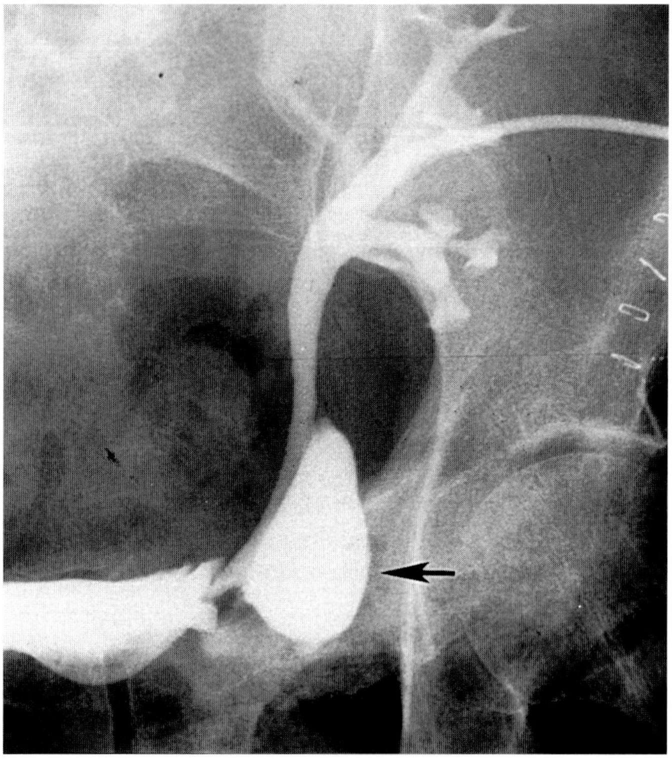

A

Figure 13–12. Nephrostomy and ureteral stent for treatment of urine leak. A. Nephrostogram after catheter insertion into bladder shows large leak (arrow) from distal ureter.

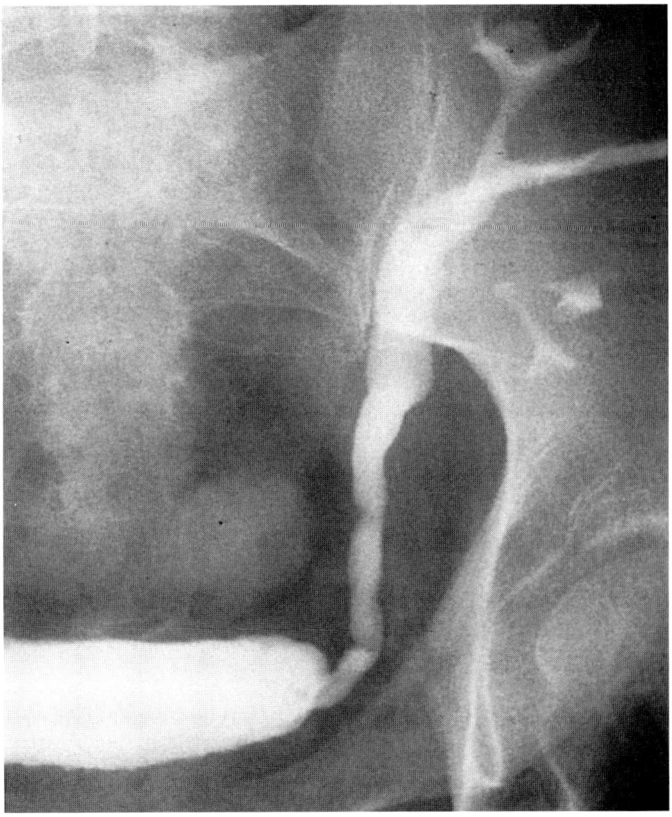

B

Figure 13–12. (*Continued*) B. Nephrostogram after 8 weeks of external drainage shows patent ureter with no leakage. Catheter was removed.

▲ REFERENCES

1. Raiss GJ, Bree RL, Schwab RE, et al: Further observations in the ultrasound evaluation of renal allograft rejection. *J Ultrasound Med* 5:439–444, 1986.
2. Letourneau JG, Day DL, Feinberg SB: Ultrasound and computed tomographic evaluation of renal transplantation. *Radiol Clin North Am* 25:267–279, 1987.
3. Maklad NF, Wright CH, Rosenthal SJ: Gray scale ultrasound appearances of renal transplant rejection. *Radiology* 131:711–727, 1979.
4. Hillman BJ, Birnholz JC, Busch GJ: Correlation of echographic and histologic findings in suspected renal allograft rejection. *Radiology* 132:673–676, 1979.
5. Frick MP, Feinberg SB, Sibley R, et al: Ultrasound in acute renal transplant rejection. *Radiology* 138:657–660, 1981.
6. Swobodnik WL, Spohn BE, Wechsler JG, et al: Real-time ultrasound evaluation of renal transplant failure during the early postoperative period. *Ultrasound Med Biol* 12:97–105, 1986.
7. Linkowski GD, Warvariv V, Filly RA, et al: Sonography in the diagnosis of acute renal allograft rejection and cyclosporine nephrotoxicity. *AJR Am J Roentgenol* 148:291–295.
8. Fleischer AC, James AE Jr, MacDonnell RC Jr, et al: Sonography of renal transplant patients. *Crit Rev Diagn Imaging* 18:197–242, 1982.
9. Berland LL, Lawson TL, Adams MB, et al: Evaluation of renal transplants with pulsed Doppler duplex sonography. *J Ultrasound Med* 1:215–222, 1982.
10. Pozniak MA, Kelcz F, Dodd GD: Renal transplant ultrasound: imaging and Doppler. *Semin Ultrasound CT MR* 12:319–334, 1991.
11. Fried AM, Woodring JH, Loh FK, et al: The medullary pyramid index: an objective assessment of prominence in renal transplant rejection. *Radiology* 149:787–791, 1983.
12. Griffin JF, Short CD, Lawler W, et al: Diagnosis of disease in renal allografts: correlation between ultrasound and histology. *Clin Radiol* 37:59–62, 1986.
13. Hoddick W, Filly RA, Blackman U, et al: Renal allograft rejection: US evaluation. *Radiology* 161:469–473, 1986.
14. Murphy AM, Robertson RJ, Dubbins PA: Duplex ultrasound in the assessment of renal transplant complications. *Clin Radiol* 38:229–234, 1987.
15. Kelcz F, Pozniak MA, Pirsch JD, et al: Pyramidal appearance and resistive index: insensitive and nonspecific sonography indicators of renal transplant rejection. *AJR Am J Roentgenol* 155:531–535, 1990.
16. Hricak H, Terrier F, Marotti M, et al: Posttransplant renal rejection: comparison of quantitative scintigraphy, ultrasound, and MR imaging. *Radiology* 162:685–688, 1987.
17. Rifkin MD, Needleman L, Pasto ME, et al: Evaluation of renal transplant rejection by duplex Doppler examination: value of the resistive index. *AJR Am J Roentgenol* 148:759–762, 1987.
18. Needleman L, Kurtz AB: Doppler evaluation of the renal transplant. *J Clin Ultrasound* 15:661–673, 1987.
19. Buckley AR, Cooperberg PL, Reeve CE, et al: The distinction between acute renal transplant rejection and cyclosporine nephrotoxicity: value of duplex sonography. *AJR Am J Roentgenol* 149:521–525, 1987.
20. Drake DG, Day DL, Letourneau JG, et al: Doppler evaluation of renal transplants in children: a prospective analysis with histopathologic correlation. *AJR Am J Roentgenol* 154:785–787, 1990.

21. Grigat KP, Leimenstoll G, Engemann R, et al: Monitoring of renal allografts by duplex ultrasound. *Transplant Int* 2:102–107, 1989.
22. Genkins SM, Sanfilippo FP, Carroll BA: Duplex Doppler sonography of renal transplants: lack of sensitivity and specificity in establishing pathologic diagnosis. *AJR Am J Roentgenol* 152:535–539, 1989.
23. Rubin JM, Platt JF, Adler RS: Applications of Doppler ultrasound in transplant and native kidney disease. *Ultrasound Q* 8:95–120, 1990.
24. Don S, Kopecky KK, Filor RS, et al: Duplex Doppler US of renal allografts: cause of elevated resistive index. *Radiology* 171:709–712, 1989.
25. Pozniak MA, Kelcz F, Stratta RJ, et al: Extraneous factors affecting resistive index. *Invest Radiol* 23:899–904, 1988.
26. Warshauer DM, Taylor KJW, Bia MJ, et al: Unusual causes of increased vascular impedance in renal transplants: duplex Doppler evaluation. *Radiology* 169:367–370, 1988.
27. Jordan ML, Cook GT, Cardella CJ: Ten years of experience with vascular complications in renal transplantation. *J Urol* 128:689–692, 1982.
28. Palleschi J, Novick AC, Braun WE, Magnusson MO: Vascular complications of renal transplantation. *Urology* 16:61–67, 1980.
29. Hohnke C, Abendroth D, Schleibner S, Land W: Vascular complications in 1,200 kidney transplantations. *Transplant Proc* 19:3691–3692, 1987.
30. Rijksen JFWB, Koolen MI, Walaszewski JE, Terpstra JL, Vink M: Vascular complications in 400 consecutive renal allograft transplants. *J Cardiovasc Surg (Torino)* 23:91–98, 1982.
31. Hanto D, Simmons R: Renal transplantation: clinical considerations in organ transplantation. *Radiol Clin North Am* 25:239–248, 1987.
32. Grenier N, Douws C, Morel D, et al: Detection of vascular complications in renal allografts with color Doppler flow imaging. *Radiology* 178:217–223, 1991.
33. Mitchell DG: Color Doppler imaging: principles, limitations and artifacts. *Radiology* 177:1–10, 1990.
34. Dodd GD, Tublin ME, Shah A, Zajko AB: Imaging of vascular complications associated with renal transplants. *AJR Am J Roentgenol* 157:449–459, 1991.
35. Roberts JP, Ascher NL, Fryd DS, et al: Transplant renal artery stenosis. *Transplantation* 4:580–583, 1989.
36. Munda R, Alexander WJ, Miller S, First MR, Fidler JP: Renal allograft artery stenosis. *Am J Surg* 134:400–403, 1977.
37. Barth MO, Gagnadoux MF, Mareschal JL, et al: Angioplasty of renal transplant artery stenosis in children. *Pediatr Radiol* 19:383–387, 1989.
38. Stanley P, Malekzadeh M, Diament MJ: Posttransplant renal artery stenosis: angiographic study in 32 children. *AJR Am J Roentgenol* 148:487–490, 1987.
39. Taylor KJW, Morse SS, Rigsby CM, Bia M, Schiff M: Vascular complications in renal allografts: detection with duplex Doppler ultrasound. *Radiology* 162:31–38, 1987.
40. Snider JF, Hunter DW, Moradian GP, Castaneda-Zuniga WR, Letourneau JG: Transplant renal artery stenosis: evaluation with duplex sonography. *Radiology* 172:1027–1030, 1989
41. Scott Samara EN, Voss BL, Pederson JA: Renal artery thrombosis associated with elevated cyclosporin levels: a case report and review of the literature. *Transplant Proc* 20:119–123, 1988.
42. Rigotti P, Flechner SM, Van Buren CT, Payne WT, Kahan BD: Increased incidence of renal allograft thrombosis under a cyclosporin immunosuppression. *Surgery* 71:38–41, 1986.
43. Aujila ND, Greenberg A, Banner BF, Johnson JR, Tzakis AG: Atheroembolic involvement of renal allografts. *Am J Kidney Dis* 12:329–322, 1989.

44. Zajko AB, McLean GK, Grossman RA, et al: Percutaneous transluminal angioplasty and fibrinolytic therapy for renal allograft arterial stenosis and thrombosis. *Transplantation* 33:447–450, 1982.
45. Bennett AR, Wiener SN: Intrarenal arteriovenous fistula and aneurysm: a complication of percutaneous renal biopsy. *AJR Am J Roentgenol* 95:372–382, 1965.
46. Altebarmakian VK, Guthinger WP, Yakub YN, Gutierrez OH, Linke CA: Percutaneous kidney biopsies: complications and their management. *Urology* 18:118–122, 1981.
47. Wickre CG, Golper TA: Complications of percutaneous needle biopsy of the kidney. *Am J Nephrol* 2:173–178, 1982.
48. Benoit G, Charpentier B, Roche A, Bellamy J, Mohamedi D, Fries D: Arteriocalyceal fistula after grafted kidney biopsy: successful management by selective catheter embolization. *Urology* 24:487–490, 1984.
49. Baquero A, Morris MC, Cope C, Raja R, Bannett AD: Selective embolization of vascular complications following renal biopsy of the transplant kidney. *Transplant Proc* 27:1751–1754, 1985.
50. Wallace S, Schwarten D, Smith D, Gerson L, Davis L: Intrarenal AV fistulas: trans-catheter steel coil occlusion. *J Urol* 120:282–286, 1978.
51. Weissman J, Giyanani VL, Landreneau MD, Kilpatrick JS: Postbiopsy arterial pseudoaneurysm in a renal allograft: detection by duplex sonography. *J Ultrasound Med* 7:515–518, 1988.
52. Hubsch PJS, Mostbeck G, Barton PP, et al: Evaluation of arteriovenous fistulas and pseudoaneurysms in renal allografts following percutaneous needle biopsy: color coded Doppler sonography vs duplex Doppler sonography. *J Ultrasound Med* 9:95–100, 1990.
53. Middleton WD, Kellman GM, Melson GL, Madrazo BL: Postbiopsy renal transplant arteriovenous fistulas: color Doppler versus US characteristics. *Radiology* 171:253–257, 1989.
54. Renigers SA, Spigos DG: Pseudoaneurysm of the arterial anastomosis in a renal transplant. *AJR Am J Roentgenol* 131:525–526, 1978.
55. Mulderije ED, Berden JHM, Buskens FGM, Raaijmakers PAM, Rosenbusch G: False and true aneurysms of the renal artery after kidney transplantation: a report of two cases. *Br J Radiol* 58:896–899, 1985.
56. Pigott JP, Sharp WV: Arteriovenous fistula involving a transplant kidney (Brief Communication). *Transplantation* 44:1, 1987.
57. Salahudeen AK, Sellars L, Srinivasa Merthy LN, et al: Extrarenal arteriovenous fistula: an unusual complication of percutaneous renal transplant biopsy. *Nephron* 37:64–65, 1984.
58. Tobben PJ, Zajko AB, Sumkin JH, et al: Pseudoaneurysms complicating organ transplantation: roles of CT, duplex sonography, and angiography. *Radiology* 169:65–70, 1988.
59. Kyriakides GK, Simmons RL, Najarian JS: Mycotic aneurysms in transplant patients. *Arch Surg* 3:472–476, 1976.
60. Reuther G, Wanjura D, Bauer H: Acute renal vein thrombosis in renal allografts: detection with duplex Doppler ultrasound. *Radiology* 170:557–558, 1989.
61. Kaveggia LP, Parrella RR, Grant EG, et al: Duplex Doppler sonography in renal allografts: the significance of reversed flow in diastole. *AJR Am J Roentgenol* 155:295–298, 1990.
62. Preston DF, Luke R: Radionuclide evaluation of renal transplants. *J Nucl Med* 20:1095–1097, 1979.
63. Lawson RS: Mathematics. In: O'Reilly H, Shields RA, Testa HJ (eds), *Nuclear Medicine in Urology and Nephrology*, ed 2. London, Butterworth, 1986:257–269.
64. Washida H, Tsuaya H, Fushimi N, et al: Evaluation of intensity of first perfusion of renoscintigram using ^{99m}Tc-DTPA in practical urology. In: Raynaud C (ed), *Proceedings of III World Congress of Nuclear Medicine and Biology*. Paris, Pergamon, 1982:1556–1559.

65. Eshima D, Taylor A Jr: Technetium-99m (^{99m}Tc) mercaptoacetyltriglycine: update on the new ^{99m}Tc renal tubular function agent. *Semin Nucl Med* 22:61–73, 1992.
66. Dubovsky EV: Primer and atlas for renal transplant scintigraphy. *Clin Nucl Med* 10:52–62, 118–133, 1985.
67. Dubovsky EV: Renal transplantation. In: Tauxe WN, Dubovksy EV (eds), *Nuclear Medicine in Clinical Urology and Nephrology.* Norwalk, CT, Appleton-Century-Crofts, 1985:231–278.
68. Dubovsky EV, Logic RJ, Diethelm AG, et al: Comprehensive evaluation of renal function in thc transplanted kidney. *J Nucl Med* 16:1115–1120, 1975.
69. Diethelm AG, Dubovsky EV, Whelchel JD, et al: Diagnosis of impaired renal function after kidney transplantation using renal scintigraphy, renal plasma flow, and urinary excretion of hippurate. *Ann Surg* 191:604–616, 1980.
70. Dubovsky EV, Diethelm AG, Tauxe WN: Differentiation of cell-mediated and humoral rejection by orthoiodohippurate kinetics. *Arch Intern Med* 137:738–742, 1977.
71. George EA, Codd JE, Newton WT, et al: Comparative evaluation of renal transplant rejection with radioiodinated fibrogen, ^{99m}Tc-sulfur colloid and ^{67}Ga-citrate. *J Nucl Med* 17:175–180, 1976.
72. George EA, Meyerovitz M, Codd JE: Renal allograft accumulation of Tc-99m sulfur colloid: temporal quantitation and scintigraphic assessment. *Radiology* 148:547–551, 1983.
73. Winston MA, Weiss ER, Blahd WH, et al: Use of I-131-fibrogen in detection of renal transplant rejects. *Invest Urol* 9:119–123, 1971.
74. Forstrom LA, Loken MK, Cook A, et al: In-111-labeled leukocytes in the diagnosis of rejection and cytomegalovirus infection in renal transplant patients. *Clin Nucl Med* 6:146–148, 1981.
75. Collier BD, Isitman AT, Kaufman HM, et al: Concentration of In-111-oxine labeled autologous leukocytes in noninfected and nonrejection renal allografts: concise communication. *J Nucl Med* 25:156–159, 1984.
76. Martin-Comin J: Kidney graft rejection studies with labeled platelets and lymphocytes. *Nucl Med Biol* 13:173–181, 1986.
77. Kirchner PT, Rosenthall L: Renal transplant evaluation. *Semin Nucl Med* 12:370–378, 1982.
78. Chen CC, Hoffer PB, Vahjen G, et al: Patients at high risk for renal artery stenosis: a simple method of renal scintigraphic analysis with Tc-99m DTPA and captopril. *Radiology* 176:365–370, 1990.
79. Miach PJ, Ernest D, McKay J, Dawborn JK: Renography with captopril in renal transplant recipients. *Transplant Proc* 21:1953–1954, 1989.
80. Myerly KF, Kirchner PT: Renal scintigraphic findings in a case of transplant renal vein thrombosis. *Clin Nucl Med* 13:426–429, 1988.
81. Curry NS, Cochran S, Barbaric ZL, et al: Interventional radiologic procedures in the renal transplant. *Radiology* 152:647–653, 1984.
82. Grossman RA, DaFoe DC, Shoenfeld RB, et al: Percutaneous transluminal angioplasty treatment of renal transplant artery stenosis. *Transplantation* 34,6:339–343, 1982.
83. Raynaud A, Bedrossian J, Remy P, Brisset JM, Angel CY, Gaux JC: Percutaneous transluminal angioplasty of renal transplant arterial stenosis. *AJR Am J Roentgenol* 146:853–857, 1986.
84. Weigele JB: Iliac artery stenosis causing renal allograft-mediated hypertension: angiographic diagnosis and treatment. *AJR Am J Roentgenol* 157:513–515, 1991.
85. Neithamer CD, Sniderman KW, Sprayregen S, et al: Transluminal angioplasty in allograft renal artery stenosis. *Semin Intervent Radiol* 3:93–103, 1986.

86. McMullin ND, Reidy JF, Koffman CG, et al: The management of renal transplant artery stenosis in children by percutaneous transluminal angioplasty. *Transplantation* 53:559–563, 1992.
87. Robinson JM, Cockrell CH, Tisnado J, Beachley MC, Posner MP, Tracy TF: Selective low-dose streptokinase infusion in the treatment of acute transplant renal vein thrombosis. *Cardiovasc Intervent Radiol* 9:86, 1986.
88. Plainfosse MC, Calonge VM, Beyloune-Mainardi C, Glotz D, Duboust A: Vascular complications in the adult kidney transplant recipient. *J Clin Ultrasound* 20:517–527, 1992.
89. Zanon E, Right D, Robotti D, et al: The percutaneous treatment of the urological complications following kidney transplantation. *Radiol Med* 84:613–618, 1992.
90. Boschiero LB, Saggin P, Galante O, et al: Renal needle biopsy of the transplant kidney: vascular and urologic complications. *Urol Int* 48:130–133, 1992.
91. Aguera Fernandez LG, Zudaire JJ, Isa WA, et al: Vascular complications in 237 recipients of renal transplant from cadaver. *Acta Urol Esp* 16:292–295, 1992.
92. Mundy AR, Podesta ML, Bewick M, Rudge CJ, Ellis FG: The urologic complications of 1000 renal transplants. *Br J Urol* 53:397–402, 1981.
93. Bennett LR, Voegeli DR, Crummy AB, McDermott JC, Jensen SR, Sollinger HW: Urologic complications following renal transplantation: role of interventional radiologic procedures. *Radiology* 160:531–536, 1986.
94. Glassock RJ, Feinstein EI, Campese VM, Finck E, Silberman H, Chandrasoma P: Hypertension in a renal transplant recipient. *Am J Nephrol* 4:262–271, 1984.
95. List A: Interventional radiology in the treatment of ureteric complications in transplant kidneys. *Australas Radiol* 33:255–258, 1989.
96. Greenstein S, Verstandig A, McLean GK, et al: Percutaneous transluminal angioplasty: the procedure of choice in the hypertensive renal allograft recipient with renal artery stenosis. *Transplantation* 43:29–32, 1987.
97. Luke RG: Hypertension in renal transplant recipients. *Kidney Int* 31:1024–1037, 1987.
98. Benoit G, Icard P, Bensadoun H, et al: Value of antegrade ureteral dilatation for later ureteral obstruction in renal transplants. *Transpl Int* 2:33–35, 1989.
99. Becker JA, Kutcher R: Urologic complications of renal transplantation. *Semin Roentgenol* 13:341–351, 1978.
100. Lieberman RP, Glass NR, Crummy AB, Sollinger HW, Belzer FO: Nonoperative percutaneous management of urinary fistulas and strictures in renal transplantation. *Surg Gynecol Obstet* 155:667–672, 1982.
101. Duckett T, Bretan PN Jr, Cochran ST, Rajfer J, Rosenthal JT: Noninvasive radiological diagnosis of renal vein thrombosis in renal transplantation. *J Urol* 146:403–406, 1991.
102. Delbeke D, Sacks GA, Sandler MP: Diagnosis of allograft renal vein thrombosis. *Clin Nucl Med* 14:415–420, 1989.
103. Herrmann T, Granjon D, Decousus M, Soler C, Rusch P: Mismatch between radionuclide and contrast angiography in the assessment of the perfusion of a transplanted kidney. *Clin Nucl Med* 16:853–854, 1991.
104. Horowitz MD, Russell E, Abitbol C, Kyriakides G, Miller J: Massive hematuria following percutaneous biopsy of renal allograft: successful control by selective embolization. *Arch Surg* 119:1430–1433, 1984.
105. Sennett CA, Messersmith RN, Yousefzadeh DK, Thistlethwaite JR: Percapsular and percutaneous embolization of renal transplant pseudoaneurysm and AV fistula: case report. *Cardiovasc Intervent Radiol* 12:270–273, 1989.
106. Talbot-Wright R, Alcaraz A, Puyol M, et al: Vascular complications of kidney transplant: stenosis of the renal artery. *Acta Urol Esp* 14:352–355, 1990.

107. Glanz S, Gordon DH, Butt K, Rubin B, Hong J, Sclafani SJA: Percutaneous transrenal dilatation of the ureter. *Radiology* 149:101–104, 1983.
108. Benoit G, Alexandre L, Moukarzel M, Yataghene Y, Charpentier B, Jardin A: Percutaneous antegrade dilatation of ureteral strictures in kidney transplants. *J Urol* 150:37–39, 1993.
109. Jones JW, Hunter DR, Matas AJ: Successful percutaneous treatment of ureteral stenosis after renal transplantation. *Transplant Proc* 25:1038, 1993.
110. Viron B, Lacombe M, Raynaud A, Bindi P, Thibault P, Mignon F: Delayed extensive arterial dissection after percutaneous transluminal angioplasty for transplant renal artery stenosis. *Nephron* 58:351–353, 1991.

14

Renal Transplantation in Infants and Children

Demetrius Ellis / Nisan Gilboa / Mark Bellinger / Ron Shapiro

Improvements in organ preservation and surgical technique, development of more effective immunosuppressive and antirejection regimens, and close long-term medical supervision have been the principal reasons for the excellent outcomes currently obtainable after renal transplantation in infants and children. In addition, a comprehensive approach to the management of urologic disorders and meticulous attention to the special perioperative fluid and electrolyte requirements in children have resulted in a marked reduction in perioperative morbidity and early allograft failure. This chapter focuses on the unique aspects of renal transplantation in children and addresses the issues that affect outcome and overall rehabilitation.

The database on pediatric transplantation was greatly expanded by the establishment of the North American Pediatric Renal Transplant Cooperative Study (NAPRTCS) in 1987. Much of the information and statistics quoted in this chapter are from the 1993 report from this registry, which comprises more than 2600 children from 82 centers in the United States and Canada.[1] Compared with adults, children undergoing renal transplantation are more likely to have congenital disorders with a urologic component as the cause of end-stage renal disease (ESRD). Conversely, because systemic disorders and acquired glomerulopathies are relatively less common causes of ESRD in children, the overall number of graft losses due to disease recurrence or systemic multiorgan involvement after transplantation is lower in children than in adults.

Over the past decade there has been a decisive shift in favor of renal transplantation over dialysis in the treatment of children with ESRD. This change is due both to the improving results of renal transplantation and the greater potential of transplantation to support normal growth, development, function, and other important measures of quality of life. These issues are of particular importance in younger infants and children, whose development is inherently rapid and who can, therefore, be more adversely affected by uremia than can older children. Failure of intensive nutritional and medical management to deal with these issues is often a more important indication for transplantation than specific levels of blood urea nitrogen (BUN) and serum creatinine. Technical concerns related to small body size are of secondary importance in determining the timing of transplantation. A goal of early transplantation is to minimize the adverse effects of ESRD and medical therapy and to spare the child and the family the time commitment and emotional burden associated with dialysis.

The issues of renal transplantation can be subdivided into short- and long-term. The former include preoperative evaluation and perioperative surgical and medical management, including perfusion of the allograft, fluid and electrolyte disturbances, immunosuppression, and the diagnosis and management of acute rejection, hypertension, and infection. Long-term issues include chronic rejection, recurrence of the original disease, management of persistent urologic disorders, physical growth, neurologic function, adverse effects of medications, and overall rehabilitation.

▲ PRESENTATION AND ETIOLOGY OF ESRD IN CHILDREN

An increasing number of congenital genitourinary disorders are identified by prenatal ultrasonography. This often has led to earlier surgical, medical, and educational intervention and to prospective monitoring of such children for urinary tract symptoms and for biochemical disturbances. In contrast, a delay in the diagnosis of renal disease in children can result from the fact that the symptoms associated with renal insufficiency are nonspecific and often occur when renal failure is far advanced, with a glomerular filtration rate (GFR) less than 20 mL/min per/1.73 m^2. Common symptoms that lead to an evaluation for renal disease include anorexia, recurrent emesis, and rickets, which are often accompanied by short stature. Other signs include hypertension, edema, and pallor or exercise intolerance due to severe anemia. Metabolic acidosis due to build up of titratable acid together and uremia are responsible for much of the anorexia and malnutrition. Impaired synthesis of $1,25(OH)_2$-vitamin D_3 (calcitriol) and erythropoietin are largely responsible for the rickets and anemia, respectively.

The diagnosis of the specific pathologic entity responsible for renal insufficiency is important in providing a basis for genetic counseling for hereditary disorders. It also helps to predict the probability of disease recurrence in the allograft and may thereby influence the decision of whether to use a kidney from a related donor. Determining the cause of renal failure also allows the team to formulate strategies for pretransplantation surgical intervention, such as urinary tract diversion or bladder augmentation.

The causes of ESRD are markedly different in children compared with adults. Of the 96% of children who had classifiable renal disease in the NAPRTCS registry, nearly 45% had renal hypoplasia or dysplasia, obstructive uropathy, reflux nephropathy, agenesis of the abdominal musculature (prune belly syndrome), or pyelonephritis (Table 14–1). Predictably, ESRD in younger children is more likely due to congenital or hereditary disorders, whereas glomerulonephritis is more prevalent among older children or adolescents. Posterior urethral valves is the single most common cause of obstructive uropathy and of ESRD in children and contributes to the overall

TABLE 14–1 ▲ RECIPIENT CHARACTERISTICS (NAPRTCS)

	Number	%
Sex		
Male	1559	60.0
Female	1041	40.0
Race and Ethnicity		
White	1777	68.2
Black	370	14.2
Hispanic	318	12.2
Other	139	5.3
Diagnosis		
Aplastic, hypoplastic, dysplastic kidneys	447	17.2
Obstructive uropathy	444	17.1
Focal segmental glomerulosclerosis	288	11.1
Reflux nephropathy	147	5.6
Systemic immunologic disease	121	4.6
Chronic glomerulonephritis	113	4.3
Congenital nephrotic syndrome	82	3.2
Syndrome of agenesis of abdominal musculature	76	2.9
Medullary cystic disease, juvenile nephronophthisis	76	2.9
Cystinosis	72	2.8
Hemolytic uremic syndrome	71	2.7
Polycystic kidney disease	69	2.7
Renal infarct	57	2.2
Pyelonephritis, interstitial nephritis	55	2.1
Familial nephritis	54	2.1
Membranoproliferative glomerulonephritis type I	53	2.0
Idiopathic crescentic glomerulonephritis	42	1.6
Membranoproliferative glomerulonephritis type II	24	0.9
Oxalosis	22	0.8
Wilms tumor	14	0.5
Drash's syndrome	14	0.5
Membranous nephropathy	11	0.4
Sickle cell nephropathy	2	0.1
Diabetic glomerulonephritis	1	0.0
Other	150	5.8
Unknown	98	3.8

NAPRTCS 1992 data. Published with permission.

male predominance (60%) of ESRD in the pediatric population. Other congenital and hereditary disorders, such as congenital nephrotic syndrome, nephronophthisis, polycystic kidney disease, familial nephritis, cystinosis, and oxalosis, account for another 15% of diagnoses. All acquired glomerulopathies and systemic disorders account for only 23% of cases; of these, focal segmental glomerulosclerosis (FSGS) accounts for nearly half of this group. These relative disease frequencies are similar to those reported by single centers[2,3] and are in striking contrast to ESRD in adults. In the latter, adults, diabetic nephropathy, hypertensive nephrosclerosis, and acquired glomerulopathies account for 79% of cases of ESRD, whereas congenital, hereditary, and acquired urologic disorders together constitute less than 10% of cases. Autosomal dominant polycystic kidney disease, although frequently detected in childhood, rarely causes ESRD before adulthood.

▲ INDICATIONS AND CONTRAINDICATIONS

Contrary to the situation in adults, less than 25% of whom are potential candidates for transplantation, most children with ESRD should be considered for candidacy. The decision to perform transplantation should be based on the prospects for both prolongation and improvement in the quality of life.[4] There are few absolute contraindications to renal transplantation in children. A child with multiple congenital anomalies associated with severe mental retardation requires a careful evaluation by a multidisciplinary team, with proper developmental assessment, input from ethicists and, most importantly, informed input from the child's family. Absolute contraindications to transplantation include untreated malignancy and active infection. The presence of antiglomerular basement membrane antibodies requires waiting until the antibody level has become undetectable for at least 6 months. ABO incompatibility and a positive T-cell crossmatch preclude a given donor organ from being used for a specific patient. Finally, although transplantation of infants younger than 15 months previously was associated with poor outcomes, recent results from various centers have been encouraging and compare well with the 16% annual mortality associated with dialysis in such infants.

▲ UROLOGIC DISORDERS

Impact on Transplantation

It is estimated that about 30% (range 17–54%) of all children who undergo transplantation have some form of ureteral or bladder dysfunction. Churchill et al[5] evaluated the outcome of 300 pediatric cadaveric renal transplantations as a function of the cause of ESRD. The 5-year graft survival rate was approximately 70% in the group with cystic or acquired renal disease and only 30% in patients with obstructive uropathy. This study suggested that transplantation into a poorly functioning bladder reduced allograft function and survival after transplantation. Diversion of the transplanted ureter has fallen into general disfavor because of the potential for ureteral anastomotic leak, urosepsis, and deterioration of upper tract function.[6–8] Other studies have confirmed lower allograft survival rates[9] or worse renal function[10] in children with posterior urethral valves; in contrast, vesicoureteral reflux in the absence of vesical dysfunction is not associated with a worse outcome.[11] These data have led to the realization that uncorrected dysfunction of the lower urinary tract may both cause renal failure and contribute to graft dysfunction. The data underscore the need to formulate an evaluation and management plan before renal transplantation.[12]

Evaluation

Investigation must be tailored to the cause of renal failure and a history or suspicion of lower urinary tract dysfunction. A complete evaluation is needed in all patients with a history of genitourinary anomaly or dysfunction such as urethral valves, vesicoureteral reflux, prune belly syndrome, neurovesical dysfunction, imperforate anus, Hinman-Allen syndrome, exstrophy-epispadias complex, incontinence or urinary diversion, recurrent urinary tract infection, or renal failure of unknown causation. The role of the urologist is to define the presence and nature of lower-tract dysfunction, to correct or compensate for the dysfunction (improving or stabilizing renal function if possible), and to provide a plan for satisfactory management and long-term monitoring. An individualized urologic evaluation is especially important for infants and young children, because inability to cooperate with procedures or verbalize concepts such as sensation of bladder filling may influence the results of testing. Furthermore, evaluation must address both structure and function.

For all patients screening should include a complete history and physical examination, including evaluation of the external genitalia, lower spine, perineum, neurologic examination, and inspection of stomas or surgical scars. Urinalysis and urine culture should be performed in patients who are not anuric, and urinary tract infections should be treated before any testing is conducted that involves instrumentation of the urethra. A voiding diary may be helpful in the assessment of incontinence. Postvoid sonography provides a noninvasive assessment of anatomic detail and residual urine volume. If the evaluation is normal in the absence of a history of urologic disease or voiding symptoms, further urologic evaluation is usually unnecessary.

All children with a history of urinary tract infection, lower urinary tract disorder, or an abnormal renal ultrasound should undergo further urologic evaluation. Because a contrast voiding cystourethrogram (VCUG) defines urethral and bladder anatomy, confirms the presence or absence of vesicoureteral reflux, and provides information about bladder emptying, it is an essential study for all children with urologic disorders. Noninvasive information about bladder function may be obtained by uroflow or uroflow-electromyographic (EMG) studies. A formal urodynamic evaluation (cystometrogram) should be performed if neurovesical dysfunction is suspected. Cystoscopy and retrograde contrast studies may be performed if further anatomic detail is required.

Management

The approach to pre-, peri-, or posttransplant urologic management or reconstruction is highly individualized. It requires understanding of the diseases involved, the natural history of renal failure, the resources and abilities of both children and caretakers to comply with specific interventions, such as intermittent catheterization, the potential short and long-term requirements imposed by urologic reconstruction, and the proposed timing of transplantation. For example, if the date of transplantation is known, urinary undiversion to refunctionalize the bladder or augmentation cystoplasty may best be performed 3–6 months prior to transplantation.

Table 14–2 lists specific functional and urodynamic concerns that are associated with dysfunctional bladder states and that are known causes of upper urinary tract deterioration. In many specific diseases, several functional disorders may combine to hasten renal injury if uncorrected. Vesicoureteral reflux resulting from urethral obstruction, neurovesical dysfunction, or prune belly syndrome may also cause renal failure or may be associated with renal dysplasia. Low-grade primary reflux (grades 1, 2) without a history of urinary tract infection may require no treatment. However, if recurrent urinary tract infection or high-grade reflux is documented, a surgical approach may be necessary. Grade 3 and 4 reflux without marked ureteral tortuosity or upper tract stasis may best be managed by ureteroneocystostomy before transplan-

TABLE 14–2 ▲ Urodynamic and Clinical Aspects of Bladder Dysfunction

Functional Concern, etiologies	Potential Therapies

Vesicoureteric reflux (native kidney)
  Urethral valves
  Neurogenic dysfunction
  Hinman-Allen syndrome
  Exstrophy-epispadias
  Prune belly syndrome
	Prophylactic antibiotics
	Ureteral reimplantation
	Subureteric injection
	Temporary diversion
	Nephrectomy
	Nephroureterectomy

Diminished bladder capacity
Diminished bladder compliance
  Urethral valves
  Urethral valves
  Neurovesical dysfunction
	Anticholinergic therapy
	Intermittent catheterization
	Bladder augmentation

Elevated postvoid residual urine volume
  Vesicoureteric reflux
  Prune belly syndrome
  Neurovesical dysfunction
  Hinman-Allen syndrome
	Treatment of reflux (above)
	Timed voiding
	Pharmacotherapy
	Intermittent catheterization
	Urinary diversion

tation.[13] Correction of reflux by transurethral subureteric injection of polytetrafluoroethylene (PTFE; Teflon) or collagen may be applicable in certain patients, although no long-term experience has been recorded in patients who have subsequently undergone renal transplantation.[14,15] Nephrectomy or nephroureterectomy may be appropriate for patients with huge refluxing megaureters and poorly functioning kidneys, if the ureter is not needed for bladder augmentation. Management of the lower ureter varies. Leaving a ureteral stump in situ avoids perivesical scarring, which may increase the difficulty of the subsequent transplant procedure. Problems due to ureteral stumps are rare and may be managed by subsequent transurethral fulguration or removal at the time of transplantation.

The significance of a high residual urine volume is related to the general state of bladder function and the presence of reflux. If bladder compliance is good and postvoid residual volume is moderate, only prophylactic antibiotic therapy may be needed, and timed voiding or double-voiding may improve bladder emptying. In severe cases, intermittent catheterization may be appropriate. When it is necessary, it is important to document before transplantation that the patient and family are capable of complying with a catheterization regimen. Intermittent catheterization is associated with asymptomatic bacteriuria in 35–60% of patients after renal transplantation and clinical pyelonephritis in less than 10%.[16] Because vesicoureteral reflux is often present after transplantation, patients are likely to benefit from chronic antibacterial prophylaxis and aggressive treatment of symptomatic infection.

Diminished bladder compliance and intravesical pressures greater than 35–40 cm H_2O promote hydronephrosis, vesicoureteral reflux, and diminished GFR.[17,18] Many children have a combination of several of the following: diminished compliance, elevated postvoid residual volume, diminished bladder volume, vesicoureteral reflux, and incontinence. In patients with both diminished bladder compliance and massive reflux, the exact dynamics of the detrusor mechanism may be masked by the additional volume of the refluxing ureters. Considerations for management include intermittent catheterization or anticholinergic medication. Bladder augmentation with detubularized ileum or stomach,[19] native ureteral augmentation (ureterocystoplasty),[20] or "autoaugmentation" (detrusorrhaphy) as described by Cartwright and Snow,[21] is increasingly advocated for many of these children to help reduce intravesical pressure and hyperreflexic contractions, especially in children with neurogenic bladders. Children with augmentation cystoplasty often require intermittent catheterization. Consequently, we do not recommend this procedure for children younger than 5 years.

Patients with prior cutaneous urinary diversion need complete radiologic and urodynamic evaluation. The potential for rehabilitation of the defunctionalized bladder (undiversion) can frequently be assessed by bladder cycling using intermittent or indwelling suprapubic catheterization to evaluate bladder storage characteristics. If undiversion is possible, it should be performed with the goal of establishing a bladder reservoir with adequate compliance, capacity, and emptying.

Posttransplant urologic monitoring is necessary to ensure that reconstructive and bladder management efforts are adequate to maintain upper tract stability. If urinary infection, secondary reflux, hydronephrosis, or other dysfunction develops, reevaluation and prompt alteration of management strategy must be undertaken.

▲ PRETRANSPLANT BLOOD TRANSFUSIONS

The frequency of random blood transfusions has been decreasing in recent years. More than one third of all children who underwent transplantation in 1992 did not receive any pretransplant transfusions. The need for transfusions is predicated on the severity of the anemia and its symptoms. The current practice of erythropoietin usage has virtually eliminated this need. Newer, more effective immunosuppressive regimens have obviated the older practice of deliberate transfusions or donor-specific transfusions to enhance allograft survival.[22] Thus the rate of donor-specific transfusions fell from 40% in 1987 to 12% in 1991.[23] It is noteworthy however, that the frequency of blood transfusions received by all children has not changed as much over time. Although the number of children who receive a lifetime total of five units of blood or more fell from 44% in 1987 to 22% in 1992, the proportion of those receiving one to five units has increased from 39% to 47% and of those receiving no transfusions has increased from 17% to 30% over this same period (NAPRTCS data).

▲ "PREEMPTIVE" TRANSPLANTATION

The median waiting time for children already on dialysis is 11 months, according to NAPRTCS data. Over the past decade, an increasing number of children have undergone transplantation prior to going on dialysis (preemptive transplantation). NAPRTCS data show that 27% of transplants were performed without prior dialysis in 1993 and in 1990, up from 18% in 1987. This trend toward an increasing percentage of preemptive transplantation has been paralleled by the increased number of living-related donor (LRD) transplants from 43% in 1987 to 51% in 1992. In 1992, a disproportionate number (70%) of patients who underwent preemptive transplantation received kidneys from living donors. Overall, one third of LRD and 13% of cadaveric donor transplantations were preemptive.

▲ ORGAN SOURCE AND MATCHING

Of 2819 transplants registered in NAPRTCS through 1992, 54.2% were from cadaveric donors. Compared with 1987 and 1990, the number of LRD kidneys increased in 1992 by 7–9% to a rate of 50%. Nearly 87% of the LRD kidneys came from parents; five live donors were between 13 and 18 years of age, and three of these were identical twins. Only two cadaveric kidneys were transplanted into 406 children younger than 2 years during 1991 and 1992. The cold ischemia time for cadaveric kidneys was less than 48 hours in 99.2% of the cases.[1] Aside from the usual need for ABO blood group compatibility and a negative pretransplant cross match, there has been less emphasis on histocompatibility antigen matching in children.

▲ SURGICAL ASPECTS AND MEDICAL MANAGEMENT

Surgical Technique

The surgical plan must be established before transplantation so that urologic procedures, including cystoscopic examination with fulguration of residual posterior urethral valve leaflets, vesicostomy closure, or nephrectomy with or without ureterectomy, may be performed at the time of transplantation. Attention to the technical aspects of renal transplantation in children is critical. These issues are almost entirely a function of the recipient's size. Pediatric patients with a body weight over 30 kg can be treated surgically as adults using the standard pelvic retroperitoneal approach (see Chapter 6); smaller children need an individualized approach.[24–27] The key issue is appropriate matching of vessel size and anticipation of circulatory volume requirements.

For infants and children with a body weight less than 10 kg, the transplant incision is a midline laparotomy, with mobilization of the right colon and terminal ileum to the left side of the abdomen. The distal aorta and inferior vena cava and their respective iliac branches are mobilized. Lumbar branches are divided as necessary. An adult donor kidney is often used, and an anastomosis at the level of the inferior vena cava and aorta is required (Fig. 14–1). For toddlers and older children with a body weight between 10 and 30 kg, there is some variability with regard to the incision and placement of the kidney. Our personal bias is to anastomose to the largest appropriate recipient vessel; the external iliac vessels are, in our view, sometimes too small until body weight exceeds 30 kg. For children with a body weight less than 15–20 kg we almost always make a midline incision and anastomose at the level of the inferior vena cava and aorta or right common iliac artery. For children weighing between 20 and 30 kg, using the inferior vena cava or right common iliac vein and the right common iliac artery (the left side can be used in a retransplant setting) with either a midline or a retroperitoneal exposure is least likely to risk narrowing of or damage to the native vessels. This view is not universal; some surgeons prefer to use and can achieve excellent results with the standard retroperitoneal external iliac approach for patients who weigh more than 20 kg. A few even use this approach for children who weigh 10–20 kg. Whatever the approach, the surgical technique must be meticulous and gentle.

In contrast to the variability surrounding the selection of vessels for anastomosis, ureteral reimplantation is not particularly different from the standard approach (see Chapter 6). With intraabdominally placed kidneys, it is not necessary to make a retroperitoneal tunnel for the ureter, although some surgeons may prefer to do so.

In small children or infants, an adult kidney may occupy the entire right side of

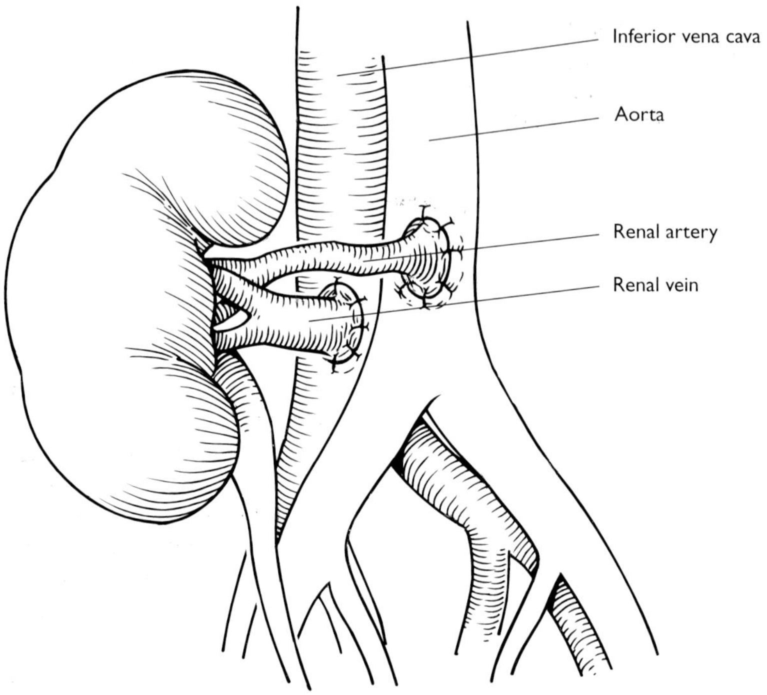

FIGURE 14–1. An adult donor kidney is often used for renal transplantation in children. An anastomosis at the level of the inferior vena cava and the aorta may be necessary, especially very small recipients (<10 kg).

the abdomen, displacing the large and small intestines toward the left side of the abdomen. In this circumstance, abdominal wound closure is generally not a problem. However, prolonged ileus occasionally may result, and therefore removal of the nasogastric tube or institution of enteral feedings may be delayed. Should a biopsy of the allograft be required, intraabdominal placement is usually not a problem. The lateral edge of the allograft is almost always accessible to an ultrasound-guided percutaneous approach (see Chapter 7).

Perioperative Medical Management

General Preparation

The medical preparation of a child for renal transplantation begins well before the actual operation. Many children are maintained on either peritoneal dialysis or hemodialysis for months and sometimes years while awaiting a suitable kidney. During this period it is necessary to optimize the child's general health, nutrition, and growth and to avoid the complications of ESRD, such as poor physical growth, decline in neurologic and mental function, renal osteodystrophy, severe anemia, cardiomegaly, and hypertension. Potential sources of infection must be eradicated, and urinary tract abnormalities that may hinder graft function should be corrected. Patients with severe, uncontrollable hypertension or proteinuria in spite of adequate dialysis may need to undergo bilateral native nephrectomy. In children already on dialysis, a treatment immediately before transplantation may be needed to optimize serum electrolytes, correct acid-base disturbances, and improve hemostasis. However, excessive removal of fluid should be avoided to prevent the risk of early graft dysfunction secondary to inadequate intravascular volume and suboptimal graft perfusion.

Intraoperative Management

The most important issue during intraoperative management of a pediatric recipient is to expand the circulatory volume to allow for adequate perfusion of the allograft. An adult graft may sequester up to 250 mL of blood, and in infants, nearly 50% of the cardiac output may be directed toward perfusion of the allograft kidney. The anesthesiologist actually needs to volume overload the child while closely monitoring the central venous pressure (CVP) and mean arterial pressure (MAP) of the recipient during vessel anastomosis to ensure adequate perfusion of the allograft. During completion of the anastomoses 20% mannitol (0.5–1.0 g/kg) and intravenous furosemide, 1 mg/kg, are given before the cross clamps are released. Before cross clamp release, CVP should be maintained at 8–12 cm H_2O, and the systolic pressure and MAP above 120 mm and 70 mm Hg respectively. If the MAP is inadequate to achieve good renal perfusion of an adult kidney, dopamine infusion of up to 5 μg/kg per minute may be started.[28] Intraoperative blood gases may have to be monitored frequently, because clamping of the aorta and accumulation of lactic acid can result in metabolic acidosis and vasoconstriction. The critical issue is to obtain immediate function; hypotension after cross-clamp release in an infant with inadequate circulatory volume and an underperfused allograft is a potential catastrophe.

Intravenous furosemide (1–2 mg/kg per dose), sodium bicarbonate (1.0 mEq/kg), 25% salt-poor albumin (0.5 g/kg per dose), and 20% mannitol (0.3–0.5 g/kg per dose), or 0.9 normal saline solution (10 mL/kg bolus) may be given to help promote urine output in the immediate postoperative period.

Postoperative Management

Attention to the volume and composition of intravenous fluid during the first 48 postoperative hours is essential to ensure good renal function. The CVP should be maintained in the range of 5–10 cm H_2O and MAP greater than 70 mm Hg. Urine output is replaced milliliter for milliliter. The initial diuresis is usually sufficiently large that insensible losses are quantitatively less important. Although fluids of different chemical composition are often used, our preference is for an initial solution consisting of 5% dextrose, 0.45 normal saline solution, and 10–20 mEq sodium bicarbonate per liter. During the first 24–48 postoperative hours, urine output frequently exceeds 5 mL/kg per hour; for such patients, we reduce the concentration of dextrose to 1.0% to prevent hyperglycemia and excessive osmotic diuresis. During the first 24–36 hours, additional fluid boluses of 10 mL/kg of normal saline solution or 5% albumin in saline solution may be given if there is a reduction in the urine output below 1.5 mL/kg per hour. In conjunction with such fluid boluses, we also administer intravenous furosemide (1 mg/kg). After 36–48 hours fluid replacement and diuretic administration are gradually reduced.

We initially monitor serum electrolytes (Na, K, Cl, HCO_3, Ca, P, Mg) at 4–6 hour intervals. Potassium chloride is given separately as needed when the serum K is 3.5 mEq/L or less. In infants and young children, close monitoring of fluid balance and physical examination are essential to prevent electrolyte imbalance and fluid overload, which may result in severe hypertension or pulmonary edema or reduction of intravascular volume and acute tubular necrosis (ATN). A bladder catheter inserted intraoperatively is necessary for accurate measurement of urine volume. Unless there are specific urologic indications, the catheter is removed after 3–4 days to diminish the risk of urinary tract infection.

Postoperative oliguria is worrisome, and immediate measures must be undertaken to improve urine output. Besides the easily correctable problems such as hypovolemia or a malfunctioning catheter, other possible causes include early rejection, vascular occlusion, ATN, urinary extravasation, or obstruction. In patients with oxalosis, precipitation of calcium oxalate crystals in the graft may cause acute graft failure.

A child with delayed graft function, congestive heart failure, or marked electrolyte abnormalities may need hemodialysis or peritoneal dialysis. Fluid removal should be performed cautiously to avoid exacerbation of renal hypoperfusion. Hypertension in the postoperative setting is usually due to fluid overload, partial ischemia of the graft, high dosages of corticosteroids, or incisional pain. If appropriate preventive measures are inadequate to relieve the hypertension in the early postoperative period, sublingual nifedipine 0.25 mg/kg per dose (maximum 10 mg) is often effective without compromising renal function. Use of angiotensin converting enzyme (ACE) inhibitors or β_1-adrenergic blocking agents should be avoided.

Perioperative Immunosuppression

Children not only are strong immunologic responders but also are particularly susceptible to early cyclosporine nephrotoxicity. Therefore a sequential immunosuppressive protocol has been popular (Table 14–3). It consists of withholding cyclosporine for 1 week, or until good graft function has been obtained, while azathioprine, corticosteroids, and muromonab-CD3 (Orthoclone OKT3, Ortho, Raritan, NJ), antithymocyte globulin (ATG), or another antilymphocyte antibody preparation is given to prevent rejection. Delayed introduction of cyclosporine is believed by some authors to be associated with better renal function, and antilymphocyte preparations can be stopped after 14 days.[28] During this time in the hospital, the family is instructed on the use of immunosuppressive and other medications (see Table 14–3).

Children appear to metabolize cyclosporine differently than adults. Because the half-life of cyclosporine is directly proportional to age, younger children may require higher doses on a mg/kg basis or shorter dosing intervals to maintain adequate immunosuppressive blood levels.[28] Moreover, cyclosporine absorption is partly

TABLE 14–3. ▲ OUTLINE OF IMMUNOSUPPRESSION IN CHILDREN

Preoperative

Cyclosporine: 10 mg/kg orally 6–12 h preoperatively. Cyclosporine use may be delayed for 4–7 d if ATG is to be used, if OKT3 is to be used, or if the allograft procurement history suggests an increased likelihood of DGF.

Postoperative Induction

ATG 15 mg/kg a day IV for 14 days

or

OKT3 5.0 mg/day (or 2.5 mg for body weight <30 kg)

Continue OKT3 until serum creatinine level is ≤2 mg/dL (180 μmol/L) or for 10 days.

Azathioprine 1–2 mg/kg a day orally

Methylprednisolone 10 mg/kg IV intraoperatively and 1–3 h before OKT3 dose for days 1–3; then IV methylprednisolone recycle, 5→1 mg/kg/d over 5 days; then prednisone 0.5 mg/kg a day (minimum dose 20 mg)

If OKT3 is to be used, give cyclosporine 6 mg/kg a day orally in 2 divided doses; dose may be increased when serum creatinine level ≤2 mg/dL (180 μmol/L).

Maintenance Therapy

Cyclosporine 10–12 mg/kg a day divided two or three times a day starting on day 8. For children ≤6 y give 500 mg/m^2 surface area divided two or three times a day (the cyclosporine and antilymphocyte preparation should be overlapped for 1–3 days until therapeutic levels of cyclosporine are achieved

Adjust cyclosporine dosage to achieve target 12-h trough levels that diminish over time

Weeks 0–4: 500–750 ng/mL (polyclonal TDX) assay for cyclosporine

Weeks 4–8: 350–500 ng/mL (TDX) or 125–175 ng/mL (HPLC)

Weeks 8–12: 300–450 ng/mL (TDX) or 100–150 ng/mL (HPLC)

Weeks 12–16: 250–350 ng/mL (TDX) or 80–125 ng/mL (HPLC)

Weeks 16–26: 200–300 ng/mL (TDX) or 75–100 ng/mL (HPLC)

Azathioprine: 1–2 mg/kg a day

Prednisone: start with 0.5 mg/kg and taper to about 0.15 kg/day by 6 months

ATG, antithymocyte globulin; OKT3, muromonab-CD3; DGF, delayed graft function.

dependent on the length of the small intestine. Therefore, small children may have a reduced capacity for gastrointestinal absorption of this agent. Diarrhea, which may either result from or be exacerbated by the use of cyclosporine, may also reduce absorption. A host of medications may alter cyclosporine pharmacology (see Chapter 8). Of particular importance in children are barbiturates and diphenylhydantoin (potent activators of the P450 hepatic enzyme system), which reduce blood levels of cyclosporine. These factors contribute to the high variability of cyclosporine pharmacokinetics in children and occasionally require more frequent dosing and close monitoring of blood levels. That such monitoring is important was shown by Hoyer et al,[29] who documented that cyclosporine blood levels less than 400 ng/mL were observed in 74% of children with acute rejection episodes.

It is important to keep in mind that the nephrotoxicity of cyclosporine is enhanced in patients with early graft dysfunction. Improper adjustment in dosing may contribute to an irreversible reduction in graft function and graft loss. Neurotoxicity is a second important side effect. Apart from tremor and insomnia, cyclosporine may trigger convulsions, possibly because of a direct toxic effect or hypomagnesemia caused by magnesuria and decreased intracellular magnesium concentrations, which lower the seizure threshold. Therefore, oral magnesium supplements may be helpful during the first months after transplantation. Intravascular volume expansion and hypertension associated with concomitant use of cyclosporine and prednisone also exacerbate the risk for seizures. Other side effects of cyclosporine are mostly cosmetic but may be very important because of potential noncompliance. Common changes induced by cyclosporine are the coarsening of facial features, gingival hypertrophy (particularly if nifedipine is also administered), and hypertrichosis.

A review of more than 2000 pediatric renal transplants since 1987 registered with NAPRTCS found that cyclosporine dosages decreased from a median of 9.0 mg/kg per day at 1 month after transplantation to 4.3 mg/kg a day at 36 months.[30] Between 6 and 36 months after transplantation, patients who experienced rejection or graft loss had lower median cyclosporine dosages than those without such complications. Lower dosages of cyclosporine were especially associated with late rejections, and median blood levels were lower at the time of rejection episodes. The conclusion of this study was that cyclosporine dosages should not be excessively lowered after renal transplantation in children.

Over the past 5 years, we have routinely used tacrolimus (FK 506, Prograf), rather than cyclosporine, at Children's Hospital of Pittsburgh. The protocol is shown in Table 14–4. Unlike typical cyclosporine regimens, our FK 506 regimen does not include induction with an antilymphocyte preparation. For patients with stable renal function with no rejection or a reversible episode of rejection during the first postoperative month, azathioprine, if it is used (and it is usually unnecessary), can be tapered after two to three months, whereas prednisone is routinely tapered and stopped by the sixth to twelfth posttransplant month. Seventy-three percent of our

TABLE 14–4 ▲ TACROLIMUS IMMUNOSUPPRESSIVE PROTOCOL

Preoperative	Tacrolimus 0.15 mg/kg orally; Methylprednisolone 15 mg/kg IV (1 g maximum) (Intraoperatively)
Postoperative	Tacrolimus 0.05–0.1 mg/kg IV per day as a continuous infusion
	Tacrolimus 0.15 mg/kg orally twice a day
	Prednisone or prednisolone 3 mg/kg per day starting on postoperative day 1 tapered to 0.75 mg/kg a day by postoperative day 6
	Prednisone 0.25–0.5 mg/kg per day orally by 1 month with subsequent tapering, with or without azathioprine 2–3 mg/kg per day orally (selectively, if there is recurrent rejection), or mycophenolate mofetil 250–500 mg qd-BID
Target tacrolimus whole blood level	20–25 ng/mL for first 2 weeks
	15–20 ng/mL at one month
	10–15 ng/mL at 3 months
	5–10 ng/mL chronically

patients taking tacrolimus are on monotherapy with stable renal function and with improved growth over a follow-up time of 32 ± 20 months.[31,31a]

In our experience, tacrolimus has nephrotoxic, neurotoxic, and diabetogenic side effects similar to those of cyclosporine, but seizures, hypertension, gingival hypertrophy, and hirsutism are markedly attenuated.[32] The combination of excessively high prednisone dosages and elevated tacrolimus levels beyond the first month after transplantation may be associated with an increased risk of posttransplant lymphoproliferative disorder (PTLD) in children[31, 31a, 32]; therefore, it is important to taper the immunosuppressive medications aggressively beginning 6–8 weeks after transplantation.

Corticosteroids

The multiple known side effects of corticosteroids, such as cushingoid changes, hypertension, effects on bone health, and growth retardation, are particularly detrimental to growing children. With the possible exception of tacrolimus–treated renal allograft recipients,[32] a high rate of late rejection has dissuaded caretakers from withdrawing prednisone in children on cyclosporine-based regimens.[33] However, recent studies have shown a beneficial effect of long-term alternate-day prednisone therapy on growth.[34] Twenty-seven percent of the children in the NAPRTCS have had their prednisone regimens modified to an alternate-day schedule. These children have demonstrated an improved growth rate compared with children receiving prednisone daily. Another study of 48 patients who were treated with cyclosporine, azathioprine, and prednisone followed by prednisone withdrawal by 6 to 9 months after transplantation concluded that this regimen was associated with excellent patient and graft survival and good catch-up growth among prepubertal patients.[35] No renal graft was lost after the prenisone withdrawal. Similarly, a study of 107 adults showed that steroid withdrawal was more successful among patients in whom prednisone was discontinued at least 6 months after transplantation compared with those in whom prednisone was withdrawn soon after transplantation.[36] Black recipient race and donor-recipient racial mismatch were significant predictors of rejection associated with steroid withdrawal.

Length of Hospitalization

The hospitalization time for transplantation in the NAPRTCS registry varied by age. The median length of initial hospital stay for infants was 25 days. This progressively decreased; children older than 13 years were hospitalized for an average of 17 days.

POSTOPERATIVE COMPLICATIONS

Surgical Complications

Advances in organ harvesting, preservation, and surgical techniques have reduced the risk of graft loss due to technical reasons.[37] However, after acute or chronic rejection and disease recurrence, vascular thrombosis is the third leading cause of graft loss, accounting for 14% of all graft failures in the NAPRTCS registry. An analysis of the causes of vascular thrombosis has demonstrated that different risk factors are associated with LRD and cadaveric grafts.[38] In all recipients, the risk of thrombosis is inversely related to recipient age, suggesting that hemodynamic or technical problems may play a role. Prolonged cold ischemia also increases the risk of thrombosis. Other vascular complications include renal artery stenosis (see Chronic Hypertension) and bleeding from vascular anastomoses. The incidence of wound infection or ureteral ischemia or leakage is quite low. The incidence of the latter has been diminished by the use of the extravesical ureteroneocystostomy (see Chapter 6).[39]

Medical Complications

Acute Rejection

Acute and chronic rejection together account for 23% of all renal allograft losses and are the most important causes of graft failure in children.[40] More than half of all patients in the NAPRTCS had experienced an episode of rejection by 10 weeks after transplantation. The rate of acute rejection declined from 69% and 67% for the years 1987 and 1990 to 54% in 1992. By the end of the second year, 57% of living donor organ recipients and 73% of cadaveric recipients had experienced rejection. Rejection within 2 weeks after transplantation occurred in 24% of patients. Nearly 47% of 1673 children having a total of 3160 rejection episodes had two or more rejections. Rejection rates are higher in cadaveric recipients and in recipients between 6 and 12 years of age. Of 700 children who had no rejections during the first year, 17% subsequently experienced a "late" rejection. Late rejection was more frequent among nonwhite children and those older than 6 years of age.

Contrary to prevailing conceptions, newer data indicate that infants do not have a higher rate of rejection or an earlier time to initial rejection than older children. However, NAPRTCS data revealed that the rate of graft failure or death associated with first acute rejections is higher in infants younger than 1 year of age than children 13 years or older (11% vs 4% for LRD and 21% vs 7% for cadaveric donor recipients). This is probably due to the difficulty in diagnosing rejection in a timely manner for infants and a general tendency not to institute aggressive management of rejection with antilymphocyte preparations.

In the past, symptoms and signs of acute rejection frequently included fever, malaise, abdominal pain, graft tenderness, hypertension, decrease in urine output, and increase in serum creatinine and BUN level. However, since the introduction of cyclosporine and tacrolimus, the clinical manifestations of acute rejection are much more subtle, making it more difficult to establish the diagnosis. The diagnosis may be even more difficult in small children with small muscle mass and large grafts in whom serum creatinine elevation may be substantially blunted. A small rise in the serum creatinine level of only 0.1–0.2 mg/dL (9–18 μmol/L) or 10% above baseline in small children may reflect a substantial decline in graft function. Although renal ultrasound and radionuclide scanning are used in the diagnosis of acute rejection, a percutaneous graft biopsy is the most reliable indicator of rejection. Some conditions that simulate acute rejection are primary cytomegalovirus (CMV) infection and urinary tract infections, making urinalysis and urine culture important tools in establishing the correct diagnosis. In addition, nephrotoxicity secondary to cyclosporine or tacrolimus may be difficult to differentiate from acute rejection without a biopsy. Although the first acute rejection typically occurs within 4 weeks after transplantation and usually responds to treatment, drug nephrotoxicity often occurs more than 1 month after transplantation and is commonly associated with cyclosporine blood levels greater than 200 ng/mL (HPLC) or tacrolimus levels greater than 20 ng/mL (whole blood).

A protocol for management of rejection in children is shown in Table 14–5. The different steroid and antilymphoctye regimens reflect individual center preference. Intravenous or oral corticosteroids are the initial therapy for acute rejection; antilymphocyte preparations generally have been reserved for steroid-resistant rejection. NAPRTCS data indicate that complete reversal of rejection occurred in 55% and partial reversal in 38% of all children; overall success rates were higher for a first re-

TABLE 14–5 ▲ TREATMENT OF REJECTION

	Steroids
A. Methylprednisolone	15 mg/kg (1 g max) IV on day 1, then 0.75 mg/kg IV every 6 h for 4 doses, then 0.60 mg/kg IV every 6 h for 4 doses, then 0.45 mg/kg IV every 6 h for 4 doses, then 0.30 mg/kg IV every 6 h for 4 doses, then 0.30 mg/kg IV every 12 h for 2 doses, then
Prednisone	0.30 mg/kg orally once a day
B. Methyprednisolone	15 mg/kg (1 g max) IV daily for 3 days, then
Prednisone	0.30 mg/kg orally once a day
C. Methylprednisolone (or oral prednisone)	
	2.0 mg/kg (80 mg max) in 4 divided doses for 2 days, then 1.75 mg/kg in 4 divided doses for 3 days, then 1.50 mg/kg in 4 divided doses for 3 days, then 1.25 mg/kg in 4 divided doses for 3 days, then 1.0 mg/kg in 4 divided doses for 3 days, then 0.75 mg/kg in 2 divided doses for 3 days, then 0.5 mg/kg in 1–2 divided doses for 3 days
	Antilymphocyte preparations
A. OKT3	5 mg per day IV for 10–14 days (2.5 mg per day for weight <30 kg)
B. ALG	10–15 mg/kg per day IV for 14 days

OKT3, muromonab-CD3-ALG, antilymphocyte globulin.

jection episode. Late rejection was reversed in 41% of patients, partially reversed in 57%, and resulted in graft failures in 2% of patients.

Although OKT3 was used in 31% of patients in the NAPRTCS and proved successful in the reversal of steroid-resistant first episodes of acute rejection, there has been concern about an increased risk for serious infections associated with its use. Using OKT3 early as primary therapy for the first episode of acute rejection, Tesi et al[41] showed better graft survival without an increased risk for either symptomatic CMV infection or death. The study, which involved 665 adult recipients of cadaveric kidney transplants who were treated with cyclosporine, also demonstrated that patients did not experience chronic rejection if they did not experience acute rejection.[41,42] Tacrolimus has also been used successfully at our center to overcome recurrent corticosteroid and ALG-resistant rejection in children.[31]

Disease Recurrence

De novo glomerulonephritis is extremely rare in children, so development of persistent proteinuria or hematuria at any time during the posttransplant course should alert clinicians to the possibility of recurrence of a primary disorder. Disease recurrence accounts for 7% of overall allograft loss in children.[1] Because this topic is reviewed in Chapter 3, only two important disorders in which a strategy for prevention or reversal of recurrence in children has been developed, are discussed.

Focal segmental glomerulosclerosis (FSGS) (and its possible precursor, mesangial proliferative glomerulonephritis) accounts for about 50% of ESRD and transplantation in children with acquired glomerulopathy. This disorder has a recurrence rate of 30–50% and leads to graft loss in 50–85% of patients within 2–5 years.[43–46] Children with disease onset after 6 years of age and those with development of renal failure less than 3 years after onset have a high rate of recurrence.[47] Moreover, the recurrence rate of FSGS in children who have lost a prior allograft because of this disorder is 80%. Earlier studies showed that high dosages of cyclosporine could improve the proteinuria while preserving renal function; however, such therapy did not halt the progression of FSGS.[43] Two newer approaches have shown considerable success in reducing graft loss due to recurrent FSGS: (1) plasma exchange or plasmapheresis to remove a putative circulating factor responsible for the increased glomerular protein permeability and (2) aggressive immunosuppression. Institution of plasma exchange or plasmapheresis, cyclophosphamide, and intensive immunosuppression showed promise in reversing this process in a small group of children treated with this regimen.[45,47,48] Another recent report found a benefit to plasmapheresis, intravenous immunoglobulin, methylprednisolone pulses, and cyclophosphamide (instead of azathioprine) together with prednisone and cyclosporine in achieving remission in three adults with posttransplant FSGS.[49]

Primary hyperoxaluria type 1 recurs after transplantation because of persistent oxalate overproduction secondary to hepatic deficiency of peroxisomal alanine glyoxylate aminotransferase and because of mobilization of large stores of tissue oxalate. Two main strategies have been advocated for pyridoxine-resistant forms of this disorder. For a child who is losing renal function despite aggressive medical management but with a GFR greater than (30 mg/min per 1.73 m^2), isolated liver transplantation may be performed in the hope of averting the need for renal transplantation.[50] Resorption of the oxalate deposits and improvement of the calcium oxalate nephrocalcinosis may occur.[51] Acceptance of this strategy is often difficult because of the replacement of an otherwise healthy liver and the risk of orthotopic liver transplantation. In a child with already established ESRD due to this disorder, we favor intensive hemodialysis to deplete the bone and tissue oxalate burden as much as possible while pursuing aggressive medical management of the disorder.[52] Liver transplantation is then performed and is followed by renal transplantation after several months of intensive dialysis to deplete stored oxalate. Dialysis together with forced diuresis and sodium citrate to inhibit crystalization may be continued after renal transplantation until urinary oxalate concentrations fall to less than 300 μmol/L. The latter approach has dramatically improved the outlook for patients with this disorder.[53,54]

Infectious Complications

Specific aspects of viral, bacterial, fungal, protozoan, and other infections encountered after renal transplantation are discussed in Chapter 11. Only a few viral infections are discussed in this section because of their prominent role in producing morbidity and mortality in children.

Infection remains a leading cause of morbidity and mortality in children throughout the posttransplant course. A study of 171 patients younger than 18 years transplanted between 1986 and 1992 showed that infection occurred at one time or another in 76% of patients and was the cause of death in 1.2%.[47] Bacterial infections occurred in 68% of patients, fungal infections in 6%, and symptomatic CMV infection in 11%. Non-CMV viral infections occurred in 22% and urinary tract infections in 37% of patients. In that study, no significant differences were found between recipients of cadaveric and LRD kidneys.[55]

In our series of 63 consecutive kidney transplants performed on 62 children between 1988 and 1993 (mean age 9.8 ± 4.8 years, [range 0.8–17.4 years] 33 patients received cyclosporine and 30 received tacrolimus), six patients (10%) contracted CMV infection.[56] Five of these six patients were on tacrolimus, and five of the six patients were at high risk for CMV infection (seropositive donor/seronegative recipient). PTLD associated with primary Epstein-Barr virus (EBV) infection occurred in six children (10%), one receiving cyclosporine and five receiving tacrolimus ($P = 0.07$). These PTLDs behaved like viral infections; cessation or diminution of immunosuppression together with intravenous therapy with acyclovir or ganciclovir resulted in disappearance of the PTLD with maintained renal function. With a more rapid reduction in prednisone and tacrolimus dosages after the first 4–6 weeks posttransplantation, we have seen a diminution in the incidence of PTLD from 17% to 5% in our patients who more recently underwent transplantation (see Table 4–6).[31a]

Cytomegalovirus Infection. CMV is the single most common infection and occurs in 40–60% of patients during the first three posttransplant years.[57,58] It is most commonly seen

1–4 months after transplantation. In about 90% of the cases, primary CMV infection is transmitted from a CMV-seropositive donor to a CMV-seronegative child. Leukocyte-containing blood products can also transmit the virus. Although it might be preferable to use kidneys from seronegative donors to prevent CMV infection, this is not practical or realistic.

The most important complication of CMV infection is the associated immunosuppressed state that can lead to opportunistic superinfections. The notion that CMV infection adversely affects renal allograft survival by causing a glomerulitis is controversial and in any event less important. Recent studies in recipients of other (particularly thoracic) organs support the contention that CMV infection shortens allograft survival,[59] but this has not been the case in children (or adults) with renal transplants.[57]

The current treatment of symptomatic CMV disease is ganciclovir 5 mg/kg (adjusted for renal function) twice a day intravenously for 2–3 weeks. CMV hyperimmune globulin in addition to ganciclovir may be helpful in patients with severe CMV pneumonia or relapsing CMV disease. Oral acyclovir at a dosage of 650 mg/m^2 per day for 4–6 months and CMV hyperimmune globulin (eg, Cytogam infused initially at 150 mg/kg with biweekly tapering of dosage over 4 months) have been moderately effective in decreasing the severity and perhaps the incidence of CMV disease.[60] An additional approach is to administer a prophylactic course of ganciclovir during the course of antilymphocyte antibody treatment.[61] The recent ability to detect CMV (pp65) antigenemia in blood or CMV viremia by polymerase chain reaction (PCR) before the appearance of clinical symptoms may also allow the initiation of preemptive CMV therapy. It should be emphasized, however, that relatively few children with CMV who seroconvert have fever, neutropenia, a positive blood culture, or systemic symptoms and frequently seroconvert while taking acyclovir or acyclovir combined with immune globulin prophylaxis.[57,62] Truly asymptomatic infections with seroconversion but without viremia or shedding do not require therapy with ganciclovir or immune globulin.

Epstein-Barr Virus Infection. EBV infection in a transplant patient differs from EBV-induced mononucleosis in a normal individual by the lack of a positive heterophile test, the low level of atypical lymphocytes, and usually by the absence of splenomegaly and pharyngitis. Therefore, it can be difficult clinically to differentiate this syndrome from CMV disease and to detect the frequency and the effects of combined CMV and EBV infection. Primary EBV infection plays a critical role in the pathogenesis of EBV-associated PTLD.[62] The usual site of EBV proliferation is pharyngeal epithelial cells. Secondary infection of B lymphocytes results in their transformation and immortalization. Normally the EBV-specific cytotoxic T cells destroy these immortalized B cells. In transplant patients receiving antilymphocyte antibody therapy, the incidence of EBV replication in the pharynx rises to 70–80%, increasing the risk for secondary infection of B cells.[63] Cyclosporine and tacrolimus, by blocking interleukin-2 synthesis (see Chapter 8), can decrease the number of virus-specific cytotoxic T cells, which can lead to facilitation of viral replication and proliferation of transformed B cells.[64–68] The replication of EBV can be interrupted by an antiviral strategy similar to that for CMV, especially during periods of increased immunosuppression in general and with antilymphocyte preparations in particular.

Clinical manifestations of PTLD are quite varied. Children may have tonsillitis, fever, hepatocellular dysfunction, focal brain or pulmonary disease, focal gastrointestinal tumors with bleeding or perforation, or infiltration of the allograft.[64,69] PTLD is frequently extranodal. EBV-associated PTLD may vary from polyclonal, which is relatively benign and responds readily to antiviral therapy and decreased immunosuppression, to monoclonal, which can behave more like a true malignant lesion. At present there are no reliable markers to differentiate benign from highly malignant disease. As noted earlier, in most instances reduction or discontinuation of immunosuppression is sufficient to reverse PTLD. The value of high-dose intravenous acyclovir or ganciclovir after the onset of PTLD has been debated; we have found it extremely useful. The value of chemotherapy, radiation therapy, or anti–B-cell monoclonal antibody therapy also is controversial; some centers advocate it, and others oppose it strongly. We have tended to reserve it for ganciclovir-resistant cases.

Varicella-Zoster Infection. Primary varicella-zoster virus (VZV) infection is usually a mild illness, but in a small percentage of patients may result in disseminated visceral infection, fulminant hepatic failure, hemorrhagic pneumonia, encephalitis, disseminated intravascular coagulation (DIC), and death. To prevent this infection, children who are seronegative for VZV antibody should be given zoster immune globulin (V-ZIG) immediately and in any event within 72–96 hours of any exposure to the virus. In contrast to primary VZV infection, reactivated VZV causes only mild manifestations usually in the form of typical zoster. Pediatric renal transplant recipients who may be exposed frequently to chicken pox may need repeated administration of V-ZIG. The development of an effective varicella vaccine may be very useful to VZV-seronegative patients. In transplant patients, intravenous, followed by oral administration of acyclovir is always indicated for both primary varicella and herpes zoster infections.

Posttransplant Erythrocytosis

Very occasionally, children develop erythrocytosis after successful renal transplantation. The assumed cause is overproduction of erythropoietin by the allograft. The erythrocytosis can be ameliorated by treatment with an ACE inhibitor such as enalapril or captopril.[70]

▲ PATIENT AND GRAFT SURVIVAL

In recent years, there has been a dramatic fall in intraoperative morbidity and mortality from anesthetic and surgical complications. The principal cause of death after renal transplantation is systemic infection, particularly during the first posttransplant year.[23] Two other causes of death beyond 10 years after transplantation are accelerated atherosclerosis and ischemic heart disease, apparently linked to immunosuppression-related lipid abnormalities,[71,72] and malignancy often associated with EBV infection. The NAPRTCS has reported 16 malignant tumors among 2000 pediatric transplant recipients during a 5-year follow-up period.[23]

The NAPRTCS data show that the 1-year actuarial patient survival rate is 96% for LRD and 94% for cadaveric graft recipients. The 1-, 2-, and 5-year actuarial graft survival rates for LRD transplants are nearly 90%, 85%, and 75%; for cadaveric transplants, they are 76%, 71%, and 62% (Fig. 14–2). The 2-year graft survival rate in LRD recipients younger than 2 years is 71%, whereas the 1-year graft survival rate among recipients of cadaveric donors in the same age group is only 46%. The half-life has been estimated at 14 and 11 years for LRD and cadaveric grafts, respectively. Although transplantation outcome in infants and younger children has varied

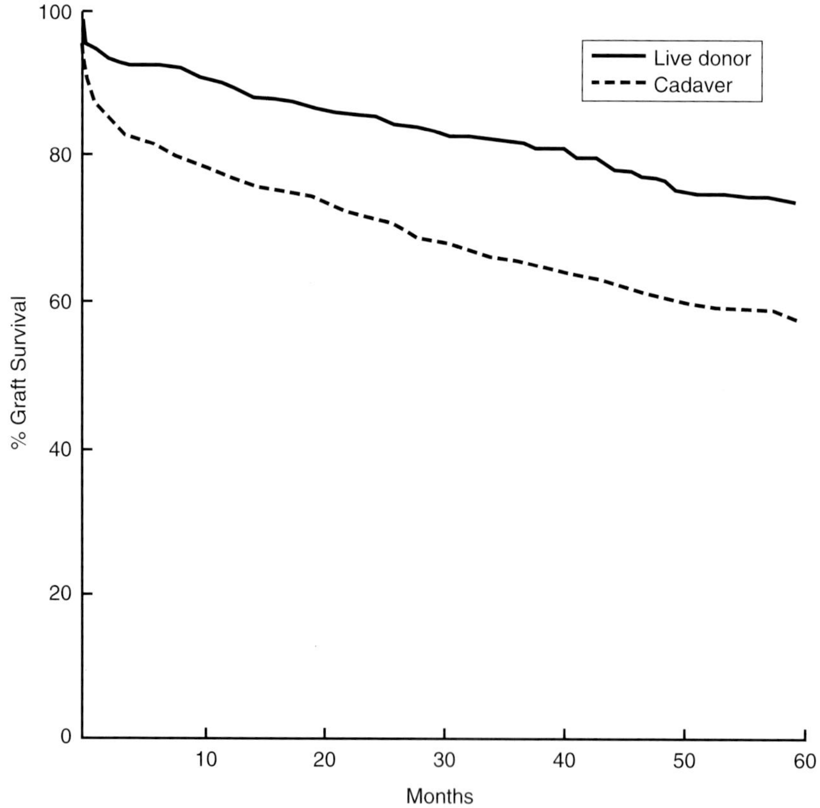

Numbers at Risk at:	Baseline	12	Months 24	36	48	60
Live donor	1533	1050	776	518	303	162
Cadaver	1641	994	713	479	284	162

FIGURE 14–2. Graft survival rate according to allograft source. *(From NAPRTCS 1994 data.)*

markedly from center to center, recent reports demonstrate excellent results even with cadaveric kidneys in recipients weighing less than 10 kg.[73–79] Preemptive transplantation is not associated with increased graft loss.[80,81]

Over the past 6.5 years, we have used tacrolimus as the primary immunosuppressive agent after renal transplantation in 69 cases at the Children's Hospital of Pittsburgh; 57% were with cadaveric grafts, and 25% of the patients were undergoing retransplantation.[31] Table 14–6 shows the general features and outcome for these children. With a mean follow-up of 32 ± 20 months, the 1- and 4-year actuarial patient survival rates were 100 and 95%, and the 1- and 4-year actuarial graft survival rates were 99% and 85%. This regimen was associated with less hypertension and no

TABLE 14–6 ▲ GENERAL FEATURES AND COMPLICATIONS IN 69 PEDIATRIC RENAL TRANSPLANT RECIPIENTS TREATED WITH TACROLIMUS

Actuarial Graft Survival	
1 year	99%
4 years	85%
Allograft loss	Disease recurrence 3 Rejection 3 Infection/Death 1 Noncompliance 1
Delayed Graft Function	4.3% (3/69)
Acute rejection	49% (34/69) 1/1/94–6/30/95 27% (7/26)
Steroid resistant	6% (4/69)
Renal function (n = 61)	
Serum creatinine level	1.2 ± 0.8 mg/dL (106 ± 70 μmol/L)
Creatinine clearance (Schwartz)	82 ± 26 mL/min/1.73 m^2
BUN	25 ± 13 mg/dL (9.3 ± 3.9 μmmol/L of urea)
Off steroids	73%
Viral infection	CMV 13% (9/69) Early PTLD 10.1% (7/69) 12/89–12/92 17% (5/29) 1/93–6/95 5% (2/40)
Transient diabetes mellitus	10.1% (7/69)
Hypertension	21%
Cholesterol	158 ± 54 mg/dl
Gingival hypertrophy	None
Hirsutism	None

LRD, living-related donor; CMV, cytomegalovirus; PTLD, posttransplant lymphoproliferative disease.

hirsutism or gingival hypertrophy. With the possible exception of an increased incidence of EBV-related PTLD, which has since declined with our modified immunosuppressive regimen (see Table 14–4), the side-effect profile of the tacrolimus regimen compares favorably with that of cyclosporine–based regimens. Although patient and allograft survival rates from centers that use cyclosporine immunosuppression may exceed outcome figures reported by NAPRTCS, only tacrolimus has allowed withdrawal of steroids in 73% of successfully transplanted children.[31a]

The proportion of children receiving different immunosuppressive regimens is shown in Figure 14–3. Two years after transplantation, the combination of prednisone, cyclosporine, and azathioprine was the most common immunosuppressive regimen and was used by 69% of LRD and in 80% of cadaveric donor recipients; 27% of all children were receiving alternate-day prednisone.[23] Children who received only azathioprine and prednisone (mainly after LRD transplantation) received the highest dosages of corticosteroids. By 3 years posttransplantation, the median prednisone dosage for all patients was 0.17 mg/kg a day.

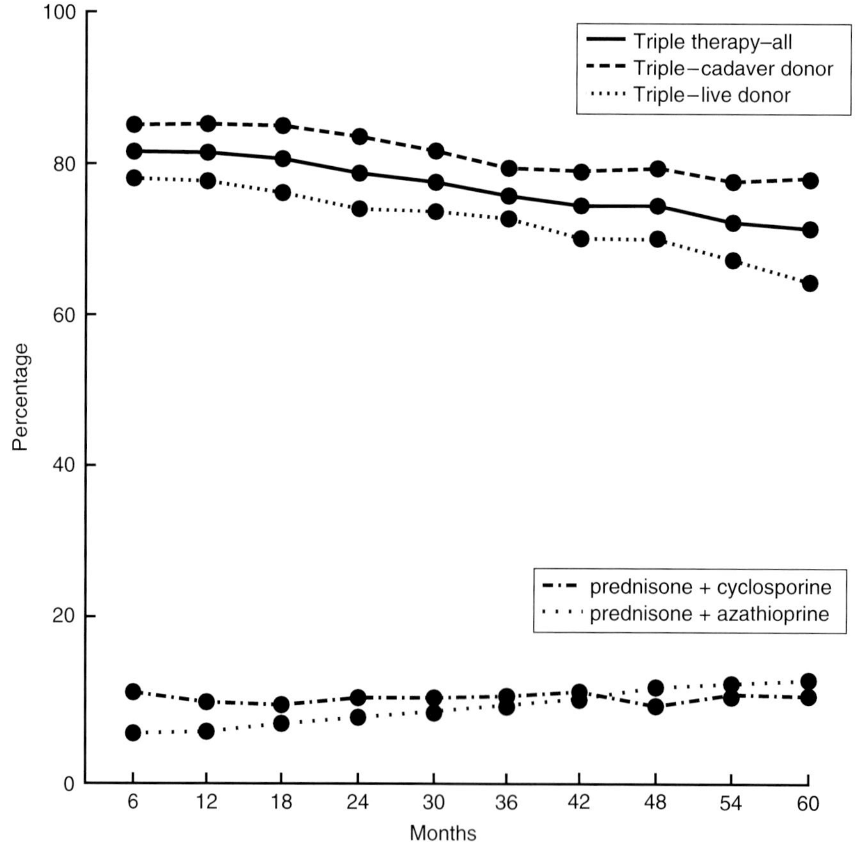

FIGURE 14–3. Percentage of patients receiving designated maintenance immunosuppression regimens according to month of follow-up study. *(From NAPRTCS 1994 data.)*

▲ ALLOGRAFT FUNCTION

Several factors may affect allograft function in children. Delayed graft function (DGF) necessitating dialysis support beyond the first week after transplantation predicts a 45% graft survival 3 years posttransplantation, compared with 70% in patients with immediate function.[23] This complication is more common in cadaveric grafts, 20.3, vs 6.0% in LRD grafts; additional risk factors for DGF included ischemia time greater than 24 hours, more than five blood transfusions prior to transplantation, native nephrectomies, recipient younger than 1 year, and the use of cyclosporine on day 0 as opposed to sequential immunosuppression with antilymphocyte preparations.[23]

Another important factor influencing long-term function of the allograft is the age of the recipient and the donor. Cadaveric kidneys from donors younger than 5 years are associated with a worse outcome, particularly in recipients younger than 5 years (parenthetically, under tacrolimus-based immunosuppression, we have observed 100% 1- and 4-year actuarial graft survival with donors under 5 years of age[31a]). Figure 14–4 shows allograft function as a function of recipient age and follow-up time after transplantation. The younger children have the lowest serum creatinine concentrations and the highest calculated creatinine clearance values. Donor source is also important, because both short-term[23] and long-term[82] function are decidedly better in children with kidneys from living donors.

Administration of antilymphocyte antibody is used in over 50% of children in the perioperative period. It is associated with lower serum creatinine and higher creatinine clearance values at discharge in both LRD and cadaveric recipients, although the creatinine clearance over the next 2.5 years remains improved only in LRD recipients.[23,83] Other factors, including the number of rejection episodes,[84,85] a prior failed transplant, and more than five pretransplant blood transfusions also correlate with worse graft function. In addition, renal function may be suboptimal in children with oxalosis.

Allograft function in younger recipients may be improved by avoiding very young donors and multiple blood transfusions, by the use of induction regimens with antilymphocyte preparations for both living and cadaveric donor graft recipients, and by making all possible efforts to make the first transplant a successful one.

▲ REHABILITATION AFTER SUCCESSFUL RENAL TRANSPLANTATION

The goals of renal transplantation in children are not merely to avoid dialysis and improve school attendance (the equivalent of employment in an adult). Other objectives include maximizing physical growth, neurologic and psychosocial development, and promoting as normal a life as possible. This includes attempts to minimize the use of antihypertensive and other medications, the undesirable effects of which may be difficult to assess, especially in younger children and infants. Unfortunately, with the exception of the recent experience with tacrolimus-based immunosuppression[31a] (see below), progress in these areas has not paralleled the success in allograft

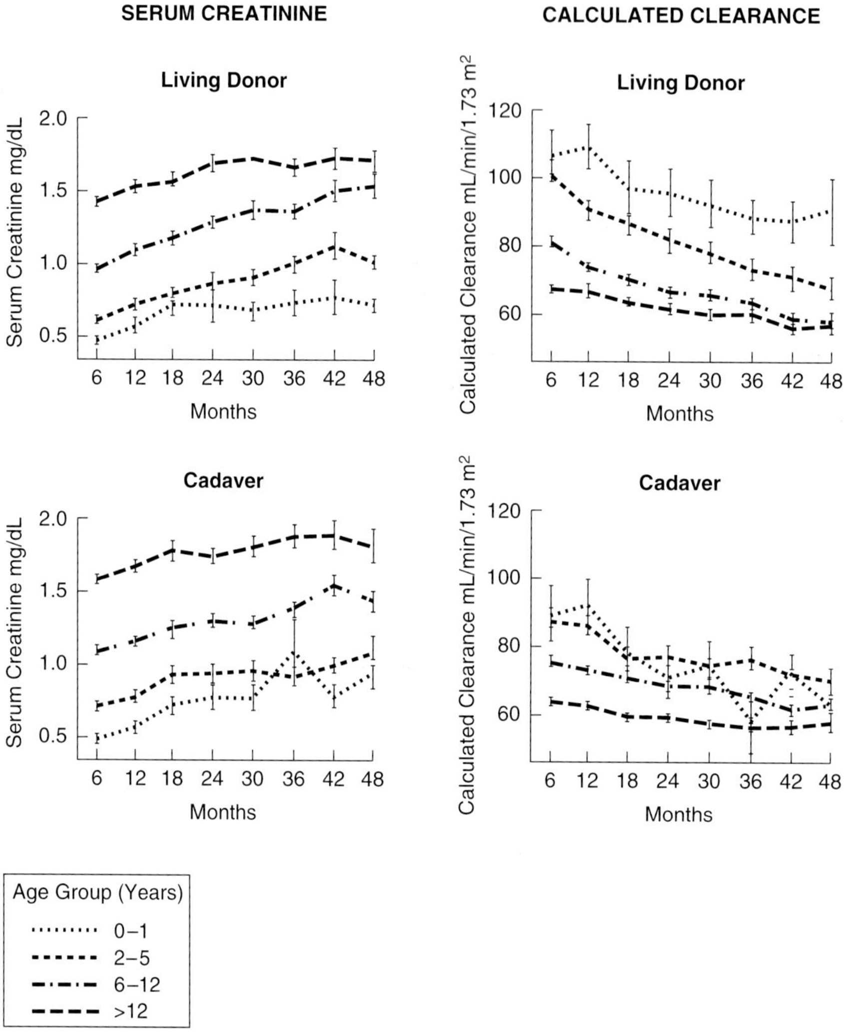

FIGURE 14–4. Serial serum creatinine and calculated creatinine clearance measurements (mean ± SE) for functioning grafts according to age at transplantation. *(From NAPRTCS 1994 data.)*

survival and function. Both better understanding and management of factors limiting the rehabilitation of children are essential to realize the benefits of transplantation.

Physical Growth

Long-term growth of children after renal transplantation falls well below expectations.[86] Much of the growth deficit usually precedes transplantation. Apart from syndromatic disorders, such as Jeune's syndrome, in which orthopedic abnormalities constitute an integral part, growth deficit occurs in most children who develop chronic renal failure before puberty. The greatest loss of growth potential occurs in infants with a GFR less than 25 mL/min per 1.73 m^2.[87–89] With a GFR above this level and with optimal medical management, infants and children often maintain a stable growth rate along a given percentile and may also exhibit a growth spurt during puberty.[88,89] However, catch-up or accelerated growth is the exception in older children with severe chronic renal failure (CRF) or after transplantation,[89] so that achievement of normal adult height or height consistent with the child's genetic potential is rarely achieved. The deficit in linear growth is highest in infants and in children younger than 5 years, is proportional to the time of exposure to the uremic environment, and begins to manifest itself when the GFR falls to less than 60 mL/min per 1.73 m^2.[38,90] The average height standard deviation score, or Z score, in 300 children with ESRD entering the NAPRTCS was -2.41 ± 0.09, and the change in Z score 2 years after transplantation was 0.18 ± 0.06.[91] Z score is calculated as follows:

$$\text{Z score}^{92} = \frac{\text{Observed height (cm)} - \text{Expected mean height for age}^{93}}{\text{Standard deviation of the height for age}}$$

The mechanisms underlying growth failure in children with uremia include undernutrition, renal osteodystrophy, and deficiency of anabolic and growth-promoting hormones.[94] Newer data, however, ascribe a key role to growth hormone (GH) insensitivity as the main cause of growth failure in CRF.[95–97] It is fairly well established that plasma GH levels are elevated in patients with CRF because of increased secretion or decreased clearance of GH. In addition, insulin-like growth factors (IGF) are normal in children with uremia. Bioavailable IGF may be reduced in uremia, however, possibly because of accumulation of plasma IGF-binding proteins. The administration of exogenous recombinant human GH (rh-GH) has been effective in increasing growth velocity in children with CRF by increasing plasma IGF levels.[95–97]

Successful renal transplantation leads to reversal of the "uremia" and metabolic acidosis and promotes general well-being and improved appetite so that dietary intake is more supportive of growth. However, corticosteroids exert important catabolic actions and suppress secretion of GH. Despite improved renal function and reduction in plasma IGF-binding protein levels, growth failure after transplantation persists in most children older than 7 years at the time of transplantation.[1,98] A serious problem in most of these children is lack of catch-up growth.

The mechanisms of catch-up growth are incompletely understood. Clinical studies have shown that as long as bone age does not exceed 12 years, daily prednisone dosage is 6 mg/m^2 or less, and serum creatinine level is 2 mg/dL (180 μmol/L) or less, most children who receive transplants will maintain linear growth along a given percentile or may even demonstrate catch-up growth.[90,99–101] Children younger than 7 years at transplantation may show good catch-up growth if renal function is excellent and steroids are administered on alternate days.[98,102,103] However, catch-up growth is observed more frequently with cyclosporine or tacrolimus monotherapy regimens.[31a,104–109] Two years after transplantation, 60–80% of prepubertal children in whom corticosteroids are discontinued have an accelerated growth velocity and return to near-normal skeletal growth.[99,100,106,108,109] As many as 77% of children on cyclosporine monotherapy exhibit catch-up growth, compared with 12% on regimens that include prednisone[109] (Fig. 14–5). Despite such benefit, decreased renal function or allograft loss to rejection has deterred attempts at steroid withdrawal.[33,100,109] Our data have shown that prednisone can be discontinued in most children transplanted under tacrolimus-based immunosuppression (Table 14–6). The mean gain in height Z score of preadolescents on such a regimen was significantly higher than that of children receiving corticosteroids or of children older than 12 years with either regimen ($+3.62$ vs $\leq +1.48$, $P < 0.01$)[31] (Table 14–7). Furthermore, improved growth occurred without compromise of renal function.

Data from NAPRTCS[91] have confirmed results of other studies showing that children younger than 6 years at the time of transplantation experience an accelerated growth rate regardless of corticosteroid use provided that renal function is good.[32,98,110] The largest recovery in potential linear growth was attainable in these younger children and infants with maximal growth deficit, a fact that argues for earlier transplantation in this age group. As these small children often have a higher GFR because of an adult-sized renal mass relative to small body size, it would seem that improved renal function may be very important in promoting growth in such children.[111] This idea is supported by data from our center that indicate 9 of 10 (90%)

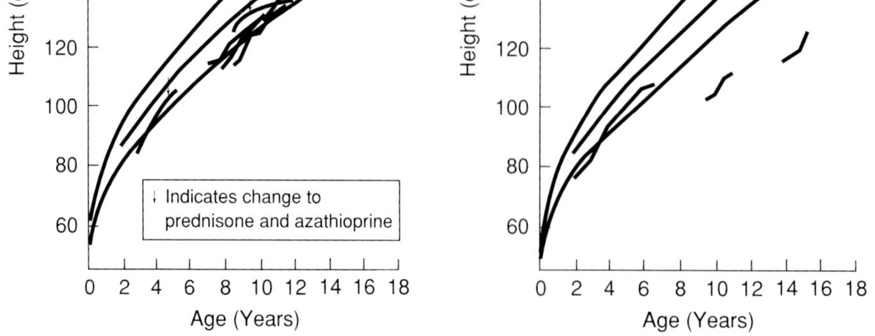

FIGURE 14–5. Linear growth curves for nine boys (A) and four girls (B) who underwent maintenance cyclosporine therapy alone for 1 year or more after renal transplantation. Curves represent the 3rd, 50th, and 97th percentiles for age. *(From Hodson EM, et al: Cyclosporine A as sole immunosuppressive agent for renal transplantation in children: effect on catch-up growth.* Transplant Proc *21:1687–1692, 1989.)*

TABLE 14–7 ▲ GROWTH PATTERNS (Z SCORE MEAN ± SD) AMONG RENAL TRANSPLANT RECIPIENTS TREATED WITH FK 506

	Steroids		No Steroids	
Time	*≤12 Years of Age n = 11*	*>12 Years of Age n = 4*	*≤12 Year of Age n = 15*	*>12 Years of Age n = 9*
At transplant	−1.9 (±12)	−3.0 (±1.1)	−2.7(±1.3)	−2.3 (±2.6)
6 months	1.2 (±1.2)	−2.7 (±1.1)	−0.8 (±0.8)	−2.1 (±2.5)
1 year	−0.4 (±1.1)	−2.1 (±1.1)	−0.02 (±1.7)	−1.6 (±2.4)
Follow-up 12 ± 14 months (mean ± SD)	−0.42 (±1.7)	−2.0 (±1.1)	+0.92 (±1.64)	−1.4 (±2.3)
Mean change in height Z score	+1.48	+1.0	+3.62[a]	+0.9

[a]$P < 0.01$ compared with other groups.

children younger than 6 years, most of whom had accelerated growth after transplantation, had estimated GFRs over 60 mL/min per 1.73m^2 at 1-year follow-up examinations compared with 20 of 34 (59%) of children 6 years or older who had GFRs in this range and who, as a group, exhibited a lower growth rate.[32] The effect of optimal renal function on growth was confirmed in another study of 68 renal allograft recipients.[112] Thus, preservation of renal function may be just as important as avoidance of high dosages of corticosteroids in promoting growth. Finally, there are data from the NAPRTCS suggesting that children who receive antihypertensive agents during the first posttransplantation month have a lower rate of linear growth in the first two posttransplantation years and that these differences persist at 3 years. These findings are intriguing and remain unexplained.

Despite improvement in height velocity and Z score in selected groups of children with successful renal transplantation, only a third of these children achieve an adult height that exceeds 2 standard deviations below the mean; about 70% of prepubertal children do not experience significant catch-up growth.[113] Such children may be candidates for the use of growth hormone (rh-GH). Studies evaluating the risk-to-benefit ratio of rh-GH injections in counteracting the catabolic and IGF-inhibiting effects of steroids appear promising.[114–119] rh-GH can lead to both increased insulin secretion and insulin resistance, with the effect of elevating blood sugar levels; one must therefore be vigilant for an exacerbation of the diabetogenic effects of steroids and other immunosuppressive agents that patients are already receiving.[119] There are also data suggesting that rh-GH is associated with a deterioration of renal allograft function and with rejection. However, other studies, including one that had a retrospective control group, did not find a reduction in insulin or creatinine clearances in short children with renal allografts who received rh-GH and found no deterioration in renal function due to rejection.[119,120] Thus rh-GH treatment may be very effective in the management of growth failure of pediatric renal allograft recipients, especially those older than 6 years. A controlled study stratifying for renal function, rh-GH and prednisone dosage, muscle mass, and rh-GH and IGF-I levels is needed to help determine the efficacy and safety associated with long-term use of this promising agent. Furthermore, the strategy of preventing growth deficit in infants undergoing dialysis may also include rh-GH, since the great deficit in linear growth in this group may never be recovered. Another important challenge for the future is the elucidation of the mechanisms that mediate catch-up growth so that more rational intervention strategies can be developed, especially for infants and very young children.

Osteopenia

Musculoskeletal disorders occur among 70% of long-term survivors of pediatric kidney transplantation.[121] Preexisting bone disease may be an important precursor to disturbed linear growth and poor bone health after renal transplantation, but bone density also falls to 60–70% of normal within 1–2 years after heart transplantation.[122] Treatment of uremic children with effective vitamin D_3 analogues, phosphate binders, and improved dialytic techniques has been effective in ameliorating the biochemical abnormalities in serum calcium, phosphate, magnesium and hydrogen ion, improving hydroxyapatite composition and reversing secondary hyperparathyroidism. Despite such treatment, as many as 30% of children with ESRD have genu valgum, scoliosis, and other bone deformities at the time of transplantation. Many of these patients have clinical evidence of osteopenia that is not readily apparent on radiologic or even histologic assessment. This disorder is better defined by special bone density measurements and has been found in 32% of children despite the fact that the parathyroid hormone level falls and the $1,25(OH)_2$ vitamin D_3 level increases after transplantation. Indeed, bone formation may decrease by 50% after transplantation.[123]

In adults, the prevalence of osteopenia contributing to avascular necrosis (especially of the femoral head) has decreased to less than 5%. Autonomous (ie, tertiary) hyperparathyroidism and posttransplant hypercalcemia also are seen in less than 5% of patients.[124,125] These complications have been practically eliminated in the pediatric population during the cyclosporine era. The beneficial effects of cyclosporine and perhaps tacrolimus on bone may be due to not only a steroid-sparing effect compared with azathioprine-prednisone regimens but also enhanced bone formation, which has been demonstrated experimentally in a rat model of bone transplantation.[126,127] However, prednisone is still the major inhibitor of growth of children after transplantation. Corticosteroids are known to enhance osteoblastic activity and hypercalciuria, interfere with gastrointestinal absorption of calcium, increase parathyroid hormone secretion, and decrease bone remodeling. The use of a new antiinflammatory steroid, deflazacort, devoid of the adverse effects of prednisone on bone, has been associated with decreased hypercalciuria and increased serum osteocalcin levels, decreased cancellous bone formation, and decreased osteopenia.[128] Diphosphonates, calcitonin, and rh-GH may also improve osteopenia. However, these agents have not been adequately studied in humans. Finally, the avoidance of hypercalciuric diuretics, such as furosemide, may also decrease the risk of posttransplantation osteopenia.

Neurologic and Mental Function

Several studies have assessed the cognitive and developmental function of infants and children with chronic renal failure and after transplantation.[110,129–134] Disturbances in these areas affect 64–100% of patients. Children younger than 2–3 years with uremia frequently exhibit irritability, decreased attention span, sleep disorders, and cognitive and motor dysfunction. Speech and hearing disorders and visuomotor dysfunction are common. In addition, one study found that 20 of 23 infants with severe renal failure starting before 1 year of age manifested profound neurologic impairment, including developmental delay, hypotonia, ataxia, seizures, brain atrophy, and acquired microcephaly.[129] Similarly high rates of severe neurologic impairment were reported in two other studies of young children with a serum creatinine exceeding 1.5 mg/dL (132 μmol/L) from infancy.[130,131] Seizures due to "uremic encephalopathy" are seen in 10% of older children undergoing renal transplantation.

Although uremic encephalopathy in adults is reversed by transplantation, the pathophysiologic features of the progressive and often irreversible neuronal injury of infants and small children are not understood.[130,131] Disturbed osmotic and nonosmotic cell volume homeostasis and neurotransmitter release may be especially deleterious to the normal development of the immature brain.[135–138]

In recent years, greater attention to nutritional supplementation, avoidance of aluminum-containing phosphate binders (to prevent aluminum encephalopathy), and intensive dialytic management with continuous cyclic peritoneal dialysis have improved the neurologic function of young infants.[139] However, clinical data suggest that perhaps the greatest benefit of transplantation lies in prevention or amelioration of permanent neurologic impairment due to prolonged uremia in the first 2 years of life. This benefit of early transplantation was demonstrated in nine infants who underwent successful transplantation during the first year of life.[110,140] After 2–7.5 years of follow-up care, most had improvement in cognitive and motor development. Moreover, head circumference normalized, and seizures, experienced by five of the infants before transplantation, stopped completely.[110] Recovery of neurologic function is much less likely when transplantation is delayed beyond early childhood.[129,130] Nevertheless, older children with transplants also demonstrate improvement in cognitive function, whereas those undergoing dialysis do not improve.[140–144] Sequential assessment of head circumference and auditory evoked potentials, and routine evaluation of developmental milestones in uremic infants are essential and may influence the decision to perform transplantation earlier.

Chronic Hypertension

Two years after transplantation, 50% of recipients of LRD kidneys and 65% of recipients of cadaveric kidneys in the NAPRTCS registry were taking antihypertensive medications 62% needed multiple agents.[145] A 78% prevalence of hypertension was reported with cyclosporine/prednisone immunosuppression in another study.[146] Children with chronic rejection leading to worsening renal function and higher corticosteroid dosages are also more likely to become hypertensive. Other risk factors and causes of hypertension include recurrence of the original disease, segmental allograft infarction, ischemia of the remaining native kidneys, drug toxicity, and renal artery stenosis.[145,147,148] In addition, severe vascular rejection may cause accelerated hypertension.

Unlike single-center reports, in which renal artery stenosis (RAS) occurred in 8–13% of patients,[149,150] RAS accounted for a small fraction of the causes of hypertension in the NAPRTCS. This disorder rarely develops in LRD allografts[149,150] and is more common in grafts from donors younger than 2 years of age.[150]

Although intrinsic renal disease appears to be an important determinant of hypertension, corticosteroids may play an important role independent of other immunosuppressive agents. Discontinuation of prednisone in children and adults receiving cyclosporine-based immunosuppression or in children receiving tacrolimus immunosuppression has resulted in resolution or marked improvement in hypertension.[30,31,31a,32,151,152]

Hypertension caused by ischemia of the native kidneys is difficult to diagnose even if there is a history of pretransplant hypertension. This form of hypertension usually behaves as if mediated by the renin-angiotensin system and responds to ACE inhibitors such as captopril or enalapril. However, in spite of high renin production by native kidneys, selective renal renin measurements are not reliable as a diagnostic test for native kidney–induced hypertension, particularly in patients receiving cyclosporine.[148] In a child who has excellent allograft function but severe hypertension, a helpful diagnostic approach in the decision to perform native nephrectomy is the following: First, perform ACE inhibitor–linked scintigraphy. If there is a marked decline in GFR of the allograft without evidence of intrinsic disease, renal arteriography should be performed, because allograft renal artery stenosis is likely. If the patient's GFR remains good, but the blood pressure responds dramatically to captopril, the patient's native kidneys are probably the source of the hypertension. If there is little or no response to captopril in terms of renal function or blood pressure, it is possible that the hypertension is caused by intrinsic renal disease, vascular rejection, or cyclosporine or tacrolimus and steroids. Cyclosporine apparently induces hypertension by renal sodium retention related to its ability to cause afferent renal artery vasoconstriction. A reduction of cyclosporine dose can be attempted with careful monitoring to watch for acute rejection. No controlled trials have identified the best form of medical control of cyclosporine-induced hypertension, but it appears that both calcium channel blockers and volume depletion may be effective.[148] In our patients taking tacrolimus, hypertension appears to be less of a problem than with cyclosporine. This difference may be partly related to the lower corticosteroid requirements in patients treated with tacrolimus.

Although aggressive treatment of hypertension is important in reducing long-term cardiac and neurologic complications,[153] the risk-to-benefit ratio of use of antihypertensive agents is difficult to assess in children. Because of the effect of cyclosporine on intracellular binding protein,[148,154] it appears that calcium channel blocking agents may be the drug of first choice for these patients. Diuretics are often used to counteract the renal retention of sodium and water induced by cyclosporine and corticosteroids. Methyldopa and clonidine may be associated with greater neurologic dysfunction and should be avoided in the pediatric population. Similarly, nifedipine, as opposed to diltiazem or verapamil, is associated with more pronounced gingival overgrowth and may exacerbate the effects of cyclosporine.[155]

In children with renal artery stenosis at the anastomosis, surgical correction is associated with cure or improvement of the hypertension in 50–67% of patients but carries a high risk for ischemia or graft loss.[149,150] If the stenosis is distal to the anastomosis, medical management may be preferable, and hypertension may be controlled in 56% of the children.[149] Transluminal angioplasty may be less effective; it controlled the hypertension of only four of 12 children in the combined series,[149,150] although we have been impressed with its efficacy at our center.

Anemia

Control of the anemia (hemoglobin ≤12 g/dL) associated with CRF with recombinant erythropoietin has resulted in improvement in cardiac function, exercise tolerance, mental function, and other symptoms previously ascribed to a variety of uremic toxins.[156] Despite the unquestioned benefit of erythropoietin, only transplantation has the potential for full correction of the anemia and elimination of the great expense and potential untoward effects of this agent. However, mild anemia can persist after transplantation in many younger children and infants. A study of healthy infants with mild iron deficiency anemia (hemoglobin concentration less than 10.5 g/dL) showed decreased cognitive mental function and motor skills, which improved after correction of the anemia.[157] It is likely that children with anemia that persists after transplantation may also have similar problems with cognitive function.

Sexual Development

Sexual maturation is delayed in 33–50% of pubertal children with ESRD. Successful transplantation restores a higher nocturnal gonadotropin response and improves sexual development.[112,158] Adolescent girls usually begin to menstruate 6 months after transplantation. Counseling about birth control measures should include education about the interactions of oral contraceptives and cyclosporine, which can result in an increase in blood pressure, and the adverse effects of pregnancy on renal function, particularly if renal function is already impaired. Nevertheless, men can father and women can carry and deliver babies, although the rate of prematurity and fetal loss is higher than in the general population (see Chapter 16).

Obesity

In our experience, when dietary restrictions imposed before transplantation are lifted, many children have calorie intakes that exceed the amounts needed even for catch-up growth, and may become obese. Corticosteroids exacerbate this problem and may lead to disproportionate increases in body weight. Calorie control and an exercise program are essential in limiting weight gain and in enhancing the general appearance of pediatric kidney recipients.

Psychologic Function, Medical Noncompliance, and Overall Rehabilitation

Successful transplantation markedly improves the emotional and social well-being of the child and his or her family. The family no longer experiences the stress associated with daily dialysis. About 6 months after transplantation, when medications, biochemical monitoring, and visits to physicians are reduced, and the child is under fewer dietary constraints and less parental supervision, the family's routine becomes more manageable. Once the child resumes full school activities, the parents can devote more time and attention to themselves and to the other children at home. It is after this early period that the family can begin to focus on the other emotional and social concerns of the pediatric transplant recipient.

The side effects of medications, such as cushingoid appearance, obesity, gingival hypertrophy, acne, and hirsutism, are important to the perception of body image, especially for adolescent girls, and may adversely influence medical compliance and lead to allograft loss. Medical noncompliance is prevalent in 43–50% of the pediatric transplant population and is believed to account for about 25% of pediatric allograft losses, more than twice the rate in adults.[159] The highest incidence of noncompliance is in adolescent girls with unstable family structure, inadequate emotional support, and poor overall supervision.[78,160–162] Information obtained at social service assessment and a pattern of noncompliance before transplantation may alert caretakers to the need for intensive counseling or psychiatric intervention for patients at high risk. For some patients transplantation may be postponed until the noncompliance is rectified. It is critical that patients at high risk for noncompliance or who have previously lost an allograft because of noncompliance be examined frequently for ongoing family stress, low blood drug concentrations of medications, and physical signs (ie, absence of side effects of immunosuppressive medications), which may indicate noncompliance. A caring and supportive attitude on the part of the medical team is important in modifying noncompliant behavior.

Adults who have received transplants have near normal and higher rates of employment, life satisfaction, well-being, and general psychologic health than patients who continue dialysis.[163] This gap has been narrowed by the wide use of human recombinant erythropoietin, which has substantially improved quality of life measurements in the dialysis population.[129,164–166] For children, who depend on an adult caretaker to meet their dialysis needs and are faced with the special problems of mental development, physical growth, sexual maturation, bone deformities, and psychosocial adjustments imposed by puberty and adolescence, the challenges after transplantation may be substantial. Nevertheless, with awareness of and attention to these problems, 86–88% of long-term survivors of pediatric transplantation assess their health as good or excellent on the basis of their ability to obtain full-time employment, attend school, marry, or rear a family.[121,123]

Immunizations

In general, children with CRF respond well to immunizations with minimal modification in the type or dosage of vaccine used. Therefore, attempts should be made to bring up to date all immunizations before transplantation. There is no formal immunization protocol, and there is no consensus on the approach to immunization of children after transplantation. Our general guidelines for those not previously immunized is to begin diphtheria-pertussis-tetanus (DPT) about 1 year after transplantation, when the prednisone dosage has been tapered or discontinued. An inactivated polio vaccine (IPV or Salk vaccine) should be given by injection rather than a live oral polio vaccine (OPV). Such a vaccine is also recommended for siblings; contacts with children who have had OPV vaccinations should be avoided for 2 weeks. DPT, IPV, and conjugate vaccines against *Haemophilus influenzae* type b may be given 13 months, and DPT and IPV boosters 14 and 24 months and 5 years after transplantation. Although the use of measles-mumps-rubella vaccine is controversial, this live trivalent vaccine has been given to our patients without serious adverse effects. Tetanus/diphtheria may be given 10 years after transplantation. A hepatitis vaccine may be especially helpful in a child with a transplant (40 μg 1 month apart for 3 months). The attenuated varicella virus vaccine may be useful in children prior to transplantation. Early reports indicate a good antibody response, with about 20% of patients developing a mild clinical varicella infection.[167,168] An influenza vaccine should be given on an annual basis. There is as yet no effective vaccine available for the prevention of CMV infection.

▲ REFERENCES

1. North American Pediatric Renal Transplant Cooperative Study (NAPRTCS): NAPRTCS 1993 Annual Report. Brooklyn, New York, SUNY-Health Science Center, 1994.
2. Garcia C, Goldani J, Garcia V: Paediatric dialysis and renal transplantation in the state of Rio Grande do Sul, Brazil. *Pediatr Nephrol* 6:74–77, 1992.
3. Foreman JW, Chan JCM: Chronic renal failure in infants and children. *J Pediatr* 113: 793–800, 1988.
4. Mauer SM, Nevins TE, Ascher N: Renal transplantation in children. In: Edelmann CM (ed), *Pediatric Kidney Disease,* ed 2. Vol 1. Boston, Little Brown, 1992:941–981.
5. Churchill BM, Sheldon CA, McLorie GA, Arbus GS: Factors influencing patient and graft survival in 300 cadaveric pediatric renal transplants. *J Urol* 140:1129–1133, 1988.
6. Firlit CF, Merkel FK: The application of ileal conduits in pediatric renal transplantation. *J Urol* 118:647–650, 1977.

7. Schwarz GR, Jeffs RD: Ileal conduit urinary diversion in children: computer analysis of follow up from 2 to 16 years. *J Urol* 114:285–288, 1975.
8. Cairns HS, Leaker B, Woodhouse CR, Rudge CJ, Neild GH: Renal transplantation into abnormal lower urinary tract. *Lancet* 338:1376–1379, 1991.
9. Reinberg Y, Gonzalez R, Fryd D, Mauer SM, Najarian JS: The outcome of renal transplantation in children with posterior urethral valves. *J Urol* 140:1491–1983, 1988.
10. Bryant JE, Joseph DB, Kohaut EC, Diethelm AG: Renal transplantation in children with posterior urethral valves. *J Urol* 146:1585–1587, 1991.
11. Reinberg Y, Manivel JC, Fryd D, Najarian JS, Gonzalez R: The outcome of renal transplantation in children with the prune belly syndrome. *J Urol* 142:1541–1542, 1989.
12. Marshall FF, Smolev JK, Spees EK, Jeffs RD, Burdick JF: The urological evaluation and management of patients with congenital lower urinary tract anomalies prior to renal transplantation. *J Urol* 127:1078–1081, 1982.
13. Bouchot O, Guillonneau B, Cantarovich D, et al: Vesicoureteric reflux in the renal transplant candidate. *Eur Urol* 20:26–28, 1991.
14. O'Donnell B: Endoscopic correction of vesicoureteric reflux (the sting): six years experience. *Pediatr Surg Int* 6:266–268, 1991.
15. Leonard MP, Canning DA, Peters CA, Gearhart JP, Jeffs RD: Endoscopic injection of glutaraldehyde cross-linked bovine dermal collagen for correction of vesicoureteric reflux. *J Urol* 145:115–119, 1991.
16. Gill IS, Hayes JM, Hodge EE, Novick AC: Clean intermittent catheterization and urinary diversion in the management of renal transplant recipients with lower urinary tract dysfunction. *J Urol* 148:1397–1400, 1992.
17. Houle A, Gilmour RF, Churchill BM, Gaumond M, Bissonnette B: What volume can a child normally store in the bladder at a safe pressure? *J Urol* 149:561–564, 1993.
18. McGuire EJ, Woodside JR, Borden TA, Weiss RM: Prognostic value of urodynamic testing in myelodysplastic patients. *J Urol* 126:205–209, 1981.
19. Nguyen DH, Reinberg Y, Gonzales R, Fryd D, Najarian J: Outcome of renal transplantation after urinary diversion and enterocystoplasty: a retrospective, controlled study. *J Urol* 144:1349–1351, 1990.
20. Bellinger MF: Ureterocystoplasty: a unique method for vesical augmentation in children. *J Urol* 149:811–813, 1993.
21. Cartwright PC, Snow BW: Bladder autoaugmentation early clinical experience. *J Urol* 142:505–508, 1989.
22. Opelz G, Senger DPS, Mickey MR, Terasaki PI: Effect of blood transfusion on subsequent kidney transplants. *Transplant Proc* 4:253–259, 1973.
23. McEnery PT, Alexander SR, Sullivan K, Tejani A: Renal transplantation in children and adolescents: the 1992 Annual Report of the North American Pediatric Renal Transplant Cooperative Study. *Pediatr Nephrol* 7:711–720, 1993.
24. Starzl TE, Marchioro TL, Morgan WW, Waddell WR: A technique for use of adult renal homografts in children. *Surg Gynecol Obstet* 119:106, 1994.
25. Simmons R, Najarian JS: Kidney transplantation. In: Simmons R, Finch ME, Ascher NL, Najarian JS (eds), *Manual of Vascular Access, Organ Donation, and Transplantation.* New York: Springer-Verlag 1984:292–328.
26. Sheldon CA, Elick B, Najarian JS, Mauer SM: Improving survival in the very young renal transplant recipient. *J Pediatr Surg* 20:622–626, 1985.
27. Shapiro R, Simmons R: Renal transplantation. In: Starzl TE, Shapiro R, Simmons R (eds), *Atlas of Organ Transplantation.* New York, Gower, 1992:4.2–4.21.

28. Ettenger RB, Grimm P, Firtzli ES: Kidney transplantation in children. In: Danovitz GM (ed), *Handbook of Kidney Transplantation.* Boston, Little Brown, 1992:305–325.
29. Hoyer PF, Offner G, Krohn HP, Brodehl J: Acute rejection episodes after renal transplantation in children under cyclosporine A treatment. *Pediatr Nephrol* 1:253–259, 1987.
30. Harmon WE, Sullivan EK: Cyclosporine dosing and its relationship to outcome in pediatric renal transplantation. *Kidney Int* 44 (Suppl 43):S50–S55, 1993.
31. Shapiro R, Scantlebury VP, Jordan ML, et al: FK-506 in pediatric kidney transplantation: primary and rescue experience. *Pediatr Nephrol* 9:S43–S48, 1995.
31a. Shapiro R, Scantlebury VP, Jordan ML: Tacrolimus in pediatric renal transplantation. *Transplantation* 62(12):1752, 1996.
32. Ellis D, Shapiro R, Jordan ML, et al: Comparison of FK-506 and cyclosporine regimens in pediatric renal tranplantation. *Pediatr Nephrol* 8:193–200, 1994.
33. Ingulli E, Tejani A, Markell M: The beneficial effects of steroid withdrawal on blood pressure and lipid profile in children posttransplantation in the cyclosporine era. *Transplantation* 55:1029–1033, 1993.
34. Broyer M, Guest G, Gagnadoux MF: Growth rate in children receiving alternate-day corticosteroid treatment after kidney transplantation. *J Pediatr* 120:721–725, 1992.
35. Francis DM, Walker RG, Jones C, Powell H: Cessation of steroids in pediatric renal transplant recipients treated with cyclosporine, azathioprine and prednisolone. *Transplant Proc* 26:99–101, 1994.
36. Hricik DE, Whaleu CC, Lautman J, et al: Withdrawal of steroids after transplantation: clinical predictors of outcome. *Transplantation* 53:41–45, 1992.
37. Chavers BM, Kim E, Matas AJ, Gillingham KJ, Najarian JS, Mauer SM: Causes of kidney allograft loss in a large pediatric population at a single center. *Pediatr Nephrol* 8:57–61, 1994.
38. Harmon WE, Stablein D, Alexander SR, Tejani A: Graft thrombosis in pediatric renal transplant recipients: a report of the North American Pediatric Renal Transplant Cooperative Study. *Transplantation* 51:406–412, 1991.
39. Benoit G, Blanchet P, Moukarzel M, et al: Surgical complications in kidney transplantation. *Transplant Proc* 26:287–288, 1994.
40. Harmon WE: Pediatric renal transplantation. *Transpl Immunol Letter* 9:3, 1993.
41. Tesi RJ, Elkhammas EA, Henry ML, Ferguson RM: OKT3 for primary therapy of the first rejection episode in kidney transplants. *Transplantation* 55:1023–1029, 1993.
42. Tesi RJ, Elkhammas EA, Henry ML, Davies EA, Salazar DA, Ferguson RM: Acute rejection episodes: best predictor of long-term primary cadaveric renal transplant survival. *Transplant Proc* 25:901–902, 1993.
43. Ingulli E, Tejani A, Butt KMH, Rajpoot D, Gonzalez F, Pomrantz A, Ettenger R: High-dose cyclosporine therapy in recurrent nephrotic syndrome following renal transplantation. *Transplantation* 49:219–221, 1990.
44. Cameron JS: Recurrent primary disease and de novo nephritis following renal transplantation. *Pediatr Nephrol* 5:412–421, 1991.
45. Artero M, Biava C, Amend W, Tomlanovich S, Vincenti F: Recurrent focal glomerulosclerosis: natural and history and response to therapy. *Am J Med* 92:375–383, 1992.
46. Stephanian E, Matas AJ, Mauer SM, et al: Recurrence of disease in patients retransplanted for focal segmental glomerulosclerosis. *Transplantation* 53:755–757, 1992.
47. Mowry J, Marik J, Cohen A, Hogg R, Sahney S, Ettenger R: Treatment of recurrent focal segmental glomerulosclerosis with high-dose cyclosporine A and plasmapheresis. *Transplant Proc* 25:1345–1346, 1993.
48. Laufer J, Ettenger RB, Ho WG, Cohen AH, Marik JL, Fine RN: Plasma exchange for recurrent nephrotic syndrome following renal transplantation. *Transplantation* 46:540–542, 1988.

49. Cochat P, Kassir A, Colon S, et al: Recurrent nephrotic syndrome after transplantation: early treatment with plasmapheresis and cyclophosphamide. *Pediatr Nephrol* 7:50–54, 1993.
50. Cochat P, Scharer K: Should liver transplantation be performed before advanced renal insufficiency in primary hyperoxaluria type 1? *Pediatr Nephrol* 7:212–218, 1993.
51. Danpure CJ: Scientific rationale for hepato-renal transplantation in primary hyperoxaluria type I. *Transplant Clin Immunol* 22:91–98, 1991.
52. Scheinman JI: Primary hyperoxaluria: therapeutic strategies for the 90's. *Kidney Int* 40:389–399, 1991.
53. Watts RW, Morgan SH, Danpure CJ, et al: Combined hepatic and renal transplantation in primary hyperoxaluria type I: clinical report of nine cases. *Am J Med* 90:179–192, 1991.
54. Schurmann G, Scharer K, Wingen A-M, Otto G, Herfarth C: Early liver transplantation for primary hyperoxaluria type I in an infant with chronic renal failure. *Nephrol Dial Transplant* 5:825–827, 1990.
55. Granger DK, Burd RS, Schmidt WJ, Dunn DL, Matas AJ: Incidence and timing of infections in pediatric renal transplant recipients in the cyclosporine era. *Transplant Proc* 26:64, 1994.
56. Scantlebury VP, Shapiro R, Tzakis A, et al: Pediatric kidney transplantation at the University of Pittsburgh. *Transplant Proc* 26:46–47, 1994.
57. Iragorri S, Pillay D, Scrine M, Trompeter RS, Rees L, Griffiths PD: Prospective cytomegalovirus surveillance in paediatric renal transplant patients. *Pediatr Nephrol* 7:55–60, 1993.
58. Marker SC, Howard RJ, Simmons TL, et al: Cytomegalovirus infection: a quantitative prospective study of three hundred twenty consecutive renal transplants. *Surgery* 89:660, 1981.
59. Rubin RH: Impact of cytomegalovirus infection on organ transplant recipients. *Rev Infect Dis* 12(Suppl 7):S754–S766, 1990.
60. Syndman DR, Werner BG, Heinz-Lacey B, et al: Use of cytomegalovirus immune globulin to prevent cytomegalovirus disease in renal-transplant recipients. *N Engl J Med* 317:1049–1054, 1987.
61. Bailey TC, Ettinger NA, Storch GA, et al: Failure of high-dose oral acyclovir with or without immune globulin to prevent primary cytomegalovirus disease in recipients of solid organ transplants. *Am J Med* 95:273–278, 1993.
62. Stephanian E, Gruber SA, Dunn DL, Matas AJ: Posttransplant lymphoproliferative disorders. *Transplant Rev* 5:120–129, 1991.
63. Preiksaitis JK, Dias-Mitoma F, Mirzayans F, Roberts S, Tyrell DLJ: Quantitative or pharyngeal Epstein-Barr virus shedding in renal and cardiac transplant recipients: relationship to immunosuppressive therapy, serological responses and the risk of post-transplant lymphoproliferative disorder. *J Infect Dis* 166:986–994, 1992.
64. Hanto DW, Frizzera G, Purtilo DT, et al: Clinical spectrum of lymphoproliferative disorders in renal transplant recipients and evidence for the role of Epstein-Barr virus. *Cancer Res* 41:4253–4261, 1981.
65. Hanto DW, Gajl-Peczalska KJ, Frizzera G, et al: Epstein-Barr virus (EBV) induced polyclonal and monoclonal B-cell lymphoproliferative diseases occurring after renal transplantation. *Ann Surg* 198:356–369, 1983.
66. Hanto DW, Frizzera G, Gajl-Peczalska KJ, Simmons RL: Epstein-Barr virus, immunodeficiency, and B cell lymphoproliferation. *Transplantation* 39:461–472, 1985.
67. Kay JE, Benzie CR, Goddier MR, Wick CJ, Doe SE: Inhibition of T-lymphocyte activation by the immunosuppressive drug FK-506. *Immunology* 67:473–477, 1989.

68. Tocci MJ, Matkovich DA, Collier KA, et al: FK-506 selectively inhibits expression of early T cell activation genes. *J Immunol* 143:718–726, 1989.
69. Rubin RH: Infectious disease complications of renal transplantation. *Kidney Int* 44:221–230, 1993.
70. Rostaing L, Demur C, Huyn A, Durand D, Lloveras JJ, Suc JM: Erythrocytosis after renal transplant: study of erythroid progenitors and response to enalapril. *Transplant Proc* 26:280–281, 1994.
71. Kim MS, Jabs K, Harmon WE: Long-term patient survival in a pediatric renal transplantation program. *Transplantation* 51:413–417, 1991.
72. Pirsch JD, D'Alessandro AM, Sollinger HW, et al: Hyperlipidemia and transplantation: etiologic factors and therapy. *J Am Soc Nephrol* 2:S238–242, 1992.
73. Najarian JS, Frey DJ, Matas AJ, et al: Renal transplantation in infants. *Ann Surg* 212:353–367, 1990.
74. Briscoe DM, Kim MS, Lillehei C, Eraklis AJ, Levey RH, Harmon WE: Outcome of renal transplantation in children less than two years of age. *Kidney Int* 42:657–662, 1992.
75. Potter D, Feduska N, Melzer J, et al: Twenty years of renal transplantation in children. *Pediatrics* 77:465–470, 1986.
76. Arbus GS, Rochon J, Thompson D: Survival of cadaveric renal transplant grafts from young donors and in young recipients. *Pediatr Nephrol* 5:152–157, 1991.
77. Fitzpatrick MM, Duffy PG, Fernando ON, Barratt TM, Dillon MJ, Trompeter RS: Cadaveric renal transplantation in children under 5 years of age. *Pediatr Nephrol* 6:166–171, 1992.
78. Ettenger RS, Rosenthal JT, Marik JL, et al: Improved cadaveric renal transplant outcome in children. *Pediatr Nephrol* 5:137–142, 1991.
79. Cochat P, Castelo F, Glastre C, et al: Outcome of cadaver kidney transplantation in small children. *Acta Pediatr* 83:78–83, 1994.
80. Flom LS, Reisman EM, Donovan JM, et al: Favorable experience with pre-emptive renal transplantation in children. *Pediatr Nephrol* 6:258–261, 1992.
81. Offner G, Hoyer PF, Meyer B, Pichlmayr R, Brodehl J: Pre-emptive renal transplantation in children and adolescents. *Transplant Int* 6:125–128, 1993.
82. Brazy PC, Pirsch JD, Belzer FO: Factors affecting renal allograft function in long-term recipients. *Am J Kidney Dis* 19:558–566, 1992.
83. Berg UB, Bohlin AB, Tyden G: Adaptation and long-term function of transplanted kidneys in children. *Transplant Proc* 25:1324–1328, 1993.
84. Hoyer PF, Krohn HP, Offner G, et al: Renal function after kidney transplantation in children. *Transplantation* 43:489–493, 1987.
85. Berg UB, Bohlin AB: Renal function following kidney transplantation in children treated with cyclosporine. *Pediatr Nephrol* 6:339–344, 1992.
86. Harmon WE, Jabs K: Factors affecting growth after renal transplantation. *J Am Soc Nephrol* 2 (Suppl 12):S295–303, 1992.
87. Betts PR, Magrath G: Growth pattern and dietary intake of children with chronic renal insufficiency. *Br Med J* 2:189–193, 1974.
88. Kleinknecht C, Broyer M, Huot D, Marti-Henneberg C, Dartois AM: Growth and development of nondialyzed children with chronic renal failure. *Kidney Int* 15(Suppl):S40–47, 1983.
89. Rizzoni G, Basso T, Setari M: Growth in children with chronic renal failure on conservative treatment. *Kidney Int* 26:52–58, 1984.
90. Pennisi AJ, Costin G, Phillips LS, et al: Linear growth in long term renal allograft recipients. *Clin Nephrol* 8:415–421, 1977.
91. Tejani A, Fine R, Alexander S, Harmon W, Stablein D: Factors predictive of sustained growth in children after renal transplantation. *J Pediatr* 122:397–402, 1993.

92. Krick J: Using the Z score as a descriptor of discrete changes in growth. *Nutr Suppl Serv* 6:14–16, 1986.
93. Hamill PV, Drizd TA, Johnson CL, Reed RB, Roche AF, Moore WM: Physical growth: National Center for Health Statistics percentiles. *Am J Clin Nutr* 32:607–629, 1979.
94. Potter D, Greifer I: Statural growth of children with renal disease. *Kidney Int* 14:334–339, 1978.
95. Tonshoff B, Schaefer F, Mehls O: Disturbance of growth hormone-insulin-like growth factor axis in uraemia: implications for recombinant human growth hormone treatment. *Pediatr Nephrol* 4:654–662, 1990.
96. Fine RN, Pyke-Grimm K, Nelson PA, et al: Recombinant human growth hormone treatment of children with chronic renal failure: long-term (1- to 3-year) outcome. *Pediatr Nephrol* 5:477–481, 1991.
97. Hokken-Koelega AC, Stijnen T, de Muinck Keizer-Schrama SM, et al: Placebo-controlled, double-blind, cross-over trial of growth hormone treatment in prepubertal children with chronic renal failure. *Lancet* 338:585–590, 1991.
98. Ingelfinger JR, Grupe WE, Harmon WE, Fernbach SK, Levey RH: Growth acceleration following renal transplantation in children less than 7 years of age. *Pediatrics* 68:255–259, 1981.
99. Aschendorff C, Offner G, Winkler L, Schirg E, Hoyer PF, Brodehl J: Adult height achieved in children after kidney transplantation. *Am J Dis Child* 144:1138–1141, 1990.
100. Guest G, Broyer M: Growth after renal transplantation: correlation with immunosuppressive therapy. *Pediatr Nephrol* 5:143–146, 1991.
101. Grushkin CM, Fine RN: Growth in children following renal transplantation. *Am J Dis Child* 125:514–516, 1973.
102. Rees L, Greene SA, Adlard P, et al: Growth and endocrine function after renal transplantation. *Arch Dis Child* 63:1326–1332, 1988.
103. Broyer M, Guest G: In: Schirer K (ed), *Growth and Endocrine Changes in Children and Adolescents with Chronic Renal Failure.* Basel, Krager, 1989.
104. Klare B, von Walter J, Hahn H, Emmrich P, Land W: Cyclosporin in renal transplantation in children. *Lancet* 2:692, 1984.
105. Knight JF, Roy LP, Sheil AG: Catch-up growth in children with successful renal transplants immunosuppressed with cyclosporin alone. *Lancet* 1:159–160, 1985.
106. Tejani A, Butt KMH, Rajpoot D, et al: Strategies for optimizing growth in children with kidney transplants. *Transplantation* 47:229–233, 1989.
107. Klare B, Strom TM, Hahn H, et al: Remarkable long-term prognosis and excellent growth in kidney-transplant children under cyclosporine monotherapy. *Transplant Proc* 23:1013–1017, 1991.
108. Reisman L, Lieberman KV, Burrows L, Schanzer H: Follow-up of cyclosporine-treated pediatric renal allograft recipients after cessation of prednisone. *Transplantation* 49:76–80, 1990.
109. Hodson EM, Knight JF, Sheil AG, Roy LP: Cyclosporin A as sole immunosuppressive agent for renal transplantation in children: effect on catch-up growth. *Transplant Proc* 21:1687–1692, 1989.
110. So SKS, Chang P-N, Najarian JS, Mauer SM, Simmons RL, Nevins TE: Growth and development in infants after renal transplantation. *J Pediatr* 110:343–350, 1987.
111. Ettenger RB, Blifeld C, Prince H, et al: The pediatric nephrologist's dilemma: growth after renal transplantation and its interaction with age as a possible immunologic variable. *J Pediatr* 111:1022–1025, 1987.

112. van Diemen-Steenvoorde R, Donckerwolcke RA, Brackel H, Wolff ED, de Jong MCJW: Growth and sexual maturation in children after kidney transplantation. *J Pediatr* 110:351–356, 1987.
113. Hokken-Koelega ACS, Van Zaal MAE, deRidder MAJ, et al: Growth after renal transplantation in prepubertal children: impact of various treatment modalities. *Pediatr Res* 35:367–371, 1994.
114. Yadin O, Kamil ES, Koch VH, Ettenger RB, Pyke-Grimm K, Fine RN: Accelerated growth following recombinant human growth hormone (met-hGH) therapy (Rx) in children after kidney transplantation. *Kidney Int* 37:616A, 1990.
115. Johansson G, Sietnieks A, Janssens F, et al: Recombinant human growth hormone treatment in short children with chronic renal disease, before transplantation or with functioning renal transplants: an interim report on five European studies. *Acta Paediatr Scand* 370:36–42, 1990.
116. Bartosh S, Kaiser B, Rezvani I, et al: Effects of growth hormone administration in pediatric renal allograft recipients. *Pediatr Nephrol* 6:68–73, 1992.
117. Van Dop C, Jabs KL, Donohoue PA, Bock GH, Fivush BA, Harmon WE: Accelerated growth rates in children treated with growth hormone after renal transplantation. *J Pediatr* 120:244–250, 1992.
118. Benfield MR, Parker KL, Waldo B, Overstrete SL, Kohaut EC: Treatment of growth failure in children after renal transplantation. *Transplantation* 55:305–308, 1993.
119. Tonshoff B, Haffner D, Mehls O, et al: Efficacy and safety of growth hormone treatment in short children with renal allografts: three year experience. *Kidney Int* 44:199–207, 1993.
120. Janssen F, Van Damme-Lombaerts R, Van Dyck M, et al: Effects of recombinant human growth hormone on graft function in renal-transplanted children and adolescents: the three year experience of a Belgian study group. *Transplant Proc* 25:1049–1050, 1993.
121. Lee HM, Mendez-Picon G, Posner MP: The status of rehabilitation, morbidity, and mortality of long term survivors of pediatric kidney transplants. *Transplant Proc* 21:1989–1991, 1989.
122. Muchmore JS, Cooper DK, Ye Y, Schlegel VT, Zuhdi N: Loss of vertebral bone density in heart transplant patients. *Transplant Proc* 23:1184–1185, 1991.
123. Offner G, Aschendorff C, Hoyer PF, et al: End stage renal failure: 14 years' experience of dialysis and renal transplantation. *Arch Dis Child* 63:120–126, 1988.
124. Parfrey PS, Farge D, Parfrey NA, Hanley JA, Guttman RD: The decreased incidence of aseptic necrosis in renal transplant recipients: a case control study. *Transplantation* 41:182–187, 1986.
125. Alsina J, Gonzalez MT, Bonnin R, et al: Long-term evolution of renal osteodystrophy after renal transplantation. *Transplant Proc* 21:2151–2158, 1989.
126. Ekelund A, Nilsson OS: Effects of cyclosporin A on experimental new bone formation in rats. *Clin Orthop* 284:288–298, 1992.
127. Hsu M, Umeda H, Nishijima K: An experimental study of the osteogenicity of free periosteal allografts with cyclosporine A administration. *Int J Oral Maxillofac Surg* 21:178–182, 1992.
128. Ferraris JR, Day PF, Gutman R, Granillo E, Ramirez J, Ruiz S, Pasqualini T: Effect of therapy with a new glucocorticoid, deflazacort, on linear growth and growth hormone secretion after renal transplantation. *J Pediatr* 121:809–813, 1992.
129. Rotundo A, Nevins TE, Lipton M, Lockman LA, Mauer SM, Michael AF: Progressive encephalopathy in children with chronic renal insufficiency in infancy. *Kidney Int* 21:486–491, 1982.

130. McGraw ME, Hake-Ikse K: Neurologic developmental sequelae of chronic renal failure in infancy. *J Pediatr* 106:579–583, 1985.
131. Kohaut EC, Alexander SR, Mehls O: The management of the infant on CAPD. In: Fine RN, Scharer K, Mehls O (eds), *CAPD in Children*. Heidelberg, Springer-Verlag, 1985:97.
132. Geary DF, Haka-Ikse K: Neurodevelopmental progress of young children with chronic renal disease. *Pediatrics* 84:68–72, 1989.
133. Bock GH, Conners K, Ruley J, Samango-Sprouse CA, et al: Disturbances of brain maturation and neurodevelopment during chronic renal failure in infancy. *J Pediatr* 114:231–238, 1989.
134. Fennell RS, Fennell EB, Carter RL, Mings EL, Klausner AB, Hurst JR: A longitudinal study of the cognitive function of children with renal failure. *Pediatr Nephrol* 4:11–15, 1990.
135. Strange K: Regulation of solute and water balance and cell volume in the central nervous system. *J Am Soc Nephrol* 3:12–27, 1992.
136. Coyle JT, Puttfarcken P: Oxidative stress, glutamate, and neurodegenerative disorders. *Science* 262:689–695, 1993.
137. Fraser CL, Arieff AI: Nervous system complication in uremia. *Ann Intern Med* 109:143–153, 1988.
138. Garthwaite J: Glutamate, nitric oxide and cell-cell signalling in the nervous system. *Trends Neurol Sci* 14:60–67, 1991.
139. Elzouki A, Carroll J, Butinar D, Moosa A: Improved neurological outcome in children with chronic renal disease from infancy. *Pediatr Nephrol* 8:205–210, 1994.
140. Davis ID, Chang P, Nevins TE: Successful renal transplantation accelerates development in young uremic children. *Pediatrics* 86:594–600, 1990.
141. Fennell III RS, Rasbury WC, Fennell EB, Morris MK: The effects of kidney transplantation on cognitive performance in a pediatric population. *Pediatrics* 74:273–278, 1984.
142. Rasbury WC, Fennell RS III, Morris MK: Cognitive functioning of children with end stage renal disease before and after successful transplantation. *J Pediatr* 102:589–592, 1983.
143. Rasbury WC, Fennell RS III, Eastman BG, Garin EH, Richard GA: Cognitive performance of children with renal disease. *Psychol Rep* 45:231–239, 1979.
144. Rasbury WC, Fennell RS III, Fennell EB, Morris MK: Cognitive functioning in children with end stage renal disease: pre and post-dialysis sessions. *Int J Pediatr Nephrol* 7:45–50, 1986.
145. Baluarte HJ, Gruskin AB, Ingelfinger JR, Stablein D, Tejani A: Analysis of hypertension in children post renal transplantation: a report of the North American Pediatric Renal Transplant Cooperative Study (NAPRTCS). *Pediatr Nephrol* 8:570–573, 1994.
146. Hoyer PF, Offner G, Oemar BS, Brodehl J, Ringe B, Pichlmayr R: Four years' experience with cyclosporine A in pediatric kidney transplantation. *Acta Paediatr Scand* 79:622–629, 1990.
147. Fontaine E, Beurton D, Barthelemy Y, Quentel P, Cukier J, Broyer M: Renal artery stenosis following pediatric renal transplantation. *Transplant Proc* 26:293–294, 1994.
148. First MR, Neylan JF, Rocher LL, Tejani A: Hypertension after renal transplantation. *J Am Soc Nephrol* 4(Suppl 8):S30–S36, 1994.
149. Broyer M, Guest G, Gagnadoux MF, Beurton D: Hypertension following renal transplantation in children. *Pediatr Nephrol* 1:16–21, 1987.
150. Malekzadeh M, Grushkin CM, Stanley P, Brennan LP, Stiles QR, Liberman E: Renal artery stenosis in pediatric transplant recipients. *Pediatr Nephrol* 1:22–29, 1987.
151. Hricik DE, Lautman J, Bartucci MR, Moir EJ, Mayes JT, Schulak JA: Variable effects of steroid withdrawal on blood pressure reduction in cyclosporine-treated renal transplant recipients. *Transplantation* 53:1232–1235, 1992.

152. Fontana J, Verrina E, Basile G, et al: Arterial hypertension in the transplanted child: frequency and analysis of the causes. *Transplant Proc* 26:79–80, 1994.
153. Tejani A: Post transplant hypertension and hypertensive encephalopathy in renal allograft recipients. *Nephron* 34:73–78, 1983.
154. Feehally J, Walls J, Mistry N, et al: Does nifedipine ameliorate cyclosporin A neprotoxicity? *BMJ* 295:310, 1987.
155. Bokenkamp A, Bohnhorst B, Beier C, Albers N, Offner G, Brodehl J: Nifedipine aggravates cyclosporine A-induced gingival hyperplasia. *Pediatr Nephrol* 8:181–185, 1994.
156. Amerling R, Levin NW: Erythropoietin update. In: Humes HD (ed), *The Kidney,* vol 26, 1993:1–8.
157. Idjradinata P, Pollitt E: Reversal of developmental delays in iron-deficient anaemic infants treated with iron. *Lancet* 341:1–4, 1993.
158. Fennell RS, Moles M, Iravani A, et al: Growth in children following kidney transplantation. *Pediatr Nephrol* 4:335–339, 1990.
159. Schweizer RT, Rovelli M, Palmeri D, Vossler E, Hull D, Bartus S: Noncompliance in organ transplant recipients. *Transplantation* 49:374–377, 1990.
160. Korsch BM, Fine RN, Negrete VF: Noncompliance in children with renal transplants. *Pediatrics* 61:872–876, 1978.
161. Beck DE, Fennell RS, Yost RL, Robinson JD, Geary D, Richards GA: Evaluation of an educational program on compliance with medication regimens in pediatric patients with renal transplants. *J Pediatr* 96:1094–1097, 1980.
162. Foulkes LM, Boggs SR, Fennell RS, Skibinski K: Social support, family variables and compliance in renal transplant children. *Pediatr Nephrol* 7:185–188, 1993.
163. Evans RW, Manninen DL, Garrison LP, et al: The quality of life of patients with end-stage renal disease. *N Engl J Med* 312:553–559, 1985.
164. Levin NW: Quality of life and hematocrit level. *Am J Kidney Dis* 20 (Suppl 1):16–20, 1992.
165. Marsh JT, Brown WS, Wolcott D, et al: rHuEPO treatment improves brain and cognitive function of anemic dialysis patients. *Kidney Int* 39:155–163, 1992.
166. Nissenson AR: Epoetin and cognitive function. *Am J Kidney Dis* 20 (Suppl 1):21–24, 1992.
167. Lynfield R, Herrin JT, Rubin RH: Varicella in pediatric renal transplant recipients. *Pediatrics* 90:216–220, 1992.
168. Zamora I, Simon JM, Da Silva ME, Piqueras AI: Attenuated varicella virus vaccine in children with renal transplants. *Pediatr Nephrol* 8:190–192, 1994.

15

Concomitant or Sequential Kidney Transplantation with Other Organs

Jerry McCauley

Concomitant or sequential renal transplantation in patients with other transplanted organs is becoming increasingly common. Improvements in immunosuppression and in patient care have produced an atmosphere in which more ambitious transplants are being attempted. There are several categories. The first is patients who require life-saving extrarenal transplantation and who have concomitant end-stage renal disease (ESRD). A second category relates to the nephrotoxicity of cyclosporine and tacrolimus, which has produced a group of patients who have undergone successful transplantation with an extrarenal organ but who have developed chronic and at times progressive renal failure, leading to ESRD and the need for renal transplantation. In addition, a growing number of patients with liver, kidney, heart, and bone marrow transplants have required kidney transplants because of primary renal diseases, such as glomerular disease associated with hepatitis. Finally, a subset of patients with Type I diabetes and ESRD are candidates for combined or sequential kidney-pancreas or kidney-islet transplantation. This chapter discusses all four groups of patients.

Determining the need for renal transplantation in these settings can be challenging. Functional renal failure, such as hepatorenal syndrome (HRS) or severe prerenal azotemia due to end-stage heart disease, should improve after transplantation of the primary organ. Similarly, patients with acute renal failure without preexisting renal insufficiency can be expected to regain normal renal function after transplantation, but may have a rocky postoperative course and require temporary dialysis.

The number of renal transplantations performed in combination with transplantation of other organs has grown steadily since the introduction of cyclosporine (Table 15–1).[1] Combined kidney-pancreas transplantation is the most common, followed by liver-kidney and heart-kidney.

TABLE 15–1 ▲ MULTIORGAN TRANSPLANT PROCEDURES IN THE UNITED STATES (1988–1992)

Procedure	1988	1989	1990	1991	1992	Total
Kidney-pancreas	170	331	459	451	491	1902
Kidney-liver	23	30	46	43	56	198
Kidney-heart	3	5	12	5	9	34
Kidney-liver-pancreas	0	2	0	1	0	3
Kidney-pancreas-heart	0	0	0	0	1	1
Kidney-liver-heart	0	1	0	0	0	1

Data from the United Network of Organ Sharing.

The need for renal transplantation in a given patient is based on the determination that the loss of renal function is permanent and severe. Patients with primary renal diseases, with or without failing extrarenal organs, meet these criteria relatively easily. These patients usually have a history of progressive loss of renal function that has been well documented with serial serum creatinine or creatinine clearance studies. Other patients have less straightforward situations. Functional renal insufficiency is common among patients with end-stage liver and heart disease before and after transplantation. Before transplantation, end-organ failure leads to a reduction in the effective circulating volume (ECF) in heart failure and liver failure. After transplantation, cyclosporine and tacrolimus both cause vasoconstriction, reduction in renal blood flow, and renal insufficiency. In each case serum creatinine and blood urea nitrogen (BUN) levels may be markedly elevated. The use of other nephrotoxic drugs further compromises renal function in the pre- and posttransplantation period. Careful laboratory investigation of renal function can usually help to determine if a patient has progressive, irreversible renal failure.

Candidates for liver, heart, or small-intestinal transplantation typically have very low muscle mass and consequently, low serum creatinine (Scr) values. This is primarily due to decreased muscle mass resulting from chronic organ failure. The 24-hour creatinine clearance is the most commonly available method of estimating glomerular filtration rate (GFR) in the clinical setting. However, it may not be completely accurate in patients with severely reduced muscle mass. For these patients, two to three consecutive 24-hour collections may be needed to assure that the analysis is reproducible and complete. In addition, it is possible to estimate GFR with the Gault-Cockcroft equation, as follows.

For men

$$\text{Creatinine clearance} = \frac{(140 - \text{age}) \times (\text{weight})}{(\text{Scr}) \times 72}$$

For women

$$\text{Creatinine clearance} = \frac{(140 - \text{age}) \times (\text{weight} \times 0.85)}{(\text{Scr}) \times 72}$$

These formulas are useful clinically when creatinine clearance determinations or other studies are not available. They are reasonable approximations of GFR in most settings. The utility of both creatinine clearance determinations and the Gault-Cockcroft equation recently has been called into question for renal transplantation candidates, and alternative formulas have been proposed.[2] Whether these formulas will be more useful than the conventional methods requires additional evaluation. Finally, the use of alternate filtration markers (DTPA or iothalamate) may be useful in estimating renal function when creatinine clearance studies are likely to be inaccurate.[3]

▲ KIDNEY AND LIVER TRANSPLANTATION

Candidates for Liver Transplantation

Preexisting renal insufficiency is common prior to liver transplantation. When patients present with previously undiagnosed hepatic failure and renal failure, it is important to determine if they are suffering from acute renal failure or have a chronic process that may require simultaneous renal and hepatic replacement. For such patients, none of the estimates of renal function is useful. A history of renal insufficiency is extremely helpful but may be lacking, because the patient may not be conscious or may not have been seen by a physician prior to this event. Demonstration of a reduction in renal mass that suggests chronic renal disease is helpful. A renal ultrasound for kidney size is the most useful study. Patients with small kidneys can be assumed to have long-standing renal insufficiency. This study also rules out obstruction and, if a Doppler ultrasound is obtained, may also reduce the likelihood of renal artery stenosis.

Once an accurate assessment of renal function has been made, the decision to perform combined kidney/liver transplantation must be based on the current estimated GFR and, for patients with preexisting renal failure, the natural history of renal disease. In general, patients with creatinine clearance values of 20–30 mL/min or less are likely to need combined kidney/liver transplantation. Measures directed at improving renal function should be attempted before this value is accepted. For patients with volume depletion, rehydration should be performed before the 24-hour collection is started. Medications that might reduce GFR or compete for creatinine excretion should be stopped before the study. Despite these measures, it is possible to have a reversibly reduced GFR related to end-stage liver failure. Because no patient with reversible renal failure should be offered a renal transplant, it is important to search for antecedent events that may have caused acute renal failure even in patients with preexisting renal failure.

Acute Renal Failure

Acute renal failure is common in candidates for liver transplantation.[4] Evaluation of such patients must begin with an understanding of the causes of renal insufficiency in patients with liver failure. Severe hepatic failure produces an environment that increases renal vasoconstriction. Proposed mechanisms include activation of the renin-angiotensin system, increased activity of the sympathetic nervous system resulting in increased circulating catecholamines, increases in vasopressin levels, decreases in vasodilators such as prostaglandins and kinins, and increases in vasoconstricting substances, including thromboxane A_2, endotoxin, and endothelin.[5] When acute renal failure can be proved by prior documentation of normal renal function before the acute rise in serum creatinine level, the decision against offering a combined liver-kidney transplant is relatively easy. In this setting, acute tubular necrosis (ATN) is the most common cause.[4,6] Recovery from ATN may be delayed after liver transplantation because of the use of cyclosporine or tacrolimus and the associated renal vasoconstriction caused by these agents and delayed regeneration of renal epithelial cells. Proliferation of renal epithelial cells has been demonstrated to be inhibited in a dose-dependent manner by cyclosporine and tacrolimus.[7] We have treated many patients who have been dialysis dependent for 3–6 months before recovering renal function. Prolonged acute renal failure requiring dialysis also may be complicated by intermittent hypotension, which can accompany hemodialysis. It is important to minimize hypotension on dialysis, and attempts to remove volume aggressively over short periods of time should be avoided. Selection of more biocompatible dialysis membranes may reduce the risk of prolonged acute renal failure and improve survival.

Hepatorenal Syndrome

Hepatorenal syndrome (HRS) is defined as acute renal failure that develops in patients with severe hepatic dysfunction in the absence of other definable causes of renal failure. It is a functional form of acute renal failure that is the direct result of hepatic failure and is by definition reversible with improvement in hepatic function. The pathogenesis of HRS has not been fully delineated, but some of the factors that contribute to this syndrome have been identified.[8–10] Although patients with HRS have decreased systemic vascular resistance, the renal vasculature undergoes vasoconstriction related to factors described earlier.[11] In patients with liver failure without HRS, these factors are balanced against increasing vasodilating compounds such as stimulation of the kallikrein-kinin system and vasodilating prostaglandins. Nitric oxide is being increasingly recognized in the pathogenesis of portal hypertension and HRS.[11] Reductions in nitric oxide may be an important cause of renal vasoconstriction and also may mediate the changes in other hormonal systems such as the renin-angiotensin, kallikrein-kinin, and others. These abnormalities result in intense renal vasoconstriction in HRS, which reduces renal blood flow and causes a drastic fall in GFR. These changes are functional and develop despite normal renal architecture and are potentially reversible with restoration of normal hepatic function.

The functional nature of HRS was first demonstrated clinically by Kopple et al[12] when the kidneys obtained from a patient with HRS functioned normally after being transplanted into a patient with normal hepatic function (Fig. 15–1). Iwatsuki et al[13] later confirmed the functional nature of HRS by demonstrating that restoring nor-

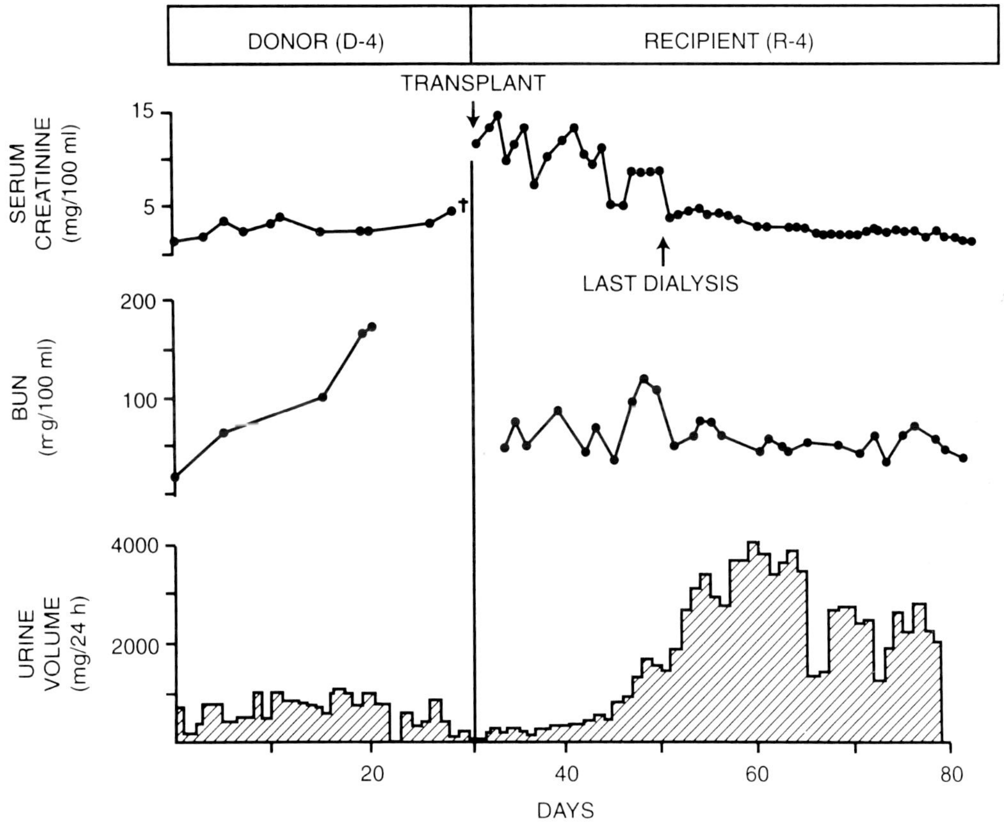

Figure 15–1. Clinical course of donor with hepatorenal syndrome and subsequent renal function after transplantation of kidney into a patient with end-stage renal disease and normal hepatic function. *(From Kopple MH, et al. Transplantation of cadaveric kidneys from patients with hepatorenal syndrome: evidence for the functional nature of renal failure in advanced liver disease.* N Engl J Med *280:1367–1371, 1969.)*

mal hepatic function by liver transplantation led to recovery of renal function (Fig. 15–2). Both of these studies were conducted with azathioprine- and prednisone-based immunosuppression, so the added nephrotoxicity of cyclosporine or tacrolimus was not a complicating factor. Despite this, recovery of renal function was not instantaneous, and the patient in the report by Iwatsuki needed approximately 6–7 days before renal function returned toward baseline. Patients with HRS treated with cyclosporine or tacrolimus also recover renal function, although they may experience concomitant nephrotoxicity, which may delay the recovery process. Renal transplantation is not indicated in these patients. It is very important, however, to establish that HRS is present by performing studies that rule out other forms of acute renal failure (Table 15–2). Confirming the diagnosis of HRS not only eliminates the need for renal transplantation but also may change the patient's status on the waiting list to a more critical level, because HRS implies terminal he-

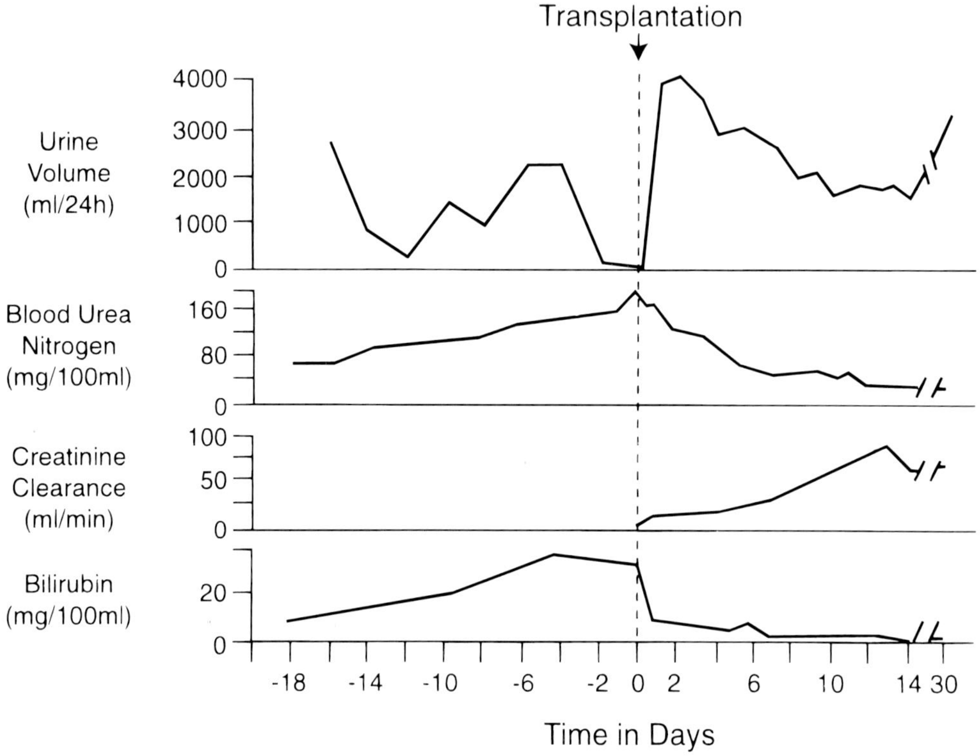

Figure 15–2. Renal function of patient with hepatorenal syndrome before and after successful hepatic transplantation. Note the lag in recovery of renal function in this patient associated with azathioprine and prednisone immunosuppression. *(From Iwatsuki S, et al: Recovery from hepatorenal syndrome after orthotopic liver transplantation.* N Engl J Med *289:1159–1173, 1973.)*

TABLE 15–2 ▲ URINARY FINDINGS IN HEPATORENAL SYNDROME AND OTHER FORMS OF ACUTE RENAL FAILURE

Laboratory Parameter	Prerenal Azotemia	Hepatorenal Syndrome	Acute Tubular Necrosis
Urinary Sodium	<10	<10	>30
Urine to Plasma Creatinine Ratio	>30:1	>30:1	<20:1
Urine Osmolality	100 mOsm ≥ plasma	100 mOsm ≥ plasma	Equal to plasma
Urine Sediment	Normal	Unremarkable except for bile pigmented casts	Muddy brown casts, renal tubular cells and casts

Modified from Epstein M: Hepatorenal syndrome: emerging perspectives of pathophysiology and therapy. *J Am Soc Nephrol* 4:1735–1753, 1994.

patic failure. In general, patients with HRS have urinary indices identical to those of prerenal azotemia.

Although patients with HRS typically recover renal function after liver transplantation, they tend to be more severely ill than patients without HRS and may be at greater risk for the development of ESRD.[14] The reasons for the increased risk for progressive renal failure have not been fully elucidated.

Renal Diseases Associated with Liver Failure

Glomerulonephritis and Liver Failure

Many liver transplant patients have liver disease that may be associated with glomerulonephritis and chronic renal insufficiency. Hepatitis B has been associated with membranoproliferative glomerulonephritis (MPGN), membranous glomerulonephritis (MGN), and polyarteritis nodosa.[15,16] Hepatitis C has been demonstrated to lead to cryoglobulinemia and MPGN.[17,18]

Many patients with advanced liver failure have deposits of immunglobulin A (IgA) in the skin, hepatic sinusoids, and in the mesangium of the kidney.[19] These deposits have been found in patients with liver failure of most causes. Renal biopsies performed on 18 patients at the time of liver transplantation disclosed mesangial proliferation or MPGN in all patients.[20] Most patients also had IgA deposition. Impaired removal of IgA by Kupffer cells in the liver may be an important pathogenetic factor. Clinically important manifestations of Berger's disease are rare, however. Apparently, restoration of normal hepatic function after liver transplantation is sufficient to allow clearing of these deposits from the kidney and other sites. The presence of IgA deposits in renal biopsies prior to liver transplantation can thus generally be viewed as a benign finding.

Primary Oxalosis

Renal transplantation in combination with liver transplantation is being performed with greater frequency in patients with oxalosis (see Chapter 3). Transplantation before extensive oxalate deposition occurs appears to be preferable to waiting until patients are debilitated by cardiac, bone, and renal disease. Staged transplantation of the liver and then the kidney approximately 6 months later may be the most successful approach. However, when survival statistics are examined for combined liver-kidney transplantation, the increased risk inherent with oxalosis must be taken into consideration. Patients with extensive deposition of oxalate in heart and bone are at greater risk for serious complications than patients with primary renal disease and hepatic failure.

Other Primary Renal Diseases

Patients with hepatic failure may have chronic renal failure from causes unrelated to their liver disease. Diabetic nephropathy, hypertensive nephrosclerosis, and glomerular diseases not associated with viral hepatitis probably occur with the same incidence as in the general population. When such patients are evaluated, it is important to consider the natural history of their specific disease when deciding to offer a concomitant renal transplant. Hypertensive disease may progress to ESRD but may improve after successful liver transplantation, with good blood pressure control. For such a patient, early renal transplantation (creatinine clearance >30 mL/min) is probably not appropriate. For patients with diseases that are likely to progress to ESRD within 1 year of transplantation of the liver and with a creatinine clearance less than 30 mL/min, early combined transplantation should be considered. A functional reduction in renal function due to hepatic failure often makes this decision difficult. It is not uncommon for stage 1 patients with severe reductions in effective circulating volume without obvious HRS to have improved renal function after transplantation even under cyclosporine or tacrolimus immunosuppression. The decision to perform combined liver-kidney transplantation can thus be difficult. Some authors have recommended offering only the liver, because the functional contribution of end-stage liver disease to renal insufficiency cannot be clearly determined. A renal transplant can be offered later if renal function does not improve after approximately 6 months of dialysis. This approach is limited by the fact that the patient may be forced to wait a long period of time for a renal transplant. In addition, the immunologic benefit obtained from simultaneous liver and kidney transplantation is lost.

Results after Combined Liver-Kidney Transplantation

Most series of combined liver-kidney transplantation have been small, with less than ten patients in each report. A summary of potential indications is listed in Table 15–3.

TABLE 15–3 ▲ INDICATIONS FOR COMBINED LIVER AND KIDNEY TRANSPLANTATION

Disease of Renal and Hepatic Failure
Polycystic kidney disease with associated "lethal fatigue" secondary to massive polycystic liver
Hepatitis B–related cirrhosis and MGN or MPGN
Hepatitis C–related cirrhosis and MGN, cryoglobulinemia, or MPGN
Primary oxalosis (PHO types I and II)
Unrelated Liver and Kidney Disease
Primary renal disease (eg, hypertension, diabetes)
Primary liver disease (eg, alcoholic liver disease, primary biliary cirrhosis)
Immunosuppression Related to Prior Extrarenal Organ Transplantation
Cyclosporine, Tacrolimus
Renal Transplantation Candidate with Liver Failure or Liver Transplantation Candidate with Renal Failure
Prior kidney transplant with failing kidney and hepatic failure

MGN, membranous glomerulonephritis; MPGN, membranoproliferative glomerulonephritis; PHO, primary hyperoxaluria.

Margreiter et al[21] reported on one of the first combined procedures in 1984. In this and a subsequent report,[22] chronic glomerulonephritis was the sole cause of renal failure. Five of six patients had viral hepatitis (hepatitis B or non-A, non-B hepatitis) as the cause of liver disease. In these reports, both the liver and kidney were derived from the same donor. The authors suggested that the liver transplant may have protected the kidney from rejection. A later study by Fung et al[23] further suggested that the liver is capable of converting a positive cross match to negative in a patient with preformed lymphocytotoxic antibodies, allowing successful renal transplantation after completion of the liver transplantation procedure. Hyperacute rejection of the kidney predictably develops if patients undergo transplantation in the presence of a positive cross match without prior hepatic transplantation from the same donor. The liver, in contrast, appears to be resistant to hyperacute rejection even in the presence of a positive cross match. Immunoabsorption studies demonstrated that the positive cross matches were entirely due to anti-human leukocyte antigen (HLA) class I antibodies.[24] Flye et al[25] confirmed these findings in a highly sensitized patient who received simultaneous liver and kidney transplants. Small case series by Gonwa et al,[26] Shaked et al,[27] Vogel et al,[28] and Gil-Vernet et al[29] suggested that acute renal rejection and graft loss occur less after combined liver-kidney transplantation in patients with varying degrees of presensitization. A recent report by Rasmussen et al[29a] demonstrated that rejection of the kidney grafts decreased markedly when the combined procedure was performed, but the rate of hepatic rejection was not improved. These authors also suggested that renal allograft survival was superior with the combined procedure. Four of the 21 (19%) patients in the series died (with good renal function) between 3 and 28 weeks after transplantation. Starzl et al[30] suggested that renal rejection may be a harbinger of a hostile immunologic environment for the liver and termed it "the case of the canary kidney."[30]

Polycystic liver and kidney disease has been an uncommon indication for the combined liver-kidney procedure. In most cases, patients have had severe liver failure in addition to progressive renal insufficiency. These have been relatively unusual cases; most patients with the autosomal dominant form of polycystic kidney disease (PCKD) seldom have severe hepatic failure. Because hepatic insufficiency has been a principal contributor to mortality in dialysis units (because of viral hepatitis and other diseases), it is likely that more patients with PCKD and combined hepatic and renal failure will undergo transplantation in the future. Some patients have required transplantation for a condition called *lethal exhaustion* by Starzl et al,[31] who performed hepatic transplantation in four patients with massive disabling hepatomegaly (liver volumes 7120–12,790 mL). Three of four patients had long-term survival with symptomatic improvement that allowed them to return to more active lives. Two of these patients received combined liver and kidney transplants, and one subsequently died of fulminant hepatic failure from hepatitis B. Taylor et al[32] subsequently reported successful transplantation of a similar patient. This patient experienced pulmonary insufficiency related to the size of the liver, which limited her to a wheelchair and caused severe abdominal pain during dialysis. In addition to severe fatigue, this patient became suicidal as a result of her physical limitations. After transplantation her activity level returned essentially to normal. Reduction of hepatic mass by other methods has been reported. Attempts at partial hepatectomy described by Lin et al,[33] have been attempted, with only limited success.[31] Combined liver-kidney transplantation in polycystic liver and kidney disease should be reserved for patients who are unable to obtain relief by nonsurgical means.

▲ SEQUENTIAL EXTRARENAL-RENAL TRANSPLANTATION

With the introduction of cyclosporine, liver and other extrarenal solid organ transplants have become increasingly successful.[4] The improvement in patient survival, coupled with the nephrotoxicity of cyclosporine, has led to a large number of patients with chronic yet stable renal dysfunction. A small number of these patients have progressed to end stage renal disease. The precise role of cyclosporine in the deterioration in renal function has not been fully elucidated. Case reports of a glomerulopathy similar to focal sclerosing glomerulonephritis have been reported to be related to long-term cyclosporine administration.[34] In addition, viral hepatitis-associated glomerulonephritis, progression of known pre-transplant renal disease, development of diabetic nephropathy, and other renal diseases not associated with the transplant process all may develop after transplantation. Kidney transplantation may thus become necessary.

The evaluation of patients with a prior extra-renal organ transplant for sequential renal transplantation is similar to that described above. When the function of the prior non-renal transplant is essentially normal, the assessment of renal function is usually much easier, since functional changes from the failing liver or heart are not present. In such patients, a creatinine clearance greater than 30 mL/min obviates the need for renal transplantation. The rate of progression can usually be assessed with serial creatinine determinations. A renal biopsy may be helpful in determining both the cause of progressive renal failure and the degree of renal impairment. Biopsies are most helpful in patients with nephrotic range proteinuria but may also be useful in progressive unexplained renal failure. Cyclosporine or tacrolimus may not necessarily be the cause of the progressive renal failure.

▲ HEART-KIDNEY AND BONE MARROW–KIDNEY TRANSPLANTATION

Recipients of extrarenal transplants are receiving renal transplants at an increasing rate (see Table 15–1). As with liver recipients, heart, lung, small intestine, and bone marrow recipients are also potentially exposed to many risks to their renal function. Infection with viral hepatitis from blood transfusions and resulting glomerulonephritis may be a common risk for all of these patients. Likewise, after transplantation, all of these patients are exposed to potentially nephrotoxic drugs, which may result in acute or chronic renal failure. As with liver transplant patients, preexisting renal failure has been associated with increased mortality and morbidity after transplantation. Given the shortage of organs, many heart transplantation centers have restricted access to heart transplantation to patients with normal renal function. Even moderate levels of renal insufficiency (serum creatinine level >2.0 mg/dL [180 μmol/L]) have been sufficient to reject such patients for heart[35] and bone marrow transplants.[36]

In spite of these conservative acceptance criteria, an increasing number of simultaneous kidney and heart transplants have been performed. The first combined heart and kidney transplantation of organs from the same donor was performed under the direction of Starzl in 1968, but the report was not published.[37] This patient survived for 3 1/2 months but died of apparent rejection, which occurred in the organs at different times. The second case was reported by Norman et al in 1978.[38] This patient died after 2 weeks of multiple organ failure. Few if any of these procedures were repeated until cyclosporine became available. Successful combined procedures have been reported by Faggian et al[39] and Livesey et al.[40] Two additional cases were reported by Bahnson and Gordon.[37]

Combined kidney–bone marrow transplantation has been performed recently in an attempt to augment chimerism but not with the intention of replacing or totally reconstituting the recipient's bone marrow (see Chapters 1 and 9). Patients undergoing conventional bone marrow transplantation are at risk for chronic renal failure due to total body irradiation, chemotherapy, and cyclosporine nephrotoxicity.[41] Chronic renal failure developed in 25% of patients in a study by Cohen et al[42] and was associated with mesangial expansion, endothelial cell dropout, and glomerular basement membrane thickening. These changes were consistent with radiation nephropathy and have been termed bone marrow transplant nephropathy.[43] Most patients experienced stabilization of renal function, but others had progression of renal insufficiency. Angiotensin converting enzyme inhibitors have been shown to attenuate this nephropathy in experimental models.[43] Hemolytic-uremic syndrome is a relatively common complication of cyclosporine after bone marrow transplantation and may lead to chronic renal failure.[44,45] Despite these potential insults to renal function, ESRD appears to be very uncommon in the bone marrow transplant population. Because these patients are at risk for hepatitis C and its related glomerular diseases in addition to chronic cyclosporine toxicity, it is possible that these patients may require renal transplantation years after obtaining a functioning bone marrow graft. There has been at least one case of a bone marrow donor subsequently donating a kidney (which functioned perfectly without need for immunosuppression). Patient selection should be similar to that for liver transplant recipients but must take into account the history of prior malignant disease. Because renal insufficiency is a contraindication to bone marrow transplantation (except in the chimerism augmentation protocols) it is unlikely that patients with leukemia or breast cancer would ever be offered simultaneous bone marrow–kidney transplantation.

Renal and Pancreatic Transplantation

Annika Tibell / Carl G. Groth

In the early days of renal transplantation, diabetes was actually regarded as a contraindication to candidacy. However, the excellent results subsequently achieved in patients with diabetes led to their routine acceptance for renal transplantation over the past 15 years. More recently, in an attempt to deal with the underlying metabolic disorder, selected patients have received a pancreas in addition to the kidney. The goal has been to render the patients normoglycemic and discontinue exogenous insulin administration, with the hope of stopping the progression of or even reversing the secondary complications of diabetes. The first attempt at combined kidney-pancreas transplantation was carried out by Kelly and Lillehei more than 25 years ago.[46] At present, a number of centers perform this procedure, and some 5000 patients have undergone renal and pancreatic transplantation around the world.

The pancreas can be transplanted simultaneously with a kidney from the same donor; alternatively, it can be transplanted from a third-party donor after a successful kidney transplant. With simultaneous kidney-pancreas transplantation, the recipient undergoes one operation and receives induction immunosuppression only once. Because the kidney and the pancreas are from the same donor, the kidney can serve as a marker for rejection. A potential disadvantage of the simultaneous procedure is that surgical or other complications related to the pancreas might cause problems with the kidney. The staged procedure involves two separate operations and thus two courses of induction immunosuppression. In addition, because the kidney is from a different donor, it cannot serve as a marker for rejection of the pancreas. At present, most groups perform the simultaneous procedure.

This section discusses recipient and donor selection, technical aspects related to pancreatic transplantation, issues of postoperative management, complications, and results.

▲ RECIPIENT SELECTION

Potential candidates for simultaneous kidney-pancreas transplantation are a subset of patients with diabetes and end stage renal disease (ESRD) who would otherwise be candidates for renal transplantation alone. Recipients are almost always younger than 50 years of age and in reasonably good health. Patients who have substantial problems with blood glucose control may be particularly appropriate candidates. Ongoing peripheral gangrene, severe coronary insufficiency with angina, cardiac decompensation, or severely incapacitating autonomic or peripheral neuropathy are contraindications to combined kidney-pancreas transplantation. Borderline patients may be candidates for renal transplantation alone.

There may be a place for staged kidney-pancreas transplantation in patients receiving a kidney from a living-related donor. In such cases, kidney transplantation is performed first, followed after successful engraftment by a cadaveric pancreas. Some patients originally deemed too sick to tolerate the simultaneous procedure, but who recover well after cadaveric kidney transplantation, might also be given a subsequent pancreas.

Pancreas transplantation is not a life-saving operation and is associated with a number of potential postoperative complications. It is important that the patient have a good understanding of the risks and a high level of motivation. Candidates for pancreatic transplantation undergo a more extensive preoperative evaluation than do candidates for renal transplantation alone. The preoperative evaluation at our hospital is outlined in Table 15–4. Pretransplant assessment of the retina is manda-

TABLE 15–4 ▲ PREOPERATIVE EVALUATION

System	Procedure
Cardiovascular	Exercise electrocardiogram
	Noninvasive evaluation of the peripheral vessels
	Coronary arteriography (optional)
	Iliac artery angiography (optional)
Gastrointestinal	Upper gastrointestinal radiographic series
	Gastroscopy
Urinary tract	Residual urine volume
	Cystoscopy (optional)
	Cystometry (optional)
Neurologic	Electroneurography of peripheral nerves and cardiac beat-to-beat variation on provocation
Ophthalmologic	Fundus photography
	Fluorescein angiography
Renal	Cr-EDTA clearance
	Renal biopsy (optional)

tory. When indicated, photocoagulation should be performed before transplantation. Unless the retina is in stable condition, the sudden improvement in glycemic control after pancreatic transplantation may cause a deterioration in the retinopathy.[47]

▲ DONOR AND RECIPIENT OPERATIONS

The pancreas is recovered in continuity with a short duodenal segment from the cadaveric donor.[48] Usually, the liver and pancreas are removed en bloc. The pancreatoduodenal graft is then separated from the liver on the back table. The celiac axis and a good length of the portal vein are kept with the liver, and iliac artery and vein extension grafts are used to lengthen the vessels of the pancreatoduodenal graft (Fig. 15–3). The pancreatoduodenal graft is placed intraperitoneally in the lower part of the abdomen in the recipient. Arterial anastomosis is to the iliac artery, and venous anastomosis is to the iliac vein or lower inferior vena cava (Fig. 15–4). In the case of simultaneous kidney-pancreas transplantation, the pancreas is usually placed on the right and the kidney on the left side. If the patient has undergone renal transplantation previously, the pancreas is placed on the opposite side. The systemic venous drainage of the pancreatic graft results in peripheral hyperinsulinemia. To avoid the unphysiologic state, some groups have advocated performing the venous anastomosis to the portal vein or to one of its tributaries, so that the venous drainage is to the liver. Although peripheral hyperinsulinemia has been avoided with portal drainage,

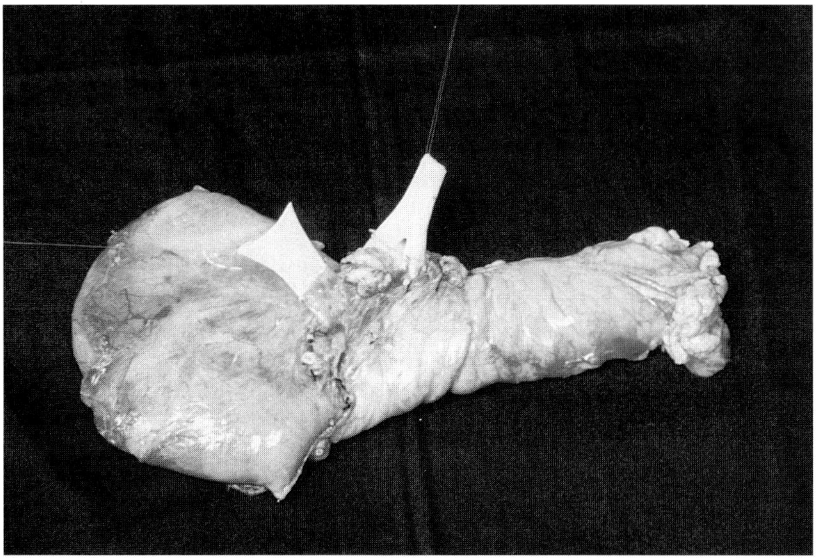

Figure 15–3. Pancreatoduodenal graft. The splenic artery and superior mesenteric artery of the graft have been connected with a Y graft consisting of the donor iliac bifurcation. The graft portal vein has been extended with the donor common iliac vein.

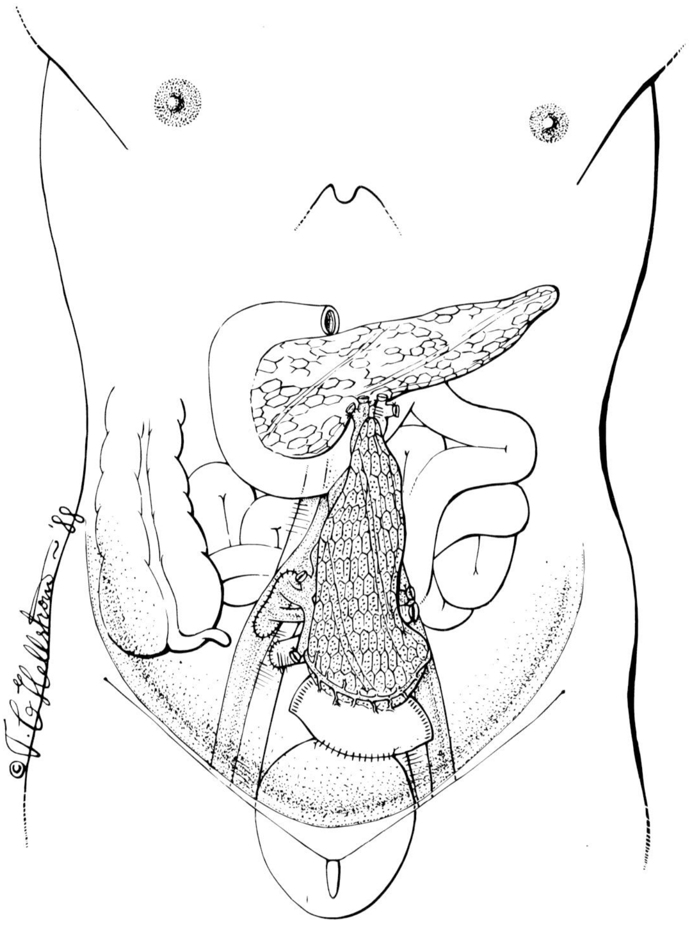

Figure 15–4. Pancreatoduodenal transplantation with exocrine diversion to the recipient bladder.

no advantage has been seen in blood glucose control.[49,50] In addition, the portal drainage techniques are surgically more demanding.

Diversion of graft exocrine secretion is often performed to the recipient's urinary bladder (see Fig. 15–4).[51] Urinary tract diversion originally was used as a means of avoiding enteric contamination of the wound,[52] which had occurred in some early recipients of pancreatic grafts with enteric exocrine drainage.[53] Another more recently perceived advantage is that urinary diversion allows daily monitoring of the graft by measurement of urinary amylase levels.[54] There are, however, some problems associated with bladder drainage. The loss of alkaline pancreatic juice in the urine may result in metabolic acidosis, and oral supplementation with bicarbonate has been required in a number of patients.[55] Urinary tract infections, and in some cases severe urinary tract symptoms, probably caused by activation of the digestive pancreatic enzymes in the urine, have occurred in some patients.[56,57] If the requirements for bicarbonate supplementation are excessive, or if the symptoms from the urinary tract are severe enough, conversion to enteric drainage might be indicated. In practice, 10–15% of patients with bladder-drained grafts require such conversion.[57]

Some groups use enteric exocrine diversion primarily (Fig 15–5).[58] In that situation, allograft amylase secretion cannot be monitored unless an exteriorized pancreatic duct catheter is placed.[59] Such a catheter can be left in place for the first several weeks after transplantation, when the risk of rejection is highest. However, the use of a pancreatic duct catheter may contribute to the development of acute graft pancreatitis.[60] The use of an enteric anastomosis has been believed to carry an increased risk for intraabdominal sepsis, although local septic complications also may occur with bladder drainage.[61] Work by our group[60] and more recently by Corry et al[62] at the University of Pittsburgh, however, has indicated that routine enteric drainage can

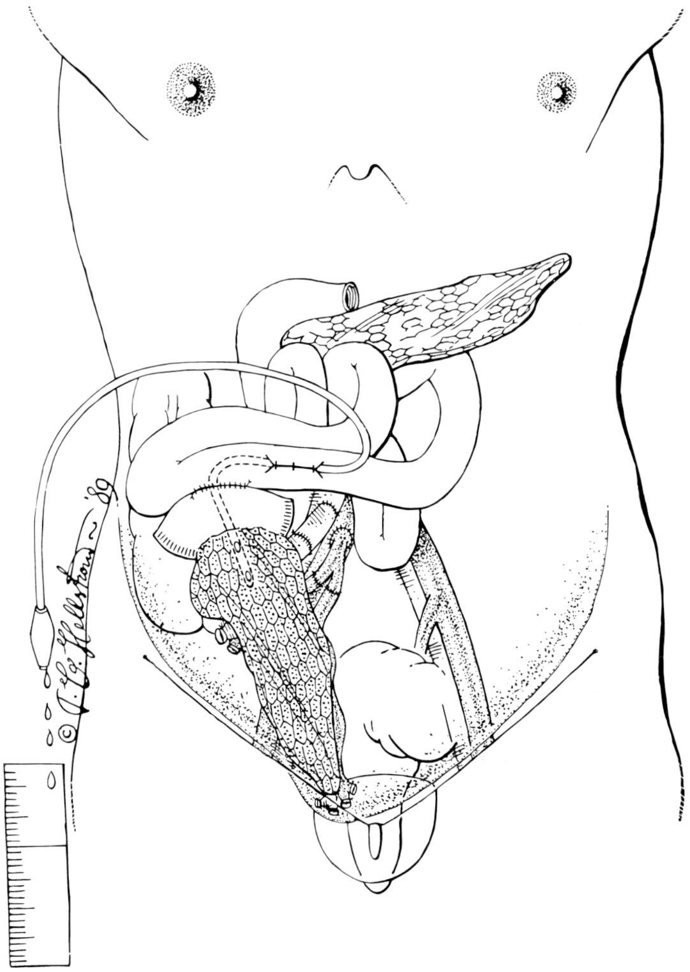

Figure 15–5. Pancreatoduodenal transplantation with enteric exocrine diversion.

be performed safely with few serious complications.[62] With either procedure, the duodenal segment is used and is anastomosed to the recipient's bladder or jejunum (see Figs. 15–4 and 15–5).

In the early 1980s, segmental body and tail pancreatic grafts were commonly used. Many groups used the ductal occlusion technique, filling the pancreatic duct with a synthetic polymer.[63] The procedure results in fibrosis and destruction of the exocrine part of the pancreas. Unfortunately, the potential surgical advantages are offset by the loss of exocrine pancreatic markers, which can be important in the diagnosis of rejection. In addition, peripancreatic fluid collections and pancreatic fistulas were not uncommon. Today, ductal occlusion is used rarely, and only for recipients of combined renal and pancreatic grafts; the diagnosis of rejection then depends on the kidney.

▲ POSTOPERATIVE MANAGEMENT

After transplantation, the exocrine part of the pancreatic graft is monitored by daily measurement of serum amylase. For recipients of bladder-drained pancreatic grafts, the amylase level in the urine is also recorded daily. For patients with an exteriorized pancreatic duct catheter, measurement of the flow of juice and its amylase content provides hourly information concerning the condition of the graft.

The endocrine function of the graft is monitored by frequent measurement of the blood glucose and changes in the recipient's insulin requirement. Measurement of serum C-peptide provides direct information about allograft insulin production. Hemoglobin A_{1c} also is measured regularly. Intravenous and oral glucose tolerance tests occasionally are performed.

Usually, blood glucose levels become normal or near normal within hours after transplantation, and exogenous insulin administration can be discontinued. In some instances, blood glucose control is poor, and insulin therapy has to be maintained. Inadequate blood glucose control and marked hyperamylasemia soon after transplantation are usually a reflection of severe damage to the graft from ischemia, acute rejection, or vascular thrombosis.

Ultrasonography may be used both to diagnose peripancreatic fluid collections and to assess arterial and venous flow by Doppler. Radionuclide scans, computed tomography (CT), and magnetic resonance imaging (MRI) also have been used, but the findings often are inconclusive. Angiography is indicated when partial or complete graft thrombosis is suspected.

Postoperative ileus is more common after pancreatic transplantation than after renal transplantation, presumably because of the intraperitoneal placement of the pancreatic graft. As a result, patients are usually kept NPO for 4–5 days, until complete recovery of gastrointestinal function has occurred.

For immunosuppression, most groups use sequential four-drug immunosuppression. Acute rejection episodes are treated similarly to renal transplant rejection, although primary treatment with monoclonal CD3 antibodies (Orthoclone OKT3, Ortho, Raritan, NJ), antilymphocyte globulin (ALG), or antithymocyte globulin (ATG) is more often used to treat recipients of pancreatic transplants. There has been some encouraging experience with tacrolimus-based therapy without induction ALG therapy. In the first 60 consecutive cases reported by Corry et al[62], 97% 1-year actuarial renal allograft survival, and 83% 1-year actuarial pancreatic allograft survival were recorded.

Graft thrombosis occurs more commonly in pancreatic grafts than in renal grafts. As a consequence of this, many groups use various anticoagulant protocols; low-molecular-weight dextran and aspirin are the drugs most commonly used.

Prophylactic antibiotics are routinely given during the operation and for the first few postoperative days. The drugs used should be effective against staphylococci and enteric and urinary tract bacteria.

▲ GRAFT-RELATED COMPLICATIONS

The usual surgical complications, such as bleeding and wound infection, are more common after pancreatic transplantation than after renal transplantation. A contributing factor may be the use of anticoagulant drugs. To reduce the risk of bleeding, meticulous hemostasis is essential. The increased incidence of wound infection may be related to contamination from the recipient's intestine or bladder, or from the duodenal segment of the graft.

A number of other complications related to the pancreatic graft may occur. A list of these complications, the symptoms and signs observed, and the respective therapies, is given in Table 15–5. In an immunosuppressed patient, many of these complications may become life threatening. Because the pancreatic graft is not a life-saving organ, prompt allograft removal may be the most prudent treatment alternative.

Patients who have undergone combined transplantation often require longer hospitalization than patients who have received a kidney transplant only. Recovery from complications related to the pancreatic graft usually accounts for the prolonged hospital stay.

▲ DIAGNOSIS OF REJECTION

For reasons not understood, kidneys transplanted simultaneously with the pancreas have a higher incidence of rejection than kidneys transplanted alone.[65,66] It is surprising that pancreatic graft function usually remains unaffected while the kidney is experiencing rejection. Sometimes symptoms and signs of rejection occur in both grafts. In some rare instances, isolated pancreatic graft rejection has been encountered.[66] However, when a pancreas is transplanted after a kidney or is transplanted alone in a nonuremic diabetic patient, pancreatic graft rejection is commonly seen.[67,68]

Although the diagnosis of rejection in recipients of simultaneous grafts can generally be based on changes in the kidney, the diagnosis of rejection in a pancreas transplanted after a kidney depends on changes in the pancreatic markers. An increase in the serum amylase level may occur at the time of rejection, but the level

TABLE 15-5 ▲ GRAFT RELATED SURGICAL COMPLICATIONS AFTER PANCREATIC TRANSPLANTATION

Complication	Time When Complication Usually Occurs	Main Symptoms	Suggested Treatment
Arterial graft thrombosis	Days to weeks	Sharp rise in blood glucose Drop in serum amylase level No amylase output in pancreatic juice or urine	Graft removal
Venous graft thrombosis	Days to weeks	Rise in serum amylase level Blood staining of pancreatic juice or urine Tenderness and swelling of the graft	Graft removal
Pancreatic exocrine "sweating"	Days to weeks	Wound problems	Drainage
Anastomotic leaks and intraabdominal sepsis	Weeks	Fever Leukocytosis Tenderness at graft site Endocrine function intact	Drainage Surgical repair
Pancreatic fistula	Weeks	Discharge of clear fluid with high amylase content Reddening of skin due to digestion	Repair of damage
Early graft pancreatitis	Days to weeks	High serum amylase level Tenderness at graft site Fever Endocrine function maintained	Conventional measures, in severe cases removal of graft
Late graft pancreatitis	Several months or years	Hyperamylasemia with or without local symptoms	If treatment is required, conventional measures Identify and avoid trigger factors
Intrapancreatic abscess	Weeks to months	Fever Abdominal discomfort Impaired endocrine function	Graft removal

also may remain unaffected. Assays for more specific plasma markers, such as anodal trypsin or pancreas-specific protein have been found to correlate somewhat better with rejection, but even with these tests, the discrimination is poor.[69,70]

In recipients of bladder-drained pancreatic grafts, a drop in urinary amylase excretion is commonly used as a marker of acute rejection.[54] It originally was believed that a decline in amylase excretion correlated closely with the rejection process. The reliability of the test has come into question, because urinary amylase excretion may vary for other reasons.

In grafts with an exteriorized pancreatic duct catheter, a decrease in the amylase content of the pancreatic juice has been found to correlate closely with graft rejection.[71] Cytologic examination of the juice has proved to be helpful in this context.[70,72] Lymphoblasts have been found to appear in the juice 1 or 2 days before the decrease in amylase output.

Elevated blood glucose levels usually occur late in the rejection process, when it might be difficult or even impossible to reverse rejection.[73] This discrepancy in the timing of rejection has been observed in animal experiments with nonimmunosuppressed dogs. Cellular infiltrates appeared early in the exocrine tissue at a time when the endocrine tissue was still unaffected.[74]

Fine-needle biopsy and core-needle biopsy have been used to diagnose rejection.[75–77] In the case of bladder-drained grafts, a cystoscope can be advanced into the duodenal segment, and a transmural biopsy can be taken from the pancreatic parenchyma.[76] With enterically drained grafts, a small laparotomy is often made; ultrasound-guided percutaneous biopsy also can be attempted. Pancreatic graft biopsies entail a risk of pancreatitis and pancreatic fistula formation and should therefore be performed with caution.

In chronic rejection, a progressive deterioration in blood glucose control is the most characteristic finding. Episodes of hyperamylasemia can occur weeks or months earlier. These changes presumably reflect inflammation and perhaps outflow obstruction in the exocrine part of the graft.

▲ PATIENT AND GRAFT SURVIVAL

The International Pancreas Transplant Registry maintained at the University of Minnesota has for many years provided information on patient and graft survival after pancreatic transplantation. Patient survival once was higher in patients receiving a pancreas after a kidney. This was not surprising; these patients represented a selected population who had done well after renal transplantation. This difference has disappeared. The 1-year patient survival after simultaneous pancreas and kidney transplantation is 90%; after staged kidney-pancreas transplantation it is 92%.[78] These patient survival figures are similar to those after renal transplantation alone in patients with diabetes.

The question of whether pancreatic transplantation has an impact on the life expectancy of patients with diabetes has not been settled. Data from the University of Minnesota indicate that in patients with diabetes with abnormal autonomic function, those with a functioning pancreatic transplant have better survival rates than patients with failed pancreatic transplants or patients not given a pancreatic transplant.[79]

With simultaneous pancreatic and renal transplantation with bladder drainage, the registry figure for 1-year pancreatic graft survival is about 75%. The corresponding figures for grafts with enteric drainage and duct occlusion are 54% and 63%, respectively. Individual groups have reported 1-year graft survival rates in the 70–80% range with the latter two techniques.[60,80]

With staged kidney-pancreas transplantation, the pancreatic graft survival rate is inferior to that with the simultaneous procedure, the 1-year outcome being about 45%. However, the Minnesota group has shown that it is possible to improve the results in these patients by using both better human leukocyte antigen (HLA) matching and an intensified treatment of rejection as soon as the urinary amylase level declines.[78] For the latest series of patients undergoing pancreas-after-kidney transplantation, the 1-year pancreas graft survival rate was 72%.

Data concerning long-term graft survival are also emerging. In a recent analysis of the Stockholm series, it was found that of 65 pancreatic grafts that had been transplanted in combination with a kidney more than 5 years previously, 20 (31%) were functioning 5–9 years after transplantation.[81]

There has been concern that renal allograft survival in simultaneous kidney-pancreas transplantation might be inferior to that after kidney transplantation alone because of immunologic or other problems. Comparison of the data from the Pancreas Transplant Registry and the United Network of Organ Sharing (UNOS) Kidney Transplant Registry revealed, however, comparable graft survival whether the kidney was transplanted in conjunction with a pancreas or alone into diabetic recipients with diabetes.[78,82]

▲ METABOLIC CONTROL

After successful pancreatic transplantation, the patient becomes insulin independent and blood glucose levels and glycosylated hemoglobin levels are normal or near normal.[83–85] Oral and intravenous glucose tolerance tests show normal findings in most but not all patients. One important explanation for glucose tolerance not being completely normal is the diabetogenic effect of the immunosuppressive agents. Steroids induce insulin resistance because of their effect on peripheral tissues.[86] Cyclosporine is toxic to the β cells and may cause impaired insulin production.[87] Some findings indicate that cyclosporine may induce peripheral insulin resistance.[88,89] Studies have shown that in recipients of pancreatic grafts, the insulin response to various stimuli is blunted compared with the response in renal allograft recipients given similar immunosuppression.[90] Because this blunting is most pronounced among recipients of segmental grafts, an insufficient β cell mass may be implicated.[91]

▲ EFFECTS ON SECONDARY COMPLICATIONS

It initially was hoped that normoglycemia after successful pancreatic transplantation would result in a lack of progression or even reversal of the secondary complications of diabetes. Today, with follow-up results available for a rather large number of patients, it is clear that the results are disappointing in this regard.

After combined renal and pancreatic transplantation, a clear improvement in neuropathy occurs, but comparisons with the findings in recipients of renal grafts alone indicate that this improvement is due mainly to the reversal of uremia.[92] With longer follow-up periods, a small additional advantage has been demonstrated in patients who have received a pancreas.[93–95]

Similar observations have been made about retinopathy. No improvement was noted initially, and for some patients the retinopathy actually worsened.[96,97] Three to four years after transplantation, stabilization or even improvement has been observed by some groups. Other groups have been unable to find any beneficial effect.

Studies with vital microscopy and laser techniques indicate that pancreatic transplantation may have a favorable impact on the microvascular reactivity of the skin. Thermoregulatory behavior and reoxygenization time also improved after transplantation.[98,99]

The finding that pancreatic transplantation has only a small or no effect on established diabetic neuropathy and retinopathy probably has its explanation in the fact that most of the patients who have received transplants have suffered from end-stage diabetes. The secondary complications have therefore been far advanced, the tissue destruction probably being beyond recovery. Beneficial effects on the secondary complications will probably occur only if pancreatic transplantation is performed earlier in the natural history of diabetes.

This reasoning derives strong support from observations about the effects of pancreatic transplantation on diabetic nephropathy. In diabetic patients who received a kidney and a pancreas transplant, either simultaneously[100] or as staged procedures,[101] the renal graft has been protected from the glomerular lesions characteristic of diabetes. However, when patients with long standing diabetes (15–29 years) were given a pancreas transplant only, it was found that the glomerular lesions present in their native kidneys did not improve even 5 years after transplantation.[102] Thus while the development of diabetic lesions in a normal kidney were prevented by pancreatic transplantation, established diabetic lesions were not affected.

▲ QUALITY OF LIFE

After successful pancreatic transplantation, insulin can be discontinued, and dietary restrictions can be eliminated. These changes have considerable social and psychological implications for the patient. Several groups of investigators have performed formal analyses concerning the quality of life after pancreatic transplantation. Although the findings concerning performance parameters have been conflicting,[103–106] in most of these studies, the measurements of subjective health perception showed improvement. There is no question that most patients feel an almost miraculous sense of relief after pancreatic transplantation, in the belief that their diabetes has ended.

▲ CONCLUSION

Simultaneous kidney-pancreas transplantation has emerged as a successful therapeutic option for good-risk patients with ESRD secondary to diabetes mellitus. Although the procedure is not without serious complications, 1-year patient and pancreatic graft survival rates of 90% and 75% have been achieved. Improved immunosuppression with tacrolimus-based therapy may further improve the outcome. Patients who have undergone successful transplantation have discontinued insulin and are normoglycemic; unfortunately, there has been little corresponding improvement in the secondary complications of diabetes. With increasingly better outcomes, it should be possible eventually to intervene earlier in the natural history of this disease and perhaps have more impact on the long-term complications.

Renal and Pancreatic Islet Cell Transplantation

Camillo Ricordi

Islet cell transplantation in patients with type I diabetes mellitus is limited by the requirement for chronic recipient immunosuppression, the side effects of which are potentially more harmful to the patient than the administration of exogenous insulin. Islet cell transplantation has therefore been available only to patients who are already receiving immunosuppressive agents for a previous or concurrent solid organ transplant, such as a kidney.

The recipient categories for islet and kidney transplantation are (1) Simultaneous islet/kidney, in which islets (either from the same donor or from multiple donors) are infused at or around the time of renal transplantation (generally postoperative day 0–7); (2) islet after kidney, in which the islet allograft, generally from a different donor or donors, is performed months to years after the original renal allograft.

In both cases, the preferred islet transplant site is the liver, by catheterization of the portal vein either at the time of renal transplantation, or by percutaneous catheterization of the portal vein. The latter is the preferred modality for islet infusion in islet-after-kidney transplantation and whenever islet transplantation is delayed, ie, after induction treatment with antilymphocyte globulin (ALG) or muromonab-CD3 (Orthoclone OKT3, Ortho, Raritan, NJ). We have performed only one renal subcapsular islet transplantation (beneath the renal capsule of the transplanted kidney), which did not result in substantial posttransplant C-peptide secretion. Unlike the situation in small animal experimental models, in which the renal subcapsular site is an excellent location for implantation of insulin-producing tissue, in humans, the characteristics of the renal capsule and the mechanical stress to the implanted islets may render this location unsuitable.

Insulin independence has been achieved in several patients who received intrahepatic islet allografts and has persisted in some instances for years. However, most recipients of islet allografts have either never become insulin independent or after a temporary interval without insulin have returned to insulin therapy.[107–112] Rejection, recurrence of autoimmunity, insufficient β cell mass, and problems related to islet engraftment at a heterotopic site have been postulated to play a role in islet graft failure.

Results indicate that patients who have maintained islet allograft function, even in the absence of complete insulin independence, have excellent glycemic control compared with the pretransplant period. In fact, islet allografts with partial graft function (C-peptide secretion >1 ng/mL) can be associated with long-term metabolic control that appears superior to that observed in patients undergoing intensive insulin therapy, such as in the insulin regimens used in the Diabetes Control and Complications Trial.[113] Reports from several centers indicate that patients with long-term partial graft function have maintained normal or near normal glycosylated hemoglobin levels for more than 4 years without the occurrence of severe hypoglycemic episodes associated with intensive insulin therapy. In addition, the hyperinsulinemia that accompanies systemic venous drainage in whole-organ pancreatic transplantation is eliminated.

The International Islet Transplant Registry[114] reported a detailed analysis involving 75 patients with type I diabetes who received transplants between 1990 and 1993, who were C-peptide–negative before islet cell transplantation. At 1 year the patient survival rate was 95%, and the graft survival rate (defined as a basal C-peptide level >1 ng/mL) was 28%; 11% of patients were insulin independent. In patients who became insulin independent, four common factors were identified: (1) the mean preservation time of the pancreas was less than 8 hours, (2) patients received more than 6000 islet equivalents per kilogram body weight, (3) islets were transplanted into the liver via the portal vein, and (4) induction immunosuppression was given and consisted of antithymocyte globulin (ATG) and ALG (but not OKT3). Recipient age, sex, or duration of diabetes, and number of donor pancreata and islet purity did not appear to affect 1-year graft survival rate. The number of patients with a C-peptide level greater than 1 ng/mL more than 1 year after transplantation was higher when all four criteria were met (46%) than when only one was met (20%). Similarly, the percentage of insulin independent patients was significantly higher ($P = 0.001$) when all four criteria were met (29%) versus only one (1%). This can be compared with the overall 1-year insulin independence rate achieved in recipients of islet allografts who have undergone pancreatectomy (43%) (these patients also received livers from the same donors after removal of the upper abdominal organs for cancer), and for all categories of islet allotransplants combined (14%).

The true potential of islet cell transplantation will not be realized until it is possible to infuse islets in the absence of immunosuppression or with agents that do not have harmful side effects. Ultimately, of course, patients with diabetes would receive transplants early in the course of the disease.

The field of islet cell transplantation has progressed rapidly over the past decade. As we look to the future, it may be necessary to question the paradigms that have limited the application of islet transplantation as therapy for type I diabetes. An adequate number of islets can be isolated to reverse diabetes, and even in the absence of insulin independence, metabolic control can be achieved. This alone may be an important achievement for patients with diabetes, even if complete insulin independence has not occurred. Maintaining normoglycemia without intensive insulin therapy (and without a greatly restricted lifestyle), eliminating severe hypoglycemia and diabetic ketoacidosis, and maintaining normal or near-normal hemoglobin A_{1C} levels are goals within reach of combined kidney-islet transplantation procedures. The real challenge for the future may be to achieve similar goals without the requirement for chronic recipient immunosuppression and to perform islet transplantation in the early stages of disease, perhaps obviating the need for renal transplantation.

▲ REFERENCES

Concomitant or Sequential Kidney Transplantation with Other Organs

1. UNOS: Single and Multiorgan US Transplant Procedures (data table). *UNOS Update* 9:36, 1993.
2. Nankivell BJ, Gruenewald SM, Allen RDM, Chapman JR: Predicting glomerular filtration rate after kidney transplantation. *Transplantation* 59:1683–1689, 1995.
3. Rolin HA, Hall PM, Wei R: Inaccuracy of estimated creatinine clearance for prediction of iothalamate glomerular filtration fraction rate. *Am J Kidney Dis* 4:48–54, 1984.
4. McCauley J, Van Thiel DH, Starzl TE, Puschett JB: Acute and chronic renal failure in liver transplantation. *Nephron* 55:121–128, 1990.
5. Schrier R, Caramelo C: Hemodynamics and hormonal alterations in hepatic cirrhosis. In: Epstein M (ed), *The Kidney in Liver Disease,* ed 3. Baltimore, 1988.
6. McCauley J, Gaynord M, Hrinya M, Starzl TE: Dialysis in liver failure and liver transplantation. *Transplant Proc* 25:1740, 1993.
7. McCauley J, Farkus SJ, Prasad HA, Murray SA: Cyclosporine and FK 506 induced inhibition of renal epithelial cell proliferation. *Transplant Proc* 23:2829–2830, 1991.
8. Badalamenti S, Graziani G, Salerno F, Ponticelli C: Hepatorenal syndrome: new perspectives in pathogenesis and treatment (review). *Arch Intern Med* 153:1957–1967, 1993.
9. Bernardi M, Trevisani F, Gasbarrini A, Gasbarrini G: Hepatorenal disorders: role of the renin-angiotensin-aldosterone system (review). *Semin Liver Dis* 14:23–34, 1994.
10. Gines A, Escorsell A, Gines P, et al: Incidence, predictive factors, and prognosis of the hepatorenal syndrome in cirrhosis with ascites (comments). *Gastroenterology* 105:229–236, 1993.
11. Epstein M: Hepatorenal syndrome: emerging perspectives of pathophysiology and therapy (editorial). *J Am Soc Nephrol* 4:1735–1753, 1994.
12. Kopple MH, Coburn JW, Mims MM, et al: Transplantation of cadaveric kidneys from patients with hepatorenal syndrome: evidence for the functional nature of renal failure in advanced liver disease. *N Engl J Med* 280:1367–1371, 1969.
13. Iwatsuki S, Popovtzer MM, Corman JL, et al: Recovery from hepatorenal syndrome after orthotopic liver transplantation. *N Engl J Med* 289:1159–1173, 1973.
14. Gonwa TA, Klintmalm GB, Levy M, Jennings LS, Goldstein RM, Husberg BS: Impact of pretransplant renal function on survival after liver transplantation. *Transplantation* 59:361–365, 1995.
15. Johnson RJ, Couser WG: Hepatitis B infection and renal disease: clinical, immunopathogenetic and therapeutic considerations. *Kidney Int* 37:663, 1990.

16. Lai KN, Lai FM-M: Clinical features and natural history of hepatitis B virus related glomerulopathy in adults. *Kidney Int* 40:s–40, 1991.
17. Davis CL, Gretch DR, Carithers RL: Hepatitis C virus in renal disease (review). *Curr Opin Nephrol Hypertens* 3:164–173, 1994.
18. Misiani R, Bellavita P, Fenili D, et al: Hepatitis C virus infection in patients with essential mixed cryoglobulinemia. *Ann Intern Med* 117:573, 1992.
19. Van del Weil A, Valentijn TM, Schuurman HJ, et al: Circulating IgA immune complexes and skin IgA deposits in liver disease: relation to liver histology. *Dig Dis Sci* 33:679, 1988.
20. Noble-Jamieson G, Thiru S, Johnston P, et al: Glomerulonephritis with end stage liver disease in childhood. *Lancet* 339:706, 1992.
21. Margreiter R, Kramer R, Huber C, et al: Combined liver and kidney transplantation. *Lancet* 1:1077, 1984.
22. Margreiter R, Kornberger R, Koller J, et al: Preliminary results with combined hepatorenal transplantation. *Transplant Proc* 19:3552, 1987.
23. Fung J, Griffin M, Duquesnoy R, Shaw B, Starzl TE: Successful sequential liver-kidney transplantation in a patient with preformed lymphocytotoxic antibodies. *Transplant Proc* 19:767, 1987.
24. Fung J, Makowka L, Tzakis A, et al: Combined liver-kidney transplantation: Analysis of patients with preformed lymphocytotoxic antibodies. *Transplant Proc* 20:88, 1988.
25. Flye NW, Duffy BF, Phelan DL, et al: Protective effect of liver transplantation on a simultaneously transplanted kidney in a highly sensitized patient. *Transplantation* 50:1051, 1990.
26. Gonwa TA, Nery JR, Husberg BS, et al: Simultaneous liver and renal transplantation in man. *Transplantation* 46:690–693, 1988.
27. Shaked A, Thompson M, Wilkinson AH, et al: The role of combined liver/kidney transplantation in end stage hepato-renal disease. *Am Surg* 59:606–609, 1993.
28. Vogel W, Steiner E, Koller J, et al: Preliminary results with combined hepatorenal allografting. *Transplantation* 45:491–493, 1988.
29. Gil-Vernet S, Prieto C, Grino JM, et al: Combined liver-kidney transplantation. *Transplant Proc* 24:128–129, 1992.
29a. Rasmussen A, Davies HF, Jamieson NV, Evans DB, Calne RY. Combined transplantation of liver and kidney from the same donor protects the kidney from rejection and improves kidney graft survival. *Transplantatio*n 1995;59(6):919–921.
30. Starzl TE, Demetris AJ, Todo S, et al: Evidence for hyperacute rejection of human liver grafts: the case of the canary kidneys. *Clin Transpl* 3:37–45, 1989.
31. Starzl TE, Reyes J, Tzakis A, et al: Liver transplantation for polycystic liver disease. *Arch Surg* 125:575–577, 1990.
32. Taylor JE, Calne RY, Stewart WK: Massive cystic hepatomegaly in a female patient with polycystic kidney disease treated by combined hepatic and renal transplantation. *Q J Med* 81:771–775, 1991.
33. Lin TY, Chen CC, Wang SM: Treatment of non-parasitic cystic disease of the liver: a new approach to therapy with polycystic liver. *Ann Surg* 168:921–927, 1968.
34. Takeda A, Morozumi K, Uchida K, et al: Is cyclosporine-associated glomerulopathy a new glomerular lesion in renal allografts using CyA? *Transplant Proc* 25:515–517, 1993.
35. Gallegher RC, Kormos RL: Heart transplantation. In: Makowka LRG (ed), *The Handbook of Transplantation Management.* Austin TX, Landes, 1991.
36. Managan KF, Klumpp TR, Rosenfeld CS, Shadduck RK: Bone marrow transplantation. In: Makowka L (ed), *The Handbook of Transplantation Management.* Austin TX, Landes, 1991.

37. Bahnson HT, Gordon RD: Transplantation of other organs with the heart. *Cardiovasc Clin* 20:237–248, 1990.
38. Norman JC, Cooley DA, Kahan DB, et al: Total support of the circulation of a patient with post-cardiotomy stone-heart syndrome by a partial artificial heart (ALVAD) for 5 days followed by heart and kidney transplantation. *Lancet* 1:1125, 1978.
39. Faggian G, Bortolotti V, Stellin G, et al: Combined heart and kidney transplantation: a case report. *J Heart Transplant* 5:480, 1986.
40. Livesey SA, Rolles K, Calne RY, et al: Successful simultaneous heart and kidney transplantation using the same donor. *Clin Transpl* 2:1, 1988.
41. Antignac C, Gubler MC, Leverger G, Broyer M, Habib R: Delayed renal failure with extensive mesangiolysis following bone marrow transplantation. *Kidney Int* 35:1336–1344, 1989.
42. Cohen EP, Lawton CA, Moulder JE, Becker CG, Ash RC: Clinical course of late-onset bone marrow transplant nephropathy. *Nephron* 64:626–635, 1993.
43. Moulder JE, Cohen EP, Fish BL, Hill P: Prophylaxis of bone marrow transplant nephropathy with captopril, an inhibitor of angiotensin-converting enzyme. *Radiat Res* 136: 404–407, 1993.
44. Wassmann B, Martin H, Elsner S, et al: Microangiopathic hemolytic anemia and renal impairment following autologous bone marrow transplantation: a case of hemolytic uremic syndrome? *Bone Marrow Transplant* 14:849–851, 1994.
45. Silva VA, Frei-Lahr, D, Brown RA, Herzig GP: Plasma exchange and vincristine in the treatment of hemolytic uremic syndrome/thrombotic thrombocytopenic purpura associated with bone marrow transplantation. *J Clin Apheresis* 6:16–20, 1991.

Renal and Pancreatic Transplantation

46. Kelly WD, Lillehei RC, Merkel FK, et al: Allotransplantation of the pancreas and duodenum along with the kidney in diabetic nephropathy. *Surgery* 61:827–837, 1967.
47. Kroc Collaborative Study Group: Diabetic retinopathy after two years of intensified insulin treatment. *JAMA* 260:37–41, 1988.
48. Yanaga K, Podesta L, Broznick B: Multiple organ recovery for transplantation. In: Starzl TE, Shapiro R, Simmons R (eds), *Atlas of Organ Transplantation.* New York, Gower, 1991: 3.2–3.49.
49. Brons IGM, Calne RY, Trolles K, et al: Glucose control after simultaneous segmental pancreas and kidney transplantation. *Transplant Proc* 19:2288–2289, 1987.
50. Sutherland DER, Goetz FC, Moudry KC, et al: The use of recipients mesenteric vessels for revascularization of segmental pancreas grafts: technical and metabolic considerations. *Transplant Proc* 19:2300–2304, 1987.
51. Sollinger HW, Ploeg RJ, Eckhoff DE, et al: 200 consecutive simultaneous pancreas-kidney (SPK) transplants with bladder drainage. *Surgery* 114:736–744, 1993.
52. Gliedman ML, Gold M, Whittaker J, et al: Pancreatic duct to ureter anastomoses for exocrine drainage in pancreatic transplantation. *Am J Surg* 125:245–252, 1973.
53. Lillehei RC, Simmons RL, Najarian JS, et al: Pancreatico-duodenal allotransplantation: experimental and clinical experience. *Ann Surg* 172:405–436, 1970.
54. Prieto M, Sutherland DER, Fernandez-Cruz L, et al: Experimental and clinical experience with urinary amylase monitoring for early diagnosis of rejection in pancreas transplantation. *Transplantation* 43:73–79, 1987.
55. Nghiem DD, Gonwa TA, Corry RJ: Metabolic effects of urinary diversion of exocrine secretions in pancreatic transplantation. *Transplantation* 43:70–73, 1987.

56. Stephanian E, Gruessner RWG, Brayman KL, et al: Conversion of exocrine secretions from bladder to enteric drainage in recipients of whole pancreaticoduodenal transplants. *Ann Surg* 216:663–672, 1992.
57. Sollinger HW, Messing EM, Eckhoff DE, et al: Urological complications in 210 consecutive simultaneous pancreas and kidney transplant with bladder drainage. *Ann Surg* 218:561–570, 1993.
58. Tydèn G, Tibell A, Groth CG: Pancreaticoduodenal transplantation with enteric exocrine drainage: technical aspects. *Clin Transplant* 5:36–39, 1991.
59. Groth CG, Lundgren G, Klintmalm G, et al: Successful outcome of segmental human pancreatic transplantation with enteric exocrine diversion after modifications in technique. *Lancet* 2:522–524, 1982.
60. Tibell A, Brattström C, Wadström J, et al: Improved results using whole-organ pancreaticoduodenal transplants with enteric drainage. *Transplant Proc* 26:412–413, 1994.
61. Hesse UJ, Sutherland DER, Simmons RL, et al: Intra-abdominal infections in pancreas transplant recipients. *Ann Surg* 203:153–162, 1986.
62. Corry RJ, Egidi MF, Shapiro R, et al: Enteric drainage of pancreas transplants revisited. *Transplant Proc* 27:3048–3049, 1995.
63. Dubernard JM, Traeger J, Neyra P, et al: A new method of preparation of segmental pancreatic grafts for transplantation: trials in dogs and man. *Surgery* 84:633–640, 1978.
64. Shapiro R, Jordan ML, Scantlebury VP, et al: The superiority of tacrolimus in renal transplant recipients: the Pittsburgh experience. *Clin Transpl* 1995.
65. Nakache R, Mainetti L, Tydén G: Renal transplantation in diabetes mellitus: influence of combined pancreas-kidney transplantation on outcome. *Transplant Proc* 22:624, 1990.
66. Gruessner RWG, Dunn DL, Tzardis PJ, et al: Simultaneous pancreas and kidney transplantation versus single kidney transplantation and previous kidney transplants in uremic patients and single pancreatic transplants in non-uremic diabetic patients: comparison of rejection, morbidity and long-term outcome. *Transplant Proc* 22:622–623, 1990.
67. Sutherland DER, Gruessner A, Moudry-Munns K: Report on results of pancreas transplantation in the United States, October 1987 to October 1991 from the United Network for Organ Sharing Registry. *Clin Transpl* 31–38, 1991.
68. Tydén G, Tibell A, Bolinder J, et al: High incidence of late rejections in preuremic recipients of pancreas transplants given alone or in combination with renal transplants. *Transplant Proc* 22:1582–1583, 1990.
69. Brattström C, Tydèn G, Reinholt F, et al: Markers for pancreas graft rejection in humans. *Diabetes* 38(Suppl 1):57–62, 1989.
70. Kubota K, Reinholt FR, Tydén G, et al: Pancreas cytology for monitoring pancreatic grafts in the early postoperative period. *Transplant Int* 5:133–138, 1992.
71. Brattström C, Tydèn G, Lundgren G, et al: Studies of the exocrine secretion of segmental pancreatic grafts with special reference to the diagnosis of rejection and to the penetration of drugs into the pancreatic juice. *Transplant Proc* 19:2332–2336, 1987.
72. Steiner E, Klima G, Niederwisser D, et al: Monitoring of the pancreatic allograft by analysis of exocrine secretion. *Transplant Proc* 19:2336–2338, 1987.
73. Sutherland DER, Goetz FC, Najarian JS, et al: One-hundred pancreas transplants at a single institution. *Ann Surg* 200:414–440, 1984.
74. Florack G, Sutherland DER, Sibley RK, et al: Combined kidney and segmental pancreas allotransplantation in dogs. *Transplant Proc* 17:374–377, 1985.
75. Allen RD, Wilson TG, Griersson JM, et al: Percutaneous biopsy of bladder-drained pancreas transplants. *Transplantation* 51:1213–1216, 1991.
76. Casanova D, Gruessner R, Brayman K, et al: Retrospective analysis of the role of pancre-

atic biopsy (open and transcystoscopic technique) in the management of solitary pancreas transplants. *Transplant Proc* 25:1192–1193, 1993.
77. Egidi MR, Shapiro R, Khanna A, Fung JJ, Corry RJ: Fine-needle aspiration biopsy in pancreatic transplantation. *Transplant Proc* 27:3055–3056, 1995.
78. Sutherland D: Pancreatic transplantation: an update. *Diabetes Metab Rev* 1:152–165, 1993.
79. Navarro X, Kennedy WR, Loewenson RB, et al: Influence of pancreas transplantation on cardiorespiratory reflexes, nerve conduction and mortality in diabetes mellitus. *Diabetes* 39:802–806, 1990.
80. Martin X, Lefrancois N, Marechal JM, et al: Pancreas transplantation in Lyon: overall results. *Diabetologia* 34:8–10, 1991.
81. Brattström C, Tibell A, Tydèn G, et al: Outcome in 22 patients with pancreas transplants functioning beyond 5 years. *Transplant Proc* 26:414–415, 1994.
82. Cats S, Galton J: Effect of original disease in kidney transplant outcome. In: Terasaki PI (ed), *Clinical Kidney Transplantation* Los Angeles, UCLA Press, 1985:III.
83. Robertson RP, Abid M, Sutherland DER, et al: Glucose homeostasis and insulin secretion in human recipients of pancreas transplantation. *Diabetes* 38(Suppl 1):97–98, 1989.
84. Pozza G, Bosi E, Secchi A, et al: Metabolic control of type 1 (insulin dependent) diabetes after pancreas transplantation. *Br Med J* 291:510–513, 1985.
85. Tibell A, Bolinder J, Tydèn G, et al: Long term glucose control after pancreatic transplantation with enteric exocrine diversion. *Transplant Proc* 24:856, 1992.
86. Pagano G, Cavallo-Perin P, Cassader M, et al: An in vivo and in vitro study of the mechanism of prednisone-induced insulin resistance in healthy subjects. *J Clin Invest* 72:1814–1820, 1983.
87. Andersson A, Borg H, Hallberg A, et al: Longterm effects of cyclosporine A on cultured mouse pancreatic islets. *Diabetologia* 27:66–69, 1984.
88. Reboldi GP, Ruggeri A, Quintaliani G, et al: Cyclosporine induces a defect in insulin independent and dependent glucose disposal in kidney transplanted patients: a minimal model assessment. *Diabetologia* 34(Suppl 2):A76, 1991.
89. Gunnarsson R, Klintmalm G, Lundgren G, et al: Deterioration in glucose metabolism in pancreatic transplant recipients after conversion from azathioprine to cyclosporine. *Transplant Proc* 16:709–712, 1984.
90. Christiansen E, Tibell A, Rasmussen K, et al, and the Danish-Swedish Study Group of Metabolic Effect of Pancreas Transplantation (DSSGMEPT): Defects in quantitative and qualitative β-cell function following successful segmental pancreas transplantation. *Transplant Proc* 25:1186–1189, 1993.
91. Christiansen E, Tibell A, Vølund A, et al and the Danish-Swedish Study Group of Metabolic Effect of Pancreas Transplantation (DSSGMEPT): Insulin secretion, insulin action and non-insulin-dependent glucose uptake in pancreas transplant recipients. *Clin Endocrinol Metab* 79:1561–1569, 1994.
92. Solders G, Wilczek H, Gunnarsson R, et al Effects of combined pancreatic and renal transplantation on diabetic neuropathy. *Lancet* 2:1232–1235, 1987.
93. Solders G, Tydén G, Persson A, et al: Improvement in diabetic neuropathy four years after successful pancreatic and renal transplantation. *Diabetologia* 34:125–127, 1991.
94. Kennedy WR, Navarro X, Goetz F, et al: Effects of pancreatic transplantation on diabetic neuropathy. *N Engl J Med* 322:1031–1037, 1990.
95. Müller-Felber W, Landgraf R, Scheuer F, et al: Diabetic neuropathy 3 years after successful pancreas and kidney transplantation. *Diabetes* 42:1482–1486, 1993.
96. Ulbig N, Kampick A. Landgraf R, et al: The influence of combined pancreatic and renal transplantation on advanced diabetic retinopathy. *Transplant Proc* 19:3554–3556, 1987.

97. Ramsey RC, Goetz FC, Sutherland DER, et al: Progression of diabetic retinopathy after pancreas transplantation for insulin dependent diabetes mellitus. *N Engl J Med* 318: 208–214, 1988.
98. Jörneskog G, Östergren J, Tydén G, et al: Dose combined kidney and pancreas transplantation reverse functional diabetic microangiopathy? *Transplant Int* 3:167–170, 1990.
99. Abendroth P, Landgraf R, Milner WD, et al: Course of diabetic microangiopathy after simultaneous pancreas and kidney transplantation. *Transplant Proc* 20:874–875, 1988.
100. Wilczek H, Jaremko G, Tydèn G, et al: Evolution of diabetic neuropathy in kidney grafts. Evidence that a simultaneously transplanted pancreas exerts a protective effect. *Transplantation* 59:51–57, 1995.
101. Bilous RW, Mauer SM, Sutherland DER, et al: The effects of pancreas transplantation on the glomerular structure of renal allografts in patients with insulin dependent diabetes. *N Engl J Med* 321:80–85, 1989.
102. Fioretto P, Mauer SM, Bilous RW, et al: Effects of pancreas transplantation on glomerular structure in insulin-dependent diabetic patients with their own kidneys. *Lancet* 342:1193–1196, 1993.
103. Nakache R, Tydén G, Groth CG: Quality of life in diabetic patients undergoing combined pancreas-kidney transplantation and kidney transplantation only. *Diabetes* 38(Suppl 1):40–42, 1989.
104. Pichlmeier W, Bollinger M, Nusser J: Quality of life in type 1 (insulin-dependent) diabetic patients prior to and after pancreas and kidney transplantation in relation to organ function. *Diabetologia* 34:150–157, 1991.
105. Secchi A, DiCarlo V, Martinenghi S: Effects of pancreas transplantation on life expectancy, kidney function, and quality of life in uraemic type-1 (insulin dependent) diabetic patients. *Diabetologia* 34(Suppl 1):141–144, 1991.
106. Gross CR, Zehrer CL: Health-related quality of life outcomes of pancreas transplant recipients. *Clin Transplant* 6:165–171, 1992.

Renal and Pancreatic Islet Cell Transplantation

107. Ricordi C, Tzakis AG, Carroll PB, et al: Human islet transplantation in 22 consecutive cases. *Transplantation* 53:407, 1992.
108. Scharp DW, Lacy PE, Santiago JV, et al: Results of our first nine intraportal islet allografts in type I, insulin-dependent diabetic patients. *Transplantation* 51:76, 1991.
109. Warnock GL, Kneteman NM, Ryan E, Seelis REA, Rabinovitch A, Rajotte RV: Normoglycemia after transplantation of freshly isolated and cryopreserved pancreatic islets in Type I (insulin-dependent) diabetes mellitus. *Diabetologia* 34:55, 1991.
110. Socci C, Falqui L, Davalli AM, et al: Fresh human islet transplantation to replace pancreatic endocrine function in type I diabetic patients. *Acta Diabetol* 28:151, 1991.
111. Warnock G, Kneteman NM, Ryan EA, Rabinovitch A, Rajotte RV: Long-term follow-up after transplantation of insulin-producing pancreatic islets into patients with Type I (insulin-dependent) diabetes mellitus. *Diabetologia* 35:89, 1992.
112. Ricordi C. (ed): *Pancreatic Islet Cell Transplantation.* Austin, TX, Landes, 1992.
113. DCCT Research Group: The effect of intensive treatment of diabetes on the development and progression of long-term complications in insulin-dependent diabetes mellitus *N Engl J Med* 329:977, 1993.
114. International Islet Transplant Registry: Newsletter. Vol 5, No. 1, June 1995.

16

Pregnancy after Kidney Transplantation

Velma P. Scantlebury

As described in previous chapters, there have been ongoing improvements in survival and quality of life after renal transplantation. These have been accompanied by an improvement in reproductive function and reversal of the relative infertility that occurs despite maintenance hemodialysis. Chronic renal failure has been known to be associated with sexual dysfunction and, for many women, infertility and/or menstrual irregularities. Conception is rare for women on dialysis, and occurs at a rate of one in every 200 patients. There have been a few reports of pregnancies occurring in patients on dialysis[1,2] and, in most cases, abortions have been recommended because of the risks from exacerbation of hypertension and superimposed preeclampsia.[3] Successful live births have occurred in fewer than 20% of these patients. Renal failure is often associated with hypogonadotropic hypogonadism, which may be the cause of the low incidence of successful pregnancies.[4]

Since the initial case report in 1963 of a successful pregnancy 5 years following kidney transplantation, there have been hundreds of successful pregnancies reported in renal transplant recipients.[5,6] In spite of improving outcomes, pregnancy after renal transplantation remains a high-risk endeavor and mandates a cooperative effort involving the nephrologist, surgeon, obstetrician, and patient, to minimize the short- and long-term complications to both mother and child.

In this chapter we will review the experience of women undergoing childbirth after kidney transplantation, with a focus on outcomes and suggested management strategies.

▲ HISTORICAL BACKGROUND

The first reported successful pregnancy occurred in a recipient of a kidney transplant from an identical twin sister performed in 1958.[7] The first successful pregnancy in a recipient of a cadaveric kidney transplant did not occur until 1970. The use of immunosuppressive agents following kidney transplantation and the continued need for these medications during pregnancy have raised justifiable concerns about the adverse effects of such drugs on the offspring of these patients.

The effects of corticosteroids and azathioprine in pregnancy are relatively well known. The intrauterine growth retardation associated with steroid use in animal studies has not been substantiated in humans when low doses are used, ie, less than 15 mg/day of prednisone. Steroids may be implicated in the increased frequency of premature rupture of membranes in transplant recipients and can aggravate hypertension in the mother. Adrenal insufficiency in two infants has been reported by Penn, and this may have been the cause of death in a set of twins born to a mother on steroids and azathioprine.[8,9] Overall, however, the treatment of rejection with steroids, if necessary, should not be avoided during pregnancy.

The use of azathioprine has been associated with a slight increase in the frequency of congenital anomalies in the offspring. Hou has summarized the neonatal problems seen with the use of azathioprine in transplant recipients, with one third having significant complications.[10] The incidence of prematurity has been high, ranging from 20% to 60%. Of newborns, 20% to 50% have been small for gestational age, and congenital anomalies have been seen in 3%. Leukopenia and thrombocytopenia have been reported with azathioprine use, but reducing the dose to 1–2 mg/kg has resulted in a lower incidence of these complications.[11] Chromosome studies on lymphocytes from an infant born to a mother on azathioprine have demonstrated chromatin gaps and chromosome deletions, which disappeared after 1 year. Studies in rats have shown normal offspring, but increased infertility in the second generation.[12] This has not been reported clinically in the adult offspring of recipients treated with azathioprine.

▲ PREGNANCY AND CYCLOSPORINE

The first successful pregnancy in a renal transplant recipient on cyclosporine was recorded in 1982. Since then, hundreds of female recipients have undergone successful pregnancies while taking cyclosporine. Earlier reports documented low birth weights similar to those seen under azathioprine-based immunosuppression, but an increased number of live births were observed.[13–15] Severe intrauterine growth retardation with cyclosporine was described by Pickrell, implicating a direct effect of cyclosporine on fetal growth. Over 50% of infants had growth retardation, and the incidence was higher in the presence of renal dysfunction and hypertension.[16] However, nearly one third of infants had growth retardation in the absence of maternal hypertension or renal dysfunction. This direct effect of cyclosporine is thought to be dose related, and it is thus necessary to maintain cyclosporine levels as low as possible during pregnancy.

Studies of cyclosporine concentration in the blood, as well as its metabolities in maternal and cord blood, have shown that the highest concentrations of cyclosporine are in the umbilical cord and placenta. Venkataramanan has documented the concentration of cyclosporine and its metabolities in mother and child, with no specific harmful effects observed.[17] Claris also reported on the pharmacokinetics of cyclosporine in 16 newborns of transplant mothers and reported no correlations between maternal and cord levels, or between peripheral blood and cord blood levels. No detectable level in the infants was found 3–5 days after birth in most cases.[18] In addition, there were no toxic effects on the offspring. Cyclosporine is not known to be mutagenic or carcinogenic; it does cross the placental barrier, but there is no evidence of direct harm to the fetus.

A national transplantation pregnancy registry has been compiled by Armenti and his associates, and they have reported on the outcome of pregnancies in kidney transplant recipients treated with cyclosporine.[19,20] Spontaneous abortions occurred in 16.4%, with a live birthrate of 68%. Of 137 live births, 54% were premature, and 50% had low birth weights. The risks to the mother included a high incidence of preeclampsia (29%), premature delivery, and an increased rate of caesarian sections (64%). Other maternal factors present in cyclosporine patients were (1) an increased incidence of drug-treated hypertension prior to pregnancy (56%), (2) an increased incidence of maternal diabetes, and (3) a shorter time interval between transplantation and pregnancy. All three of these risk factors have been shown to affect the newborn adversely and are predictors of lower birth weight.

Sturgiss et al reported on the impact of hypertension on perinatal outcome and emphasized that adverse outcomes (stillbirths, growth retardation, and death) were more likely when hypertension was seen prior to 28 weeks gestation; hypertension was noted in 73% of pregnancies.[21] They also showed that pregnancy itself had no adverse effect on renal function or blood pressure in renal allograft recipients.[22]

Since a significant number of patients on cyclosporine are hypertensive, it is important to try to maintain good blood pressure control in order to decrease the risk to the fetus. While it is tempting to reduce the cyclosporine dose to control this side effect, trough levels during pregnancy are often lower than prepregnancy values.[23] At the same time, the serum creatinine improves during the first and second trimester in patients with good graft function. During the third trimester, there can be a rise in the serum creatinine back to a prepregnancy level. A rising serum creatinine above baseline with a falling cyclosporine level may be a sign of rejection. Dosage requirements as much as 50% higher have been reported, especially during the third trimester. Changes in the levels may be due to the increased distribution of pregnancy and/or the increase in metabolic degradation of cyclosporine. Maintaining appropriate levels is necessary to prevent rejection, especially in the perinatal period.

▲ PREGNANCY AND TACROLIMUS

Tacrolimus was first used at the University of Pittsburgh in 1989 as a primary immunosuppressive agent after transplantation. Jain reported on nine female liver transplant recipients who became pregnant while using tacrolimus.[24] Five of these patients had been switched to tacrolimus from cyclosporine because of chronic rejection. The length of time on tacrolimus ranged from 6 to 22 months. One fetal death was reported: an infant born at 22 weeks, having been conceived within 1 month after transplantation. None of the other babies were considered small for gestational age, but all had low birth weights. A successful pregnancy born to a liver transplant patient on tacrolimus alone was also reported by Winkler.[25] This infant was delivered at 36 weeks by caesarian section and had a normal birth weight for gestational age.

So far, there have been no published reports of pregnancies in kidney transplant recipients on tacrolimus. Within our own center, there are data from six kidney recipients who became pregnant while on tacrolimus. A preterm delivery occurred at 28 weeks, with subsequent normal growth and development. One infant delivered at 38 weeks was stillborn, without any abnormal pathology on autopsy. Two patients who had normal renal function prior to their pregnancies developed acute rejection in the early postpartum period, which was treated with steroids and an increased dose of tacrolimus. Though not on dialysis, they have evidence of chronic rejection on biopsy, and have serum creatinine levels of 1.7 mg/dL and 3.1 mg/dL, 1 and 2.5 years after delivery.

In this small experience, the long-term use of tacrolimus in females after transplantation has not had negative impact on their offspring. There are no reports to date of any teratogenicity of this drug. Reports from murine pregnancies using low-dose tacrolimus have not shown any detrimental effects.[26] At high doses, there was resorption of all fetuses. It is essential that patients on tacrolimus be weaned to the lowest possible dose prior to conception. The added advantage of the ability to discontinue steroids in many patients taking tacrolimus may lead to fewer steroid-related side effects in pregnancies. It is even possible that as these patients conceive on tacrolimus monotherapy, there may be a trend toward normal-birth-weight babies and less prematurity, but no data are yet available. More time is needed to assess the effects of tacrolimus on offspring long term, but for the short term, patients have given birth to normal, healthy babies.

▲ GRAFT FUNCTION

Although pregnancy can cause an increase in the glomerular filtration rate, which could theoretically lead to hyperfiltration and resultant glomerulosclerosis, the hyperfiltration of pregnancy may be flow related, with no concomitant increase in intraglomerular pressure. Glomerular hypertension, on the other hand, can cause glomerulosclerosis. In one study of non-cyclosporine-treated patients, when pregnant and nonpregnant kidney transplant recipients were compared, there was no evidence of an adverse effect of pregnancy on long-term renal function or the development of hypertension,[22] with a mean follow-up of 12 years (range 4–23). In cyclosporine-treated patients, Armenti[20] found that graft dysfunction after pregnancy was seen in patients with higher mean serum creatinine levels and lower mean cyclosporine doses prior to conception. It was postulated that the higher baseline creatinine may have prompted a reduction in the cyclosporine dosage, which could be detrimental. It was also noted that while the serum creatinine decreased during pregnancy in patients with stable graft function, cyclosporine blood levels also tended to drop during pregnancy. This may be due to the changes in volume distribution, as previously discussed.

Hypertension and declining renal function may cause patients to be at risk for subsequent graft loss and also for low-birth-weight infants. The success of the pregnancy and the graft is related to good prepregnancy graft function, the absence of hypertension, and an interval from the time of transplantation to conception of at least 2–3 years. However, waiting 5 or more years may result in impaired renal function postpartum which fails to recover, because of gradually deteriorating renal function secondary to chronic rejection.

There is other evidence to suggest that long-term graft survival in patients after pregnancy is inferior to that of matched controls. Salmela reported 29 pregnancies in 22 recipients, most of whom were on ozathioprine-based immunosuppression.[27] Though only one patient lost her graft at 1 month after delivery, seven (32%) patients lost their grafts after the first year postpartum. Three of these occurred at 13, 25, and 39 months postdelivery respectively; in four patients graft losses to chronic rejection were seen after 3–11 years. More recent data from Armenti[20] suggest that graft loss after delivery occurred within 2 years when there was associated graft dysfunction or rejection during pregnancy. The incidence of graft dysfunction during pregnancy was higher under cyclosporine–based immunosuppression when compared with azathioprine-based therapy.

Davison[11] suggested that chronic rejection may occur with a progressive subclinical course, which may or may not be immunologically based. Rejection is often difficult to diagnose, but should be suspected if there is any deterioration in renal function. It is known that there is a transient reduction in GFR during the third trimester, but such changes are not necessarily representative of renal impairment. Proteinuria is also present in 30–40% of pregnancies, but in the absence of hypertension is not significant.

Compromised renal function prior to conception can be associated with a greater possibility of irreversible renal impairment postpartum. While reports show that the existence of hypertension preconception can lead to significant adverse outcomes such as neonatal death, stillbirths, and severe growth retardation, serum creatinine levels and 24-hour creatinine clearances in these patients were no different when compared with good-outcome pregnancies.[21] This report suggests that the existence of prepregnancy hypertension, even if adequately treated, or hypertension occurring prior to 28 weeks' gestation, may contribute to covert microvascular changes that could led to compromised development of the uteroplacental circulation. It is interesting that in this series of 22 pregnancies in recipients treated with prednisone and azathioprine, there were no acute rejections, and only 1 patient experienced deteriorating renal function at 31 weeks; this patient progressed to graft failure by 11 months postpartum, having conceived 9 years after a living donor transplant.

▲ INFECTION

Cytomegalovirus (CMV) remains the most frequent cause of viral infection posttransplantation. The donor kidney is known to be a major source of CMV in primary infections. Reactivation of CMV is also possible in the postoperative period. For transplant recipients, the early diagnosis and treatment of CMV disease has resulted in markedly reduced morbidity and mortality. However, there is a risk of congenital CMV infection in the offspring of a renal transplant recipient; this was first reported in 1975.[28] With the use of cyclosporine, there has been no reported increased incidence of congenital CMV infections as the cause of neonatal deaths or spontaneous abortions.

The risk of urinary tract infection in the pregnant immunosuppressed female should always be a focus of concern, with careful monitoring throughout the pregnancy. If there is a need for invasive procedures such as fetal monitoring with scalp electrodes or intrauterine pressure monitoring, prophylactic antibiotics are recommended.

▲ OFFSPRING OF MALE RECIPIENTS

For many male patients with renal failure, impotence and loss of libido have been seen frequently, with less than 10% experiencing any improvement in sexual function after the initiation of dialysis. Moderate recovery of sexual function has been noted after successful transplantation.[29]

The outcome of pregnancies with fathers on immunosuppression after transplantation has not been different from that seen in the general population. Penn reported on 19 male recipients responsible for 28 pregnancies.[5,30] Nineteen live births occurred, 18 of which were normal. There was one spontaneous abortion and 3 unborn pregnancies. One neonate had congenital abnormalities. Salmela[27] reported on 65 children born to 39 male kidney recipients, with a mean age of 26 years at time of transplantation. Mean gestational age was 40 weeks, with only one stillborn infant. Mean weights were normal for age, with normal growth and development in all children after 1–8 years of follow-up. Ahlswede et al analyzed the outcomes of pregnancies fathered by 204 transplant recipients who received kidney, heart, liver, or kidney/pancreas grafts.[31] Although there was a 3.3% incidence of neonatal malformations, this was not different from that seen in the general population.

Overall, children born to male transplant recipients are essentially at no increased risk for developing abnormalities. For patients with familial diseases as the cause of their renal disease, there will of course be a higher risk of transmitting renal disease to their offspring (eg, polycystic kidney disease).

▲ RECOMMENDATIONS FOR PATIENTS DURING PREGNANCY AFTER KIDNEY TRANSPLANTATION

Pregnancy management should begin with the establishment of guidelines for all premenopausal female patients undergoing transplantation. Patients should understand that the guidelines are meant to offer them the best possible outcome for both mother and child and to minimize any potential risks that are inherent due to the presence of the graft and the use of immunosuppressive agents.

Good general health and stable renal function should be present before any consideration of pregnancy. A minimum of 2 years following transplantation will allow for tapering of the dosage of immunosuppressive agents. This interval will also allow for better control or perhaps elimination of posttransplant hypertension and/or diabetes. Patients should understand that there are greater risks associated with hypertension and elevated serum creatinine levels, but the majority of these women can still have successful pregnancies. Some 25% of transplant recipients are diabetic, and this places a significant proportion of females at risk for the associated complications of diabetes and pregnancy. Any pregnant transplant recipient should be managed at a high-risk center, where the transplant surgeon, nephrologist, and obstetrician can work together. It is reasonable to expect, prior to the consideration of pregnancy, that there be no evidence of graft rejection or hydronephrosis. Proteinuria should be absent or minimally present. Patients should be of a reasonable stature compatible with a good obstetric outcome.

Breast-feeding is discouraged for patients taking any immunosuppressive drugs. Cyclosporine levels in breast milk were reported to be greater than 200 ng/mL.[10] These levels can be toxic to a newborn. Similar recommendations exist for tacrolimus or any other immunosuppressive agent.

▲ REFERENCES

1. Rizzoni G, Ehrich JHH, Broyer M, et al: Successful pregnancies in women on renal replacement therapy: Report from the EDTA Registry. *Nephrol Dial Transplant* 7:279–287, 1992.
2. Pregnancy after renal replacement (Editorial). *Br Med J* 1:733–734, 1976.
3. Davison JM: Dialysis, transplantation, and pregnancy. *Am J Kidney Dis* 17(2):127–132, 1991.
4. Tagatz GE, Simmons RL: Pregnancy after renal transplantation. *Ann Intern Med* 82:113, 1975.
5. Penn I, Makowski EL, Harris P: Parenthood following renal and hepatic transplantation. *Transplantation* 30:397, 1980.
6. Davison JM: Pregnancy in renal allograft recipients: Prognosis and management. *Balliere's Clin Obstet Gynecol* 1:1027–1045, 1987.

7. Murray JE, Reid DE, Harrison JH, et al: Successful pregnancies after human renal transplantation. *N Engl J Med* 269:346, 1963.
8. Penn I, Makowski EL, Harris P: Parenthood following renal transplantation. *Kidney Int* 18:221, 1980.
9. Lower GD, Stevens LE, Najarian JS, Reemtsma K: Problems from immunosuppressives during pregnancy. *Communications in Brief* 111(8):1120–2212, 1971.
10. Hou S: Pregnancy in organ transplant recipients. *Med Prob Pregnancy* 73:667–683, 1989.
11. Davison JM, Dellagrammatikas H, Parkin JM: Maternal azathioprine therapy and depressed haemopoiesis in the babies of renal allograft patients. *Br J Obstet Gynecol* 92:233–239, 1985.
12. Reiners TS, Sluss PM: 6-Mercaptopurine treatment of pregnant mice: Effect on second and third generation. *Science* 201:65, 1978.
13. Cockburn I, Krupp P, Monka C: Present experience of sandimmum in pregnancy. *Transplant Proc* 21(4):3730–3732, 1989.
14. Burrows DA, O'Neil TJ, Sorrells TL: Successful twin pregnancy after renal transplant maintained on cyclosporine A immunosuppression. *Obstet Gynecol* 72(3):459–461, 1988.
15. Lewis GJ, Lamont CA, Lee HA, Slapak M: Successful pregnancy in renal transplant recipient taking cyclosporine A. *Br Med J* 286:603, 1983.
16. Pickrell MD, Sawers R, Michael J: Pregnancy after renal transplantation: Severe intrauterine growth retardation during treatment with cyclosporine A. *Br Med J* 296–825, 1988.
17. Venkataramanan R, Koneru B, Chung-Chiee PW, et al: Cyclosporine and its metabolites in mother and baby. *Transplantation* 46(3):468–469, 1988.
18. Claris O, Picaud JC, Brazier JL, Salle BL: Pharmacokinetics of cyclosporine A in 16 newborn infants of renal or cardiac transplant mothers. *Dev Pharmacol Ther* 20:180–185, 1993.
19. Armenti VT, Ahlswede KM, Ahlswede A, et al: National transplantation pregnancy registry—outcomes of 154 pregnancies in cyclosporine-treated female kidney transplant recipients. *Transplantation* 579(4):502–506, 1994.
20. Armenti VT, Ahlswede KM, Ahlswede A, et al: Variables affecting birthweight and graft survival in 197 pregnancies in cyclosporine-treated female kidney transplant recipients. *Transplantation* 59(4):476–479, 1995.
21. Sturgiss SN, Davison JM: Perinatal outcome in renal allograft recipients: Prognostic significance of hypertension and renal function before and during pregnancy. *Obstet Gynecol* 78(4):573–577, 1991.
22. Sturgiss SN, Davison JM: Effect of pregnancy on long-term function of renal allografts. *Am J Kidney Dis* 19(2):167–172, 1992.
23. Burrows L, Knight R, Thomas A, Panico M: Cyclosporine levels during pregnancy. *Transplant Proc* 26(5):2820–2821, 1994.
24. Jain A, Venkataramanan R, Lever J, et al: FK506 and pregnancy in liver transplant patients. *Transplantation* 56(6):1588–1589, 1993.
25. Winkler ME, Niesert S, Ringe B, Pichlmayr R: Successful pregnancy in a patient after liver transplantation maintained on FK506. *Transplantation* 56(6):1589–1590, 1993.
26. Farley DE, Shelby J, Alexander D, Scott JR: The effect of two new immunosuppressive agents, FK506 and Didemnin B, in murine pregnancy. *Transplantation* 52(1):106–110, 1991.
27. Salmela KT, Kyllonen LEF, Holmberg C, Gronhagen-Riska C: Impaired renal function after pregnancy in renal transplant recipients. *Transplantation* 56(6):1372–1375, 1993.
28. Evans TJ, McCollum JP, Valdimarsson H: Congenital cytomegalovirus infection after maternal renal transplantation. *Lancet* 1:1359, 1975.

29. Salvatierra O, Jr, Fortmann JL, Belzer FO: Sexual function in males before and after renal transplantation. *Urology* 5(1):64–66, 1975.
30. Penn I, Makowski EL: Parenthood in kidney and liver transplant recipients. *Transplant Proc* 13(1Pt1):36–39, 1981.
31. Ahlswede KM, Armenti VT, Moritz MJ, et al: Premature births in female renal transplant recipients: Degree and effect of immunosuppressive regimen. *Surg Forum* 43:524–525, 1992.

17

Xenogeneic Renal Transplantation

Donald V. Cramer / Leonard Makowka

The use of cross-species transplants (xenografts) in clinical renal transplantation offers the potential for an unlimited supply of donor organs for the treatment of patients with end-stage kidney failure. At present, the most critical problem restricting the widespread use of transplantation as a therapeutic procedure is the shortage of human donor organs.[1] This shortage of organs limits transplantation to a relatively small number of patients, produces higher health care costs because of the need for continued dialysis for patients with end-stage renal disease (ESRD), and is associated with a certain dialysis-related mortality rate.

The development of nonhuman species as kidney xenograft donors would provide an important source of organs. One of the primary limitations in the current application of xenografting to resolve the problem of kidney donor shortages, however, is an incomplete lack of understanding of the nature of the xenograft reaction and the therapeutic techniques required to control adequately rejection of the donor graft.[2,3] Rejection of xenografts is more vigorous than rejection of allografts; the greater degree of genetic disparity between the donor and recipient species, the more rapid is the rejection.[4] Recipients of xenografts from genetically distant donors have performed circulating ("natural") antibody to the donor tissue before transplantation. The response is immediate because it is the result of a simple set of chemical reactions between preformed reactants. These pairs are called *discordant species.* For example, pig-to-human xenografts are destroyed within a few minutes or hours (hyperacute rejection).[5] In contrast, recipients of grafts from more closely related (*concordant*) species do not exhibit high titers of natural antibodies to donor tissues, and the grafts are rejected within a few (2–4) days (a delayed reaction compared with hyperacute reaction). Although preformed antibody is not traditionally believed to play an important role in this type of reaction, rejection of the xenograft is, in fact, mediated by antibody that is rapidly produced after transplantation.[6–8] Baboon-to-human xenografts are an example of a concordant pair in which rejection of the graft occurs in a delayed manner.

This chapter focuses on four areas. First, it provides an overview of the immunologic mechanisms involved in the rejection of xenografts, particularly those that might be seen in a future clinical application of kidney xenotransplantation. Second, it describes the characteristics of two species of potential xenograft donors for humans, baboons and pigs. Third, it summarizes the clinical experience with kidney xenotransplantation in humans. Finally, it describes areas of future experimentation that may lead to important advances in our ability to use xenografts to address the shortage of renal allografts.

▲ IMMUNOLOGIC CHARACTERISTICS OF THE XENOGRAFT REACTION

Antibody

The primary reason for failure of xenografts is the aggressive rejection of the graft by the host immune system. The present classification system divides xenograft reactions into those mediated by natural or preformed antibody (discordant) and those that are not (concordant). This classification has had an important influence on the choice of potential donors for human xenografting.[4] The implicit assumption is that the lack of natural antibody in a concordant reaction leads to the development of a T cell–mediated rejection reaction that may be more easily managed with traditional forms of immunosuppressive therapy. Humans do not exhibit high levels of natural antibody to closely related species, such as baboons and other nonhuman primates, and these species have served as the preferred donors in human xenografting.[2] Xenografts from these species are rejected aggressively but not immediately. Other potential donor species, such as pigs and sheep, are genetically more distant, and the role of preformed natural antibody is apparent early in the rejection process.[2] The presence of preformed anti-donor xenoantibodies precipitates violent, hyperacute rejection of the graft by the recipient because of deposition of the antibody on the graft endothelium and activation of the complement and coagulation systems. This type of xenograft rejection is difficult to control, and these species pose difficult problems in terms of their potential as organ donors for humans.

The characterization of xenograft rejection has produced substantial evidence that antibody plays an important role in the pathogenesis of both concordant and discordant xenograft rejections. The pathologic features of unmodified concordant rejection are those of antibody-mediated vascular injury. Rejection of both discordant and concordant xenografts therefore, is associated with evidence of humorally mediated damage rather than accumulation of inflammatory cells characteristic of T cell–mediated rejection. In instances of human xenografting in which the grafts are rejected late[9,10] or in experimental animals when sequential examination has been conducted,[6,11,12] the pathologic changes present in the grafts are consistent with antibody-mediated damage to the vessels of the grafts. The primary pathologic changes include endothelial cell swelling, necrosis, interstitial edema, platelet and fibrin thrombi, and hemorrhage.[13–15] Although the exact nature of the humoral response and target antigens that mediate the reaction is largely unknown, the changes are compatible with antibody binding to antigens expressed on the endothelium of the donor graft vessels with activation of the complement cascade.

Species that normally exhibit concordant reactions can also be shown to display hyperacute rejection after immunization with donor tissues. Immunization of rats with hamster lymphocytes[16] or cardiac grafts[17] results in an antibody-mediated hyperacute rejection of hamster xenografts. As described below, low levels of immunoglobulin M (IgM) antibody that react with hamster lymphocytes and vascular endothelium are normally present in rat sera. Immunization with hamster tissues stimulates the rapid rise of hamster-specific IgM antibodies and graft rejection. Passive transfer of the antibodies to naive animals precipitates a hyperacute rejection of a subsequent xenograft.

At present, the nature of the antibodies produced in response to either discordant or concordant grafts is not known. One possibility is that for both types of xenograft reactions, anti-donor IgM antibody is produced in response to the stimulation of precommitted B lymphocytes that are responsible for "natural" antibody present in the serum of the naive animals. Some investigators have suggested that $CD5^+$, T lymphocyte–independent B lymphocytes, similar to those that secrete polyreactive autoimmune antibodies, produce the preformed antibodies responsible for discordant xenograft reactions.[18] These antibodies react with proteins or glycoproteins in the range of 22–135 kd expressed on the surface of donor lymphocytes or endothelial cells.[19,20] Natural antibodies share with autoantibodies a broad pattern of reactivity to several antigens (ssDNA, thyroglobulin). It has been postulated that xenoantibodies are members of a family of antibodies produced by a subset of B cells, the B1 cells, including B1a ($CD5^+$) B cells and the B1b ($CD5^-$) "sister" B cells.[21–23] Antibodies eluted from xenogeneic organs perfused with human or monkey blood are thought to be polyreactive, and it has been suggested that they are produced by $CD5^+$ cells.[18,24,25] These conclusions, however, are based primarily on indirect evidence that suggests human polyreactive monoclonal antibodies (MoAb), some of which originate from $CD5^+$ B cells, react in vitro with xenoantigens expressed on porcine platelet extracts.[18] Evidence also suggests that antibodies eluted from rejected xenografts share idiotypic specificity with a human polyreactive MoAb known to bind strongly to xenogeneic (pig) endothelial cells.[25] Whether these antibodies would be directly involved in precipitating the rejection of these xenografts, however, is not known.

It also is possible that the antibody response that mediates xenograft rejection is a T lymphocyte–dependent, antigen-specific response induced after exposure of the recipient to new graft antigens. There is evidence, described below, that the xenograft response depends on $CD4^+$ helper T cells and that recognition of xenogeneic antigens in mice may involve antigen processing and presentation in the context of host major histocompatibility (MHC) antigens.[26] The rapidity of the response and the pattern of antigen recognition would require prior sensitization and evidence of restriction in the specificity of antigen recognition by the xenoreactive antibodies. At present, there is limited direct evidence to support either T cell–dependent or T cell–independent alternatives for explaining the nature of the antibody response.

Complement

Binding of anti-donor antibodies to the vascular endothelium of the xenograft is believed to result in activation of the classic complement pathway.[27] This activation may play an important role in the generation of humoral and cellular components of the coagulation-inflammatory cascades responsible for the rejection of xenografts. The exact nature of the complement activation and the relative roles that the classic and alternative pathways play in the hyperacute reaction are not clear. The primary evidence for involvement of the complement system in these reactions is the fact that xenograft survival is prolonged by prior treatment of the recipient with cobra venom factor, which depletes the C3 component of complement.[28,29] One current approach to prevent complement activation is to use a soluble form (sCR1) of human C3b/C4b receptor (complement receptor type 1 or CD35) that is found normally on endothelial cells.[30] As the complement cascade progresses, C3b and C4b are generated and bind to CD35. The product acts as a cofactor in the proteolysis of components of the C3 and C5 convertase steps. sCR1 should successfully compete for available C3b/C4b and prevent the progression of the complement cascade.

Both sCR1 and cobra venom factor prevent activation of both the classic and alternative complement pathways, which obscures the role that each pathway may play in the xenograft reaction. Other experiments, however, have demonstrated that inhibition of C1 activation prevents binding of C4b and iC3b to pig endothelium, suggesting that rejection of a pig xenograft is the result of activation of the classic pathway by the binding of natural human antibodies to the vascular endothelium.[31] There are also several reports of the precipitation of this type of response in the absence of preformed antibody, suggesting the inadvertent activation of the alternative complement pathway directly in some models of xenograft rejection.[32–34] Direct activation of the alternative complement pathway by an endothelial xenoantigen would precipitate the same type of disseminated thrombosis of small vessels that occurs with activation of the traditional pathway by preformed antibody. The guinea pig–to–rat cardiac xenograft model may represent an example of direct alternative pathway complement activation, as there is conflicting evidence for the involvement of preformed antibody early in the rejection of the grafts.[33,35] Most experiments are consistent with the concept of direct activation of complement as the initiating event in the reaction. There have been extensive and carefully executed attempts by some investigators to eliminate the existence of small amounts of preformed antibody in the guinea pig–to–rat model.[36,37] A similar lack of natural antibody (IgM) binding has been observed in the pig-to-rabbit model.[14] Direct activation of the alternative pathway may be relevant for human xenotransplantation, because the perfusion of human blood through rabbit kidneys results in complement activation, even in the absence of preformed antibody.[38]

The relative importance of the roles played by preformed antibody and complement activation for human xenotransplantation is not yet clear.[35,39] However, these reports suggest that both pathways may participate. If so, the hyperacute rejection associated with "discordant" xenografts may be the result of two or more distinct humoral pathogenetic mechanisms. It is of interest to note that the rejection of a pig liver xenograft by a patient at our hospital with fulminant liver failure exhibited evidence of activation of the alternative complement pathway in the graft as early as 2 hours posttransplantation.[5]

The therapy necessary to prevent alternative pathway–mediated rejection will be very different from that used with antibody-mediated reactions. One approach to circumventing the problem of simultaneous activation of both complement pathways is the use of agents, such as sCR1, that should compete for C3b/C4b in any complement cascade. This compound blocks both pathways and has been demonstrated to be highly effective in both rodent[40] and primate[41] models. Graft survival could be prolonged for that period of time during which effective inhibition of complement activation could be maintained. This form of therapy may well play an important role in future trials of clinical xenotransplantation.

Cells

The role that cellular immune responses play in the rejection of xenografts is less clear than that for allografts. Extensive examination of the involvement of the traditional cells that mediate allograft rejection, particularly in vitro lymphocyte responses, has demonstrated that the same cellular components of the lymphoid system participate in the xenograft reaction, albeit with reduced intensity.[26] T cell–mediated responses to xenografts are weak, apparently as a result of defective recognition of xenogeneic antigens by host T cells. The nature of this defect is not clear. In mice, xenoantigen recognition depends on host antigen-presenting cell processing and indirect presentation, whereas in humans xenoantigens may be recognized directly.

The induction phase of the immune response to xenografts is dependent on the activity of $CD4^+$ T cells. Depletion of $CD4^+$ cells has the effect of prolonging xenograft survival,[42] whereas depletion of $CD8^+$ cells has little influence on graft survival.[43] This form of graft rejection differs from the allograft response in which both T cell subsets are important. It is not clear whether the effect of CD4 T-cell depletion is related to the function of this subset of cells in cell-mediated immune responses or to the role that these cells play in the regulation of humoral antibody production. Treatment with immunosuppressive agents that are most effective for interfering with T-cell function, such as cyclosporine and tacrolimus, has little effect on the rejection of xenografts.[44–46] In contrast, combination therapy that includes one of these agents and a second immunosuppressive compound that prevents antibody production can be highly effective for preventing xenograft rejection.[44,45] This suggests that control of humoral antibody production is a key factor for effective control of the xenograft reaction and that future therapy for this form of graft rejection will include agents directed against a broad spectrum of lymphocyte functions.

It is also possible that components of the immune response to xenografts may be unique. There are, for example, several reports in which cells, particularly neutrophils and natural killer (NK) cells, may play an important role in the rejection of xenografts. This involvement of specific components of cellular immune responses is seen most clearly in models in which immunosuppression has prevented the early destruction of the graft by antibody.[7,47] The reaction of human peripheral blood cells to rat cardiac xenografts is characterized by a predominance of NK cells infiltrating the graft, because of both antibody-dependent and antibody-independent mechanisms.[48] These cells are capable of lysing rat endothelial cells in vitro, particularly when human serum that contains natural antibodies to rat tissue is used in the assay system. Similar patterns of T-cell and NK-cell reactivity of human peripheral blood leukocytes have been observed for pig class II MHC antigens expressed on B lymphoblastoid lines and primary endothelial cell cultures.[49] These studies illustrate the involvement of cellular components of the immune response, perhaps using patterns of reactivity not normally attributed to allografts, to respond to xenogeneic tissues. Immunosuppressive regimens that are designed specifically to prevent xenograft reactivity may require the application of new immunosuppressive techniques to be optimally effective.

Xenograft Target Antigens

The nature of the target antigens for xenograft reactions is largely unknown. It is well known that a variety of different types of antigen-antibody reactions are capable of precipitating accelerated or hyperacute rejection of foreign grafts. Naturally occurring antibodies against ABO antigens, antibodies that cross react with infectious agents, such as the Paul-Bunnell antibody, previous sensitization with blood transfusions, pregnancy, and previous transplants, antibodies directed at bacterial lipopolysaccharide, and Forsman antigens are all capable of precipitating a rapid loss of organ allografts, particularly kidneys and hearts.[50] Many species, particularly those distantly related genetically, have antibodies in their blood that react with potential xenograft donors. Natural antibodies against xenografts may represent antibodies directed against environmental antigens that inadvertently cross react with antigens normally expressed in the graft. Gnotobiotic dogs born in isolation do not exhibit preformed antibody to other species before exposure to environmental antigens such as solid food.[51] The antigens to which natural xenoantibodies are known to bind include cell surface–associated molecules present on erythrocytes,[52,53] vascular endothelium,[54] and lymphocytes.[55,56] The disseminated intravascular coagulation, hemorrhage, and increased vascular permeability that occur in hyperacute rejection suggest that endothelial cells expressing xenoantigens are the most important target for antibody binding.

Xenograft target antigens are believed to consist of carbohydrate-containing glycolipids or glycoproteins.[19] Platt et al[54] demonstrated the reaction of human natural antibodies with a group of potential target antigens with molecular weights of 115 to 135 kd. In addition to the 115/135 antigen complex, a number of studies demonstrate that additional pig endothelial membrane antigens of different molecular weights react with human natural antibodies. Monoclonal antibodies derived from Epstein-Barr virus (EBV)–transformed human lymphocytes against pig lymphocytes detect sulfated glycolipids[57]; natural antibodies in baboons react with 26 and 76 kd xenoantigens[58]; and human natural antibodies to pig antigens react with endothelial membrane antigens in the 25–98 kd range.[20] It remains to be established which, if any, of these molecules represent functional xenograft target antigens and whether the reaction patterns for the human antibodies are directed against one or more distinct target epitopes.

Absorption of human sera with the 115/135 antigens removes most but not all antibody activity in normal humans. Treatment of the 115/135 complex antigens with glycosidases indicates that the target antigen is a complex oligosaccharide. This is consistent with findings in several reports that indicate that this oligosaccharide may be an α-galactosyl compound. The expression of an αGal1-3Gal oligosaccharide on pig endothelial cells, and not those of humans and selected nonhuman primates, may be the basis for the reactivity of natural antibodies in this species combination. It has not, however, been directly demonstrated that this carbohydrate serves as a target for hyperacute reaction. It is likely that other epitopes and protein-CHO structures may also be targets for the reaction. There is also little information about the number of these target antigens or whether they are the same in different organs or species. It has been suggested that natural antibodies may represent the production of polyspecific IgM antibodies by T lymphocyte–independent B lymphocytes that display substantial cross reactivity with carbohydrate moieties on proteins and lipids.[53,59] It is important to note that in the pig-human and guinea pig–rat species combinations, natural antibodies can react to the protein portions of the endothelial target antigens after digestion with glycosidases.[20,60] These studies suggest that the reaction patterns observed for human antibodies with pig endothelium may not be restricted to a single carbohydrate epitope.

▲ POTENTIAL DONORS FOR CLINICAL XENOTRANSPLANTATION

The selection of the most appropriate donor species for kidney xenografts will eventually depend on a complex series of considerations, some scientific and others related to social and ethical issues. From a scientific perspective, the most important issues include the physiologic and anatomic compatibility of the donor organ with the patient, the ability of the foreign graft to function for a prolonged period in the host, and the level of difficulty encountered in providing effective, long-term immunosuppression without adverse side effects for the recipient of a xenograft donor organ. Two species, the closely related baboons and the more distantly related pig, are generally considered to be the most logical choices as xenograft donors. Each of these species, however, is burdened by serious deficiencies as a potential donor that may prevent the long-term use of organs from either animal in a clinical setting.

Nonhuman Primates

The use of nonhuman primates as xenograft donors for kidney transplantation has several clear advantages. Nonhuman primates, particularly larger species such as baboons, share close genetic and physiologic similarities with humans. In general, humans do not exhibit high titers of preformed antibodies to primate xenografts, and the immunologic rejection of grafts from these species are potentially more amenable to current treatment strategies. These considerations have led to the use of kidneys, hearts, and livers from nonhuman primates in patients early during the development of clinical organ transplantation.[2] As described later, the use of chimpanzee kidneys resulted in the demonstration that renal xenografts can function normally for several months and that relatively primitive immunosuppressive regimens allowed preservation of function and survival for as long as 9 months after transplantation.[61,62]

The close genetic and functional relationship of nonhuman primates to humans is an important advantage but is unlikely to compensate for the practical and ethical issues that will limit their use in xenotransplantation. The two most important practical issues are a lack of sufficient numbers of animals to provide a useful number of donor organs, particularly in the face of future increases in the demand for kidney transplantation. Baboons are the most appropriate species because of their large size and current availability. These animals, however, reach sexual maturity late and reproduce slowly. Their low reproductive rate and frequent problems associated with the influence of captivity on breeding behavior would severely limit the commercial development of sufficient animals to meet even current needs for transplantation. Because of their close similarity to humans, nonhuman primates also pose possible health risks for the transmission of infectious diseases, including herpesviruses, retroviruses, and parasites.[63] These scientific considerations are complicated by the belief of many concerned individuals, including workers in the field of transplantation research, that the use of potentially endangered and highly intelligent animals cannot be justified ethically.

Pigs

The use of pigs as kidney xenograft donors poses more difficult immediate problems for the control of the host immune response to a graft. Pigs are physiologically and anatomically suited to act as kidney graft donors for humans.[64] Both kidneys and livers of pigs have been used in a variety of clinical settings. The use of pig livers has included temporary extracorporeal support for patients with acute hepatic failure, bioartifical liver support devices, and in vivo transplantation.[65] The expectation is therefore that pig kidney xenografts could provide appropriate long-term function for patients. This functional compatibility is complemented by a reduction in the potential for disease transmission and ethical concerns about the use of these animals. At present, pigs are one of the most reproductively efficient of the larger farm animals and are commercially raised in large numbers for food consumption. An additional practical consideration is the recent demonstration in several laboratories of genetic manipulations in pigs, including the creation and production of transgenic lines of animals. These are complex and time-consuming manipulations that to date have not been possible in primates.

The primary difficulty associated with the choice of the pig as a xenograft donor for humans is the aggressive immunologic reaction of normal humans to pig xenografts. As described above, normal individuals, even without antigenic challenge, express preformed antibodies that can react with pig xeno-grafts.[2] These antibodies are primarily of the IgM isotype, and their binding to the endothelium of vascularized xenografts is considered to be the initial event that triggers hyperacute rejection of the graft.[3,66] Ex vivo perfusion of pig kidneys with human blood is associated with antibody and complement deposition and platelet aggregation in small vessels and glomeruli.[67,68] The disseminated lesions result in increased vascular resistance and cessation of blood flow. In discordant species, such as pigs and dogs, this immunopathologic process rapidly precipitates ischemic necrosis and subsequent loss of the graft. The use of pig kidneys for clinical transplantation clearly requires techniques to remove preformed antibody, suppress new antibody formation, and prevent cellular rejection. The kidney and heart, unlike the liver, are supplied by a single source of arterial blood, and vascular damage, combined with limited regenerative capacity, makes these organs more susceptible to injury associated with xenograft rejection.

▲ CLINICAL EXPERIENCE WITH RENAL XENOGRAFTING

The use of xenografts for renal transplantation in humans has been reported to have been attempted in 30 patients (Table 17–1).[62,69–77] These attempts were made at a time early in the development of organ transplantation (three patients) or after the introduction of immunosuppressive therapy, but before the widespread availability of dialysis (27 patients).

The early attempts at kidney xenotransplantation conducted in the 1960s included two small series comprising a total of 18 cases.[62,76] These trials were con-

TABLE 17–1 ▲ Clinical Experience in Kidney Xenotransplantation

Year	Donor Species	No. of Cases	Graft Survival Time	Reference
1906	Pig	1	3 days	Jaboulay[70]
1908	Goat	1	3 days	Unger[71]
1923	Sheep	1	9 days	Neuhof[72]
1964	Chimpanzee	12	≤9 months	Reemtsma et al[62]
	Monkey	1	10 days	
1964	Baboon	1	5 days	Hitchcock et al[75]
1964	Baboon	6	36 days (mean)	Starzl et al[76]
1964	Chimpanzee	1	1 day	Hume, unpublished[73]
1964	Chimpanzee	3	2 months	Traeger et al[73]
1965	Chimpanzee	2	4 months	Millard et al[74]
1966	Chimpanzee	1	1 month	Cortesini et al[69]

Modified from Cooper, DKC, Taniguchi S: Clinical xenotransplantation: past, present and future. *Ann R Coll Surg Eng*, in press.

ducted at a time when the techniques for surgical implantation of human renal allografts had been successfully developed and the first immunosuppressive regimens that allowed prolonged allograft survival were available. However, this also was a time when donor organ availability was limited and other support technologies, such as hemodialysis, were of limited availability and effectiveness. In both series, the kidney donors were closely related primate species, either chimpanzees or baboons.

The largest group of patients was that of Reemstma et al[61,62] at Tulane University. Patients with renal failure for whom human allografts were not available received kidneys from chimpanzee donors. The transplanted kidneys functioned well with brisk urine output during the first several days postoperatively. The early courses were frequently complicated by infection; rejection assumed a more important role in the subsequent loss of xenograft function. Immunosuppressive protocols included azathioprine, steroids, actinomycin C, and local graft irradiation. This type of treatment was capable in some cases of reversing a rejection episode, but in general the grafts were lost within a few weeks.[61] Surprisingly, one graft survived for 9 months and was functioning normally without evidence of serious pathologic change when the patient died within 24 hours of an undefined illness.

The six transplantations performed in Denver by Starzl et al[76] involved the use of baboons as kidney donors. In general, the results were similar to those of the Tulane group, the average graft survival being 36 days. The immunosuppressive protocols were similar, but graft survival was severely limited by more aggressive rejection of the grafts. In both series, the characterization of the nature of the immune response to the xenografts was limited. There was evidence of anti-chimpanzee cytotoxic antibody production in the recipients, but little characterization of the nature of the antibody response was provided.[79]

The pioneering work in the 1960s established the feasibility of the surgical techniques, demonstrated the ability of the xenografts to function normally in a foreign environment, and illustrated the potential for the reversal of rejection of the renal xenograft with immunosuppressive drugs.[61] Although the results of these early transplant studies were limited in their clinical effectiveness, it is clear that the availability of newer, more powerful immunosuppressive agents (see Chapter 8) has raised hopes that clinical renal xenotransplantation may one day become a realistic option.

▲ FUTURE DIRECTIONS

The attention directed at the potential use of xenografts for human transplantation has highlighted the complexity of this procedure as a form of medical therapy. There are serious deficiencies in our understanding of the xenograft reaction, and these deficiencies must be resolved before rational and effective use of organs from nonhuman species will be associated with long-term xenograft survival.

One of the primary issues to be addressed is the development of effective immunosuppressive therapy to provide an umbrella under which attempts at xenotransplantation can be made. The xenograft reaction, both for closely and distantly related species, has an important humoral component, including anti-donor antibody production and the involvement of complement, coagulation, and inflammatory cascades. These humoral reactions are not as important a component of the allograft reaction, and the immunosuppressive regimens so carefully developed over the last 30 years do not effectively prevent the xenograft reaction. Accordingly, there is a pressing need to develop more effective treatment protocols, including new immunosuppressive agents, that show promise for preventing the rejection of xenografts. It is unlikely that any one or even a combination of the advanced genetic manipulation techniques under development and discussed below will allow long-term graft survival in the absence of safe and effective immunosuppression.

Some combinations of traditional immunosuppressive drugs have been shown to be highly effective in experimental animals for preventing xenograft rejection. In rodents, the use of cyclosporine or tacrolimus in combination with a variety of antimetabolites can induce long-term heart and liver xenograft survival.[44,45] Combinations of some of these therapeutic agents are currently being evaluated in clinical trials, and the application of the more successful combinations of drugs to xenotransplantation is a realistic expectation. Other more aggressive therapies, including the combination of total lymphoid irradiation and cyclosporine, can be shown to induce long-term survival in xenografts exchanged between nonhuman primates.[80] Survival of heart xenografts for as long as 1 year has been reported, and these experiments are an encouraging development for the use of xenografts in humans.

It is clear that additional refinements in immunosuppressive therapy, including reagents such as sCR1, monoclonal antibodies directed against specific cell subsets, and anti-inflammatory drugs, such as platelet-activating factor antagonists and prostaglandin compounds,[81,82] will provide additional improvements in graft survival and function. Included within this group of new compounds will be those with specificity for humoral antibody production. The early involvement of antibody responses in the xenograft reaction makes it important to develop new strategies that will selectively prevent the production of anti-donor antibodies without disrupting the response to more conventional agents. Preformed natural antibodies, like those in autoimmune disease, are polyreactive. They display reactivity for multiple antigens, frequently with low avidity. This suggests that these antibodies are produced by specific subsets of B cells, including $CD5^+$ lymphocytes, and that strategies to prevent xenograft rejection in the future may include elimination of these cells.

One of the areas of current investigation that may have an important application for renal xenotransplantation is the induction of donor-specific tolerance in xenograft recipients.[83,84] Hematopoietic chimerism has been associated with long-term donor-specific tolerance of allografts in rodents. Experiments with rats and mice have suggested that it may be possible to induce this form of tolerance across species barriers.[85] Administration of pig bone marrow to cynomolgus monkeys after antibody depletion, irradiation, and treatment with antithymocyte globulin has resulted in prolongation of kidney graft survival for as long as 13 days.[86] These results are encouraging, and donor-recipient bone marrow chimerism may eventually be useful for a variety of clinical conditions. Development of clinically acceptable conditioning regimens and procedures for donor bone marrow transplantation could be incorporated into xenograft treatment protocols without precluding other manipulations of the graft or the donor.

The experimental manipulation of the donor graft to improve the possibility of xenograft survival in the face of an active host immune response will have substantial impact on xenotransplantation in the future.[87] The creation and production of lines of pigs transgenically modified for regulation of donor gene expression is technically possible and is being performed in many laboratories.[88] Of particular interest to several investigators is the potential manipulation of complement regulatory proteins to prevent or interfere with the participation of complement in the hyperacute rejection process. Membrane cofactor protein (MCP, CD46), decay accelerating factor (DAF, CD55), and protectin (CD59) are examples of complement regulatory proteins that act as protection from endogenous complement activation. Human forms of these proteins can be transfected into xenogeneic cells and may protect these tissues from damage related to activation of the human complement system. Several laboratories are now attempting to develop transgenic pigs that express human regulatory proteins to disrupt complement activation after xenotransplantation. The complexity of the complement system, however, may require that multiple gene transfections may be necessary for effective prevention of activation.[89]

The genetic manipulation of donor organs will also eventually extend to the antigens expressed on the xenogeneic tissues that serve as the targets for the xenograft reaction. If the number of xenogeneic target antigens is small, perhaps consisting of a restricted number of carbohydrate-protein-lipid epitopes, this approach offers the most direct and potentially effective method of preventing xenograft rejection. Downregulation of antigen expression or transfection with genes that encode the human equivalent of the target antigen may avoid the immediate binding of preformed antibody and the stimulation of host anti-donor responses after transplantation. This approach may be less effective if the number of target antigens is large or if the expression of the target antigen is developmentally important. MHC antigens, for example, serve as a principal target for the allograft reaction, and disruption of their expression to prevent graft rejection is not associated with increases in embryonic or neonatal mortality. This may not prove to be true for xenografts, and many potential target antigens may be required for normal embryologic development. One alternative to the production of a transgenic animal could include the ex vivo transfection of the donor organ at the time of xenotransplantation to regulate antigen expression.

Despite enthusiastic predictions to the contrary, regular use of xenogeneic organs for human transplantation is not likely to occur in the near future. Although the appropriate surgical techniques have been developed and new immunosuppressive agents are in advanced stages of experimental testing, the development of safe and effective strategies for preventing the xenograft reaction in the clinical setting has not yet occurred. The aggressive nature of the xenograft response will require extensive experimental testing of one or more of these technologies before xenotransplantation can be applied to patients.

▲ REFERENCES

1. Starzl TE, Demetris AJ, Van Thiel DH: Liver transplantation. *N Engl J Med* 321:1014, 1989.
2. Auchincloss H Jr: Xenogeneic transplantation: a review. *Transplantation* 46:1, 1988.
3. Makowka L, Cramer DV: The pathogenesis of the xenograft reaction. In: Hackel B, Aubuchon J (eds), *Advances in Transplantation*. Bethesda, MD, American Association of Blood Banks, 1993:93.
4. Calne RY: Organ transplantation between widely disparate species. *Transplant Proc* 2:550, 1970.
5. Makowka L, Cramer DV, Hoffman A, Sher L, Podesta L: Can pig liver xenografts be used as a temporary bridge for human allografting? *Xenobiotica* 1:1, 1993.
6. Rosengard BR, Adachi H, Ueda K, et al: Differences in the pathogenesis of first-set allograft rejection and acute xenograft rejection as determined by sequential morphologic analysis. *J Heart Transplant* 5:263, 1986.
7. Cramer DV, Chapman FA, Jaffee BD, et al: The prolongation of concordant hamster-to-rat cardiac xenografts by brequinar sodium. *Transplantation* 54:403, 1992.
8. Hasan R, Van den Bogaerde JB, Wallwork J, White DJG: Evidence that long-term survival of concordant xenografts is achieved by inhibition of antispecies antibody production. *Transplantation* 54:408, 1992.
9. Bailey LL, Nehlsen-Cannarilla SL, Concepcion W, Joiley WB: Baboon-to-human cardiac exnotransplantation in a neonate. *JAMA* 254:3321, 1985.
10. Linn BS, Jensen JA, Pardo V, Davies D, Franklin L: Relationship between structural and functional changes in rejecting renal xenografts. *Transplant Proc* 3:527, 1971.
11. Bogman MJJT, Berden JHM, Hagemann JFHM, Maass CN, Koene RAP: Patterns of vascular damage in the antibody-mediated rejection of skin xenografts in the mouse. *Am J Pathol* 100:727, 1980.
12. Ertel W, Reichenspurner H, Hammer C, et al: Heart transplantation in closely related species: a model for humoral rejection. *Transplant Proc* 16:1259, 1984.
13. Larsen S, Starklint H: Histopathology of kidney xenograft rejection. In: Cooper DKC, Kemp E, Reemtsma K, White DJG (eds), *Xenotransplantation: The Transplantation of Organs and Tissue Between Species*. Berlin, Springer-Verlag, 1991:181.
14. Marino JR, Celli S, Ferla G, Stieber A, Maggiano N, Musiani P: Histopathological, immunofluorescent, and electron-microscopic features of hyperacute rejection in discordant renal xenotransplantation. In: Cooper DKC, Kemp E, Reemtsma K, White DJG (eds), *Xenotransplantation: The Transplantation of Organs and Tissues Between Species*. Berlin, Springer-Verlag, 1991:207.
15. Rose AG: Histopathology of cardiac xenograft rejection. In: Cooper DKC, Kemp E, Reemtsma K, White DJG (eds), *Xenotransplantation: The Transplantation of Organs and Tissues Between Species*. Berlin, Springer-Verlag, 1991:231.
16. Marquet RL, Heystek GA, van Leersum RH: Xenogeneic heart transplantation from the hamster to the rat: the effect of nonspecific and specific immunosuppressive treatment. *Int J Microsurg* 2:113, 1980.
17. Wu GD, Cramer DV, Chapman FA, et al: Cardiac hyperacute rejection in concordant xenograft combinations induced by immunization. *Transplant Proc* 24:691, 1992.
18. Turman MA, Casali P, Notkins AL, Bach FH, Platt JL: Polyreactivity and antigen specificity of human xenoreactive monoclonal and serum natural antibodies. *Transplantation* 52:710, 1991.

19. Platt JL, Bach FH: The barrier to xenotransplantation. *Transplantation* 52:937, 1991.
20. Tuso PJ, Cramer DV, Middleton YD, et al: Pig aortic endothelial cell antigens recognized by human IgM natural antibodies. *Transplantation* 56:651, 1993.
21. Kasaian MT, Ikematsu H, Casali P: CD5+ B lymphocytes. *Proc Soc Exp Biol Med* 197:226, 1991.
22. Casali P, Notkins AL: Probing the human B-Cell repertoire with EBV: Polyreactive antibodies and CD5+ B lymphocytes. *Annu Rev Immunol* 7:513, 1989.
23. Kantor AB, Herzenberg LA: Origin of murine B cell lineages. *Annu Rev Immunol* 11:501, 1993.
24. Platt JL, Fischel RJ, Matas AJ, Reif SA, Morton Bolman R, Bach FH: Immunopathology of hyperacute xenograft rejection in a swine-to-primate model. *Transplantation* 52:214, 1991.
25. Geller RL, Bach FH, Turman MA, Casali P, Platt JL: Evidence that polyreactive antibodies are deposited in rejected discordant xenografts. *Transplantation* 55:168, 1993.
26. Moses RD, Auchincloss H Jr: Mechanisms of cellular xenograft rejection. In: Cooper DKC, Kemp E, Reemtsma K, White DJG (eds), *Xenotransplantation: The Transplantation of Organs and Tissues Between Species.* Berlin, Springer-Verlag, 1991:101.
27. Dalmasso AP: The complement system in xenotransplantation. *Immunopharmacology* 24:149, 1992.
28. Mejia-Laguna JE, Martinez-Palomo A, Biro CE, Chavez B, Lopez-Soriano F, Garcia-Cornejo M: Morphologic study of the participation of the complement system in hyperacute rejection of renal xenotransplants. *Am J Pathol* 69:71, 1972.
29. Gewurz H, Clark DS, Cooper MD, Varco RL, Good RA: Effect of cobra venom–induced inhibition of complement activity on allograft and xenograft rejection reactions. *Transplantation* 5:1296, 1967.
30. Ryan US: Complement inhibition: the sine qua non of xenotransplantation? *Xenobiotica* 2:19, 1994.
31. Dalmasso AP, Platt JL: Prevention of complement-mediated activation of xenogeneic endothelial cells in an in vivo model of xenograft hyperacute rejection by C1 inhibitor. *Transplantation* 56:1171, 1993.
32. Cramer DW, Wu G-D, Makowka L: The pathogenesis of xenograft reactions in rodents and other small laboratory species. *Transplant Proc* 25:2846, 1993.
33. Miyagawa S, Hirose H, Shirakura R, et al: The mechanism of discordant xenograft rejection. *Transplantation* 46:825, 1988.
34. Leventhal JR, Matas AJ, Sun LH, et al: The immunopathology of cardiac xenograft rejection in the guinea pig-to-rat model. *Transplantation* 56:1, 1993.
35. Paul LC, Green B, Davidoff A, Benediktsson H: Xenoantibodies in the rat against guinea pig tissues. *Transplant Int* 3:199, 1990.
36. Leventhal JR, Flores HC, Gruber SA, et al: Evidence that 15-deoxyspergualin inhibits natural antibody production but fails to prevent hyperacute rejection in a discordant xenograft model. *Transplantation* 54:26, 1992.
37. Johnston PS, Wang M-W, Kim SML, Wright LJ, White DJG: Discordant xenograft rejection in an antibody-free model. *Transplantation* 54:573, 1992.
38. Forty J, Cary N, White DJG, Wallwork J: Hyperacute rejection of rabbit hearts by human blood is mediated by the alternative pathway of complement. *Transplant Proc* 24:488, 1992.
39. Gambiez L, Weill BJ, Chereau C, Calmus Y, Houssin D: The hyperacute rejection of guinea pig to rat heart xenografts is mediated by preformed IgM. *Transplant Proc* 22:1058, 1990.
40. Pruitt SK, Baldwin WM III, Marsh HC Jr, Lin SS, Yeh CG, Bollinger RR: The effect of soluble complement receptor type 1 on hyperacute xenograft rejection. *Transplantation* 52:868, 1991.

41. Pruitt SK, Kirk AD, Bollinger RR, et al: The effect of soluble complement receptor type 1 on hyperacute rejection of porcine xenografts. *Transplantation* 57:363, 1994.
42. Pierson RN III, Winn HJ, Russell PS, Auchincloss H Jr: Xenogeneic skin graft rejection is especially dependent on $CD4^+$ T cells. *J Exp Med* 170:991, 1989.
43. Auchincloss H Jr, Moses R, Conti D, et al: Xenograft rejection of class I-expressing transgenic skin is CD4-dependent and CD8-independent. *Transplant Proc* 22:2335, 1990.
44. Murase N, Starzl TE, Demetris AJ, et al: Hamster-to-rat heart and liver xenotransplantation with FK506 plus antiproliferative drugs. *Transplantation* 55:701, 1993.
45. Cosenza CA, Cramer DV, Tuso PJ, Chapman FA, Wang HK, Makowka L: Combination therapy with brequinar sodium and cyclosporin A synergistically prolongs hamster-to-rat cardiac xenograft survival. *J Heart Lung Transplant* 13:489, 1994.
46. McManus RP, O'Hair DP, Komorowski R, Scott JP: Immunosuppressant combinations in primate cardiac xenografts: a review. *Ann N Y Acad Sci* 696:281, 1993.
47. Cramer DV, Wu GD, Chapman FA, Wang HK, Cajulis E, Makowka L: A comparison of lymphocytic subsets participating in concordant cardiac xenograft and acute cardiac allograft rejection. *Transplant Proc* 24:533, 1992.
48. Inverardi L, Samaja M, Motterlini R, Mangili F, Bender JR, Pardi R: Early recognition of a discordant xenogeneic organ by human circulating lymphocytes. *J Immunol* 149:1416, 1992.
49. Kirk AD, Li RA, Kinch MS, Abernethy KA, Doyle C, Bollinger RR: The human anti-porcine cellular repertoire: in vitro studies of acquired and innate cellular responsiveness. *Transplantation* 55:924, 1993.
50. Paul LC: Mechanism of humoral xenograft rejection. In: Cooper DKC, Kemp E, Reemtsma K, White DJG (eds), *Xenotransplantation: The Transplantation of Organs and Tissues Between Species.* Berlin, Springer-Verlag, 1991:47.
51. Hammer C, Hingerle M: Development of preformed natural antibodies in gnotobiotic dogs and pigs: impact of food antigens on antibody specificity. *Transplant Proc* 24:707, 1992.
52. Hammer C: Isohemagglutinins and preformed natural antibodies in xenogeneic organ transplantation. *Transplant Proc* 19:4443, 1987.
53. Boyden SV: Natural antibodies and the immune response. *Adv Immunol* 5:1, 1964.
54. Platt JL, Lindman BJ, Chen H, Spitalnik SL, Bach FH: Endothelial cell antigens recognized by xenoreactive human natural antibodies. *Transplantation* 50:817, 1990.
55. Edwards N, Ott G, Berger C: Incidence of preformed antibodies against potential xenodonors in human serum. *Transplantation* 49:1022, 1990.
56. Cameron DJ, Rajagopalan PR, Fitts CT, Majeski JA: Characterization of the preformed antibodies involved in the xenograft reaction. *J Surg Oncol* 22:154, 1983.
57. Holgersson J, Cairns TDH, Breimer ME, Taube D, Welsh K, Samuelsson BE: Carbohydrate antigen specificity of pig lymphocytotoxic IgM antibodies produced by two EBV transformed human B cell lines (abstract). *Glycoconjugate J* 8:172, 1991.
58. Ratner AJ, Canhul H, Pepino P, et al: Lymphocyte xenoantigens recognized by preformed antibodies. *Transplant Proc* 24:583, 1992.
59. Platt JL, Vercellotti GM, Dalmasso AP, et al: Transplantation of discordant xenografts: a review of progress. *Immunol Today* 11:450, 1990.
60. Scherrer L, Leventhal JR, Matas AJ, Dalmasso AP: Evidence that rat xenoreactive antibodies recognize multiple protein antigens on guinea pig endothelial cells and platelets. *Transplantation* 58:458, 1994.
61. Reemtsma K: Renal heterotransplantation from nonhuman primates to man. *Ann N Y Acad Sci* 162:412, 1969.
62. Reemtsma K, McCracken BH, Schlegel JU, et al: Renal heterotransplantation in man. *Ann Surg* 160:384, 1964.

63. Michaels MG, Simmons RL: Xenotransplant-associated zoonoses: strategies for prevention. *Transplantation* 57:1, 1994.
64. Cooper DKC, Ye Y, Rolf LLJ, Zuhdi N: The pig as potential organ donor for man. In: Cooper DKC, Kemp E, Reemtsma K, White DJG (eds), *Xenotransplantation: The Transplantation of Organs and Tissues Between Species.* Berlin, Springer-Verlag, 1991:481.
65. Makowa L, Cramer DV, Hoffman A, et al: The use of a pig liver xenograft for temporary support of a patient with fulminant hepatic failure. *Transplantation.* 59(12):1654–1659, 1995.
66. Platt JL, Bach FH: Mechanism of tissue injury in hyperacute xenograft rejection. In: Cooper DKC, Kemp E, Reemtsma K, White DJG (eds), *Xenotransplantation: The Transplantation of Organs and Tissues Between Species.* Berlin, Springer-Verlag, 1991:69.
67. Otte KE, Anderson N, Jorgensen KA, et al: Xenoperfusion of pig kidney with human AB or O whole blood. *Transplant Proc* 22:1091, 1990.
68. Tuso PJ, Cramer DV, Yasunaga C, Cosenza CA, Wu GD, Makowka L: Removal of natural human xenoantibodies to pig vascular endothelium by perfusion of blood through pig kidneys and livers. *Transplantation* 55:1375, 1993.
69. Cortesini R, Casciani C, Cucchiara G: Heterotransplantation in primates: current state of affair. In: *Infection and Immunosuppression in Subhuman Primates.* 1969:239.
70. Jaboulay M: Greffe de rein au pli du coude par suture de l'artere et de la veine. *Lyon Med* 39:575, 1906.
71. Unger I: Transplantation des vaisseux et des organes. *B Chir* 46:1367, 1908.
72. Neuhof H: *The Transplantation of Tissues.* New York: Appleton, 1923.
73. Traeger J, Fries D, Perrin J: Heterotransplantation chex l'homme: premiers resultats. *Proc Eur Dial Transplant Assoc* 2:214, 1965.
74. Millard C, Shumway NE, Starzl TE, et al: Xenografts: review of the literature and current status. *JAMA* 254:2253, 1985.
75. Hitchcock CR, Kiser JC, Telander RL, Seljeskag EL: Baboon renal grafts. *JAMA* 189:934, 1964.
76. Starzl TE, Marchioro TL, Peters GN, Kirkpatrick CH: Renal heterotransplantation from baboon to man: experience with 6 cases. *Transplantation* 2:752, 1964.
77. Cooper DKC, Taniguchi S: Clinical xenotransplantation: past, present and future. *Ann R Coll Surg Eng,* in press.
78. Markmann JF, Barker CF: Basic and clinical considerations in the use of xenografts. *Curr Probl Surg* 31:387, 1994.
79. DeWitt CW, Reemtsma K, Oliver CB, Ahlschier AA: Production of anti-chimpanzee cytotoxin in human subjects. In: *Advance in Transplantation.* Copenhagen, Munksgaard, 1968:409.
80. Roslin MS, Tranbaugh RE, Panza A, et al: One-year monkey heart xenograft survival in cyclosporine-treated baboons: suppression of the xenoantibody response with total-lymphoid irradiation. *Transplantation* 54:949, 1992.
81. Makowka L, Chapman FA, Cramer DV, Qian S, Sun H, Starzl TE: Platelet-activating factor and hyperacute rejection: the effect of a platelet-activating factor antagonist, SRI 63-441, on rejection of xenografts and allografts in sensitized hosts. *Transplantation* 50:359, 1990.
82. Makowka L, Chapman F, Cramer DV, et al: The antagonism of platelet-activating factor and hyperacute organ rejection. In: Handley DA, Houlihan WJ, Saunders RN, Tomesch JC (eds), *Platelet-Activating Factor in Endotoxin and Immune Diseases.* New York, Dekker, 1990:387.
83. Ildstad ST, Sachs DH: Reconstitution with syngeneic plus allogeneic or xenogeneic bone marrow leads to specific acceptance of allografts or xenografts. *Nature* 307:168, 1984.
84. Ildstad ST, Boggs SS, Vecchini F, et al: Mixed xenogeneic chimeras (rat + mouse to mouse): evidence of rat stem cell engraftment, strain-specific transplantation tolerance, and skin-specific antigens. *Transplantation* 53:815, 1992.

85. Ildstad ST, Vacchio MS, Markus PM, Hronakes ML, Wren SM, Hodes RJ: Cross-species transplantation tolerance: rat bone marrow-derived cells can contribute to the ligand for negative selection of mouse T cell receptor Vβ in chimeras tolerant to xenogeneic antigens (mouse + rat → mouse). *J Exp Med* 175:147, 1992.
86. Tanaka M, Latinne D, Gianello P, et al: Xenotransplantation from pig to cynomologous monkey: the potential for overcoming xenograft rejection through induction of chimerism (abstract 122). Presented at the Second International Congress on Xenotransplantation, September 26–29, 1993, Cambridge, England.
87. Kearns-Jonker M, Cramer DV, Makowka L: The future of transgenic animals in transplantation. In: Sher LS, Makowka L (eds), *Intra-Abdominal Organ Transplantation 2000.* Austin, TX, Landes, 1994:95.
88. Pinkert CA: Transgenic pig models for xenotransplantation. *Xenobiotica* 2:10, 1994.
89. McKenzie IFC, Johnstone R, Szokolaik TK, Thorley B, Petris A, Loveland B: Coordinate functions of multiple complement regulating molecules CD46, CD55, and CD59. *Transplant Proc* 26:1070, 1994.

18

Future Prospects

Ron Shapiro

Any discussion of the future of renal transplantation runs the risk of degenerating into idle speculation on the one hand, and a timid presentation of obvious short-term near-certainties on the other. This chapter addresses four discrete issues—immunosuppression, organ donation, alternative sources of organs, and the impact of changes in health care delivery. The aim is to delineate the likely possible developments and assess their impact.

▲ IMMUNOSUPPRESSION

Pharmacologic Agents

As pointed out in Chapter 2, the development of the first immunosuppressive protocols using azathioprine and prednisone was critical to the initial widespread application of renal transplantation as a therapeutic modality. In the past quarter century, only cyclosporine, which essentially replaced azathioprine, has had a major impact on clinical practice. Now, however, many new drugs are becoming available, and finding the most effective combination will not be simple.

For the near- or medium-term future, some agent that inhibits T-cell function will be needed. Tacrolimus is the only new candidate in clinical use. Tacrolimus has a mode of action similar to cyclosporine, and has the same kinds of side effects[1–7] but has a more favorable therapeutic index.[8–14] It is likely that both cyclosporine and tacrolimus will retain a place in the immunosuppressive armamentarium, either in their present form or in a slightly different formulation, such as the microemulsion form of cyclosporine (Neoral),[15] cyclosporine G,[16] or liposomal tacrolimus.[17] Unfortunately, a nonnephrotoxic agent does not yet exist in this category.

With regard to so-called "third agents," the future of azathioprine is, in contrast to that of cyclosporine, in jeopardy. Mycophenolate mofetil, now approved by the

Food and Drug Administration (FDA), has a more favorable therapeutic index than azathioprine, and will likely replace it as a third agent.[18–20]

The situation with sirolimus (rapamycin) is a bit less clear. Thus far it has been used with cyclosporine, and it seems likely to become another effective third agent.[21,22] Although rapamycin and tacrolimus share the same binding protein,[23,24] they were found to be synergistic in a mouse cardiac allograft model,[25] and it is conceivable that they could be used together clinically; antagonism apparently requires a 100-fold excess of one agent or the other.[24] Whether rapamycin is a sufficiently efficacious agent to replace cyclosporine or tacrolimus is unclear; it is currently being evaluated as a main-line agent in a clinical trial in Europe.

The role of 15-deoxyspergualin remains to be established. Now unusable as a maintenance agent because of the lack of an oral formulation, it seems to have potential either as an induction agent[26–28] or as a treatment for rejection.[29–34] More evaluation of this agent is needed; thus far there appear to be relatively few trials in progress outside Japan.

Of the other new potential pharmacologic agents that have not yet entered or are just on the verge of entering into clinical transplantation trials, such as castanospermine,[35] leflunomide analogues,[36,37] phosphatidic acid-active agents,[38] LF 08-0299,[39] SK&F 105685,[40] and others, it is still too early to speculate. The fact that new agents are continuing to be developed and evaluated is encouraging. However, there are many hazards on the road to FDA approval. Recent examples include the unwillingness of the company responsible for leflunomide to develop it for transplantation and the recent decision to stop the further development of brequinar.

Biologic Agents

As noted in Chapter 8, a large number of different monoclonal antibodies have already begun to be evaluated in clinical trials, and a larger number are being studied in preclinical models. To forecast which of these new agents or even which class of agents will become useful is premature. Certainly, many researchers are hoping that these agents will be useful in attempts at tolerance induction; thus far this work has been carried out exclusively in a preclinical setting.[41–47]

Other Modalities

Bone marrow augmentation may well play an important role in future therapies. Early studies have already been published by Barber and Starzl and their colleagues,[48–53] and several single-center studies are in progress, as is a multicenter trial. Thus far these early studies have suggested that a low level of peripheral blood chimerism is achieved routinely, that patient and graft survival is not adversely affected, and that clinical graft versus host disease in kidney recipients is never seen. Important long-term questions remain: Is the chimerism durable? Is chimerism predictive of donor-specific hyporesponsiveness? What is the effect on long-term patient and graft survival? Many different protocols are being evaluated. Some utilize induction antilymphocyte therapy[54,55]; some "make space" with cytoreduction regimens with drugs or pretransplant irradiation of the recipient[56,57]; some modify the bone marrow itself (Ildstad ST, personal communication) or vary the number of doses or timing of marrow administration,[57a,b] and some utilize hematopoietic growth factors, such as granulocyte-macrophage colony-stimulating factor (GM-CSF).[58] Because the end points of these studies deal with long-term results as well as short-term freedom from rejection, resolution of these issues will take time. However, a method to establish chimerism with stem cells, with the aim of conferring tolerance, is likely to have an important place in the near- and medium-term future.

▲ ORGAN DONATION

The ever-widening gap between the relatively stagnant number of kidney donors and the increasing number of potential recipients is well established. Interestingly, even a 25% increase in the supply of kidneys could go a long way toward stabilizing the growth of the national waiting list, and a 50% increase could lead to a gradual decrease in the number of patients on the list. A number of approaches have been tried to provide organs for needy patients.

Living unrelated donation has been used successfully and is considered to be ethical in many programs around the world.[59–65] In almost all cases, only emotionally related persons—spouses, in-laws, close friends—donate organs. Employment of paid unrelated donors, as has been the practice until recently in India[66–70] (which has neither large cadaveric programs nor broad access to dialysis) and Iraq,[71] is illegal in the United States and is morally unacceptable in almost all countries.[72–75] Similarly, use of organs from executed criminals, as is practiced in China,[76,77] is viewed with sufficient moral repugnance that it is unlikely to be considered in the western world.

The concept of presumed consent, whereby cadaveric donors are used unless explicit refusal has been previously documented, has been put into practice in Belgium, Austria, Finland, France, Norway, Denmark, Portugal, and Singapore.[78–84] Presumed consent has, in fact, led to an increase in organ donation in those countries, of both renal and extrarenal organs. As a practical matter, in a country as litigious as the United States, presumed consent is unlikely to become a reality until there is a major shift in public understanding of and support for organ donation.

The experience of Spain is worth studying. In a remarkably short period of time, organ donation there increased dramatically, and Spain now has the highest per capita rate of organ donation in the world.[85–87] The Spanish model relies on a network of hospital-based coordinators composed of physicians, usually nephrologists or intensivists.[86,87] The coordinator's job is part-time and allows the physician to continue in his or her hospital-based position. This system has been extremely effective and is in the process of being developed in a number of Latin American countries. Its applicability to the U.S. system, which is composed largely of independent organ procurement organizations, is unclear but is certainly worth considering.

Another consideration, not yet adopted and still controversial, involves financial compensation to the donor's family.[88–92] The possibilities have ranged from paying for funeral expenses[88] to the establishment of a market for donated organs.[89] The argument being advanced is that altruism has failed to lead to a sufficient number of organs (although it has led to a large absolute number of donors, more than 4000 per year) and that compensation should be offered as a incentive. It is not yet clear where the national debate will go with this idea. It should, however, be noted that blood banks in the United States had a dual system of volunteer and paid blood donors in the not-so-distant past, and that use of blood from paid donors eventually was phased out because of the increased risk of disease transmission. Compensation of organ donors, although not entirely analogous, might cause more problems than it solves.

The only available and generally accepted modality that could be used to increase organ donation is the obvious (but perhaps still underutilized) one—public and professional education. Targeting particular groups, such as Callender's program to increase awareness about organ donation within the African-American community,[93–97] has had demonstrated effectiveness. There is still room in the community at large for additional efforts of this type.

▲ ALTERNATIVE SOURCES OF ORGANS

Xenografts

The prospects for the near-term clinical use of xenogeneic organs in renal transplantation is addressed in Chapter 17. At present, clinical xenotransplantation is not a realistic option. It may be feasible in the medium-term future, but this depends on advances in immunobiology and the development of new pharmacologic and biologic agents.

Bioartificial Kidney

Although perhaps not of immediate practical relevance to renal transplantation, it is nonetheless still worth noting that there has been a certain amount of research on the development of a bioartificial kidney.[98–100] Some of this work has studied the culture of monolayers of renal tubular cells on semipermeable synthetic (cellulose nitrate or acetate) membranes coated with various attachment substrates, extracellular matrix being the most effective.[98] In such a system, renal tubular cells exhibited reabsorption of glucose and secretion of tetraethylammonium in either tissue culture fluid or hemofiltrate from a patient with uremia.[99] It is not difficult to envision this work leading to the development of a self-contained unit that mimics the function of the renal tubules.[100] This could be coupled with already existing technologies. For example, commercially available ultrafiltration is being used clinically, albeit in an ex vivo system.[101,102] Endothelial seeding of artificial surfaces has already been accomplished for artificial blood vessels, such as polytetrafluoroethylene (PTFE) grafts.[103–105] Endothelial seeding of an ultrafiltration device could allow for its use without chronic anticoagulation. The use of an ultrafiltration unit and a renal tubular epithelium unit in series could lead to an effective bioartificial kidney, and with further refinements, this could be implanted permanently with appropriate ureteral or bladder drainage of the resulting "urine" produced by the system. A totally implantable bioartificial kidney could conceivably provide renal replacement comparable to that seen with a successful transplant, without the need for waiting time or chronic immunosuppression.

Renal Organogenesis

Although the ability to grow a kidney in a test tube is neither at hand nor is likely to occur in the near future, there has been some interesting research in the area of renal tubulogenesis, an important initial step. Simultaneous addition of transforming growth factor-β_1 (TGFβ_1), epidermal growth factor (EGF), and retinoic acid to a confluent monolayer of renal proximal tubule cells was shown to lead to the formation of a three-dimensional polarized cell cluster containing lumens, microvilli, and tight junctional complexes.[106,107] Addition of triiodothyronine (T_3) was shown to lead to increased cell replication, and the effect was mediated by EGF.[108] Adenosine triphosphate (ATP), by contrast, did not promote cell growth.[109] TGFβ_1 was found to promote proteoglycan synthesis and lead to rearrangement of actin fibers.[110] Thus the role of specific growth factors in renal organogenesis is starting to be elucidated. Again, it is not impossible to envision this research maturing, eventually, into the production of a kidney in the laboratory.

▲ THE IMPACT OF HEALTH CARE REFORM

Although the issues in this section are perhaps intellectually less challenging than those raised in the other sections of this chapter, they are at least as important and may well have much more of an effect on the future of transplantation. The rhetoric of health care reform has emphasized improving access to and maintaining the quality of health care, while at the same time reducing its costs. Clearly, health care professionals engaged in transplantation have an important obligation to reduce expenditures by helping to promote greater efficiency and cost effectiveness in patient care. In the process, however, it is important to remember that the most important obligation is to the patient, not to the health maintenance organization or the insurance company. A kidney transplant is conceptually different from a cholecystectomy or a joint replacement, and it is not always clear that managed care organizations understand that difference. The procedure marks the beginning of a lifelong relationship between the transplant team and the patient. Issues of posttransplant immunosuppression, infection prophylaxis, and other matters are often complex. In our own experience, the patients' primary care physicians have generally preferred to defer to us in the management of these issues, out of a mutually shared concern for the patients' best interest. Conversely, it is generally our preference to have the patient's primary care physicians take care of all the nontransplant-related issues.

There are real dangers that managed care will lead to an erosion of these standards of posttransplant care at several levels. First, it is likely that cost, not outcome, will be the primary factor. A possible result might be that less expensive programs with somewhat worse results will profit at the expense of programs with better results but higher costs. Second, long-term patient management may be taken out of the hands of the transplant team and given to individuals with little understanding of the long-term issues related to transplantation. Finally, innovations in immunosuppression, which are critical to ongoing efforts to improve results after transplantation, may be less likely to be viewed favorably by organizations whose principal goal is to deliver a cost-effective health care "product." The fact that the long-term costs may be higher, ie, an earlier return to dialysis or retransplantation, may not be understood by individuals or institutions whose concerns are measured quarterly.

Transplantation, like other branches of medicine, is driven primarily by the needs of patients, and, to be sure, one of those needs is affordable care. To the extent that health care providers have not appreciated this need, they have contributed to the problem of rising costs. It is incumbent on health care professionals in transplantation to help keep the focus of managed health care on the patients' special requirements and at the same time keep costs under control. Earlier hospital discharge; performance of more transplantation-related procedures, such as biopsies and administration of intravenous medications on an outpatient basis; and the use of outpatient in place of inpatient facilities when feasible, will help keep costs down without sacrificing patient care. At the same time, maintaining quality control over transplant-related management issues will ensure that patients receive the best possible care. Health-care reform need not lead to a deterioration in the quality of care of renal transplant patients, but therapeutic decision making will have to remain in the hands of transplant professionals to ensure this. Given the well-established cost effectiveness of transplantation compared with dialysis,[111,112] optimizing the outcomes after transplantation would seem to be the most economically sensible course.

▲ REFERENCES

1. McCauley J, Takaya S, Fung J, et al: The question of FK506 nephrotoxicity after liver transplantation. *Transplant Proc* 23:1444, 1991.
2. Starzl TE, Abu-Elmagd K, Tzakis A, Fung JJ, Porter KA, Todo S: Selected topics on FK506, with special references to rescue of extrahepatic whole organ grafts, transplantation of "forbidden organs," side effects, mechanisms, and practical pharmacokinetics. *Transplant Proc* 23:914, 1991.
3. Starzl TE: FK506 versus cyclosporine. *Transplant Proc* 25:511, 1993.
4. Demetris AJ, Banner B, Fung JJ, Shapiro R, Jordan M, Starzl TE: Histopathology of human

renal allograft function under FK506: a comparison with cyclosporine. *Transplant Proc* 23:944, 1991.

5. Randhawa PS, Shapiro R, Jordan ML, Starzl TE, Demetris AJ: The histopathological changes associated with allograft rejection and drug toxicity in renal transplant recipients maintained on FK506: clinical significance and comparison with cyclosporine. *Am J Surg Pathol* 17:60, 1993.
6. Shapiro R, Fung JJ, Jain AB, Parks P, Todo S, Starzl TE: The side effects of FK506 in humans. *Transplant Proc* 22:35, 1990.
7. Scantlebury V, Shapiro R, Fung JJ, et al: New onset of diabetes in FK506 vs. cyclosporine-treated kidney transplant recipients. *Transplant Proc* 23:3169, 1991.
8. Shapiro R, Jordan M, Scantlebury V, et al: A prospective randomized trial of FK506 in renal transplantation—a comparison between double and triple drug therapy. *Clin Transplant* 8:508, 1994.
9. Shapiro R, Jordan ML, Scantlebury VP, et al: A prospective, randomized trial of FK506-based immunosuppression after renal transplantation. *Transplantation* 59:485–490, 1995.
10. Shapiro R, Jordan ML, Scantlebury VP, et al: A prospective, randomized trial of FK506/prednisone vs. FK506/azathioprine/prednisone in renal transplant patients. *Transplant Proc* 27:814–817, 1995.
11. Shapiro R, Scantlebury V, Jordan ML, et al: FK506 in pediatric kidney transplantation: primary and rescue experience. *Pediatr Nephrol* 9:S43–S48, 1995.
12. Jordan ML, Shapiro R, Vivas CA, et al: FK506 salvage of renal allografts with ongoing rejection failing cyclosporine immunosuppression. *Transplant Proc* 25:638–640, 1993.
13. Jordan M, Shapiro R, Vivas C, et al: FK506 rescue for resistant rejection of renal allograft under primary cyclosporine immunosuppression. *Transplantation* 57:860–865, 1994.
14. Gjertson DW, Cecka JM, Terasaki PI: The relative effects of FK506 and cyclosporine on short- and long-term kidney graft survival. *Transplantation* 1995, submitted.
15. Mueller EA, Kallay Z, Kovarik JM, Arns W, Renner E, Kutz K: Assessment of glomerular filtration rate after multiple administration of a new oral formulation of cyclosporine in clinically stable renal transplant patients. *Transplant Proc* 27:834–836, 1995.
16. Henry ML, Tesi RJ, Elkhammas EA, Ferguson RM: Trial of cyclosporine vs OG37-325 in cadaveric renal transplantation: a preliminary report. *Transplant Proc* 25:689–690, 1993.
17. Ko S, Nakajima Y, Kanehiro H, et al: Significance of newly developed liposomal FK 506 in canine liver transplantation. *Transplant Proc* 27:351–353, 1995.
18. Sollinger HW, Deierhoi MH, Belzer FO, Diethelm AG, Kauffman RS: RS-61443-A phase I clinical trial and pilot rescue study. *Transplantation* 53:428, 1992.
19. Young CJ, Sollinger HW: RS-61443: A new immunosuppression agent. *Transplant Proc* 26:3144–3146, 1994.
20. Sollinger HW: RS-61443 (mycophenolate mofetil). Plenary address at the XVth World of Congress of the Transplantation Society, August 29, 1994, Kyoto, Japan.
21. Kahan BD: Concentration-controlled immunosuppressive regimens using cyclosporine with sirolimus or brequinar in human renal transplantation. *Transplant Proc* 27:33–38, 1995.
22. Kahan BD: Brequinar and rapamycin trials. Presented at the ASTP/ASTS Joint Symposium, May, 1994.
23. Schreiber SL: Chemistry and biology of the immunophilins and their immunosuppressive ligands. *Science* 251:283–287, 1991.
24. Thomson AW, Shapiro R, Fung JJ, Starzl TE: New immunosuppressive drugs: mechanisms of action and early clinical experience. In: *Immunology of Renal Transplantation.* Sevenoaks, Kent, England, Edward Arnold, 1993.

25. Morris RE, Meiser BM, Wu J, Shorthouse R, Wang J: Use of rapamycin for the suppression of alloimmune reactions in vivo: schedule dependence, tolerance induction, synergy with cyclosporine and FK 506 and effect on host-versus-graft and graft-versus-host reactions. *Transplant Proc* 23:521–524, 1991.
26. Takahashi K, Tanabe K, Ooba S, et al: Prophylactic use of a new immunosuppressive agent, deoxyspergualin, in patients with kidney transplantation from ABO-incompatible or preformed antibody-positive donors. *Transplantation* 23:1078–1082, 1991.
27. Okazaki H, Sato T, Jimbo M, Senga S, Amada N, Oguma S: Prophylactic use of deoxyspergualin in living related renal transplantation. *Transplant Proc* 23:1094–1095, 1991.
28. Koyama I, Amemiya H, Taguchi Y, et al: Prophylactic use of deoxyspergualin in a quadruple immunosuppressive protocol in renal transplantation. *Transplant Proc* 23:1096–1098, 1991.
29. Ameniya H, Suzuki S, Kazuo O, et al: A novel rescue drug, 15-deoxyspergualin. *Transplantation* 49:337–343, 1990.
30. Takahashi K, Ota K, Tanabe K, et al: Effect of a novel immunosuppressive agent, deoxyspergualin, on rejection in kidney transplant recipients. *Transplant Proc* 22:1606–1612, 1990.
31. Suzuki S, Hayashi R, Kenmochi T, Shimatani K, Fukuoka T, Amemiya H: Clinical application of 15-deoxyspergualin for treatment of acute graft rejection following renal transplantation. *Transplant Proc* 22:1615–1617, 1990.
32. Amemiya H, Dohi K, Otsubo O, et al: Markedly enhanced therapeutic effect of deoxyspergualin on acute rejection when combined with methylprednisolone in kidney recipients. *Transplant Proc* 23:1087–1089, 1991.
33. Groth CG, Ohlman S, Ericzon BG, Barkholt L, Reinhold FP: Deoxyspergualin for liver graft rejection (letter). *Lancet* 336:626, 1990.
34. Amemiya H, Japanese Collaborative Transplant Study Group of NKT-01: Immunosuppressive mechanisms and action of deoxyspergualin in experimental and clinical studies. *Transplant Proc* 27:31–32, 1995.
35. Hibberd AD, Grochowicz PM, Smart YC, et al: Castanospermine down regulates membrane expression of adhesion molecules in heart allograft recipients. *Transplant Proc* 27:448–449, 1995.
36. Morris RE, Huang X, Cao W, Zhend B, Shorthouse RA: Leflunomide (HWA 486) and its analog suppress T- and B-cell proliferation in vitro, acute rejection, ongoing rejection, and antidonor antibody synthesis in mouse, rat, and cynomolgus monkey transplant recipients as well as arterial intimal thickening after balloon catheter injury.
37. Xiao F, Chong AS-F, Bartlett RR, Williams JW: Leflunomide: a promising immunosuppressant in transplantation, 203–212.
38. Thomson AW, Starzl TE: Immunosuppressive drugs: developments in anti-rejection therapy, 37–40, 1994.
39. Dutartre P, Annat J, Derrepas P: LF 08-0299 induces tolerance after short-term treatment in a fully major histocompatibility mismatched rat cardiac allograft model. *Transplant Proc* 27:440–442, 1995.
40. Kupiec-Weglinski JW, Schmidbauer G, Badger AM: SK&F 105685: a novel azaspirane with immunosuppressive activities in animal models of autoimmune diseases and organ transplantation, 213–220.
41. Stepkowski SM, Uy Y, Condon TP, Bennett CF: Induction of transplantation tolerance by treatment with ICAM-1 antisense oligonucleotides and anti-LFA-1 monoclonal antibodies. *Transplant Proc* 27:113, 1995.

42. Binder J, Hancock WW, Wasowska B, et al: Donor-specific transplantation unresponsiveness in sensitized rats following treatment with a nondepleting anti-CD4 MAb is associated with selective intragraft sparing of TH2-like cells. *Transplant Proc* 27:114–116, 1995.
43. Saitovitch D, Bushell AR, Morris PJ, Wood KJ: Induction of transplantation tolerance using a nondepleting anti-CD4 MAb and donor-specific transfusion before transplantation: evidence that a critical period of time is required for the development of immunological unresponsiveness. *Transplant Proc* 27:117–118, 1995.
44. Saitovitch D, Morris PJ, Wood KJ: Donor-type single MHC locus products combined with anti-CD4 MAb can induce tolerance to cardiac allografts which is dependent on active suppression. *Transplant Proc* 27:119–120, 1995.
45. Lehmann M, Hvlickova J, Risch K, et al: Role of the spleen in the establishment and maintenance of anti-CD4-induced transplant nonresponsiveness. *Transplant Proc* 27:121–122, 1995.
46. Watson CJE, Davies HFFS, Cobbold SP, et al: CD4 and CD8 monoclonal antibody therapy in the dog: strategies to induce tolerance to renal allografts. *Transplant Proc* 27:123–124, 1995.
47. Lacha J, Chadimova M, Havlickova J, et al: A short course of cyclosporin A combined with anti-CD4 and/or anti-TCR MAb treatment induces long-term acceptance of kidney allografts in the rat. *Transplant Proc* 27:125–126, 1995.
48. Barber WH, Mankin JA, Laskow DA, et al: Long-term results of a controlled prospective study with transfusion of donor specific bone marrow in 57 cadaveric renal allograft recipients. *Transplantation* 51:70–75, 1991.
49. McDaniel DO, Naftilan J, Hulvey K, et al: Peripheral blood chimerism in renal allograft recipients transfused with donor bone marrow. *Transplantation* 57:852–856, 1994.
50. Fontes P, Abdul R, Demetris AJ, et al: Bone marrow augmentation of donor-cell chimerism in kidney, liver, heart, and pancreas islet transplantation. *Lancet* 344:151–155, 1994.
51. Rao AS, Fontes P, Zeevi A, et al: Combined bone marrow and whole organ transplantation from the same donor. *Transplant Proc* 26:3377–3378, 1994.
52. Rao AS, Fontes P, Zeevi A, et al: Augmentation of chimerism in whole organ recipients by simultaneous infusion of donor bone marrow cells. *Transplant Proc* 27:210–212, 1995.
53. Shapiro R, Rao AS, Fontes P, et al: Combined kidney/bone marrow transplantation: evidence for augmentation of chimerism. *Transplantation* 59:306–309, 1995.
54. Caridis DT, Liegeois A, Barrett I, Monaco AP: Enhanced survival of canine renal allografts of ALS-treated dogs given bone marrow. *Transplant Proc* 5:671–674, 1973.
55. Monaco AP, Clark AW, Brown RW: Active enhancement of a human cadaver renal allograft with ALS and donor bone marrow: case report of an initial attempt. *Surgery* 79:384–392, 1976.
56. Ildstad ST, Sachs DH: Reconstitution with syngeneic plus allogeneic or xenogeneic bone marrow leads to specific acceptance of allografts or xenografts. *Nature* 307:168–170, 1984.
57. Slavin S, Strober S, Fuks Z, Kaplan HS: Induction of specific tissue transplantation tolerance using fractionated total lymphoid irradiation in adult mice: long-term survival of allogeneic bone marrow and skin grafts. *J Exp Med* 146:34–48, 1977.
57a. Ricordi C, Karatzas T, Nery J, et al: High-dose donor bone marrow infusions to enhance allograft survival: the effect of timing. *Transplantation* 63(1):7–11, 1997.
57b. Garcia-Morales R, Carreno M, Mathew J, et al: The effects of chimeric cells following donor bone marrow infusions as detected by PCR-flow assays in kidney transplant recipients. *J Clin Inv* 99(5):1118–1129, 1997.

58. Lu L, Woo J, Rao AS, et al: Propagation of dendritic cell progenitors from normal mouse liver using GM-CSF and their maturational development in the presence of type-1 collagen. *J Exp Med* 179:1823, 1994.
59. Sollinger HW, Kalayoglu MK, Belzer FO: Use of the donor specific transfusion protocol in living-unrelated donor-recipient combinations. *Ann Surg* 204:315, 1986.
60. Pirsch JD, Sollinger HW, Kalayoglu M, et al: Unrelated living donor kidney transplantation: results of 40 patients. *Am J Kidney Dis* 12:499, 1988.
61. Squifflet JP, Pirson Y, Poncelet A, et al: Unrelated living donor kidney transplantation. *Transplant Int* 3:32, 1990.
62. Elick BA, Sutherland DER, Gillingham K, et al: Use of distant relatives and living unrelated donors: a strategy to increase the application of kidney transplantation to treat chronic renal failure. *Transplant Proc* 22:343, 1990.
63. Haberal M, Gulay H, Tokyay R, et al: Living unrelated donor kidney transplantation between spouses. *World J Surg* 16:1183, 1992.
64. Park K, Kim YS, Lee EM, Lee HY, Han DS: Single center experience of living-unrelated donor renal transplantation in the cyclosporine era. *Clin Transpl*, 249, 1993.
65. Terasaki PI, Cecka JM, Gjertson DW, Takemoto S: High graft survival rates of spousal and living-unrelated donor kidney transplants. *N Engl J Med,* in press.
66. Patel CT: Live renal donation: a viewpoint. *Transplant Proc* 20(Suppl 1):1068, 1988.
67. Reddy KC, Thiagarajan CM, Shunmugasundaram D, et al: Unconventional renal transplantation in India: to buy or let die. *Transplant Proc* 22:910, 1990.
68. Reddy KC: Organ donation for consideration: an Indian view point. In: Land, W, Dossetor JB (eds), *Organ Replacement Therapy: Ethics, Justice and Commerce.* Berlin: Springer-Verlag, 1991:173.
69. Thiagarajan CM, Reddy KC, Shunmugasundaram D, et al: The practice of unconventional renal transplantation in a single centre in India. *Transplant Proc* R2:912–914, 1990.
70. Sells R, Daar A: Unrelated renal transplantation. *Transplant Rev* 4:128–140, 1990.
71. Little PJ, McMullin JP, Macdonald A: Live donor renal transplantation in Iraq. *Transplant Proc* 21:1400, 1989.
72. Council of the Transplantation Society: Commercialization in transplantation: the problem and some guidelines for practice. *Lancet* 2:715, 1985.
73. Council of the Transplantation Society: Ruling of the Council. *Transplantation* 41:1, 1986.
74. Daar A, Sells RA: The problem of paid organ donation in India: Report on behalf of the Ethical Committee of the Transplantation Society to the President and Council of the Transplantation Society, 1990.
75. Morris PJ, Sells R: Paying for organs from living donors. *Lancet* 1:1510, 1985.
76. Guttmann RD. On the use of organs from executed prisoners. *Transplant Proc* 6:189–193, 1992.
77. Human Rights Watch/Asia: Organ procurement and judicial execution in China. *Newsletter* 6 (9), 1994.
78. Roels L, Michielsen P: Altruism, self-determination and organ procurement efficiency: the European experience. *Transplant Proc* 23:2514, 1990.
79. Soh P, Lim SML: Impact of the opting-out system on kidney procurement in Singapore. *Transplant Proc* 23:2523, 1991.

80. Pena JR, Pena R, Gomes da Costa A: Legal aspects/post mortem organ donation and psychological. In: Land W, Dossetor JB (eds), *Organ Replacement Therapy: Ethics, Justice and Commerce.* Berlin, Springer-Verlag, 1991:276–279.
81. Mendes A, Alves H: Organ donation by presumed consent: consequences and duties to the society that legalizes it. In: Land W, Dossetor JB (eds), *Organ Replacement Therapy: Ethics, Justice and Commerce.* Berlin, Springer-Verlag, 1991:280–283.
82. Roels L, Coosemans W, Christiaens R, Waer M, Vanrenterghem Y: The relative impact of legislative incentives on multi–organ donation rates in Europe. *Transplant Proc* 27:795–796, 1995.
83. Vathsala A, Lee WT, Li MK, Woo KT, Lim CH: Transplantation in Singapore. *Transplant Proc* 27:1472–1475, 1995.
84. Dennis JM, Hanson P, Hodge EE, Kroom RAF, Veatch RM: An evaluation of the ethics of presumed consent and a proposal based on required response. *UNOS Update* 16–21, 1994.
85. Navarro A, Escalante JL, Andres A, and Group of Transplant Coordinators of the Region of Madrid: Donor detection and organ procurement in the Madrid region. *Transplant Proc* 25:3130–3131, 1993.
86. Matesanz R: Organ procurement in Spain: the importance of a transplant coordinating network. *Transplant Proc* 25:3132–3135, 1993.
87. Matesanz R: The Spanish model of obtaining organs. Presented at the 8th Latin-American Congress of Transplantation. April 25, 1995, Havana, Cuba.
88. Dossetor JB, Manickavel V: Ethics in organ donation: contrasts in two cultures. *Transplant Proc* 23:2508–2511, 1991.
89. Jacksonville Transplant Center: Life or death: the issue of payment in cadaveric organ donation. *JAMA* 265:1302–1305.
90. Cohen LR: Financial incentives in post mortem organ donation: the ethical virtues of a futures market in cadaveric organs. In: Land W, Dossetor JB (eds), *Organ Replacement Therapy: Ethics, Justice and Commerce.* Berlin, Springer-Verlag, 1991:302–310.
91. Peters TG: Financial incentives in organ donation current issues. *Dial Transplant* 21:270–273, 290, 1992.
92. Caplan AL, Van Buren CT, Tilney NL: Financial compensation for cadaver organ donation: good idea or anathema. *Transplant Proc* 25:2740–2742, 1993.
93. Callender CO, Bayton JA, Yeager CL, et al: *J Natl Med Assoc* 74:807, 1982.
94. Callender CO. *Transplant Proc* 21:3407, 1989.
95. Callender CO, Hall LE, Yeager CL, et al: *N Engl J Med* 325:442, 1991.
96. Hall LE, Callender CO, Yeager CL, et al: *Transplant Proc* 23:2500, 1991.
97. Callender CO, Bey AS, Miles PV, Yeager CL: A national minority organ/tissue transplant education program: the first step in the evolution of a national minority strategy and minority transplant equity in the USA. *Transplant Proc* 27:1441–1443, 1995.
98. Ip TK, Galletti PM, Aebischer P: Effects of attachment substrates on the growth and differentiation of LLC-PK 1 cells. *In Vitro Cell Dev Biol Anim* 26(2):162–168, 1990.
99. Uludag H, Ip TK, Aebischer P: Transport functions in a bioartificial kidney under uremic conditions. *Int J Artif Organs* 13:93–97, 1990.
100. Cieslinski DA, Humes HD: Tissue engineering of a bioartificial kidney. *Biotechnol Bioeng* 43:678–681, 1994.

101. Kramer P, Wigger W, Rieger J, Matthaei D, Scheler F: Arterior-venous haemofiltration: a new and simple method for treatment of overhydrated patients resistant to diuretics. *Klin Wochenschr* ff:1121–1122, 1977.
102. Golper TA: Continuous arteriovenous hemofiltration in acute renal failure. *Am J Kidney Dis* 6:373–381, 1986.
103. Shepard AD, Eldrup-Jorgesen J, Keough EM, et al: Endothelial cell seeding of small-caliber grafts in the baboon. *Surgery* 99:318–325, 1986.
104. Schnider PA, Hanson SR, Price TM, Harker LA: Durability of confluent endothelial cell monolayers of small-caliber vascular prostheses in vitro. *Surgery* 103:456–462, 1988.
105. Kadletz M, Magometschnigg H, Minar E, et al: Implantation of in vitro endothelialized polytetrafluoroethylene grafts in human beings. *J Thorac Cardiovasc Surg* 104:736–742, 1992.
106. Humes HD, Cieslinski DA: Interaction between growth factors and retinoic acid in the induction of kidney tubulogenesis in tissue culture. *Exp Cell Res* 201:8–15, 1992.
107. Humes HD, Beals TF, Cieslinski DA, Sanchez IO, Page TP: Effects of transforming growth factor-β, transforming growth factor-α, and other growth factors on renal proximal tubule cells. *Lab Invest* 64:538–545, 1991.
108. Humes HD, Cieslinski DA, Johnson LB, Sanchez IO: Triiodothyronine enhances renal tubule cell replication by stimulating EGF receptor gene expression. *Am J Physiol* 262:F540–F545, 1992.
109. Humes HD, Cieslinski DA: Adenosine triphosphate stimulates thymidine incorporation but does not promote cell growth in primary cultures of renal proximal tubule cells. *Ren Physiol Biochem* 14:253–258, 1991.
110. Humes HD, Nakamura T, Cieslinski DA, Miller D, Emmons RV, Border WA: Role of proteoglycans and cytoskeleton in the effects of TGF-β_1 on renal proximal tubule cells. *Kidney Int* 43:575–584, 1993.

Index

Figures and tables are represented by *f* and *t* respectively.